Color Doppler, 3D and 4D Ultrasound in Gynecology, Infertility and Obstetrics

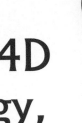

Color Doppler, 3D and 4D Ultrasound in Gynecology, Infertility and Obstetrics

Second Edition

Sanja Kupesic MD PhD
Professor of Obstetrics and Gynecology
Department of Medical Education
Paul L Foster School of Medicine
Texas Tech University at El Paso, Texas, USA

Asim Kurjak MD PhD
Professor
Department of Obstetrics and Gynecology
Medical School University of Zagreb
Sveti Duh Hospital, Zagreb, Croatia

JAYPEE BROTHERS MEDICAL PUBLISHERS (P) LTD

New Delhi • St Louis • Panama City • London

Published by

Jaypee Brothers Medical Publishers (P) Ltd

Corporate Office
4838/24 Ansari Road, Daryaganj, **New Delhi** - 110 002, India
Phone: +91-11-43574357, Fax: +91-11-43574314

Offices in India
- **Ahmedabad**, e-mail: ahmedabad@jaypeebrothers.com
- **Bengaluru**, e-mail: bangalore@jaypeebrothers.com
- **Chennai**, e-mail: chennai@jaypeebrothers.com
- **Delhi**, e-mail: jaypee@jaypeebrothers.com
- **Hyderabad**, e-mail: hyderabad@jaypeebrothers.com
- **Kochi**, e-mail: kochi@jaypeebrothers.com
- **Kolkata**, e-mail: kolkata@jaypeebrothers.com
- **Lucknow**, e-mail: lucknow@jaypeebrothers.com
- **Mumbai**, e-mail: mumbai@jaypeebrothers.com
- **Nagpur**, e-mail: nagpur@jaypeebrothers.com

Overseas Offices
- **North America Office, USA**, Ph: 001-636-6279734
  e-mail: jaypee@jaypeebrothers.com, anjulav@jaypeebrothers.com
- **Central America Office, Panama City, Panama**, Ph: 001-507-317-0160
  e-mail: cservice@jphmedical.com, Website: www.jphmedical.com
- **Europe Office, UK**, Ph: +44 (0) 2031708910
  e-mail: info@jpmedpub.com

Color Doppler, 3D and 4D Ultrasound in Gynecology, Infertility and Obstetrics

This book has been published in good faith that the material provided by contributors is original. Every effort is made to ensure accuracy of material, but the publisher, printer and editors will not be held responsible for any inadvertent error(s). In case of any dispute, all legal matters are to be settled under Delhi jurisdiction only.

First Edition: **2003**
Second Edition: **2011**

ISBN 978-93-5025-090-7

Typeset at JPBMP typesetting unit

Printed at Ajanta Offset & Packagings Ltd., New Delhi

Contributors

Badreldeen Ahmed MD
Professor
Fetomaternal Unit
Department of Obstetrics and Gynecology
Women's Hospital, Hamad Medical Corporation
Doha, State of Qatar

Baston Kirk MD
Assistant Professor of Pathology
Department of Medical Education
Paul L Foster School of Medicine
Texas Tech University at El Paso, Texas, USA

Bekavac Ivanka MD
Specialist, Obstetrics and Gynecology
Department of Obstetrics and Gynecology
Medical School University of Zagreb
Sveti Duh Hospital Zagreb, Croatia

Breyer Branko PhD
Professor of Physics
Laboratory Breyer
Zagreb, Croatia

Gersak Ksenija MD PhD
Associate Professor
Department of Obstetrics and Gynecology
University Clinical Center Ljubljana, Slovenia

Honemeyer Ulrich MD
Specialist, Obstetrics and Gynecology
Department of Obstetrics and Gynecology
Welcare Hospital EHL
Dubai, United Arab Emirates

Kupesic Plavsic Sanja MD PhD
Professor
Obstetrics and Gynecology
Department of Medical Education
Paul L Foster School of Medicine
Texas Tech University at El Paso, Texas, USA

Kurjak Asim MD PhD
Professor
Department of Obstetrics and Gynecology
Medical School University of Zagreb
Sveti Duh Hospital, Zagreb, Croatia

Patham Bhargavi MD PhD
Assistant Professor of Pathology
Department of Medical Education
Paul L Foster School of Medicine
Texas Tech University at El Paso
Texas, USA

Sparac Vladimir MD PhD
Specialist, Obstetrics and Gynecology
Cyto Clinic, Split, Croatia

Stanojevic Milan MD PhD
Neonatologist
Department of Obstetrics and Gynecology
Medical School University of Zagreb
Sveti Duh Hospital, Zagreb, Croatia

Subramanya Sandesh MS PhD
Instructor
Department of Biomedical Sciences
Center of Excellence for Infectious Disease
Paul L Foster School of Medicine
Texas Tech University at El Paso
Texas, USA

Tikvica Luetic MD
Department of Obstetrics and Gynecology
Medical School University of Zagreb
Sveti Duh Hospital, Zagreb, Croatia

Zafar Nadah MD
Assistant Professor of Emergency Medicine
Department of Medical Education
Paul L Foster School of Medicine
Texas Tech University at El Paso
Texas, USA

Preface to the Second Edition

Over the last decade impressive improvements in computer and ultrasound technology have promoted a wide use of ultrasound in clinical practice. With the advent of color and power Doppler ultrasound, and more recently three- (3D) and four-dimensional (4D) ultrasound, research expansion in the field of human reproduction, obstetrics and gynecologic oncology has occurred.

Ultrasound has simplified guided techniques such as oocyte collection and breast biopsy, but has also become an important technique in the assessment of the follicular growth and endometrial development, as well as in evaluation of the uterine and ovarian perfusion. Significant studies have been made in the gynecological application of Doppler sonography and screening for ovarian and uterine malignancy. In obstetrics, Doppler sonography has allowed unprecedented insight in the pathophysiology of human fetal development. In a relatively short period of time, 3D and 4D ultrasound has proved to be a useful clinical tool in almost all sections of gynecology and obstetrics. In this book the authors explain the significance of each of the discussed subjects in an effective way, by integrating important and updated information and illustrative examples.

The contributors of this edition have made significant improvements, included updated information and a few unique illustrations. Each chapter has been reviewed and revised to focus on the clinicians' needs in ultrasound practice. The educational impact of the book is further enhanced by adding a manual for sonographers and physicians entitled "Clinical Sonographic Pearls" that was created for better organization of important clinical presentation-based information.

With the aid of such a didactic approach it is hoped that the process of becoming capable is performing and interpreting Doppler information and 3D ultrasound images will become more enjoyable and interesting.

Sanja Kupesic
Asim Kurjak

Preface to the First Edition

Over the last decade impressive improvements in computer and ultrasound technology have promoted the widest use of ultrasound in clinical practice. With the advent of color and power Doppler ultrasound, and more recently three-dimensional ultrasound, we did phenomenal research expansion in the field of human reproduction, obstetrics and gynecologic oncology.

Ultrasound has simplified guided techniques such as oocyte collection, but has also become an ideal noninvasive technique for the assessment of the follicular growth and endometrial development, as well as for evaluation of the uterine and ovarian perfusion. Significant studies have been made in the gynecological application of Doppler sonography and screening for ovarian and uterine malignancy. In obstetrics, Doppler sonography has allowed unprecedented insight into the pathophysiology of human fetal development.

In a relatively short period of time three-dimensional ultrasound has proved to be useful clinical tool in almost all sections of gynecology and obstetrics.

The contributors in this book has tried to explain the significance of each of the discussed subjects in an effective way, by putting together important and updated information and illustrative examples. With the aid of such a didactic approach it is hoped that the process of becoming capable at performing and interpreting Doppler information and three-dimensional ultrasound images will become more enjoyable and interesting.

Asim Kurjak
Sanja Kupesic

Contents

B Breyer

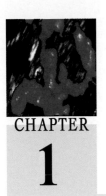

CHAPTER

1

Physical Principles of the Doppler Effect and Its Application in Medicine

INTRODUCTION

Doppler technique has been used in medicine for many years but only in the last decade this diagnostic modality has gained practical importance in obstetrics and gynecology. B-mode ultrasound gives information about morphology. Doppler ultrasound gives information about blood flow.

One must bear in mind that Doppler techniques and instruments are highly complex. Therefore, additional education and knowledge about the pelvic hemodynamics is required for correct usage. Moreover, many Doppler measurements may not be standardized. Additional complications are the cost-benefit issues (Doppler machines are usually very expensive), the question whether Doppler should be used as a screening tool or as a secondary or even tertiary test, interpretation of results, time consuming procedure and the question regarding its safety in early pregnancy.

For successful application of this technique to medical diagnosis, an understanding of Doppler physics, its possibilities and limitations is necessary. Flow can be detected even in vessels that are too small to image. Doppler ultrasound can determine the presence or absence of flow, flow direction and flow character. One of the fundamental limitations of flow information provided by the Doppler effects is that it is angle dependent. Furthermore, artifacts in Doppler ultrasound can be confusing and lead to misinterpretation of flow information. These problems will be addressed in this chapter.

THE DOPPLER EFFECT[1]

The basic principle of the Doppler effect for the case when the waves reflect from a reflector is illustrated in Figure 1.1.

If the reflector does not move (case a) the frequency of the reflected wave f_1 is equal to the transmitted frequency f_0. If the reflector moves towards the transceiver, the reflected frequency will be higher than the transmitted one, while in case the reflector moves away (case c) from the transceiver, the received frequency f_1 will be lower than the transmitted f_0. This frequency change Δf (called the Doppler shift) is proportional to the velocity v of the reflector movement.

In practice this means that we need an apparatus that transmits ultrasound waves into the body and receives their reflections from the body. The apparatus must then measure the difference between the transmitted and received frequency. The frequency difference (Doppler shift expressed in Hz) is proportional to the velocity of the movement along the line that connects the wave transceiver and the moving reflector.

In medical applications, the Doppler effect is usually used by insonating the moving blood and assessment of the Doppler shift of ultrasound scattered on erythrocytes (Figure 1.2). Single erythrocytes reflect (retransmit) ultrasound in various directions, but the total back-scattered energy is sufficient for velocity assessment.

The general method of measurement consists of transmission of bundled ultrasound into the body at a general angle α to the flow. In this case, the following equation of Doppler shift is valid to sufficient approximation.

$$\Delta f = \frac{2f_0 V}{C} \cos(\alpha)$$

It is important to note that in this approximation, the Doppler shift for $\alpha = 90°$ equals zero.

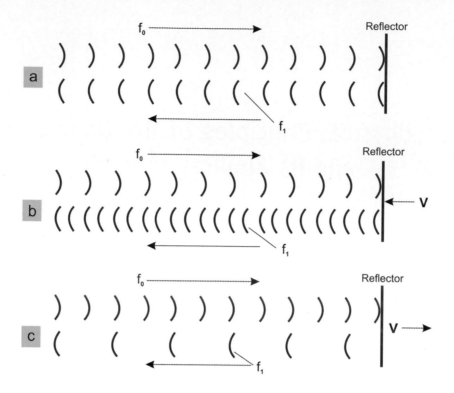

FIGURE 1.1: Illustration of the Doppler effect: change of frequency due to the movement of the reflector.

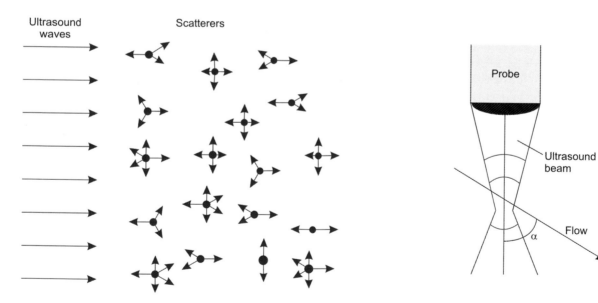

FIGURE 1.2: Scattering of ultrasound yields: multiple back scattered wavelets.

FIGURE 1.3: Relation between ultrasound beam and the flow.

It has been demonstrated that for wave beams the Doppler shift is not exactly zero at $\alpha = 90°$, but the shift is small and not used in the present commercial instrumentation (Figure 1.3). Thus, the plane wave approximation from the above equation is valid for the normal practice.

From the above Doppler shift formula we can calculate the velocity, V with the help of the following equation:

$$V = \frac{\Delta f\, gc}{2f_0 \cos\alpha}\,(m/s)$$

where c = ultrasound propagation speed; Δf = Doppler shift; f_0 = transmitted wave frequency; and α is the angle between the ultrasound beam and flow direction.

The flow in blood vessels depends on the quality of their walls and vessel dimensions. If the flow is laminar (when the walls are even and blood vessel is large enough) the flow profile is parabolic, that is, the velocity in the center is the fastest and slows down as we approach the walls. The law by which this changes is approximately a parabola (Figure 1.4). If there is an obstacle in the blood vessel (a plaque, a branching, etc.) the profile deviates from parabolic and can become turbulent. In any case, at any instance and at any cross section the blood flows at many different velocities at the same time, i.e. there is a full spectrum of flow velocities.

The results are usually shown as Doppler shift spectra in real-time according as in Figure 1.5.

The ordinate is the Doppler shift (Figures 1.5 and 1.6) and the abscissa is the running time. Doppler shift measured in Hz is proportional to flow velocity and if the angle α is known, one can put velocities onto the ordinate by using the equation for velocity calculation.

The upper spectrum (ART) has the typical shape of an arterial spectrum. It is pulsatile. The peripheral venous spectrum (VEN) in the lower part of Figure 1.5 is not pulsatile. Venous flow is not pulsatile in peripheral blood vessels but can be very pulsatile as the vessels approach the heart. Since the blood flows at each instance at different velocities, the spectra are generally filled-in. The lowest frequencies are cut off with special high-pass filters, the so-called, wall filters (wf). The filter was originally designed to eliminate the artifacts from moving blood vessel walls.

Apart from absolute velocity measurement, one can define relative indices, which are particularly useful for flow evaluation without known angle between the flow and ultrasound beam.

DOPPLER INDICES

Because of inherent difficulties in quantitatively evaluating blood flow, the blood flow velocity waveform has commonly been interpreted to distinguish patterns associated with high and low resistance in the distal vascular tree (Figure 1.6). Three indices are in common use, the systolic/diastolic ratio (S/D ratio), the pulsatility index (PI,

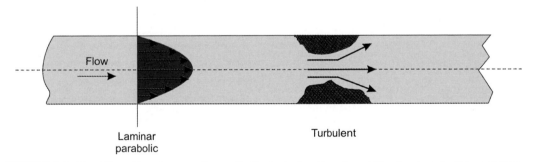

FIGURE 1.4: Real-time Doppler spectrum. Ordinate is the Doppler shift; abscissa is the real time.

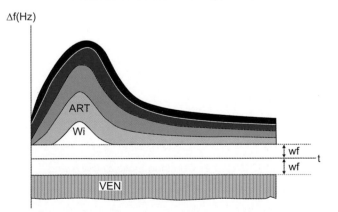

FIGURE 1.5: Illustrative arterial (ART) and venous (VEN) flow Doppler spectra.

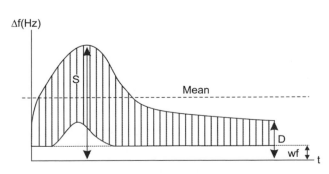

FIGURE 1.6: Spectrum part used in the calculation of RI and PI.

also called the impedance index) and the resistance index (RI, also called the Pourcelot ratio). If we designate the peak systolic Doppler shift with S and the maximal diastolic Doppler shift with D, simple indices can be defined that roughly describe some properties of the spectra (Figure 1.6).

The S/D ratio is the simplest but it is irrelevant when diastolic velocities are absent and the ratio becomes infinite. Values above 8.0 are considered "extremely high".

Definitions of RI and PI are as follows:

$$\text{Resistance index} \quad RI = \frac{S - D}{S}$$

$$\text{Pulsatility index} \quad PI = \frac{S - D}{(\text{mean})}$$

The RI is moderately complicated but has the appeal of approaching 1.00 when diastolic velocities are abnormally low and does, therefore, reflect the relative impairment of flow by high resistance. These indices are ratios, independent of the angle between the ultrasound beam and the insonated blood vessel and therefore not dependent on absolute measurement of true velocity.

The PI requires computer-assisted calculation of mean velocity, which still may be subject to very large experimental error. In a normal pregnancy, neither the S/D ratio nor PI is normally distributed across all gestational ages.

L Pourcelot and R Gossling initially derived the indices for their statistically demonstrated association with adverse clinical findings. However, the RI must not be considered independent of changes in physiologic variables, such as heart rate, cardiac contractility, blood pressure and the many other determinants of flow. This information does not depend on the measurement angle since all the parts of the spectrum change proportionally when angle α changes. However, as the angle approaches 90°, the measurement error increases drastically. In practice, it is the best compromise between the resolution of B mode image resolution and accuracy of Doppler spectroscopy is obtained at angles between 30° and 60°.

The three indices are highly correlated.[2,3] There are intrinsic errors in all that have been quantified and lie between 10% and 20%. There may be advantages to the RI or PI where flow is markedly abnormal or in early pregnancy, when a very low end-diastolic velocity can be a normal finding.

INSTRUMENTATION FOR DOPPLER MEASUREMENTS

There are two basic technological methods for application of the Doppler effect in medicine (Figure 1.7). It is possible to transmit and receive ultrasound waves continuously with a probe that contains a transmission transducer and a reception transducer (continuous wave in Figure 1.7). Another possibility is to transmit in the form of pulses whose Doppler shift is measured after the time necessary for ultrasound to reach a defined depth in the body (pulse wave in Figure 1.7).

These two systems have different properties. The CW system has no depth resolution so that the measurement results of all flows along the line-of-sight add together and mix. On the other hand, this system measures well all (fast and slow) velocities. If there is only one blood vessel along the line-of-sight or one flow is dominant, the CW system is very good for practice.

If, however, one must measure the flow in a single blood vessel, the PW system can measure within a well-defined sensitive volume. The sensitive volume has a length that depends on the pulse length (in time) and a width that depends on the beam width (and focusing) (shown as sensitive volume in Figure 1.9). The disadvantage of such a pulse Doppler system is that it cannot measure high velocities deep in the body. The reason for this is that a PW system only occasionally looks at the flow so that it cannot convey all the information at an enough high throughput. The phenomenon can mathematically be described by the sampling theorem, which results in the so-called aliasing, i.e. reverse indication of flow that is too fast. The resulting artifact is shown in Figure 1.8. The top of the pulsatile spectrum (highest velocities) are shown as

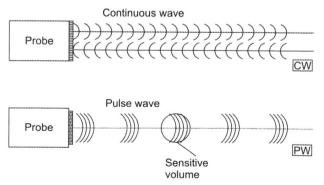

FIGURE 1.7: Continuous wave (CW) and pulse wave (PW) Doppler.

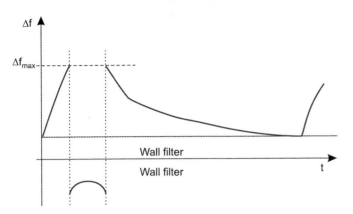

FIGURE 1.8: Aliasing.

negative (reverse flow). If the spectrum is simple like in Figure 1.8, the recognition of the aliasing artifact is easy. In complex spectra this can be hard. In such cases, it may be useful to have a combined PW and CW system or a HPRF system. The HPRF system has such a pulse rate that it violates the sampling theorem and thus yields mathematically ambiguous results. In the screen this is usually shown as multiple sampling volumes (spots, cursors). Such a system measures at multiple spots at a time. If the operator can recognize the spots with dominant flow or positions the cursors in such a way that only one of them hits flow, the system achieves a better performance for high velocity flow measurement.

Data Acquisition

The computerized generation of the flow velocity waveform is not a simple task. In addition to the modification of returned frequencies by scattering and tissue attenuation, a number of computer-based steps are required to eliminate low-frequency noise generated by tissues vibrating in response to the ultrasound beam and by nonultrasound-based movement of tissues.

Several processing mechanisms are used to modify and adjust the returned frequencies.

Both excessive low and high frequencies are filtered-out (band pass).

High-pass filtering (allowing only frequencies above a set minimum to be shown) removes unwanted low-frequency signals. Thus, interference from vessel wall vibration, or other tissue movement, is eliminated, but this mechanism will also remove low velocities representing low flow. High-pass filtering, therefore, is capable of erroneously suggesting absent flow in diastole. The operator can usually adjust this filter.

Sample volume (or "range gate") limits the area (depth-wise) to be analyzed. In duplex scanning, the range gate is adjustable for length and for position. Range gating assumes a standard time interval between pulse emission and echo return that is based on the standard tissue transmit time from the depth set by the operator. The receiving gate is open only for the anticipated moment of echo return, thus restricting information received to what is "expected" from the area designated by the calipers on the screen. The sample volume should be larger than the vessel and positioned to span it completely if we wish to have complete data on the flow within the vessel. If it is set too large, extraneous signals may be included. If it is set much smaller than the blood vessel diameter, the resulting spectrum will be narrow (i.e. it will have a "window") unless the flow is grossly turbulent.

These mechanisms, therefore, restrict the information that is returned and analyzed, in an effort to present an acceptable image. Such editing can discard some desirable data on (usually low) velocities.

Signal Processing

Since the pressure of the reflected ultrasound wave from blood is about a hundred times smaller that from the surrounding structures a substantially higher amplification is required. The data are then filtered and demodulated. Demodulation consists of comparing the transmitter carrier frequencies of the transducer's output, to reflected echoes. The so-called quadrature detector separates the demodulated signal in two channels, that is, flow toward the transducer is represented as positive Doppler shift and flow away from the transducer is represented as negative Doppler shift. The flow data are represented in real-time.

The spectral analysis is done with an algorithm called the fast Fourier transform, which makes a fast and approximate Fourier analysis of the signal.

Flow vs Velocity

The actual display is Doppler shift versus time. If the angle between the ultrasound beam and the flow is known, one can display velocity versus time. The actual measurement of the Doppler angle is often difficult. In some disciplines, the practice is to ignore the angle and speak about "velocities" (TCD, sometimes fetal echocardiography). The nature of the flow (pulsatile or steady, regular or turbulent, single or branching, parabolic or plug), impacts significantly on the frequencies returned. Thus, although volume blood flow can be calculated as the product of mean blood flow velocity and vessel area, this is fraught with variation in practical terms.

The cross-sectional area of the vessel measured from the gray scale image is very susceptible to error. Additionally, the volume flow depends on the fourth power of the vessel diameter so that any measurement error is grossly amplified.[4,5] Even the thickness of the distance measurement cursor plays a major role in measurement accuracy in blood vessels of a few millimeters in diameter.

Another major problem in measuring flow is the variation of blood velocity across the vessel cross section. Because the overall flow rate is the sum of the contributions made by the blood at every point on the cross section, it is necessary to average the velocity profile (mean blood flow velocity). Various approaches to this have been described. The calculation is different when the velocity profile is measured (with multigated pulsed Doppler) and averaged or if it is averaged using a large sample volume to encompass the whole vessel. Volume blood flow has been expressed as milliliters per minute. In fetal applications the result may be normalized to the fetal weight. Estimating the fetal weight by ultrasound measurement formulas is also error-prone. It is clear, to allow accurate or even vaguely useful volume flow measurement that Doppler interrogation must be limited to large vessels, with meticulous attention to methodology.

Figure 1.8 is an illustration of the aliasing effect on an arterial spectrum where the peak velocities have been too fast to measure with the particular pulse repetition frequency (PRF) of a pulsed Doppler system.

TWO DIMENSIONAL FLOW MEASUREMENT

2D Color Doppler Display

The flow can be shown in two dimensions (2D). In principle, comparison or subtraction of successive two-dimensional images can achieve this. Only echoes from moving structures stay in such images. The final result is a two-dimensional display of moving structures, mainly blood flowing through blood vessels.

The directions and speeds are color coded. Movements towards the probe are shown in different shades of one color, e.g. red and away from the probe in shades of another color, e.g. blue (Figure 1.9). The different shades signify relative velocity. One must always bear in mind that this system shows the component of velocity projected onto the probing ultrasound beam. This makes the display semi-quantitative. One can display the multiple Doppler shift measurement variance. In the red-blue combination code, the variance is usually shown in green. The larger the measurement variance—the more green. This gives an

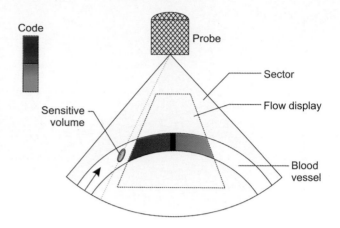

FIGURE 1.9: 2D flow mapping.

indication of turbulence. Flow at 90° to the ultrasound beam are not shown (in the image they are shown black, i.e. as if it were not there). The color code is arbitrary and in the majority of machines can be chosen from a number of different possibilities. Since the 2D, color Doppler is semi-quantitative, it is as a rule combined with a PW Doppler spectrometer. The 2D display helps in fast finding of the points where we wish to analyze the flow by spectrometry. In this way, the 2D system reduces the duration of Doppler examinations. Sometimes, however, the 2D map is characteristic enough to help with the diagnosis. The limitations of the method are equal to the pulse Doppler technique and so we got the, now ubiquitous "Color Doppler". As with any new method, the first amazement yielded its place to systematic and often controversial, but always tedious evaluation in clinical medicine. Since many of the most feared illnesses develop on a long time scale, the method is still under scrutiny but is already accepted as a useful tool.

A particular form of 2D flow mapping is the, so-called, Power Doppler (Figure 1.10).

Power Doppler Ultrasound

The shortcomings of the two-dimensional directional Doppler ("color Doppler") are many. Above all, the sensitivity to direction is a mixed blessing. It does give the much-valued information about the direction of flow, but suffers from not-very-high sensitivity and direction artifacts. Now, in many cases the directional information, if very valuable, like in echocardiography. However, there are many instances when the only relevant question is "Where are the blood vessels?" or "How many blood vessels are

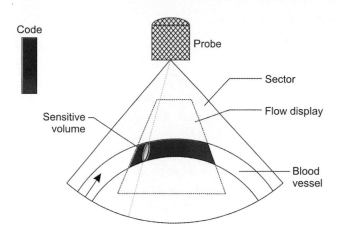

FIGURE 1.10: Doppler angiography or power Doppler.

there?" or "What is the perfusion of this area?". The direction may be of little importance or determinable with a built-in Doppler spectrometer. Basically color Doppler yields that information. However, it is not uncommon to find a clear Doppler spectrum signal from an area that is completely without any color signal or where (if we are lucky) the color appears occasionally. The reason for this is that the directional information is evaluated from a number of subsequent frames and ambiguous and low signals average out to zero.

All these considerations led the instrumentation researchers to take a step backward and develop a two-dimensional system, which just detects and displays movement; any movement, in two dimensions. The result is an instrument, which displays areas with moving structures in color. The color means that there is flow in the area and the brightness of the color qualitatively indicates the quantity of moving erythrocytes.[6]

Every normal color Doppler system has the basic capability for "power Doppler" or "Doppler Angio". Actually the power Doppler is a mode of operation in which any signal, which shows a Doppler shift (change in frequency) is tagged with color. So the direction becomes irrelevant. Unlike color Doppler where a symmetrical turbulence shows a poor signal, in power Doppler, the signal will be as strong as any. The reason for this is that when directional information is displayed, the zero mean velocity is not displayed, while in the case when the total reflection from any moving structure is displayed a turbulent flow is as indicative as any.

The decision as to what is flow and what is not is taken by looking at the frequency spectra and high enough frequency shifts are considered to represent blood flow. The color-coding is made proportional in brightness to the total power of reflected ultrasound from moving structures. Structures which do not move or move slowly are not color-coded.

The displayed color indicates the quantity of moving blood, but not the volume flow of blood per unit time. Actually the virtue of this display mode is that it shows about equally fast and slow flow so that we can get a feeling of the general blood perfusion in some area. However, if actual blood velocity or volume per unit time is of any interest, we must revert to other display and measurement modes.

The returned signal depends, in addition, on the attenuation of ultrasound in the intervening tissue. This means that the flow in deeper blood vessels or the flow in the same blood vessel that changes the depth will be shown with different brightness, depending on the depth. The density of the moving blood cells depends on the concentration of blood cells and local flow situation. The sampling volume depends on the length of ultrasound pulse and beam width. If the sampling volume is larger than the blood vessel, the average number of red blood cells in it will be smaller and the returned signal will be thus relatively weaker, showing a dimmer color on the display.

BASIC LIMITATIONS OF DOPPLER EXAMINATIONS

In Doppler measurements one encounters problems of **accuracy, precision and artifacts** like in any measurement and imaging method. The peculiarities of this method are as follows:

Accuracy

- Doppler spectrometry operates adequately for angles between ultrasound beam and flow less than 60°. The theoretical measurement error tends asymptotically towards infinity when the angle approaches 90°. The raw result of the measurement is a spectrum, which illustrates well the general behavior, but has the data on velocity hidden by an additional unknown factor— the angle. However, even with the angle a known, data like mean velocity can be calculated only by way of a fairly complicated numerical integral of the weighted spectrum. The automaton, which picks up the respective weights of single velocities within the spectrum at each instant operates fairly autonomously, usually without intervention of the operator. The intervention by way of changing measurement sensitivity can change the result of the calculation. One must continuously bear in mind that we measure Doppler shift only, while the rest of the data is derived from it. The accuracy of assessment of the Doppler shift really depends on the knowledge and control of the frequency content of the ultrasound pulses. This is often not well controlled. An exception is operation with CW Doppler systems where the measurement can be made more accurate.

- Color Doppler itself is not designed as an accurate measurement method, but mainly a semiquantitative guiding method for Doppler shift spectroscopy. In spite of this, the significance of different colors must be known and in particular one must carefully adjust the base-line shift since this can essentially change the velocity-color map.

  There exists, however, a possibility to extract the accurate data on the Doppler shift by using a cursor, which helps in reading the frequency shift from the computer memory.

  Fourier power spectra, where available, give quantitative data but are often not well understood. This spectrum is not a real-time spectrum but a graph with Doppler shift on the abscissa and the energy in frequency range on the ordinate. Its width and symmetry properties contain ample information about the nature of the flow (which is harder to read from a usual real-time spectrum). One should not confuse this power spectrum with the "Power Doppler".

- Power Doppler display method has a slightly better geometrical accuracy in showing the blood vessel lumen than the normal "color Doppler". This happens at the cost of image repetition rate.

Precision

- The quantitative functional dependence of the velocity measurement error on the knowledge of the angle α is known. However, the usual method of measurement of the angle is very crude and thus one should try to avoid using absolute values whenever possible.

- Since the color map scale is virtually continuous there is only marginal accuracy in the judgment of the velocity by way of color assessment. However, the variance map, although not accurately assessable gives a very useful clue as to where one ought to do spectroscopic measurements. Again, the Fourier power spectra capability enables a precise variance calculation and the Power Doppler modality increases observation sensitivity at the cost of loosing directional information.

CONTRAST MEDIA

The energy reflected (scattered) back from the erythrocytes is about 10,000 times smaller than the energy reflected from the blood vessel walls. This presents serious technological sensitivity problems. One of the possibilities to increase the sensitivity is to use contrast particles as scatterers instead of erythrocytes. The contrast media are basically composed of bubbles of gas or liquid enclosed in thin nontoxic, usually organic membranes. Such bubbles are of well defined size and stable enough to stay in the circulation long enough to make the required Doppler measurements before dissolving and disappearing from the circulation. They reflect ultrasound much better than erythrocytes proper and thus alleviate much of the sensitivity problems.

In addition to helping Doppler measurements, the contrast media can modify and enhance normal echographic images. A concentrated effort in research is underway to make various parameters of the contrast media more specific, e.g. resonant at specific frequencies or with biologically active membranes.

Artifacts

Several artifacts are encountered in Doppler ultrasound.[7-12] These are incorrect presentation of Doppler flow information (Table 1.1). The most common of these is aliasing. However, others occur, including range ambiguity, spectrum mirror image, location mirror image, speckle and electromagnetic interference.

Aliasing

Aliasing is the most common artifact encountered in Doppler ultrasound.[13,14] (Figure 1.8).

There is an upper limit to Doppler shift that can be detected by pulsed instruments. If the Doppler shift frequency exceeds one half the pulse repetition frequency, aliasing occurs and improper Doppler shift information (wrong direction and wrong value) results. An analogous optical form of aliasing occurs in motion pictures when wagon wheels appear to rotate in reverse direction (This happens here because the number of pictures per second is insufficient to correctly show the rotation speed). Higher pulse repetition frequencies permit higher Doppler shifts to be detected but also increase the chance of the range ambiguity artifact. Continuous-wave Doppler instruments do not have this limitation but neither do they provide depth resolution.

TABLE 1.1 Summary of Doppler artifacts

Error	Cause	Effect
Aliasing	High flow exceeds 0.5 PRF Doppler angle moving	Velocity peaks switch direction: Information lost Biphasic flow wave
Double image	Doppler angle near 90 degrees	Wave duplicated in both directions
Mirror image	Strong reflector adjacent (e.g. pelvic side wall or bone)	Inappropriate gate location Loss of Doppler information
Range ambiguity	Tissue layers (e.g. large cyst) change beam velocity	Aberrant depth resolution Incorrect gate location
Beam deflection	Tissue layers change Doppler angle	Reduced lateral spatial Incorrect gate location
Clipping	Excessive wall filter Gate inside vessel	Loss of low velocity, misperception of high resistance

Aliasing can be eliminated by increasing pulse repetition frequency, increasing Doppler angle (which decreases the Doppler shift for a given flow), or by baseline shifting. The latter is an electronic "cut and paste" technique that moves the misplaced aliasing peaks over to their proper location. It is a successful technique as long as there are no legitimate Doppler shifts in the region of the aliasing. If there are, they will get moved over to an inappropriate location along with the aliasing peaks. Other approaches to eliminating aliasing include changing to a lower frequency Doppler transducer or changing to a continuous-wave instrument, which is often built-in into specialized cardiologic units. Aliasing can occur in a pulse system since it is a sampling system, which cannot yield a correct result unless it samples often enough, that is, twice the highest Doppler shift frequency. This is called the Nyquist limit (of the sampling theorem).

Increasing the pulse repetition frequency can reduce the aliasing problem. However, this can cause localization ambiguity. This occurs when a pulse is emitted before all the echoes from the previous pulse have returned. When this happens, early echoes from the last pulse are simultaneously received with late echoes from the previous pulse. This causes difficulty with the ranging process. In effect, multiple gates or sample volumes are operating at different depths. Multiple sample gates are shown on the display to indicate this condition. Range ambiguity in color-flow Doppler, as in sonography, places echoes (color Doppler shifts in this case) that have come from deep locations after a subsequent pulse was emitted in shallow locations where they do not belong. As already said, the HPRF systems intentionally introduce this ambiguity for spectrometry, requiring sound judgment by the operator as to whether the results are correct or not. Comparison of different Doppler instruments is given in Table 1.2.

The mirror image artifact can also occur with Doppler systems. This means that an image of a vessel and a source of Doppler shifted echoes can be duplicated on the opposite side of a strong reflector (such as a bone). The duplicated vessel containing flow could be misinterpreted as an additional vessel. It will have a spectrum similar to that for the real vessel. A mirror image of a Doppler spectrum can appear on the opposite side of the baseline when, indeed, flow is unidirectional and should appear only on one side of the baseline. This is an electronic duplication of the spectral information. It can occur when receiver gain is set too high (causing overloading in the receiver and cross talk between the two flow channels) or with low gain (where the receiver has difficulty determining the sign of the Doppler shift). It can also occur when Doppler angle is near 90°. Here the duplication is usually legitimate. This is because beams are focused and not cylindrical in shape. Thus, portions of the beam can experience flow toward while other portions can experience flow away. An additional possibility is to fit a bend of a small blood vessel in the same sample volume, which then yields opposite flows in the two parts of the "hook" as opposite, nearly symmetrical spectra.

Turbulent flow measured with a small sample volume can yield a symmetrical spectrum as well.

TABLE 1.2:   Comparison of different Doppler instruments

Type	Advantage	Disadvantage	Other
SPECTROMETERS			
Pulsed wave (PW)	Has depth resolution	Poorly measures high velocities deep in the body	Higher price
HPRF (High pulse rate frequency) system	PW system which can measure fast flows	Ambiguous measurement (multiple sensitive volumes)	Requires more caution from operator
Continuous wave (CW)	Measures all velocities	Has no depth resolution—mixes flows along the US beam	Lower price
2D DOPPLER SYSTEMS			
"Color Doppler"	Yields the directional flow map and indication of turbulence. Can show fast flow changes	Does not measure at 90°, Less sensitive than spectrometer, Prone to aliasing	Quite sensitive to wrong manipulation
"Power Doppler"	Sensitive to small flows, does not confuse the operator with unclear direction data	Poorly follows fast flow changes, Color dependent on depth, No aliasing, Gives little clue about the type of flow (slow image repetition)	Insufficient clinical experience

Occasionally, a spectral trace can show one or more **straight lines** adjacent to and parallel to the baseline, often on both sides.

This is due to any electrical noise operating at multiples or whole fractions of the monitor image repetition, including 50 Hz interference from power lines or power supply. It can make determination of low or absent diastolic flow difficult. Electromagnetic interference from power lines and nearby equipment can also cloud the spectral display with lines or "snow". Improper pulse repetition frequency (PRF) settings can ultimately cause erroneous diagnosis of an absent diastolic blood flow.

In Figure 1.5, "WI" indicates the **"window"**, an empty space in the real-time spectrum. Strictly speaking, this space ought never be empty, but in the case of parabolic flow and somewhat reduced sensitivity, the space will not fill in with measurement results. This logic applies, if the sensitive volume takes up the whole blood vessel cross section. However, if we reduce the sensitive volume so as to take up only a small part of the blood vessel, a "window" will appear even at fairly irregular flows. This does not influence much the assessment of RI and PI, but disturbs our assessment of the turbulence. Very turbulent flow will show at the same time positive (towards probe) and negative (away from probe) flow spectrum. However, a similar spectrum appearance can be expected if we put the measurement angle near 90°. Therefore, we must always interpret the cause of the apparent synchronous flow in opposite directions.

Inadvertent change of the wall filter can cut off the diastolic part of arterial Doppler spectrum and lead to wrong clinical diagnosis.

How to Reduce Problems

- Use the sensitivity with caution (use as a low sensitivity as practical)
- Start examination with the standard symmetrical color map and then gradually change it to nonsymmetrical types, if needed.
- Be aware of the depth and increased aliasing probability at deeper structures and higher velocities.
- Use all the three modes (B mode, spectrum, color) for survey, but use single modality to obtain the best quality of each of them.

Acknowledgment

In writing this chapter some materials provided by Ivica Zalud, MD, PhD have been used and this is kindly acknowledged.

REFERENCES

1. Censor D, Newhouse VL, Vontz T, et al. Theory of ultrasound Doppler-spectra velocimetry for arbitrary beam and flow configurations. IEEE Trans Biomed Eng 1988; 35(9):740-51.
2. Burns PN. Principles of Doppler and color flow. Radiol Med 1993;85:3-16.
3. Taylor KJ and Holland S. Doppler ultrasound. Part I. Basic principles, instrumentation, and pitfalls. Radiology 1990; 174:297-307.
4. Mitchell DG. Color Doppler imaging: principles, limitations, and artifacts. Radiology 1990;177(1):1-10.
5. Kremkau FW. Doppler color imaging. Principles and instrumentation. Clin Diagn Ultrasound 1992;27:7-60.
6. Chen JF, Fowlkes JB, Carson PL, et al. Autocorrelation of integrated power Doppler signals and its application. Ultrasound Med Biol 1996;22(8):1053-7.
7. Zalud I and Kurjak A. Artifacts and pitfalls. In: Kurjak A (Ed). Transvaginal color Doppler, (2nd Edn), London-New York: Parthenon Publishing 1994;353-8.
8. Derchi LE, Giannoni M, Crespi G, et al. Artifacts in echo-Doppler and color-Doppler. Radiol Med 1992;83:340-52.
9. Jaffe R. Color Doppler imaging: A new interpretation of the Doppler effect. In: Jaffe R and Warsof SL (Eds). Color Doppler imaging in obstetrics and gynecology. New York: McGraw-Hill 1992;17-34.
10. Winkler P, Helmke K, Mahl M. Major pitfalls in Doppler investigations. Part II. Low flow velocities and colour Doppler applications. Pediatr Radiol 1990;20(5):304-10.
11. Suchet IB. Colour-flow Doppler artifacts in anechoic soft-tissue masses of infants. Can Assoc Radiol J 1994;45(3):201-3.
12. Pozniak MA, Zagzebski JA, Scanlan KA. Spectral and color Doppler artifacts. Radiographics 1992;12(1):35-44.
13. Maulik D. Biosafety of diagnostic Doppler ultrasonography. In: Maulik D (Ed). Doppler ultrasound in obstetrics and gynecology. New York: Springer 1997;88-106.
14. Duck F, Zauhar G. Report on experiments by Starrit H, Zauhar G and Duck F in Bath, autumn 1996.

S Kupesic Plavsic, A Kurjak, K Baston

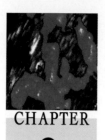

CHAPTER 2

Normal Pelvic Anatomy Assessed by 2D, 3D and Color Doppler Ultrasound

INTRODUCTION

The advantages of transvaginal over transabdominal ultrasound examination are the use of a high-frequency transvaginal transducer with better spatial resolution and no need to fill the urinary bladder. Because of these characteristics, transvaginal ultrasonography became essential in gynecologic ultrasound examination.

Two-dimensional (2D) ultrasound imaging is limited by navigation of the transvaginal transducer in the narrow space of vagina. Therefore, it allows presentation of two planes: sagittal and transverse. Three-dimensional (3D) sonography, however, permits multiplanar display of all three sections: coronal, sagittal and transverse. Using this method, it is possible to measure the volume of the studied organ or structure and evaluate it more accurately. Three-dimensional ultrasound enables storage of the data without degradation of the image quality, retrospective analysis, and application of teleconsultation in telemedicine.

Color Doppler capability of the transvaginal probes permits visualization of small intraovarian and endometrial vessels, allowing depiction of normal and pathological changes in reproductive organs.

3D color histogram measures the color percentage and flow amplitudes in the volume of interest. Therefore, the histogram enables quantification of the vascularization and blood flow within a tissue block, in contrast to 2D color histogram measurements, where only single planes can be investigated. Here, a 3D tissue block is swept through with a volume probe to obtain the 3D information and after that to enclose the volume of interest containing both the B-mode and color Doppler information resulting in an automatic delineation called "shell".

UTERUS

The transvaginal sonography transducer is pressed on the flexed cervical-corporeal junction positioned in the posterior fornix and oriented at the superior apex of the screen. The first landmark one can see is the uterus.

Adult

The normal size, shape, the length ratio of body and cervix of the uterus and appearance of the endometrium depend on the patient's age and parity. In addition, its position depends on bladder and rectal fullness.

The dimensions of the uterus can be accurately measured with transabdominal and transvaginal ultrasound. Three-dimensional ultrasound enables the estimation of the uterine volume and gives the ability to present planar sections of the uterus in three different projections: transverse, sagittal and coronal.

The fundus of the anteverted uterus is placed on the left side of the ultrasound screen, while the fundus of the retroverted uterus is placed to the right. Transvaginal scanning might be limited when the uterus is in the same axis as the cervix and vagina because the ultrasound beam and uterine position are not perpendicular.

Commonly, the uterus can be slightly deviated to the right or left side, but larger deviations might exist due to pathological lesions in the pelvis (pelvic masses or peritoneal adhesions). The importance of defining the position of the uterus is especially valuable while performing various invasive procedures, such as curettage, hysteroscopy, insertion of an intrauterine contraceptive device or embryo transfer.

The uterus consists of the body and the cervix, having a 2:1 length ratio. Dimensions of the body are commonly

7.5-9 cm (length) × 4.5-6 cm (width) × 2.5-4 cm (thickness). Sonographic studies found that the uterine size varies with parity.[1] Dimensions of the cervix are 3-5 cm (length) × 2-3 cm (width).

The uterus consists of three major portions: the endometrium, myometrium and serosa. Normal echo texture of the myometrium is homogeneously echodense. The inner layer of the myometrium can be a little less echogenic, but the junction zone with endometrium is well demarcated and smooth.

The endometrial cavity is slit-like in sagittal section with the anterior and posterior endometrial surfaces, touching one another. The triangular appearance of the endometrial cavity is imaged in a coronal section by 3D ultrasound.[2]

Multiplanar view is used to demonstrate the coronal, longitudinal and transverse sections of the same organ or structure. The coronal plane (frontal reformatted section of the uterus) is used to visualize both horns of the uterine cavity and the cervix at the same time.[2] The normal uterus usually shows a convex shape of the endometrium and myometrium in the fundus. The endometrium appears as an echogenic interface in the central part of the uterus, but the intensity of the echogenicity and the thickness depends on the phase of the menstrual cycle. 3D ultrasound enables reconstruction of the uterine cavity and measurement of the endometrial volume.[3]

During the reproductive period, all pelvic organs (their size and echogenicity) are influenced with cyclic changes in blood circulating hormone concentrations, related to the ovary function. The most obvious changes are evident in the uterus. Duration of the normal menstrual cycle is 28 days, with about equal time for the preovulatory (follicular) and postovulatory (luteal) phase. In women with normal fertility, duration of the menstrual cycle varies between 25 and 36 days. It was demonstrated that follicular phase (proliferative phase of the endometrium) is more variable, while the luteal phase (secretory phase of the endometrium) remains 14 days.[3,4] Approaching the menopause, the follicular phase becomes shorter, with earlier ovulation.

Phases of Menstrual Cycle

Proliferative phase: As menstruation ceases, the functional layer of the endometrium responds to estrogen secreted by the ovary. Simultaneously with follicular development and increased estrogen production, the endometrial glands in the basal layer start to proliferate, elongate and become tortuous.

Ultrasound findings of the endometrium are best presented on transvaginal sonography in the sagittal plane.

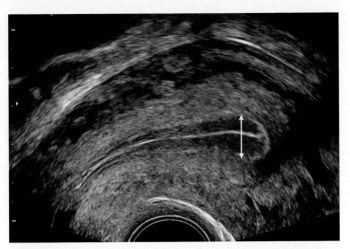

FIGURE 2.1: Transvaginal scan of a triple-line endometrium during the late proliferative phase of the menstrual cycle.

The endocervical canal is seen as continuing into the endometrial cavity. The endometrium is measured as a double-layer thickness from the proximal myometrial-endometrial junction to the distal myometrial-endometrial junction. The examiner should be careful, if intraluminal fluid is present. Measurement in that case is performed in a way that each endometrial thickness is measured separately and both layers are added.

Early proliferative phase endometrium is a thin echogenic line, measuring from 1-3 mm. With progression of the proliferative phase, the echogenicity of the endometrium decreases in comparison with the surrounding myometrium. The most characteristic sign of the late proliferative phase is the triple-line endometrium (Figure 2.1). The central echogenic line represents a zone between the anterior and posterior endometrial layers. Two outer hyperechogenic lines represent the endometrial-myometrial junction or echo of the basal layer. The endometrial tissue (functional layer) between two lines becomes hypoechoic and thick during the proliferative phase. The endometrium at the end of proliferative phase is usually thicker than 7 mm (7-14 mm).[4]

Secretory phase: Progesterone secretion during the luteal phase of the ovarian cycle, following ovulation, causes the endometrial glands to secrete glycoproteins. Increased glycoprotein secretion causes disappearance of the three lines present in the late proliferative endometrium. On ultrasound examination, the endometrium appears as an homogenous and hyperechogenic structure measuring from 8-14 mm (Figure 2.2).

Menstrual phase: Menstruation begins when circulating levels of estrogens and progesterone decrease at the end of

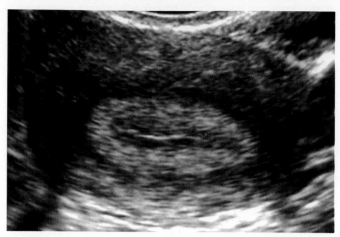

FIGURE 2.2: Transvaginal scan of a thickened and echogenic endometrium during the luteal phase of the menstrual cycle.

the ovarian cycle, causing breakdown of the functional layer. The ultrasound image varies depending on the amount of blood clots and endometrial fragments, which is visualized as echogenic debris. Basal layers are imaged as thin, irregular and hyperechogenic lines.

Postmenopausal State

The size of the cervix and body of the uterus decreases gradually as menopause progresses. The postmenopausal uterus measures approximately 4.5 cm (length) × 1.5 cm (width) × 2.5 cm (thickness). The body of the uterus shortens and the uterus body/cervix ratio decreases to almost to 1:1. There is a slight difference between women who are obese or using hormonal replacement therapy (HRT) and other postmenopausal women. The uterus body/ cervix ratio decreases much more slowly in the first group than in the second.[5] Due to the progressive decrease of the ovarian function in postmenopausal women, the endometrium becomes thin and atrophic, since it is not subjected to the cyclic changes. The mean endometrial thickness is 2.3 ± 1.8 mm.[5] In the postmenopausal state, the ovaries do not secrete estrogens, but still produce androgen hormones, which together with androgens derived from the adrenal glands are converted to estrogens in peripheral adipose cells. Estrogen production during the postmenopausal period may lead to abnormal endometrial thickening. In women taking sequential HRT, thickness of the endometrium of a maximum of 8 mm is tolerated as the result of HRT, as well as endometrium changes according to the phase of the cyclical therapy. In continuous combined regimens, the endometrium is likely to be a relatively thin. An endometrial thickness cut-off level of

< 5 mm in a symptomatic patient seems to have a high negative predictive value for the presence of endometrial cancer.[6] Once the endometrial thickness is greater than 8 mm in asymptomatic postmenopausal women not taking HRT, an outpatient biopsy is required to exclude endometrial hyperplasia or malignancy.

Cervix

The cervix constitutes the lower third of the uterus in an adult, while in childhood the cervix accounts for two-thirds of the uterine length.[7] Since the cervix connects the upper part of the vagina with the uterine cavity, it serves as a depot for spermatozoa, allowing their migration towards the uterine ostia.

The cervix of the uterus is an oval-conic shaped canal, measuring approximately 2.5 cm in length, entering the vagina vertically. The site where the uterine body turns away from the cervix marks the internal cervical os. The internal cervical os is clearly seen on ultrasound examination of the anteflexed uterus as an indentation in the anterior wall. During menstruation between the internal and external cervical os, the sonographer may visualize an echogenic stripe of bleeding.[8] At the time of ovulation and under the influence of estrogen, the cervix may be dilated from 4 to 5 mm, which is visualized as a hypoechogenic or echoless stripe within the cervix. After the rupture of the follicle and due to the drop of the estrogen level, the cervical canal closes. The mucus in the endocervical canal is viscous and echogenic, except at the time of ovulation, when it is diluted and seen as an echolucent area.

Nabothian cysts are retention cysts of the cervical glands within the vaginal portion of the cervix undergoing metaplasia from columnar to stratified squamous epithelium. They measure approximately 10 mm in diameter with thin walls and spherical shape, containing echolucent fluid. Nabothian cysts have no clinical value even when they are multiple and are large in size (> 1 cm).

Uterine Perfusion

The main uterine arteries originate from the internal iliac arteries and give off branches, which extend inward for about a third of the myometrium thickness without significant branching.[9] They subdivide into an arcuate wreath, encircling the uterus. These vessels then branch into the smaller branches, called the radial arteries, which are directed towards the uterine lumen. The radial arteries branch into the basal arteries and as they pass the myometrial-endometrial border, they become spiral arteries.

Basal arteries that are relatively short terminate in a capillary bed that serves the stratum basale of the endometrium. Spiral arteries project further into the endometrium and terminate in a vast capillary network that serves the stratum functionale of the endometrium. Only spiral arteries undergo substantial anatomical changes during the menstrual cycle.[10] At the time of menstruation, probably because of decreasing estrogen and progesterone levels, the spiral arteries constrict. Blood flow in the main pelvic vessels can be easily visualized and recognized.[11]

Color Doppler signals from the main uterine vessels is observed in a transverse plane, laterally to the cervix, at the level of the cervicocorporal junction.[12] Waveform analysis shows high to moderate blood flow velocity. Pulsed Doppler waveform profiles of the main uterine artery are characteristic, comprising a high peak-systolic component with a characteristic notch in the protodiastolic part and very low end-diastolic flow. The RI depends on the age, phase of the menstrual cycle and special conditions (pregnancy, tumor, etc.).

In most women, there is a small amount of end-diastolic flow in the uterine arteries during the proliferative phase.[13] The RI is about 0.88 ± 0.04 until day 13 of the 28th day menstrual cycle (Figure 2.3). In postmenopausal women, RI increases and in late postmenopausal period it is usually of value 1.0.

It is evident that the diastolic flow in the uterine arteries decreases or disappears during the day of ovulation.[14] An increasing RI and systolic/diastolic ratio during the postovulatory drop in serum estradiol concentration may be explained by increased uterine contractility and compression of the vessels traversing the uterine wall that decrease their diameter and cause consequently higher resistance to blood flow.[15] During the normal menstrual cycle, there is a sharp increase in end-diastolic velocities between the proliferative and secretory phases of the menstrual cycle. It is interesting that the lowest blood flow impedance occurs during the time of peak luteal function, when implantation is most likely to occur (Figure 2.4). It is expected that blood supply to the uterus should be the highest during the late luteal phase.[14-17]

In an ovulatory cycles, these changes are not present and a continuous increase in the RI is demonstrated. The persistently lower RI in the luteal phase suggests that the relaxation effects on the uterine arteries persist until the onset of menstruation. More recently a circadian rhythm of the uterine artery blood flow was documented during the periovulatory period that appears to be independent from the hormonal changes.[18]

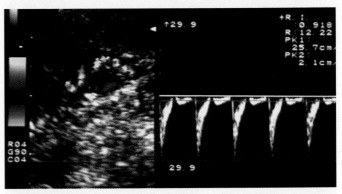

FIGURE 2.3: Transvaginal color Doppler analysis of the uterine artery blood flow in the proliferative phase of the menstrual cycle. Note a small amount of end-diastolic flow and a characteristic notch (RI = 0.92).

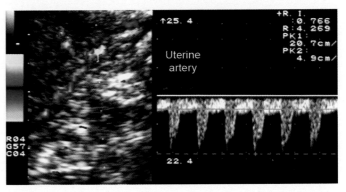

FIGURE 2.4: Uterine artery blood flow in the secretory phase of the menstrual cycle, characterized with sharp increase of an end-diastolic blood flow and decreased resistance index (RI = 0.77).

Doppler sonograms of the arcuate and radial arteries are very similar, with moderate peak-systolic and diastolic components of blood flow.

Endometrial vascularity is highly dependent upon the uterine, arcuate and radial artery blood flow. Blood flow velocity waveform changes in the spiral arteries during the normal ovulatory cycles are characterized by lower velocity and lower impedance to blood flow than are those observed in the uterine arteries (Figure 2.5).[16]

While 2D color Doppler is useful for detection of the vessels, 3D power Doppler is an excellent tool to study vascular morphology and to detect neovascularization.[19]

Uterus in Newborn and Prepuberty

The newborn uterus is tubular in shape with body and cervix length ratio 1:1. It can be 0.5-1 cm larger than the uterus in infants because of residual pregnancy hormones. Dimensions of the uterus in infants are approximately

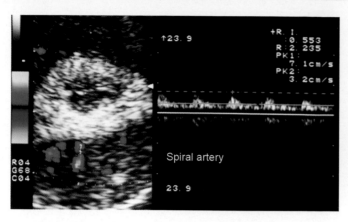

FIGURE 2.5: Spiral artery blood flow is characterized with moderate to low vascular resistance (RI = 0.55).

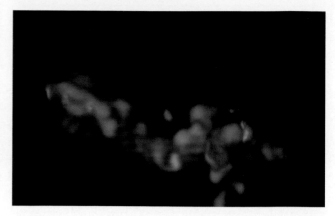

FIGURE 2.6: 3D power Doppler scan of regular tubal patency demonstrated after injection of the echo-enhancing contrast. Note regular spillage of the contrast from the fimbrial end.

3 cm (length) × 2 cm (width) × 2 cm (thickness). It is tubular shaped with the same length/cervix ratio as in newborn. During puberty, the shape of the uterus changes to pear-shaped due to the enlargement of the uterine corpus.

VAGINA

The vagina may be visualized by transabdominal ultrasound. Ultrasound determination of the vaginal length is not reliable because of the variable degree of bladder distension.

FALLOPIAN TUBE

The Fallopian tubes are approximately 10 to 12 cm long and a few millimeters wide. They spread from the lateral uterine angles toward the corresponding ovary. Fallopian tubes can only be occasionally seen on ultrasound when filled with the fluid (hydrosalpinx), during the course of the diagnostic procedures (hysterosonosalpingography), or when peritoneal fluid is present surrounding the adnexa. When visualized, the fallopian tubes are presented as tortuous echogenic structures with varying diameters from the proximal to the distal end.

By using 3D ultrasound, it is possible to visualize the fallopian tubes with more detail and differentiate them from the surrounding structures.

Kupesic and Plavsic used 3D power Doppler imaging for visualization of the tubal patency.[20] They demonstrated that 3D power Doppler imaging with surface rendering allows visualization of the flow of the contrast through the entire tubal length. Furthermore, a spill of the contrast medium may be identified in the majority of cases (Figure 2.6). This minimally invasive diagnostic method does not

require the use of ionizing radiation and enables storage of the information for off-line analysis. For additional information about hysteroncontrast-salpingography (Hy-Co-Sy), the interested reader is referred to the corresponding chapter in this book that discusses this topic.

OVARIES

Adolescence and Adulthood

This period is characterized by the appearance of the ovarian follicles and corpora lutea. The number of follicular "recruits" visible on ultrasound is proportional to the number of primordial follicles present in the ovaries and is inversely proportional to the woman's age. As one approaches menopause, the supply of such endocrine responsive follicles becomes depleted, which may be associated with menstrual cycle irregularities.

Improved resolution, closer focusing and avoiding the need for a full bladder make transvaginal ultrasound preferable for scanning the ovaries.

The ovaries are located on each side of the uterus, close to the lateral wall of the pelvis in fossa Waldeyer. The iliac vessels are a reliable landmark for their visualization, especially when using color Doppler ultrasound. Due to the mobility of the ovaries and transducer pressure, the position of the ovaries often varies (in the cul-de-sac, in front of the uterus, above the uterus or in the abdominal cavity). Sometimes, previous inflammatory disease or surgical interventions may cause pelvic adhesions that fix the position of the ovaries. This commonly occurs close to the lateral fornices of the vagina.

The ovaries are seen as homogenous, hypoechogenic ovoid structures with a slightly echogenic central part, with dimensions approximately 3 × 2 × 2 cm during the reproductive period. In postmenopausal women, detection of the ovaries is difficult due to the lack of follicles and small size.

Ovarian follicles facilitate the identification of the ovaries and are seen as containing echolucent fluid and varying in size from 2-25 mm in diameter, depending on the age and phase of the menstrual cycle. About 7 million of the follicle, containing oocytes are present in a female fetus at about 20 weeks gestation.[21] These follicles, called primordial follicles, are microscopic in size and metabolically quiescent. Later in childhood and reproductive age, they grow from primordial to primary, secondary and tertiary follicles (microscopic in size), forming a fluid-filled antrum. In adequate hormonal conditions (increased local follicle stimulating hormone-FSH levels), follicles continue to grow until they become sonographically detectable. Only 100-1000 follicles remain until the menopausal period. Most of them undergo atresia and only a fraction ovulate.

The small and transient rise in FSH serum levels at the end of each ovarian cycle affects the small antral follicles (size of 1 or 2 mm). These follicles have a potential to grow further, instead of becoming atretic. During the early follicular phase of the ovarian cycle, pituitary FSH causes follicular cells to secrete estrogen and the peptide hormone inhibin (reduces FSH production as the follicular phase progresses). Smaller follicles regress with the drop in FSH levels, while the larger ones grow regardless. One or sometimes two follicles become dominant, producing the substantial amounts of estradiol as they grow, while the others become atretic. This turnover happens by the end of the first week of the follicular phase. Atretic follicles may still be visible and can grow, especially in the dominant side, although they are undergoing atresia.

The dominant follicle, also called a Graafian follicle, is usually detected at day 10 of the menstrual cycle. At that time, it measures approximately 10 mm and increases in size 2-3 mm/day until it reaches about 18–22 mm in size. After that, growth decelerates to 1.3 mm/day.[22] Follicles grow due to increased number of follicle cells and accumulation of fluid inside the antrum. Cumulus oophorus, consisting of the oocyte and surrounding follicle cells, protrudes as a small papillary projection from the follicular wall. Cumulus oophorus can be seen by 2D and 3D ultrasound. Detection of cumulus oophorus is important because it suggests the presence of an existing oocyte. During the periovulatory period, moderate vascular resistance signals (RI = 0.49) are detected from the rim of

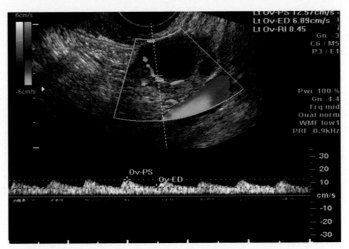

FIGURE 2.7: Transvaginal color Doppler scan of the preovulatory follicle. Note low-to-moderate vascular resistance (RI = 0.45) indicative of a high oocyte quality.

the follicle. Prominent perifollicular vascularization is an indirect sign of oocyte maturity and quality (Figure 2.7).

Dominant follicular development is not always sustained by ovulation, especially in the early reproductive age when ovulation does not occur and hence, follicular phase and consequently the entire menstrual cycle becomes longer and irregular (oligomenorrhea or amenorrhea). Multifollicular appearance of the ovaries means persistence of variable-sized developing follicles. Multifollicular appearance may be a normal finding during adolescence and recovery from weight loss, but in older women, it is usually associated with a significant ovulation disorder of primarily ovarian origin and/or beginning of the ovarian failure.

Ovulation occurs with dissolution of the part of the follicle wall, liberation of the oocyte and escape of the follicular fluid into the peritoneal cavity. It takes place about 38 hours after the luteinizing hormone (LH) surge begins, as a consequence of pituitary response to high circulating estrogen levels. At that time, the dominant follicle is 16-25 mm in diameter. The preovulatory follicle is filled with blood and forms the corpus hemorragicum. Afterwards, it luteinizes and begins to secrete progesterone, with formation of new blood vessels around the follicle, visible on color Doppler ultrasound. High-estrogen levels affect the Fallopian tube fluid secretion and transudation through the follicular wall, resulting in ultrasonically recognizable accumulation of free peritoneal fluid. In addition to the free fluid imaged on ultrasound, ovulation is presented as sudden disappearance of the echolucent dominant follicle and after several days, with formation of the corpus luteum. As a result of the corpus luteum maturation into a solid-cystic steroid-producing "organ", the progesterone concentration in serum increases.

If ovulation does not occur, the follicle continues to grow and becomes a follicular cyst. On ultrasound scanning, it is seen as a thin-walled cystic lesion filled with sonolucent fluid that is clearly demarcated from the rest of the ovary.

After ovulation, formation of the corpus luteum occurs. The follicular wall collapses, the follicular/granulosa cells luteinize, accumulating fat and secreting progesterone, and new blood vessels begin to proliferate and invade the tissue of the future corpus luteum. Proliferating capillaries invading the theca interna and granulosa layer are fragile and start to transudate serum or blood. Sometimes, the corpus luteum is hardly seen on transvaginal ultrasound due to its variable echo characteristics. Commonly, it is visualized as a structure containing thick hyperechogenic walls enclosing the hypoechoic center (Figure 2.8). Sometimes, the corpus luteum is 5-6 cm in diameter and due to its clot component can be confused with endometrioma. Because of its atypical ultrasound finding it is called "the great pretender". Corpus luteum angiogenesis starts about 24 hours after the LH surge and continues to be detectable by the means of transvaginal color Doppler through the entire functional life of the corpus luteum (Figure 2.9). Depending on its vascularization, it is possible to distinguish three phases of the corpus luteum cycle:

1. Organization and vascularization (characterized with RI = 0.43 ± 0.04) (Figure 2.10).
2. Maturation (characterized with RI = 0.46 ± 0.03)
3. Regression (characterized with RI = 0.50 ± 0.04).

If the corpus luteum is filled with serous fluid and persists for more than 2 weeks, it is called a corpus luteum cyst.

Ultrasound and color Doppler evaluation of the ovarian lesions and cysts is best done during the follicular phase of the menstrual cycle in order to avoid the diagnostic confusion that may be caused by the different appearances of a corpus luteum. If the dominant follicle does not release follicular fluid and the oocyte, but luteinization takes place with continuous growth toward a diameter of about 3 cm with echogenic or sonolucent contents, the structure is called a luteinized unruptured follicle (LUF syndrome). A luteinized unruptured follicle occurs in about 5% of normal menstrual cycles and in a higher rate in abnormal cycles. Progesterone production in LUF syndrome is less than in a normal luteal phase, leading to a shorter luteal phase of the menstrual cycle.

3D ultrasound facilitates ovarian volume calculation, determination of the antral follicle number, evaluation of

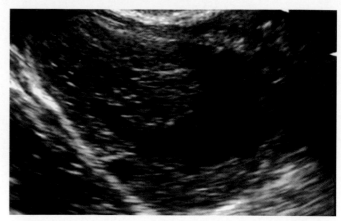

FIGURE 2.8: Transvaginal scan of an early corpus luteum. Note irregular hypoechogenic walls enclosing the hypoechoic center.

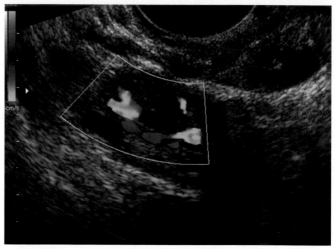

FIGURE 2.9: Transvaginal color Doppler scan of corpus luteum angiogenesis.

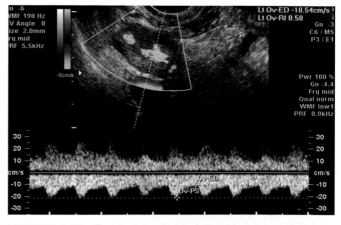

FIGURE 2.10: Transvaginal color Doppler scan of corpus luteum during the stage of organization and vascularization. Low vascular resistance indicates significant perfusion and adequate progesterone production.

the ovarian stroma and analysis of the intensity of the ovarian stromal blood flow. Advantages include a short examination time and minimal discomfort for the patient.[23,24] The average ovarian volume is between 6 and 10 cm[3].

Ovarian Circulation Presented by Color Doppler

The ovarian vascular system may be divided into extrinsic and intrinsic. The extrinsic vascular system consists of arteries that start from big abdominal trunks before they enter the ovary and homologous venous system.

Vessels entering the ovarian hilus form the intrinsic vascular system.[25] The ovary receives its arterial vascularization from two sources: the ovarian artery and the utero-ovarian branch of the uterine artery.[26] These arteries anastomose, forming an arch parallel to the ovarian hilus. The vessels sprouting from the arch pass through the central medullary part of the stroma towards the periphery (the ovarian cortex). In the ovarian cortex, the vessels form vascular arcades in the stroma, surrounding the follicles. These vessels can be seen by color Doppler ultrasound during the proliferative phase of the menstrual cycle. At this time, RI in perifollicular vessels is from 0.50-0.55 and presents an important hemodynamic parameter of the follicular growth (Figure 2.7).

Several hours before ovulation, vessels penetrate the granulosa cell layer. Reduction of the vascular resistance in perifollicular vessels is significant during the preovulatory phase and shows RI values from 0.42-0.48. The intrafollicular blood velocity increases 29 hours before the time of the follicular rupture, continues for at least 72 hours after the formation of the corpus hemorrhagicum, and is reflected in the color Doppler data obtained at this time. The mean changes in peak systolic velocity appear to follow the mean rise in circulatory LH by approximately 12 hours.[27] Following the ovulation, the RI remains at the same level for 4-5 days and then gradually rises to 0.50 ± 0.04, but remains still lower than the one measured in the proliferative phase.

This period is characterized by the proliferation of the theca vessels, which further vascularize the granulosa cell layer. Within three to four days after the follicular rupture, the corpus luteum is supplied with a dense, multilayered network of sinusoidal capillaries that are drained by numerous superficial venules. By means of color Doppler, the blood supply to the corpus luteum can be clearly seen as a bright colored ring surrounding the corpus luteum.[28]

Significantly lower vascular resistance values are detected in the dominant ovary during the luteal phase of the menstrual cycle as compared with the follicular phase. These blood flow changes reflect changes in vascularization and function of the corpus luteum. The nondominant ovary presents a slightly higher RI during the luteal and follicular phases.[29] Higher blood flow velocity and lower impedance, detected in the vessels of the dominant ovary during the late follicular and early luteal phase indicates increased blood flow to the dominant ovary. The increased blood supply to the ovary containing the dominant follicle and corpus luteum is necessary for delivery of the steroid precursors and removal of the progesterone.

In both uterine and ovarian vessels, changes in flow velocity occur before ovulation, implying that these changes are complex and not entirely related to the progesterone action. Many other vasoactive compounds (e.g. prostaglandin) are involved in the regulation of the ovarian circulation.

3D power Doppler enables the reconstruction of complete vascularization of the ovary and distinguishes normal from the pathological angiogenesis.

Newborn

During the neonatal period, the ovaries may be difficult to demonstrate with ultrasound due to their small size and the difficulty in obtaining a full bladder. Developing follicles remain small and invisible to ultrasound resolution. The ovaries continue to decrease in size for the first two years of childhood. Cohen et al.[30] demonstrated that the mean ovarian volume is 1.2 cm[3] among the girls up to 3 months old; 1.1 cm[3] among the girls 4-12 months old; and 0.7 cm[3] among the girls 13-24 months old. Failure to demonstrate the ovaries in the newborn does not imply ovarian dysgenesis.

Childhood

During childhood, transabdominal, transrectal or transperineal scanning may be performed. The ovaries grow slowly through childhood, with increases in the mean ovarian volume from 0.5 cm[3] at the age of 3 to 2.8 cm[3] at the age of 18 years.[31] There is a good correlation between the ovarian size and growth during childhood. It is documented that tall girls have ovaries larger than short girls.[31]

Perimenopausal and Postmenopausal State

During the perimenopausal phase, ovarian follicular depletion occurs diminishing the number of antral follicles for recruitment. This results in lower production of follicular inhibin and earlier rise of FSH levels (during the late luteal phase). All these events cause earlier initiation of follicular development, even before the onset of menstruation. As one approaches menopause, the follicular phase and consequently the menstrual cycle gets shorter. During the perimenopausal years, functional cysts and/or multifollicular appearance of the ovaries is commonly detected by ultrasound. In the postmenopausal period, estrogen and inhibin production falls and FSH levels increase. The ovaries become small and homogenous with no sonographic evidence of the follicles.[32,33]

In perimenopausal and postmenopausal phases of life, the shape and volume of the ovaries change. They are ovoid and significantly smaller than during reproductive life. At this time, the ovaries measure $2 \times 1.5 \times 1.5$ cm, with a maximum volume of 7 cm^3.[32,33]

CONCLUSION

3D ultrasound imaging of the gynecological structures permits more detailed evaluation of the physiological and pathophysiological changes of the reproductive organs. Color Doppler analysis enables visualization and analysis of the ovarian and uterine hemodynamic changes.

The first landmark seen by transvaginal ultrasound is the uterus. Its size, shape, the body/cervix ratio, as well as the appearance of the endometrium depend on the patient's age and parity. 3D ultrasound of the uterus enables the estimation of the uterine volume and presentation of the three orthogonal planes (multiplanar view) of the uterus. Endometrial volume and thickness measurements by 3D and 2D ultrasound, respectively, show good reproducibility. The image of the endometrium in reproductive age depends on the phase of the menstrual cycle. In postmenopausal patients, not receiving hormonal replacement therapy, the endometrium is visualized as a thin hyperechoic line usually < 5 mm. Color Doppler signals from the main uterine vessels are observed laterally to the cervix, at the level of the cervicocorporal junction. Waveform analysis shows high-to-moderate flow velocity. In most women, there is a small amount of end-diastolic flow in the uterine arteries during the proliferative phase. In postmenopausal patients RI increases and in the late postmenopausal period uterine artery blood flow is usually characterized by the absence of diastolic flow.

The fallopian tubes are seen on ultrasound if and when filled with fluid (such as in the case of hydrosalpinx), during the course of a diagnostic procedure (such as hysterosonosalpingography) or when peritoneal fluid is present surrounding the adnexa.

The ovaries are located on each side of the cervix, close to the lateral wall of the pelvis in the fossa Waldeyer. Iliac vessels are a reliable landmark for their visualization and ovarian follicles facilitate the identification of the ovaries. The follicles are visualized as sonolucent structures measuring from 2-25 mm in diameter, depending on the phase of the menstrual cycle. The dominant follicle, also called the Graafian follicle, is usually detected on the 10th day of the menstrual cycle. At that time, it measures approximately 10 mm and increases in size 2-3 mm/day until it reaches about 18–22 mm. After ovulation, formation of the corpus luteum occurs. It is visualized as a structure containing thick hyperechogenic walls, enclosing the hypoechoic center. In some cases the corpus luteum may reach 5-6 cm in diameter and due to the accompanying clot may be misinterpreted as an endometrioma. Because of its atypical ultrasound findings, it is called "the great pretender". Ultrasound and color Doppler evaluation of the ovarian lesions is best done during the follicular phase of the menstrual cycle. Application of 3D ultrasound enables measurement of the ovarian volume and assessment of its surface features.

The size and volume of the ovaries progressively decrease in postmenopausal age due to fibrotic changes.

When used together, 2D, 3D and color Doppler ultrasound give the best results in evaluation of both normal and pathological conditions of the female reproductive system.

REFERENCES

1. Ramsay PA, Jansen RPS. Ultrasonography of the normal female pelvis. In: Anderson JC (Ed). Gynecologic Imaging. London:Churchill Livingstone 1999;61-80.
2. Yaman C, Ebner T, Jesacher K, et al. Reproducibility of three-dimensional ultrasound endometrial volume measurements in patients with postmenopausal bleeding. Ultrasound Obstet Gynecol 2002;19(3):282-6.
3. Kupesic S, Kurjak A, Bjelos D. The assessment of uterine lesions. In Kurjak A, Kupesic S. (Eds). Clinical application of 3D sonography. London, New York: Parthenon Publishing 2000;55-65.
4. Abdalla HI, Brooks AA, Johnson MR, et al. Endometrial thickness: A predictor of implantation in ovum recipients? Hum Reprod 1994;9:363-5.
5. Kurjak A, Kupesic S. Ovarian senescence and its significance on uterine and ovarian perfusion. Fertil Steril 1995;64:532-7.
6. Wikland M, Granberg S. Endometrial changes as imaged by transvaginal sonography in fertile and infertile women. In: Fleischer A, Kurjak A, Granberg S (Eds). Ultrasound and endometrium. London, New York: Parthenon Publishing 1996; 17-23.

7. Suren A, Puchta J, Osmers R. Sonographic evaluation of the cervix uteri. In Osmers R and Kurjak A (Eds). Ultrasound and the Uterus. New York, London: Parthenon Publishing 1995; 13-8.

8. Hill LM, Coulam CB, Kislak SL, et al. Sonographic evaluation of the cervix during ovulation induction. Am J Obstet Gynecol 1987;157:1170-4.

9. Kurjak A, Kupesic S. Blood flow studies in normal and abnormal early pregnancy. In: Kurjak A, Kupesic S (Eds). An Atlas of Transvaginal color Doppler, (2nd edn). London, New York: Parthenon Publishing 2000;41-3.

10. Templeton AA, Penney GC. The incidence, characteristics and prognosis of patients whose infertility is unexplained. Fertil Steril 1982;37:175-81.

11. Hsieh YY, Chang FCC, Tsai HD. Doppler evaluation of the uterine and spiral arteries from different sampling sites and phases of the menstrual cycle during controlled ovarian hyperstimulation. Ultrasound in Obstet Gynecol 2000 16(2):192-6.

12. Kurjak A, Kupesic-Urek S. Normal and abnormal uterine perfusion. In: Jaffe R, Warsof LS (Eds). Color Doppler Imaging in Obstetrics and Gynecology. New York: McGraw Hill 1992; 255-63.

13. Kurjak , Kupesic-Urek S, Schulman H, et al. Transvaginal color Doppler in the assessment of ovarian and uterine blood flow in infertile women. Fertil. Steril 1991;56:870-3.

14. Steer CV, Mills CV, Campbell S. Vaginal color Doppler assessment on the day of embryo transfer (ET) accurately predicts patients in an *in vitro* fertilization programme with suboptimal uterine perfusion who fail to be pregnant. Ultrasound Obstet Gynecol 1991;1(Suppl.) 79.

15. Kurjak A, Kupesic-Urek S. Normal and abnormal uterine perfusion. In: Jaffe R, Warsof LS (Eds). Color Doppler Imaging in Obstetrics and Gynecology. New York: McGraw Hill 1992; 255-63.

16. Goswamy RK, Steptoe PC. Doppler Ultrasound studies of the uterine artery in spontaneous ovarian cycles. Hum Reprod 1988;3:721-6.

17. Battaglia C, Larocca E, Lanzani A, et al. Doppler ultrasound studies of the uterine arteries in spontaneous and IVF cycles. Gynaecol Endocrinol 1990;4:245-50.

18. Zaidi J, Jurkovic D, Campbell S, et al. Description of circadian rhythm in uterine artery blood flow during the periovulatory period. Hum Reprod 1995;10(7):1642-6.

19. Kurjak A, Kupesic S, Zodan T. The assessement of pelvic tumor angiogenesis In Kurjak A, Kupesic S (Eds). An Atlas of Transvaginal color Doppler, 2nd edn. London, New York: Parthenon Publishing 2000;149-57.

20. Kupesic S, Plavsic MB. 2D and 3D hysterosalpingo-contrast-sonography in the assessment of uterine cavity and tubal patency. Eur J Obstet Gynecol Reprod Biol. 2007;133(1):64-9.

21. Faddy MJ, Gosden RG, Gougeon A. Accelerated disappearance of ovarian follicles in mid-life: Implications for forecasting menopause. Hum Reprod 1992;7:1342-6.

22. Nugent D, Smith J, Balen AH. Ultrasound and the ovary. In: Kupesic S, de Ziegler D (Eds). Ultrasound in Infertility. London: Parthenon Publishing 2000;23-43.

23. Higgins RV, Van Nagell JR, Woods CH, et al. Interobserver variation in ovarian measurements using transvaginal sonography. Gynecol Oncol 1990;39:69-71.

24. Kupesic S. Kurjak A. Predictors of IVF outcome by 3D ultrasound. Hum Reprod 2002;17(4):950-5.

25. Reynolds SRM. Blood and lymph vascular systems of the ovary. In: Greep SR (Ed). Female Reproductive system, Part 1. Washington: American Physiological Society 1973;261-316.

26. Ginther OJ, Diersche DKJ, Walsh SW, et al. Anatomy of arteries and veins of uterus and ovaries in rhesus monkeys. Biol Reprod 1974;11:204-19.

27. Bourne TH, Athanasiou S, Bauer B. Ovulation and the Periovulatory Follicle. In: Bourne TH, Jauniaux E, Jurkovic D (Eds). Transvaginal Colour Doppler. Berlin Heidelberg: Springer-Verlag 1995;119-30.

28. Kurjak A, Kupesic-Urek S. Infertility. In: Kurjak A (Ed). Transvaginal Color Doppler. Carnforth, UK: Parthenon Publishing 1991;33-8.

29. Ratmacher RP, Andersson LL. Blood flow and progesterone levels in the ovary of cycling and pregnant pigs. Am J Physiol 1986;214:1014-8.

30. Cohen HL, Shapiro MA, Mandel FS, et al. Normal ovaries in neonates and infants: A sonographic study of 77 patients 1 day to 24 months old. Am J Roentgenol 1993;160:583-6.

31. Bridges NA, Cooke A, Healy MJR, et al. Standards for ovarian volume in childhood and puberty. Fertil Steril 1993;60:456-60.

32. Kupesic S, Kurjak A. Normal Gynecologic Anatomy (Uterus, Tubes, Ovaries). In: Kurjak A, Chervenak F (Eds). Donald School Textbook of Ultrasound in Obstetrics and Gynecology. New Delhi: Jaypee Brothers Medical Publishers (P) Ltd 2008; 783-90.

33. Kupesic S, Waldrup L, Liu JB. Normal anatomy of the female pelvis. In: Stephenson S (Ed), 3rd edn. Diagnostic Medical Sonography: A Guide to Clinical Practice. Philadelphia: Lipincott Williams & Wilkins 2010 (in press).

S Kupesic Plavsic, A Kurjak, K Baston

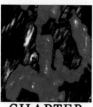

CHAPTER 3

Color Doppler and 3D Ultrasound of the Uterine Lesions

INTRODUCTION

The aim of this chapter is to investigate the role of color Doppler and three-dimensional (3D) ultrasound in the evaluation of uterine lesions. Morphological and vascular criteria assessed by different forms of ultrasound are listed for each type of uterine lesion.

The uterus lies in the middle of the pelvis with its long axis perpendicular to the ultrasound probe. Using two-dimensional (2D) ultrasound, the examination of uterine lesions is limited to transverse and sagittal planes, which give an inadequate view of the uterus and uterine pathology. 3D ultrasound provides simultaneous display of coronal, sagittal and transverse planes. Volume data are viewed using a standard anatomic orientation demonstrating the entire volume and continuity of curved structures in a single image. More accurate evaluation of numerous sections through the uterus becomes possible due to limited number and the orientation of reformatted planes. When three perpendicular planes are simultaneously displayed on the screen, the sagittal plane is chosen for volume measurements, while the other two planes are used to ensure that the entire pathology is included in the measurement. The surface rendering mode allows exploration of the outer or inner contour of the lesion, while the "niche aspect" enables detection and analysis of the selected sections of the uterine lesion. 3D ultrasound offers improved visualization of the uterine structures and lesions, more accurate volume estimation, retrospective review of stored data, assessment of tumor invasion and using rendered images, it can identify more accurately the location of abnormalities that may require surgical intervention.

3D sonohysterography is very useful in the evaluation of the uterine cavity and is more useful than hysterosonography by 2D transvaginal ultrasound in the cases of submucosal myomas and polyps.

The 3D power Doppler system improves the information on tumor angiogenesis and neovascularization, enabling visualization of the overlapping vessels and assessment of their relationship with the surrounding tissue. Power Doppler ultrasound compared to standard color Doppler has the advantage of more sensitivity to low velocity flow, overcoming the angle dependence and aliasing. Using contrast agents, it is possible to enhance the 3D power Doppler evaluation of small vessels.

In this chapter, we will compare the advantages of B mode, color Doppler, 3D and 3D power Doppler ultrasound in the assessment of uterine lesions.

NORMAL UTERUS

Two-dimensional ultrasound imaging of the uterus is limited due to the movement of the transducer allowing sagittal and transverse planes through the uterus. 3D sonography permits multiplanar display of all three perpendicular sections: Coronal, sagittal and transverse planes. The coronal plane of the uterus enables the visualization of the uterine cavity and the cervix at the same time. The normal uterus is characterized by a convex shape of the endometrium and myometrium in the fundus. Blood vessels of the uterus and endometrium can be detected by color and power Doppler ultrasound where the endometrium and myometrium constitute an anatomical and functional unit. The uterine arteries branch off the internal iliac arteries. Ultrasonically, they look like hyperechoic structures running along the cervix and the isthmic part of the uterus. Arcuate arteries are tortuous anechoic structures that spread through myometrium. Radial arteries vertically penetrate the myometrial layers of smooth muscle cells. Spiral arteries supply the functional layer of endometrium. Their shape and size change during the menstrual cycle and they shed during menstruation together with the glandular tissue. During pregnancy, these arteries become uteroplacental decidual arteries. Basal arterioles supply the basal layer of the endometrium and do not change during the menstrual cycle. Color Doppler studies have determined typical waveform signatures for each pelvic vessel. These waveform signals change under the influence of hormones, ischemia and internal or external vasoactive factors. The uterine and ovarian vessels undergo cyclic changes dictated by the hormonal cycle. During the menstrual phase, due to hormonal deprivation and alterations in the spiral arteriolar system, spiral arteries undergo increased coiling and cause a circulatory stasis which lead to tissue ischemia. Vasoconstriction of the spiral arterioles and necrosis of their walls results in menstrual bleeding. Anechoic areas that are sometimes visualized indicate endometrial breakdown. Later on, a mixed appearance with anechoic area (indicating blood) and hyperechoic parts (exfoliated endometrium and clots) may be observed. During the late menstrual phase, the endometrium appears sonographically as a thin, single-line, slightly irregular echogenic interface. In this phase, the uterine artery shows a high resistance index. In the early follicular phase, the endometrium is imaged as a hyperechoic line with an endometrial thickness of less than 5 mm, but it is not always possible to visualize the endometrial-myometrial junction. As ovulation approaches, the glands become numerous and the expected endometrial thickness is about 10 mm. A triple-line endometrium is typical of the periovulatory phase. The hyperechoic echo that represents the endometrial-myometrial junction becomes more prominent and does not produce posterior enhancement. The central echogenic interface probably represents refluxed mucus. Doppler velocimetry of the spiral arteries shows progressive diminution of resistance indices. The secretory phase is characterized by a hyperechoic and homogenous endometrium with a loss of the triple-line morphology. During this phase of the cycle the ultrasonographic image of the endometrium shows increased echogenicity with respect to the myometrium. The interface of the myometrium with the endometrium is still visible as a hypoechoic zone. Maximum echogenicity is seen in the midluteal phase, when the endometrium appears homogenously hyperechoic. Posterior enhancement is a sonographic characteristic of this phase. Doppler velocimetry demonstrates further decrease of the vascular resistance in uterine and spiral arteries being the lowest during the midluteal phase.

Since changes in the texture and volume of the endometrium can be precisely observed using 3D ultrasound, and retrospectively reviewed, this method may become a method of choice for evaluation of the endometrial pathology in a multitude of clinical conditions.

ENDOMETRIAL POLYPS

Endometrial polyps develop as solitary or multiple, soft, sessile and penduculated tumors containing hyperplastic endometrium.[1,2] Endometrial polyps may be clinically asymptomatic or patients may present with symptoms, such as vaginal spotting, intermenstrual or postcoital bleeding, infertility, infection or pain. Endometrial polyps are best imaged during the early proliferative phase of the menstrual cycle or after injection of a negative contrast medium into the uterine cavity. The vascularization of polyps is supported by already existing vessels, originating from terminal branches of the uterine arteries assessed by transvaginal color Doppler ultrasound. It is possible to identify flow in the regularly separated vessels and analyze the velocity of blood flow through them. The resistance index is moderate, usually higher than 0.45 (Figure 3.1).[1,3] Infection or necrosis of polyps may lower the impedance to blood flow ($RI_{MIN} = 0.37$). Marked reduction in blood flow impedance noted at the periphery and/or within the endometrial polyps may lead an inexperienced ultrasonographer to a false positive diagnosis of endometrial malignancy.

Tamoxifen is a nonsteroidal antiestrogen that is widely used for the treatment of breast cancer. However, the weak estrogen-like effect that tamoxifen has on the endometrium is a cause of great concern. Patients using tamoxifen should be monitored at regular intervals because several studies

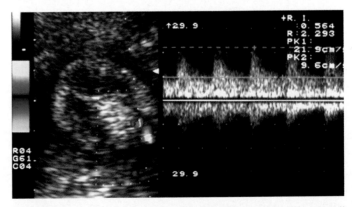

FIGURE 3.1: Transvaginal color Doppler scan of a small endometrial polyp. Note the moderate resistance (RI = 0.56) signals obtained from the periphery of the endometrial polyp (right).

have reported cases of endometrial cancer associated with this therapy. A wide spectrum of pathological uterine findings has been described in association with long-term tamoxifen therapy at a dose of 20 mg/day.[4] These findings include epithelial metaplasia, simple and atypical hyperplasia, endometrial polyps and endometrial carcinoma.[5] Endometrial changes are sonographically characterized by abnormal endometrial thickening and nonhomogenous hyperechogenicity, with multiple, small cystic structures. At least three studies have indicated that tamoxifen treatment in postmenopausal breast cancer patients is associated with a high incidence of endometrial polyps.[6-8] Gray-scale transvaginal sonography may demonstrate a peculiar endometrial honeycomb appearance in 44% patients, receiving tamoxifen therapy.[7] The effect of tamoxifen on endometrial blood flow is less understood. In asymptomatic postmenopausal patients receiving tamoxifen who have an endometrial thickness less than 5 mm, increased endometrial blood flow with significant reduction of the resistance index was detected.[7] Patients with an abnormally thickened endometrium and particularly those with endometrial polyps, presented with significantly lower vascular impedance compared to those with thin endometrium (mean resistance index, RI of 0.39 versus 0.79.[5] The RI values returned to normal values following resection of the endometrial polyps, thus supporting a benign transitory effect of long-term tamoxifen therapy on the endometrium.

Clearly, ultrasound assessment of the size and morphology of the endometrial polyps and evaluation of blood flow impedance (resistance and pulsatility index) cannot replace surgical removal and histopathologic evaluation to predict the histologic type.[9,10]

Doppler studies indicate that low vascular impedance blood flow signals (RI $\leq$ 0.50) detected within the endometrial polyps are suggestive of atypia.[9]

3D hysterosonography can better visualize the uterine cavity and the endometrial thickness than transvaginal sonography, transvaginal sonohysterography or transvaginal color Doppler.[11] Using multiplanar view polypoid structures are clearly demonstrated, allowing for the optimal plane to present their pedicle. Surface rendering mode allows visualization of the polypoid structure in continuity with the endometrial lining.[12]

Gruboeck, et al.[13] compared the measurements of endometrial thickness assessed by conventional 2D ultrasound and endometrial volume assessed with 3D ultrasound in symptomatic postmenopausal patients. The endometrial thickness was similar in patients with endometrial hyperplasia and polyps, but the endometrial volume in hyperplasia was significantly higher than the volume in patients with endometrial polyps. Since the difference between endometrial hyperplasia and polyps cannot be detected by the measurement of endometrial thickness, 3D volume measurement is the method of choice for noninvasive differentiation between these two endometrial conditions. Polyps are the localized thickenings of the endometrium not affecting the whole of the uterine cavity and therefore, their volume is much smaller, while the maximum thickness is similar to that of hyperplasia.

INTRAUTERINE SYNECHIAE (ADHESIONS)

Destruction of the basal layer of the endometrium may result in scarring and development of the bands of scar tissue (synechiae) in the uterine cavity. This damage of the endometrium may occur as a result of a too vigorous curettage of an advanced pregnancy. Tuberculosis may also cause uterine adhesions. The menstrual pattern in these patients is characterized by amenorrhea or hypomenorrhea. Ultrasound scan of a patient with Asherman's syndrome shows a mixed picture: In some parts of the uterine cavity no endometrium can be visualized and in others the endometrium appears normal. If there are adhesions in the uterine cavity, they are visualized as hyperechoic bridges. Intrauterine adhesions do not display increased vascularity on color Doppler examination (Figure 3.2). Synechiae are better visualized during menstruation, when they are outlined by intracavitary fluid. Another technique that can be used is saline infusion sonography (sonohysterography).

Sonohysterography performed with 3D ultrasound has several advantages over that with conventional 2D ultrasound. It provides more accurate information about the location of abnormalities, which is very important for preoperative assessment and differentiation of the uterine

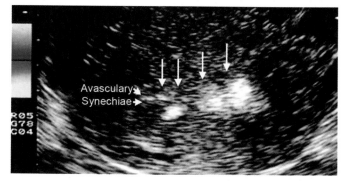

FIGURE 3.2: Transvaginal sonogram of an infertile patient with intrauterine synechiae, visualized as hyperechoic bridges within the endometrial cavity.

pathology. Furthermore, the uterus is distended during a shorter time interval, compared to the time necessary for 2D exams, which is convenient for the patient. Alternatively, echogenic contrast media (e.g. Echovist, Schering, Germany) may be used for the demonstration of intracavitary abnormalities.[14] Following distension of the uterine cavity, intrauterine synechiae are visualized as irregular hyperechogenic bridges traversing the uterine cavity.[12] Their size, volume and relationship with the surrounding structures may be analyzed in multiplanar and surface rendering view.

3D ultrasound is helpful in delineation of the intracavitary adhesions and determination of their location, which assists in surgical planning. This technique is beneficial to determine the degree of uterine cavity obliteration.

ADENOMYOSIS

Adenomyosis of the uterus is a condition in which clusters of the endometrial tissue grow into the myometrium. It may be localized close to endometrium, or it may extend through the myometrium and serosa. It is estimated that adenomyosis affects 20% of women, mainly those who are multiparous.[15] The uterus can be normal in size or enlarged, with symptoms, such as dysmenorrhea, pelvic pain and menometrorrhagia.

2D ultrasound findings include "Swiss cheese" appearance of the myometrium due to areas of hemorrhage and clots within the muscle (Figure 3.3). Disordered echogenicity of the middle layer of the myometrium is usually present in severe cases. Sometimes, the uterus is generally hypoechoic, with the large cysts rarely seen. Using hysterosonography, the contrast medium penetrates the myometrium. Color Doppler characteristics reveal increased vascularity by moderate vascular resistance within the myometrium (RI = 0.56 ± 0.12), while the RI of the uterine arteries shows a decreased value compared to controls.[15] Statistically significant differences exist between adenomyosis and uterine malignancies with respect to both RI and maximum velocity. No significant difference was noted between adenomyosis and myoma in terms of the vascular impedance, but a slight difference was observed in the assessment of maximum blood velocity.[16]

Sometimes transonic areas may not represent adenomyosis, but rather cross sections of the prominent vessels in patients with pelvic congestion syndrome. Compared to 2D transvaginal color Doppler ultrasound, 3D ultrasound coupled with power Doppler sonography is superior for the staging of adenomyosis, assessment of the

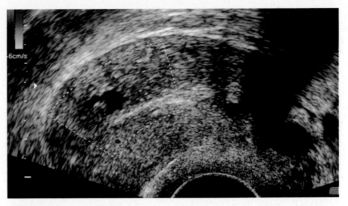

FIGURE 3.3: "Swiss cheese" appearance of the myometrium, showing increased vascularity typical of adenomyosis.

vessels' distribution and branching pattern in adenomyotic foci.[17]

ENDOMETRIAL HYPERPLASIA

The endometrial thickness in postmenopausal women usually measures between 1 to 4 mm. Abnormal endometrial thickness may be detected in benign and malignant uterine lesions. An endometrial thickness greater than 14 mm in premenopausal and greater than 5 mm in postmenopausal women should be further investigated.[1] Using B-mode transvaginal sonography alone it is not possible to distinguish endometrial hyperplasia from carcinoma. A more accurate diagnosis of endometrial pathology may be obtained with color and pulsed Doppler sonography.[2,3] Endometrial hyperplasia is characterized by peripheral distribution of the regularly separated vessels with moderate to high vascular resistance (mean RI = 0.55 ± 0.05) (Figure 3.4).[18] However, reliable differentiation between endometrial hyperplasia and carcinoma is limited due to an overlap in the endometrial thickness measurements, as well as controversial results of blood flow assessment by transvaginal color Doppler ultrasound. Since there is a positive correlation between arterial blood flow impedance and the number of years from menopause,[19] one can estimate the risk of uterine malignancy in postmenopausal patients with decreased vascular resistance.

Transvaginal color Doppler ultrasound may be used for differentiation between endometrial hyperplasia and endometrial carcinoma, as well as for prediction of the tumor spread in patients with carcinoma.[20] No significant difference was found for endometrial thickness between the patients with hyperplasia (n = 18 patients; 16.2 mm ± 15.9 mm) and patients with endometrial carcinoma (n = 53 patients; 18.7 mm ± 17.1 mm). Intratumoral blood flow was detected in a significant number of patients who

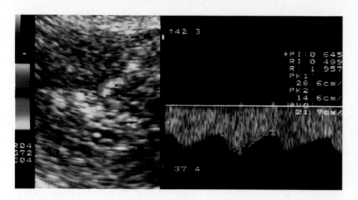

FIGURE 3.4: Transvaginal color Doppler scan of an asymptomatic postmenopausal patient with thickened endometrium. Moderate vascular resistance signals (RI = 0.48) were isolated from the periphery of the endometrium. Histopathology demonstrated endometrial hyperplasia.

had endometrial carcinoma (71.7%; 38 of 53 patients), compared with patients who had endometrial hyperplasia (5.6%; 1 of 18 patients; P < 0.0001). According to these results, transvaginal color Doppler assessment of endometrial angiogenesis and neovascularization is superior to B-mode ultrasound measurement of the endometrial thickness in differentiation between endometrial hyperplasia and carcinoma. For patients with carcinoma, the detection of intratumoral blood flow may be helpful in distinguishing between the low-grade and high-grade tumors and predicting the myometrial invasion.

In patients with endometrial hyperplasia undergoing thermal balloon endometrial ablation, transvaginal color Doppler ultrasound may be used for the evaluation of the hemodynamic changes in uterine vessels.[21] Thermal balloon endometrial ablation therapy induces an increase in the uterine blood flow impedance, but not until six months after the treatment. The rise in vascular impedance is most likely the consequence of fibrosis of the uterine cavity.

The endometrial volume measured by 3D ultrasound is significantly lower in patients with benign pathology, such as hyperplasia (mean 8.0 ml, SD 7.81 ml), than in patients with endometrial carcinoma (mean 39.0 ml, SD 34.16 ml). Normal volume of the postmenopausal endometrium in this study was 0.9 ml (SD 1.72 ml).[13]

Our group reported on the use of 3D power Doppler sonography in patients with endometrial hyperplasia.[21] Discrete, regularly separated vessels, with no evidence of penetration were detected at the periphery of the hyperplastic endometrium.

ENDOMETRIAL CARCINOMA

Endometrial carcinoma is the most common gynecological malignancy in many countries with a reported incidence of about 10% in postmenopausal patients presenting with uterine bleeding.[18] Transabdominal ultrasound studies have demonstrated that increased endometrial thickness is associated with endometrial neoplasms in postmenopausal women, but the quality of transabdominal sonographic images is affected by obesity, retroversion of the uterus and an unfilled bladder. These factors do not influence transvaginal sonographic visualization of the endometrium. Ultrasound findings assessed by conventional B-mode sonography include increased endometrial thickness >5 mm in postmenopausal women or >8 mm in perimenopausal women, hyperechogenic or inhomogeneous endometrium, free fluid in the cul-de-sac, intrauterine fluid or possible invasion in patients with a disrupted endometrial-subendometrial layer.

In addition, color and pulsed Doppler improves diagnostic accuracy because the endometrial carcinoma shows abnormal blood flow due to tumor angiogenesis.[22] Endometrial blood flow may be absent in the normal endometrium, as well as in the cases of endometrial atrophy and in most cases of endometrial hyperplasia. This contrasts with endometrial carcinoma in which 91% of the cases show areas of neovascularization in intratumoral or peritumoral region (Figure 3.5).[18] Neovascular signals obtained from the central portion of the endometrial lesion demonstrate low vascular resistance (RI = 0.42 ± 0.02). Such a pattern is typical for early stages of endometrial cancer. When there is increased vascularity surrounding the endometrial lesion, invasion by carcinoma should be suspected. If myometrial vessels are invaded, low vascular resistance is detected within the myometrial portion of the uterus due to incomplete or absent membrane and leaky

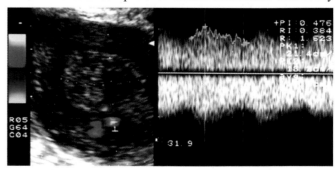

FIGURE 3.5: Transvaginal color Doppler scan of the endometrial carcinoma vessels. Peritumoral vessels demonstrate low-resistance index (RI = 0.38).

structure of the invaded radial arteries. Conventional 2D ultrasound measurements of endometrial thickness have disadvantages in distinguishing patients with benign and malignant endometrial pathology due to varying thickness and interference with other endometrial pathology like polyps or hyperplasia. In distinguishing cancer from benign pathology, endometrial volume measurements assessed by 3D ultrasound seem to be more helpful.

In the pioneering study of Gruboeck, et al[13] the mean endometrial thickness in patients with endometrial cancer was 29.5 ± 12.59 mm and the mean volume was 39.0 ± 34.16 ml. The optimal cut-off value of endometrial thickness for the diagnosis of cancer was 15 mm, with the test sensitivity of 83.3% and positive predictive value of 54.4%. With a cut-off level of 13 ml, the diagnosis of cancer was made with a sensitivity of 100%. One false-positive result from a patient with hyperplasia gave a specificity of 98.8% and a positive predictive value of 91.7%. Clearly, the endometrial volume is significantly higher in patients with carcinoma than in those with benign lesions. Volume measurement of the endometrium by 3D ultrasound is a superior diagnostic test for the detection of endometrial cancer in symptomatic postmenopausal women. Increased endometrial volume is associated with the severity or higher grade of the endometrial carcinoma and also with progressive myometrial invasion. There is a positive correlation between the depth of myometrial invasion and endometrial thickness and volume. Only patients with tumor volume larger than 25 ml had evidence of pelvic node involvement at surgery.[13]

Some authors suggest that 3D hysterosonography allows the better visualization of myometrial invasion and may play a significant role in staging of the malignant endometrial tumors.[11] Using 3D ultrasound and multiplanar view, it is possible to detect infiltration of the cervical or endometrial carcinoma into the bladder and/or rectum.

In addition to endometrial volume, our 3D power Doppler ultrasound study analyzed regularity and integrity of the subendometrial hallo, presence of intracavitary fluid, and assessment of the vessel's architecture and branching pattern (Table 3.1).[23] In patients with endometrial carcinoma, the mean endometrial volume was 37.0 ± 31.8 ml (Table 3.2). The endometrial volume in hyperplasia had a mean value of 7.82 ± 7.60 ml and was significantly higher than the endometrial volume of the patients with polyps (mean 2.63 ± 2.12 ml). In patients with normal or atrophic endometrium, the mean volume was 0.8 ± 1.51 ml. Subendometrial hallo was regular in all the patients with benign endometrial pathology, whereas 8 out of 12 patients with endometrial carcinoma had an irregular endometrial-myometrial border.

Intracavitary fluid was present in four patients with benign endometrial lesions and five patients with endometrial malignancy. Dichotomous branching and randomly dispersed vessels were detected in 91.67% of the patients with endometrial carcinoma, while single vessel arrangement and regular branching were pathognomonic for benign endometrial lesions. 3D power Doppler imaging accurately detected structural abnormalities of the malignant tumor vessels, such as microaneurysms, arteriovenous

TABLE 3.1: 3D sonographic and power Doppler criteria for the diagnosis of endometrial malignancy

3D sonographic and power Doppler criteria		Score
Endometrial volume	< 13 ml	0
	≥ 13 ml	2
Subendometrial hallo	Regular	0
	Disturbed	2
Intracavitary fluid	Absent	0
	Present	1
Vessel's architecture	Linear vessel arrangement	0
	Chaotic vessel arrangement	2
Branching pattern	Simple	0
	Complex	2
TOTAL SCORE		

(From reference 23, with permission)
Total score = sum of individual scores
Cut-off score = greater or equal to 4 is associated with a high-risk of endometrial malignancy.

TABLE 3.2: Volume and vascularity of the endometrial lesions (N = 57) obtained by 3D power Doppler imaging

Histopathology	N	V (SD) ml	Regular endometrial hallo (%)	Intracavitary fluid (%)	Neovascular signals (%)
Normal and/or atrophic endometrium	10	0.8 (1.51)	100	20.00	0
Endometrial hyperplasia	27	7.82 (7.60)	100	37.00	0
Endometrial polyp	28	2.63 (2.12)	100	35.71	3.57
Endometrial carcinoma	12	37.0 (31.8)	66.67	41.67	100

(From reference 23, with permission)

shunts, tumoral lakes, elongation and coiling.[23] Combining morphological and power Doppler criteria, the diagnosis of endometrial carcinoma had a sensitivity of 91.67%. One false positive result was obtained in a patient with endometrial hyperplasia and one false negative in a patient with endometrial carcinoma receiving tamoxifen therapy. In this case, the endometrial lesion demonstrated regularly separated peripheral vessels and was falsely interpreted as hyperplasia.

In another study we attempted to use 3D power Doppler ultrasound for staging of the endometrial carcinoma.[24] The objective of this study was to evaluate the accuracy of 3D power Doppler in determining the depth of myometrial invasion in patients with proven adenocarcinoma of the endometrium relative to the amount of myometrial invasion measured in histopathological analysis (Table 3.3).[24] Thirty four patients with histologically proven adenocarcinoma of the endometrium were analyzed. Deep myometrial invasion (>50%) was present at postoperative histology in 5/22 (22.73%) women, while superficial invasion was reported in 17/22 (77.23%). 3D power Doppler ultrasound demonstrated a sensitivity of 100% (5/5) and a specificity of 94.44% (17/18) for deep invasion, with a positive predictive value (PPV) of 83.33% (5/6) and a negative predictive value (NPV) of 100% (17/17). In only one patient with adenomyosis was invasion overestimated by 3D power Doppler. Data showed acceptable accuracy in determining the depth of myometrial invasion in patients with adenocarcinoma. 3D power Doppler can potentially detect lesions that require aggressive intervention thereby directing proper treatment.

There is a relationship between the tumoral blood flow assessed by color Doppler ultrasound, microvessel density, and vascular endothelial growth factor levels in endometrial carcinoma.[25] Significantly lower RI values were noted in

TABLE 3.3: Invasion of endometrial carcinoma assessed with the aid of 3D power Doppler imaging

Invasion	3D power Doppler	Histopathology
Superficial*	17	18
Deep**	5	4

(From reference 6, with permission)
*Invasion into less than a half of the total myometrial thickness
**Invasion into more than a half of the myometrial thickness

tumors of stage II or greater (RI = 0.37), compared with RI of 0.50 (P <0.001) in tumors with lower stages.[25] Cases with deep myometrial invasion (one-half depth or greater) had lower tumoral vascular impedance (RI = 0.39), compared with cases with proximal myometrial invasion (RI = 0.49, P = 0.002).[25] Similarly, patients with lymphovascular emboli had a lower resistance index in tumoral vessels than patients with no evidence of lymphovascular emboli (0.38 compared with 0.49, P <0.001).[25] Patients with regional lymph node metastasis were characterized by significantly lower intratumoral vascular impedance (RI = 0.30) as compared with patients having localized disease (RI = 0.49, P <0.001).[25] Increased vascular endothelial growth factor levels and microvessel density were detected in tumors of stage II or greater with lymphovascular emboli and lymph node metastasis.[25] Resistance index, microvessel density and vascular endothelial growth factor levels correlated well with the clinical and biological nature of the tumor. Blood flow assessed by color Doppler ultrasound has histologic and biologic correlations with angiogenesis and vascular endothelial growth factor levels and may play an important role for the prediction of the endometrial carcinoma behavior as well as for assessment of its metastatic potential.

Intratumoral blood flow assessed by transvaginal color Doppler ultrasound (resistance index and peak systolic velocity) may also be correlated with histopathologic characteristics, tumoral stage and risk for recurrence in endometrial carcinoma.[26] Significantly, lower RI was found in tumors with infiltrative growth pattern (infiltrating greater than or equal to 50% of the myometrium), cervical involvement, lymphvascular space invasion, lymph node metastasis and high risk for recurrence.[26] Similarly, a significantly higher peak systolic velocity was detected in grade 3 endometrial carcinoma, infiltrating more that 50% of the myometrium, stage greater than or equal to Ic and with high risk for recurrence.[26] Clearly, there is a correlation between intratumoral blood flow features and the histopathological characteristics, tumor stage and risk for recurrence exists in endometrial cancer.

Many institutions have introduced 3D ultrasound for routine the assessment of the patients presenting with postmenopausal vaginal bleeding. Yaman, et al.[27] compared the reproducibility of 2D and 3D ultrasound in the measurement of the endometrial thickness and found that the reproducibility of 3D ultrasound is significantly better.

LEIOMYOMA

Leiomyomas are the most common tumors of the female pelvis and occur in 20 to 25% of women of reproductive age, arising from the smooth muscle and soft tissue of the uterine fundus and corpus, while 3% originate from the cervix.[28] Myomas are usually multiple and of various size. Intramural tumors are the most common, while the submucosal are the least common. When leiomyomas extend outward, they become pedunculated or subserosal.[29] Symptoms of the submucsal leiomyomas include metrorrhagia, pelvic pain or infertility, whereas most subserosal leiomyomas are asymptomatic.

On gray-scale ultrasound, the uterine leiomyomas may be represented with uterine enlargement, distortion of the uterine contour and varying echogenicity depending on the amount of connective or smooth muscle tissue.

Transvaginal color Doppler sonography demonstrates increased vascularization at the periphery of the myoma (within the capsule), with the RI of 0.54 ± 0.08. Visualization of the peripheral vascularity allows better delineation of the tumor (Figure 3.6). Blood vessels in the central part of the myoma are usually demonstrated in the case of necrosis, inflammation or other degenerative changes, and demonstrate a lower RI. In patients with myomas the uterine artery blood flow presents significantly

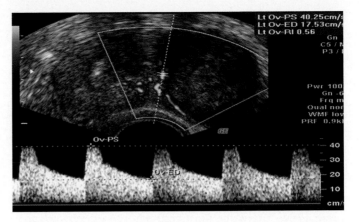

FIGURE 3.6: Transvaginal power Doppler scan of the uterus with a leiomyoma in the posterior wall and superimposed color Doppler (left). Pulsed Doppler waveform analysis (right) indicates moderate resistance of the tumoral blood flow (RI = 0.56).

lower vascular impedance (RI = 0.74 ± 0.09) compared to normal women (RI = 0.84 ± 0.09).[30]

Simultaneous display of three perpendicular planes by 3D ultrasound enables the accurate localization of the myomas, estimation of their size and relationship to the endometrium. Patients receiving medical therapy, such as gonadotropin-releasing hormone may be followed with serial 3D ultrasound scans to estimate the myoma size and effectiveness of the therapy. Hysterosonography by 3D ultrasound is valuable in the assessment of submucosal myomas.[11,12,31,32] Both positive and negative contrast media may be used for evaluation of the uterine cavity.[12,31] Negative contrast is better for the evaluation of the intracavitary surface lesions (for example, endometrial polyps), whereas positive contrast creates a cast of the uterine cavity. The most common limitation of scanning the uterus with myomas by 2D and 3D ultrasound is posterior shadowing caused by leiomyoma calcification.

In our recent 3D power Doppler ultrasound study[23] we have evaluated the morphology, volume and vascularization of the myometrial lesions. The mean volume of the leiomyomas undergoing surgery was 78.52 ± 51.8 ml. In 84.38%, 3D power Doppler detected regular vascularity at the periphery. In myomas with necrosis, inflammation, and degeneration, the irregular branching pattern of the vessels was similar to the chaotic vascular architecture of the malignant myometrial lesions. Because of the low positive predictive value of 16.67%, 3D power Doppler ultrasound was not recommended for the differentiation of benign and malignant myometrial lesions.

LEIOMYOSARCOMA

Uterine leiomyosarcoma is a rare tumor, accounting for only 1-3% of all genital tract tumors and 3-7.4% of malignant tumors of the corpus uteri and is characterized by early dissemination and poor prognosis for survival.[33] Through the years, several questions regarding these tumors have remained unanswered, and a method for its early and correct diagnosis is still unknown. Furthermore, uterine sarcoma is expected to be more common in the near future, as gynecologists are more commonly utilizing conservative treatment of uterine myomas. Abnormal vaginal bleeding is the most common presenting symptom in patients with uterine sarcoma. Lower abdominal pain or pressure and a palpable abdominal mass are additional findings. An enlarged bulky uterus is palpated and/or the tumor may be seen protruding through the cervix. Dilatation and curettage may be helpful in distinguishing benign from malignant pathology but only if the tumor is submucosal. Clinically, a rapid increase in the size of a uterine tumor after the menopause arouses suspicion of sarcoma.

Ultrasonically, leiomyosarcoma is presented as a solid or solid-cystic myometrial lesion altering the echogenicity of the myometrium. On transvaginal color Doppler neovascular signals are detected both at the border and within the center of the tumor (Figure 3.7). Pulsed Doppler waveform analysis demonstrates high blood flow velocity and low impedance to blood flow (RI = 0.37 ± 0.03), with irregular, thin, randomly dispersed vessels (Figure 3.8). When a cut-off value for RI of <0.40 is used, this method reaches the sensitivity of 90.91%, specificity 99.82%, positive predictive value 71.43% and negative predictive value of 99.96%.[34] Because of their rarity, uterine sarcomas are not suitable for screening. Transvaginal ultrasound detects differences in myometrial tissue density and therefore may be used for the detection of uterine sarcoma. Due to the low specificity this method is not appropriate as a screening procedure.[33-35]

Although the mean intratumoral vascular impedance is significantly lower and intratumoral peak systolic velocity (PSV) is significantly higher in patients with uterine leiomyosarcoma than in patients with uterine leiomyomas, transvaginal color Doppler studies have many limitations. Marked reduction of RI and PI and increased PSV may also be detected in patients with large necrotic and inflammatory changed leiomyomas. Using a cut-off value of 0.5 for RI in the myometrial vessels, the detection rate for uterine sarcoma was 67% and the false-positive rate was 11.8%.[35] These results suggest that intratumoral RI assessed by color

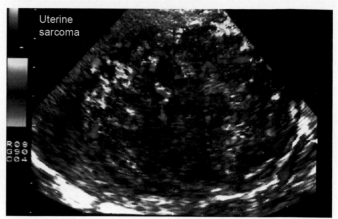

FIGURE 3.7: Transvaginal color Doppler scan of a uterine tumor. Neovascular signals are visualized within the central and peripheral parts of the uterine lesion. Histopathology revealed uterine sarcoma.

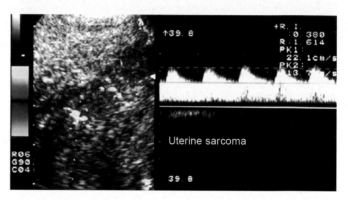

FIGURE 3.8: The same patient as in Figure 3.7. Areas of neovascularization with low-impedance to flow (RI = 0.38) are typical of uterine sarcoma.

and pulsed Doppler ultrasound could not be efficiently used for preoperative differential diagnosis of the myometrial lesions. Similarly, one patient with uterine leiomyosarcoma examined with 3D and power Doppler ultrasound had a significant volume (97.2 ml) and randomly dispersed vessels both within the central and peripheral parts of the tumor.[23] The diameter of the vessels was variable, with numerous microaneurysms and stenosis. Because of the overlap in the appearance of the leiomyoma and leiomyosarcoma vessels and low positive predictive value of 3D power Doppler imaging, this technique is not recommended for noninvasive assessment of the myometrial lesions.

CONCLUSION

Transvaginal sonography allows detailed analysis of the endometrial thickness and texture. Blood flow studies can be efficiently used to monitor the endometrial development and distinguish between benign and malignant uterine cavity lesions. It is hoped that color Doppler findings may help to reduce invasive procedures, such as dilatation and curettage or hysteroscopy for detection of the intracavitary lesions. This would decrease both the potential risks and the economic costs. Transvaginal color and pulsed Doppler sonography represents a noninvasive diagnostic tool that can be used for the assessment of the endometrial lesions' vascularity. Transvaginal color Doppler assessment of postmenopausal patients may be a viable screening option, if ovarian and endometrial carcinoma screening are performed in the same scan. In this way, the capital costs would be shared and oncologic preventive medicine for women could be initiated. The use of this technique could also result in a reduction in dilatation and curettage interventions, with considerable reduction of both the potential risks and the economic costs of the operation.

Assessment of the uterine tumor's vascularization, if used together with the analysis of the morphology and size, may increase our accuracy in differentiating between uterine sarcoma and leiomyoma. However, it is unrealistic to expect that Doppler studies may clarify confounding histological findings. Multiparameter sonographic approach, including morphology and size depicted by transvaginal ultrasonography, and color flow imaging with pulsed Doppler analysis of the neovascular signals, may aid in the diagnosis of the uterine leiomyosarcoma in high-risk groups, such as postmenopausal patients with a rapidly enlarging uterus. Serial measurements are recommended for evaluation of the myometrial density, follow-up of the tumoral growth and detection of the impedance to blood flow. Only a complex sonographic approach, such as this may lead to the accurate noninvasive diagnosis of leiomyosarcoma.

3D and power Doppler ultrasound is a new diagnostic technique, and its role in the assessment of uterine lesions has yet to be investigated. 3D ultrasound offers improved visualization of the uterine lesions providing simultaneous display of the coronal, sagittal and transverse planes. In addition, this modality offers more accurate volume estimation using standard anatomic orientation, allows retrospective review of the stored data and more complete viewing of the uterine pathology using rendered images. Also, it identifies the location of the uterine lesions and assesses their relationship with neighboring organs and/or structures. 3D hysterosonography demonstrates the exact location of the intracavitary lesions. 3D power Doppler imaging improves our understanding of malignant tumor angiogenesis. Interactive rotation of power Doppler rendered images provide improved visualization of the uterine tumor vasculature. This method permits the ultrasonographer to view the uterine lesions in three-dimensions interactively, rather than having to assemble the sectional images in his/her mind. Contrast agents are another possibility for enhancing the 3D power Doppler examination by increasing the detection rate of small vessels.[36-38]

REFERENCES

1. Kurjak A, Kupesic S, Zalud I, et al. Transvaginal color Doppler. In: Dodson MG, (Ed). Transvaginal Ultrasound. New York: Churchill Livingstone 1995;325-39.
2. Fleischer AC, Kepple DM, Entman SS. Transvaginal sonography of uterine disorders. In: Timor-Tritsch IE, Rottem S, (Eds). Transvaginal Sonography, 2nd edn. New York: Elsevier 1991;109-30.
3. Kurjak A, Kupesic S. Transvaginal color Doppler and pelvic tumor vascularity: Lessons learned and future challenges. Ultrasound Obstet Gynecol 1995;6:1-15.
4. Ismail SM. Pathology of the endometrium treated with tamoxifen. J Clin Pathol 1994;47:827-33.
5. Achiron R, Grisaru D, Golan-Porat N. Tamoxifen and the uterus: an old drug tested by new modalities. Ultrasound Obstet Gynecol 1996;7:374-8.
6. Lahti E, Blanco G, Kauppila A, et al. Endometrial changes in postmenopausdal breast cancer patients receiving tamoxifen. Obstet Gynecol 1993;81:660-4.
7. Achiron R, Lipitz S, Sivan E. Changes mimicking end, et al. Endometrial neoplasia in postmenopausal, tamoxifen-treated women with breast cancer: A transvaginal Doppler study. Ultrasound Obstet Gynecol 1995;6:116-20.
8. Exacoustos E, Zupi E, Cangi B, et al. Endometrial evaluation in postmenopausal breast cancer patients receiving tamoxifen: An ultrasound, color flow Doppler hysteroscopic and histological study. Ultrasound Obstet Gynecol 1995;6:435-42.
9. Perez-Medina T, Bajo J, Huertas MA, et al. Predicting atypia inside endometrial polyps. J Ultrasound Med 2002;21(2):125-8.
10. Goldstein SR, Monteagudo A, Popiolek D, et al. Evaluation of endometrial polyps. Am J Obstet Gynecol 2002;186(4):669-74.
11. Bonilla-Musoles F, Raga F, Osborne N, et al. Three-dimensional hysterosonography for the study of endometrial tumors: Comparison with conventional transvaginal sonography, hysterosalpingography, and hysteroscopy. Gynecol Oncol 1997; 65:245-52
12. Weinraub Z, Maymon R, Shulman A, et al. Three-dimensional saline contrast hysterosonography and surface rendering of uterine cavity pathology. Ultrasound Obstet Gynecol 1996; 8(4):277-82.

13. Gruboeck K, Jurkovic D, Lawton F, et al. The diagnostic value of endometrial thickness and volume measurements by three-dimensional ultrasound in patients with postmenopausal bleeding. Ultrasound Obstet Gynecol 1996;8(4):272-6.

14. Momtaz M, El Ebrashi A. 3D sonohysterography in the evaluation of the uterine cavity. Las Vegas: Syllabus 1999.

15. Fedele I, Bianchi S, Dorta M, et al Transvaginal ultrasonography in the diagnosis of diffuse adenomyosis. Fertil Steril 1992; 58:94-7.

16. Hirai M, Shibata K, Sagai H, et al. Transvaginal pulsed and color Doppler sonography for the evaluation of adenomyosis. J Ultrasound Med 1995;14:529-32.

17. Lee SL, Busmanis I, Tan A. 3D–Angio of Adenomyotic Uteri. Las Vegas: Syllabus 1999.

18. Kupesic-Urek S, Shalan H, Kurjak A. Early detection of endometrial cancer by transvaginal color Doppler. Eur J Obstet Gynecol Reprod Biol 1993;49:46-9.

19. Kurjak A, Kupesic S. Ovarian senescence and its significance on uterine and ovarian perfusion. Fertil Steril 1995;3:532-7.

20. Emoto M, Tamura R, Shirota K, et al. Clinical usefulness of color Doppler ultrasound in patients with endometrial hyperplasia and carcinoma. Cancer 2002;94(3):700-6.

21. Jarvela I, Tekay A, Santala M, et al. Thermal balloon endometrial ablation therapy induces a rise in uterine blood flow impedance: A randomized prospective color Doppler study. Ultrasound Obstet Gynecol 2001;17(1):65-70.

22. Folkman J, Cole D, Becker F. Growth and metastasis of tumor in organ culture. Tumor Res 1963;16:453-67.

23. Kurjak A, Kupesic S. Three-dimensional ultrasound and power doppler in assessment of uterine and ovarian angiogenesis: A prospective study. Croat Med J 1999;40(3):51-8.

24. Kupesic S, Kurjak A, Zodan T. Staging of endometrial carcinoma by 3D power Doppler. Gynecol Perinatol 1999; 8(1):1-5.

25. Lee CN, Cheng WF, Chen CA, et al. Angiogenesis of endometrial carcinomas assessed by measurement of intratumoral blood flow, microvessel density and vascular endothelial growth factor levels. Obstet Gynecol 2000; 96(4):615-21.

26. Alcazar JL, Galan JM, Jurado M, et al. Intratumoral blood flow analysis in endometrial carcinoma: Correlation with tumor characteristics and risk for recurrence. Gynecol Oncol 2002; 84(2):258-62.

27. Yaman C, Ebner T, Jesacher K, et al. Reproducibility of three-dimensional ultrasound endometrial volume measurements in patients with postmenopausal bleeding. Ultrasound Obstet Gynecol 2002;19(3):282-6.

28. Kurjak A, Zalud I. Uterine masses. In: Kurjak A (Ed). Transvaginal Color Doppler. Carnforth, UK: Parthenon Publishing 1991;123-35.

29. Fleischer AC, Entman SS, Porrath SA, et al. Sonographic evaluation of uterine malformations and disorders. In: Sanders RC, (Ed). The Principles and Practice of Ultrasonography in Obstetrics and Gynecology. Norwalk: Appleton Century Crofts 1985;531.

30. Kurjak A, Kupesic-Urek S, Miric D. The assessment of benign uterine tumor vascularization by transvaginal color Doppler. Ultrasound Med Biol 1992;18:645-8.

31. Balen FG, Allen CM, Gardener JE, et al. 3-Dimensional reconstruction of ultrasound images of the uterine cavity. Br J Radiol 1993;66(787):588-91.

32. Lev-Toaff AS, Rawool NM, Kurtz AB, et al. Three-dimensional sonography and 3D transvaginal US: A problem solving tool in complex gynecological cases. Radiology 1996;201(P):384.

33. Olah KS, Gee H, Blunt S, et al. Retrospective analysis of 318 cases of uterine sarcoma. Eur J Cancer 1991;27:1095-9.

34. Kurjak A, Kupesic S, Shalan H, et al. Uterine sarcoma: A report of 10 cases studied by transvaginal color and pulsed Doppler sonography. Gynecol Oncol 1995;59:342-6.

35. Szabo I, Szantho A, Csabay L, et al. Color Doppler ultrasonography in the differentiation of uterine sarcomas from uterine leiomyomas. EJ Gynaecol Oncol 2002;23(1):29-34.

36. Kurjak A, Kupesic S. Transvaginal color Doppler and pulsed Doppler diagnosis of benign changes in the uterine myometrium. In: Schmidt W, Kurjak A (Eds). Color Doppler sonography in Gynecology and Obstetrics. Stuttgart, New York: Thieme Verlag 2005;274-8.

37. Kupesic S, Plavsic BM. Sonography of uterine leiomyomata. U: I. Brosens (ur): Uterine fibroids: Pathogenesis and management. London, New York: Taylor and Francis 2006;139-151.

38. Kupesic S, Kurjak A. Uterine Lesions: Advances in Ultrasound Diagnosis. In: Kurjak A, Chervenak F, (Ed). Donald School Textbook of Ultrasound in Obstetrics and Gynecology. Jaypee Brothers Medical Publishers (P) Ltd 2008;791-802.

A Kurjak, S Kupesic Plavsic, U Honemeyer

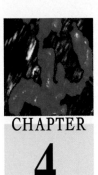

CHAPTER

4

Adnexal Masses

INTRODUCTION

Ultrasonography is accepted as the primary imaging modality in the evaluation of adnexal masses. The use of ultrasound in the detection of a suspected adnexal mass and its differentiation from uterine and nongynecologic pelvic mass has been well established. Also, ultrasound has become the main triage method before treatment. The majority of adnexal masses are benign cysts. However, 25% of ovarian neoplasms are malignant.[1] For this reason, surgical removal of a suspected ovarian neoplasm is the gold standard. In most institutions, the type of surgery performed (laparoscopy vs. laparotomy) depends on the probability of malignancy. The optimal ultrasound techniques and diagnostic criteria to be used when characterizing a suspicious adnexal neoplasm remain controversial. However, several meta-analyses revealed significantly higher performance for combined techniques using morphologic assessment and Doppler ultrasound indices than B mode evaluation alone.[2] In a multicenter European study, color Doppler evaluation was more accurate in the diagnosis of adnexal malignancies compared to gray scale sonography (kappa = 0.82 and 0.65, respectively) because of significantly higher specificity (0.94 vs. 0.84; P < 0.001). The evaluation of the cancer antigen, CA 125 serum concentration did not increase the accuracy of either method.[3] Color and pulsed Doppler sonography depicts the vascularity of the pelvic organs and can be used for the assessment of angiogenesis in tumor masses, producing insights into the tumor angiogenesis and metabolism. It has a primary role in detection of vasculature and assessment of blood flow features of the malignant pelvic lesions. Technological advances, such as three-dimensional (3D) volume acquisition and 3D power Doppler may have clinical utility in the identification of abnormal ovarian architecture, as well as vascularity. The addition of 3D power Doppler ultrasound provides a new tool for measuring the quality of tumoral vascularity and its clinical value is under clinical evaluation.

THE MAIN BASIS OF ANGIOGENESIS

All organs of human body have a physiological duty to form certain compounds and molecules while disintegrating others, with the aim of maintaining the frail molecular equilibrium. In order to perform their task, all the organ systems are connected by a single vascular network. Like any other vital tissue, vascular endothelium has the ability to regenerate and spread through other tissues in order to perfuse them. The formation of new blood vessels is called angiogenesis and if uncontrolled results in neovascularization. More than 100 years ago, Coman and Sheldon discovered that tumor angiogenesis differs from vascularity in normal tissues.[4] It was long believed that simple dilatation of existing host blood vessels was responsible for tumor hyperemia.[5] Vasodilatation was generally thought to be a side effect of tumor metabolites released from necrotic parts of the tumor. However, some authors suggested that tumor hyperemia might be related to new blood vessels growth, i.e. neovascularization, rather than to dilatation of the pre-existing vessels. A report published in 1945 revealed that new vessels in the neighborhood of a tumor implant arose from host vessels and not from the tumor itself.[6] Further experiments during 1960s with isolated perfused organs brought new and exciting concept that tumor growth is restricted in the absence of a vascular response of the surrounding host tissue.[7,8] In the following decades, scientists showed that tumors implanted into animals consistently induced the growth of new capillaries. Viable tumor cells were found to release diffusible angiogenic factors that stimulated new capillary growth and endothelial mitosis.[9,10] On the basis of these observations, Judah Folkman proposed a hypothesis that once a tumor had occurred, every further increase in the tumor cell population had to be preceded by an increase in new capillaries, which sprouted towards the early growth of the tumor.[11] Since Folkman's hypothesis, for nearly 30 years, it has been clear that the development of new blood vessels—called angiogenesis—is crucial for sustaining tumor growth, as it allows oxygenation and nutrient perfusion of the tumor and removal of waste products.[12,13] Moreover, increased angiogenesis coincides with increased tumor cell entry into the circulation and thus facilitates metastasis.[14,15]

Cancer cells activate quiescent vasculature to produce new blood vessels via an "angiogenetic switch", often during the premalignant stages of tumor development.

The concept of an "angiogenic switch" means that as the tumor grows and cells in the center of the tumor mass become hypoxic, the tumor initiates recruitment of its own blood supply, by shifting the balance between angiogenesis inhibitors and stimulators towards angioneogenesis. Thus, neovascularization precedes and promotes tumor progression and metastasis.

The density of the capillary network seems to be one of the factors determining the malignancy of a tumor. Metastases of highly vascularized tumors appear earlier than those of poorly vascularized tumors.[16,17] The reason for this is not just the capillary permeability that enables shedding of tumor cells into the blood stream, but also a current hypothesis that both the primary tumor and the distant metastases are involved in complex regulation by angiogenic and antiangiogenic factors.[18]

The first indication of its importance in tumor angiogenesis came in the early 80s from observations that tumors secreted soluble factors, which could stimulate vascular endothelial growth.[19] The basic and acidic fibroblast growth factors were among the first to be identified and were soon followed by many others, such as vascular endothelial growth factor/vascular permeability factor (VEGF/VPF) and transforming growth factors (TGF- alpha- and beta), to mention some of the most important.[20]

Investigation of these factors, powerful molecules that control the formation of new blood vessels, are still in progress.[21,22] One study reported on the expression of VEGF in the ovarian epithelial tumors (OETs) in both epithelial and stromal compartments.[23] The study showed that VEGF is significantly increased in malignant OETs compared to benign and borderline tumors and concluded that this factor might play a role in the development of ovarian cancer.

Expression of VEGF depends on tissue hypoxia, generating a feedback mechanism to reduce hypoxia by means of neoangiogenesis. The regulation of VEGF expression by hypoxia is mediated by a family of hypoxia-inducible transcription factors (HIF), which increases transcription of the VEGF gene.[24]

The ability of growth factors, such as basic fibroblast growth factor (bFGF), vascular endothelial growth factor (VEGF), the insulin-like growth factor (IGF) system and HIF-1 alpha to increase the rate of endothelial cell proliferation has been demonstrated in several animal models and is important for understanding the tumor biology to appreciate the interesting fact that proliferation is largely limited to ischemic zones, even following systemic administration of these factors.[25]

The role of the IGF system in malignancy and its oncogenic potential was reviewed in 2006 by Samani and coworkers: they found that IGF-I receptor (IGF-IR) signaling and functions are mediated through the activities of a complex molecular network of positive (e.g., type I IGF) and negative (e.g., the type II IGF receptor, IGF-IIR) effectors. Under normal physiological conditions, the balance between the expression and activities of these molecules is tightly controlled. Changes in this delicate balance (e.g., overexpression of one of the effectors) may trigger a cascade of molecular events that can ultimately lead to malignancy. In recent years, evidence has been mounting that the IGF axis may be involved in human cancer progression and can be targeted for therapeutic intervention. Because IGF targeting for anticancer therapy is rapidly becoming a clinical reality, Samani et al., stressed that understanding of this complexity is timely because it is likely to have an impact on the design, mode of action and clinical outcomes of newly developed drugs.[26]

Besides hemangiogenesis, pathways for lymph-angiogenesis have also been proposed (Figure 4.1).[13] Electron microscopy, in vitro cultures and experiments on animal models have enabled us to understand the visible part of the angiogenic development of tumor vasculature.

TUMOR NEOVASCULARIZATION— CURRENT CONCEPTS

In general, tumor vasculature consists of the vessels recruited from the pre-existing network of the host vasculature and the vessels grown from the host vessels under the influence of the angiogenic factors of cancer cells.[27-29] Although the tumor vasculature originates from

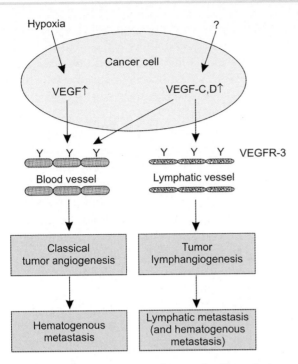

FIGURE 4.1: Dissecting tumor angiogenesis. Hypoxic tumor cells produce VEGF, which binds to and activates VEGFR-2 on vascular endothelial cells, leading to classical tumor angiogenesis. Tumors that secrete VEGF-C or VEGF-D may induce lymphangiogenesis by activating VEGFR-3 on lymphatic vessels, a process known as tumor lymphangiogenesis. Classical tumor angiogenesis has been shown to correlate with hematogenous metastasis. In the animal models, induction of lymphangiogenesis by VEGF-C or VEGF-D led to an increase in tumor metastasis via the lymphatic system.

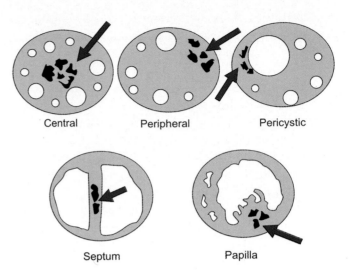

FIGURE 4.2: Schematic presentation of different types of vascularization within abnormal ovarian tissue.

the host vasculature, its organization may be completely different, depending upon the tumor type, its growth rate and its location. Macroscopically, tumor vasculature can be studied in terms of two ideal categories: peripheral and central. In tumors with peripheral vascularization, the centers are usually poorly perfused. In those with central vascularization, the opposite is expected. However, a tumor may consist of many territories, each exhibiting one or the other type of the ideal vascular pattern (Figure 4.2). Microscopically, tumor vasculature is highly heterogeneous and does not confirm to the standards of normal vascular organization. Tumor neovascularity can be differentiated from normal vascular beds by the several main characteristics:[30]

1. A single branch, varied in caliber, formed from narrow and dilated segments.
2. Elongation and coiling.
3. Nonhierarchical vascular network, vascular rings and sinusoids.

4. Abnormal precapillary architecture with dichotomous branching and no decrease in diameter of the higher-order branches.
5. Incomplete vascular wall: various gaps in the endothelium, discontinuity of the basal membrane and no muscular layer except in pre-existing vessels encased by the tumor.

A key difference between normal and tumor vessels is that the latter are dilated, saccular and tortuous, and may contain tumor cells within the endothelial lining of the vessel wall.[31] In addition, unlike normal tissue with a relatively fixed route between the arterial and venous circulation, a tumor may have blood flowing from one venule to another via a series of vessels or directly via an arteriovenous shunt.

However, the morphologic appearance of the tumor vascular bed may not necessarily allow direct assessment of the function of the tumor microcirculation. This is because only 20-80% of tumor vessels are perfused within any given tumor at a particular time. Within a particular tumor, one investigator has noted variations in flow that can be as high as tenfold.[32] Another important aspect to consider is that the microvascular permeability of the tumoral vessels is very heterogeneous and tumors have been shown to be up to eightfold more permeable than normal tissues. Vascular endothelial growth factor (VEGF) has been shown to increase vascular permeability.[17] VEGF is 50,000 times more potent in inducing vascular leakage than histamine.[33] The mechanism of this effect appears to be fenestration of the endothelium of small venules and capillaries through a Src kinase-dependent mechanism.[34]

One of the main characteristics of the tumor interstitial space is an expansion of its volume by three to five times compared to most host tissues. This results in a high interstitial fluid pressure of up to 50 mm Hg, when compared to normal tissues, in which the interstitial pressures are slightly subatmospheric. The major pathophysiologic mechanisms attributed to interstitial hypertension are absence of the functioning lymphatic vessels, high permeability of the vascular wall and rapid proliferation of tumor cells in confined spaces.[29] High interstitial pressure leads to the compression of the tumoral vessels and may even lead to local stasis. The relative perfusion of tumors resulting from these factors varies according to their growth. Initially, tumors have a hyperemic periphery with a relatively well perfused rim of tissue and later a relatively ischemic area, centrally. As the tumor enlarges, areas of central necrosis develop. Accordingly, four regions with different perfusion rates can be recognized in a tumor: an avascular (necrotic) region; a seminecrotic (ischemic) region; a stabilized microcirculation and an advancing front as a region of tumor hyperemia.[27,35] Depiction of these areas by imaging has practical importance because spatial distribution of chemotherapeutic agents varies according to the degree of tumor vascularity within different tumor regions. The multitude of data indicating that the control of angiogenesis is separate from the control of cancer cell proliferation suggests the possibility that drugs inhibiting angiogenesis could offer a treatment complementary to traditional chemotherapy, which directly targets tumor cells.[9,12,36] This exciting possibility has stimulated research on tumor angiogenesis and introduction of new 3D power Doppler evaluation of tumor vessels architecture.[37-41]

EVOLUTION OF 2D CONVENTIONAL AND COLOR DOPPLER ULTRASOUND IN IMAGING OF ADNEXAL TUMOR ANGIOGENESIS

It is clear that conflicting attitudes towards Doppler ultrasound in the evaluation of the vascular characteristics of malignant adnexal masses arise from the different results obtained from a number of studies published in the past several years. It is also important to stress that pulsed Doppler analysis and vascular resistance to blood flow were and still are one of the main features in the assessment of tumor vascular characteristics. All these studies have concentrated on differences of the vascular resistance to

blood flow between benign and malignant adnexal masses (Figures 4.3 and 4.4). It is a fact that a difference in vascularity exists and that blood vessels in malignant adnexal lesions show lower resistance to blood flow than those in benign adnexal masses (Figures 4.5A and B, 4.6A and B).

Before using any diagnostic technique related to sonographic depiction of the ovarian vascularity and flow, it is important that the investigator distinguishes the concepts of "tumor vascularity" and "tumor blood flow". Tumor vascularity refers to the number of vessels per unit volume, whereas tumor blood flow is a measure of the number of flowing blood elements over a certain period of time in a selected area of interest.[30]

Frequency-based color Doppler imaging provides information about blood flow by analyzing the changes in Doppler shift, which are proportional to velocity changes. Since the introduction of this diagnostic technique for the assessment of ovarian vascularity, opinions concerning its usefulness in the detection of adnexal malignancies have been equally divided.[42-49] Tumor blood vessels have a paucity or lack of a media muscularis, which is normally part of the vessel wall and hence are more distensible. This combined with arteriovenous shunts seen in the tumor vascular network results in low impedance to flow. However, because of the focal areas of narrowing and dilatation within the tumor vessels, focal areas of high systolic velocity can also be found.[50] Another factor that confounds this is the fact that most tumors have areas of variable perfusion. Our study reported on pre-existing vessels with normal wall structure in 60% of malignant ovarian tumors.[51]

Variable tumoral perfusion contributes to uneven tumor blood flow that makes it difficult to generalize a "characteristic" flow of ovarian tumors.[52] Diagnostic accuracy of values of flow indices in differentiating benign from malignant lesions has varied considerably, from over 96% to less than 40%.[53,54] More than 15 years of experience in multiple centers has shown that the overlap in the specific impedance values obtained by frequency-based transvaginal color Doppler imaging from vessels surrounding the ovary does not allow differentiation of benign versus malignant ovarian masses on the basis of impedance values alone.[55] Other limiting factors for this type of imaging represent slow flow and small caliber of the vessels, which are barely detectable.[56] Only vessels that are depicted by color Doppler ultrasound can be adequately studied by pulsed Doppler analysis. More precisely, it seems more important

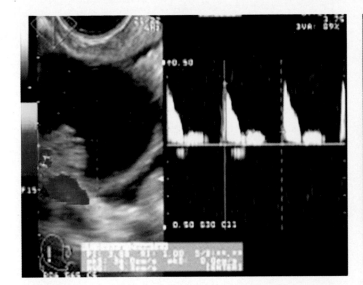

FIGURE 4.3: A transvaginal sonogram of the ovarian tumor with small echogenic formation (papilla) protruding into the lumen. Pulsed Doppler imaging demonstrates high resistance to blood flow. Benign ovarian tumor was confirmed by histology.

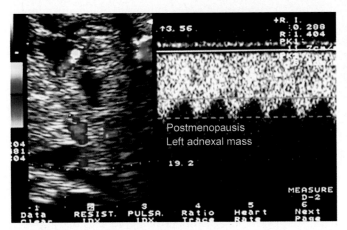

FIGURE 4.4: A malignant predominantly solid ovarian tumor in a postmenopausal patient. Pulsed Doppler waveform analysis shows low-resistance to blood flow.

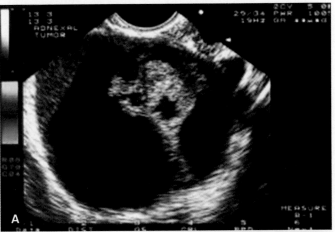

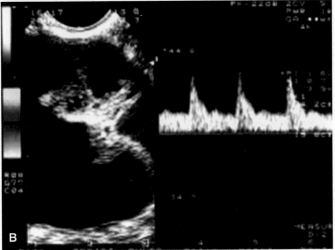

FIGURES 4.5A AND B: Complex ovarian tumor; note morphology suspicious for malignancy. Pulsed Doppler signals revealed moderate to high vascular resistance. Cystadenoma was confirmed by histology.

to provide information regarding the vascular network rather than particular vessels.[57] A solution to this problem has been offered by the introduction of amplitude-based transvaginal color Doppler imaging.[58] This imaging modality, known also as power Doppler ultrasound or Color Doppler Angiography®, takes into account the area under the curve of a spectral waveform and is related to the number of blood elements flowing over time. Power Doppler sonography has been found to be superior to frequency-based color Doppler sonography, especially in situations of low blood flow (low velocities), with the potential to detect alterations in blood flow.[59] Power

Doppler ultrasound has the advantage that it is more sensitive, less angle dependent and not susceptible to aliasing.[60,61] In this technique, the hue and brightness of the color signal represent the total energy of the Doppler signal. It displays the total flow in a confined area, giving an impression similar to that of angiography. The sensitivity of power Doppler imaging is 14 dB greater than the standard Doppler imaging.[62] Because of improved sensitivity in displaying smaller vessels, the vascularity is shown more completely. Several studies demonstrated clear correlation of the tumoral vascularity as depicted by power Doppler imaging to an estimation of vascularity seen histologically. There was a good correlation ($r = 0.82$) between Doppler parameters and number of the vessels greater than 50 micrometers in size, but poor correlation with the actual microvessel count, which typically includes vessels less than 15 micrometers.[63,64] Power Doppler

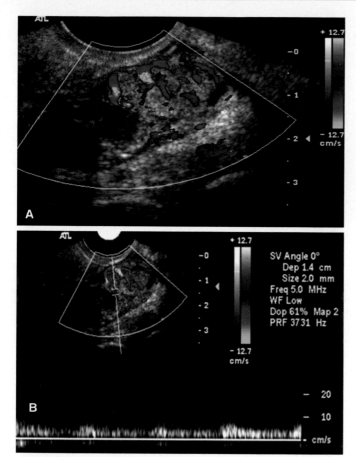

FIGURES 4.6A AND B: Ovarian carcinoma neovascularization. Randomly dispersed vessels are produced in central and peripheral parts of the tumor creating a potential for its proliferation and growth. Tumor vessels are deficient in their muscular elements and present diminished resistance to blood flow.

imaging has serious limitations in assessing temporal changes in flow and vessel size due to blooming of the color signal. This imaging modality permits depiction of even smaller vessels, but paradoxically, small intraparenchymal arterioles in benign and normal tissues may show a low impedance and a low-velocity blood flow pattern, giving rise to false-positive results.

It is clear that there is a need for further improvement in the ultrasonic assessment of pelvic tumor angiogenesis and, to this end, there has been a growing interest in 3D power Doppler ultrasound.

THREE-DIMENSIONAL ULTRASOUND AND POWER DOPPLER IMAGING OF BENIGN AND MALIGNANT ADNEXAL MASSES

Three-dimensional ultrasound (3D US) is a new, emerging technology that provides additional information to the evaluation of the adnexal masses.[65] Multiplanar and volume rendering display methods combined with the ability to rotate volume data into standard orientations are essential components of 3D US's current and future success.[66]

Patients' characteristics, CA-125 level and two-dimensional (2D) ultrasonography are commonly used to predict the probability of malignancy of an adnexal/ovarian mass. To assess the contribution of 3D ultrasonography in prediction of adnexal malignancy, Geomini and coworkers investigated 181 patients with adnexal mass using 3D ultrasound. Patients with an adnexal mass scheduled for surgery underwent 2D and 3D ultrasonographic examination during the week prior to surgery. Stepwise logistic regression was used to construct two models for the prediction of malignancy: a model based on patient's characteristics, level of CA-125 and 2D ultrasonography and a second model based on the patient's characteristics, level of CA-125, 2D and 3D ultrasonography. Out of 181 women with an adnexal mass, 144 were benign and 37 showed malignancy on histology. The 3D US model discriminated better between benign and malignant adnexal masses than the 2D US model (areas under the ROC curve of 0.92 and 0.82, respectively, p = 0.02). The calibration of both models was good. The authors concluded that in the assessment of the adnexal mass, the use of 3D ultrasonography significantly improved the prediction of malignancy as compared to 2D ultrasonography.[67]

Mansour et al. evaluated 400 patients with adnexal mass, using a risk of malignancy index (RMI). RMI consists of the following criteria: menopausal status, CA-125 serum levels and ultrasonographic morphology criteria. The authors added 3D power Doppler (3D PD) classifying parameters for the assessment of tumor vascularity, such as avascular, parallel and chaotic. The sensitivity of RMI for the prediction of malignancy was 88%, while sensitivity of 3D PD for prediction of malignancy was 75%. When RMI and 3D PD parameters were used together, the sensitivity has increased to 99%.[68]

Two months earlier Chase and Crade published a series of 66 cases undergoing preoperative assessment of the adnexal masses. They found that the positive predictive value (PPV) and the negative predictive value (NPV) of 3D vascular ultrasound were 100% and 95% respectively. The PPV and the NPV of 2D ultrasound in predicting malignancy were 37% and 100% respectively. In the same population, abnormal level of CA-125 had a PPV and NPV of 73% and 83% respectively. According to these authors, 3D ultrasound examination of the vascular architecture is discriminatory in distinguishing benign ovarian masses from malignant lesions.[69]

Multiple sections of the tumor, rotation, translation and reconstruction of 3D plastic images allow more precise evaluation of the tumor without increasing scanning time and patient discomfort.[70,71] Obvious advantages of 3D ultrasound are improved recognition of the ovarian lesion anatomy, accurate characterization of the surface features, determination of the extent of tumor infiltration through the capsule, and clear depiction of the size and volume of the mass.[40,72] The surface mode is particularly useful for the assessment of the superficial structures. If a cystic ovarian mass is found, 3D surface-rendered image offers new possibilities for evaluation and differentiation between benign and malignant lesions (Table 4.1.) (Figures 4.7A to F and 4.8A to C).[73]

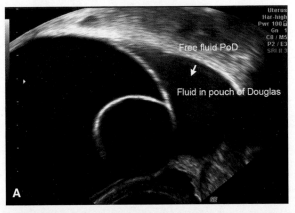

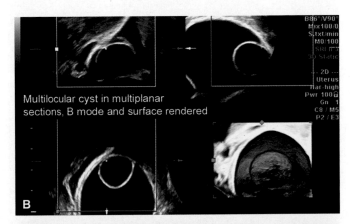

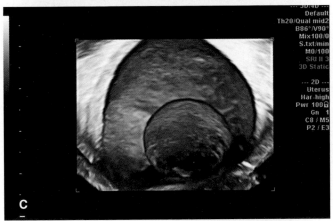

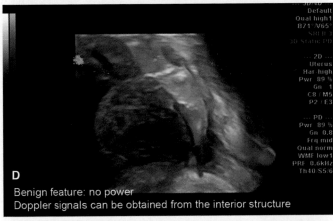

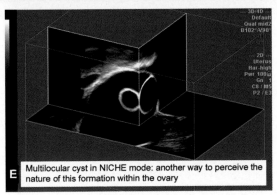

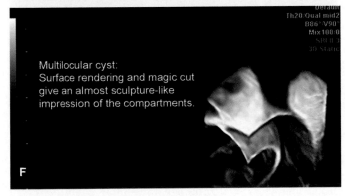

FIGURES 4.7A TO F: Ovarian multilocular cyst featured in B mode, multiplanar, 3D PD mode, "niche" mode and "magic cut".

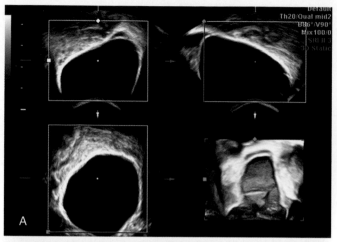

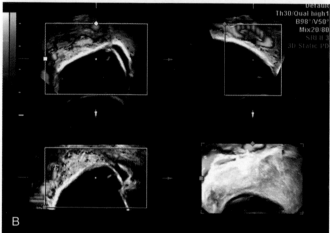

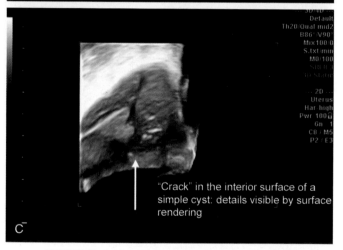

"Crack" in the interior surface of a simple cyst: details visible by surface rendering

FIGURES 4.8A TO C: Multimodel assessment of the ovarian simple cyst.

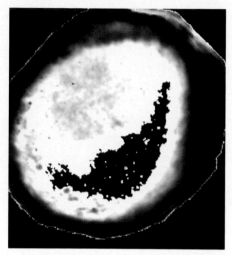

FIGURE 4.9: Three-dimensional scan of a bizarre ovarian tumor containing echogenic fluid and intracystic echoes. Dermoid cyst was confirmed by histology.

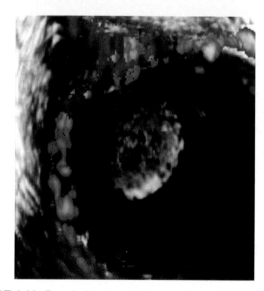

FIGURE 4.10: Regularly separated vessels are detected at the periphery of the dermoid cyst by 3D power Doppler imaging.

Application of the "transparent maximum/minimum" mode enables visualization of the tumor calcification or identification of the bone structures in dermoid cysts[74] (Figures 4.9 and 4.10).

Our team reported on five cases of the primary fallopian tube carcinoma, selected from a cohort of 520 patients with adnexal mass.[75] Using 2D ultrasound, three fallopian tube carcinomas were detected preoperatively. Three-dimensional ultrasound enabled accurate diagnosis of the Fallopian tube carcinoma by detecting intraluminal papillary projections in all five cases of tubal malignancy. Furthermore, 3D ultrasound enabled precise detection of tubal pathology by simultaneous observation of the neighboring structures: the uterus and the ipsilateral ovary. One patient had bilateral fallopian tube lesions. Preoperative

TABLE 4.1: Advantages of three-dimensional ultrasound in the assessment of adnexal masses

Authors	No of patients analyzed	Advantages of 3D US
Chan et al 1997[70]	8	- Enhanced morphologic evaluation of adnexal masses - Additional views - High-speed image acquisition - Real time analysis of the acquired image data at a later time
Weber et al 1997[71]	50	- Multiplanar view - Rotation of the stored volume - Reconstruction of the inner surface of a cystic ovarian tumor
Bonilla-Musoles et al 1995[65]	67	- Calculation of the ovarian volume - Observation of the papillary projections - Extent of capsular infiltration
Geomini et al 2007[67]	181	- Significant improvement in prediction of malignancy
Mansour et al 2009[68]	400	- Addition of 3D power Doppler imaging increases sensitivity of the *risk of malignancy index* (RMI) from 88-99%
Chase et al 2009[69]	66	- 3D power Doppler ultrasound examination of the vascular architecture is discriminatory in distinguishing benign and malignant adnexal masses

3D ultrasound imaging correctly predicted bilaterality, while 2D imaging found only unilateral changes (Table 4.2). The "niche" aspect of 3D ultrasound reveals intratumoral structures in selected sections, which is mandatory for the evaluation of the tubal pathology (Figures 4.11A to G).

Furthermore, this technique is especially useful in the evaluation of the complex ovarian lesions, such as ovarian dermoids, endometriomas, fibromas and pelvic inflammatory disease, which may give wrong impression of malignancy when using conventional transvaginal sonography

TABLE 4.2: Histopathology, 3D ultrasound morphology and vascular geometry in patients with fallopian tube carcinoma

Histopathology	3D ultrasound morphology	Vascular geometry
Adenocarcinoma	Sausage-shaped complex mass 4.0 × 2.8 × 3.2 cm with papillary projections, regular surface, no infiltration through the capsule	Chaotic vessels arrangement, disproportional calibration of the vessels and irregular branching
Adenocarcinoma	Sausage-shaped cystic mass 5.8 × 3.6 × 2.8 cm with pseudosepta and papillary projections, regular surface, thickened capsule	Chaotic vessels arrangement, demonstration of the arteriovenous shunts, tumoral lakes and microaneurysms
Adenocarcinoma	Sausage-shaped cystic mass 8.4 × 4.5 × 6.0 cm with solid parts and papillary projections, regular surface, thickened capsule	Chaotic vessels arrangement, irregular branching, visualization of numerous blind ends
Adenocarcinoma	Sausage-shaped complex mass 7.8 × 4.2 × 3.0 cm with papillary projections, irregular surface, infiltration through the capsule, bilateral tumors	Chaotic vessels arrangement, demonstration of the vascular stenosis, tumoral lakes and irregular branching
Anaplastic carcinoma	Sausage-shaped mass 4.0 × 3.0 × 2.6 cm with papillary projections, regular surface, no infiltration through the capsule	Chaotic vessels arrangement, visualization of the arteriovenous anastomosis, microaneurysms and irregular branching

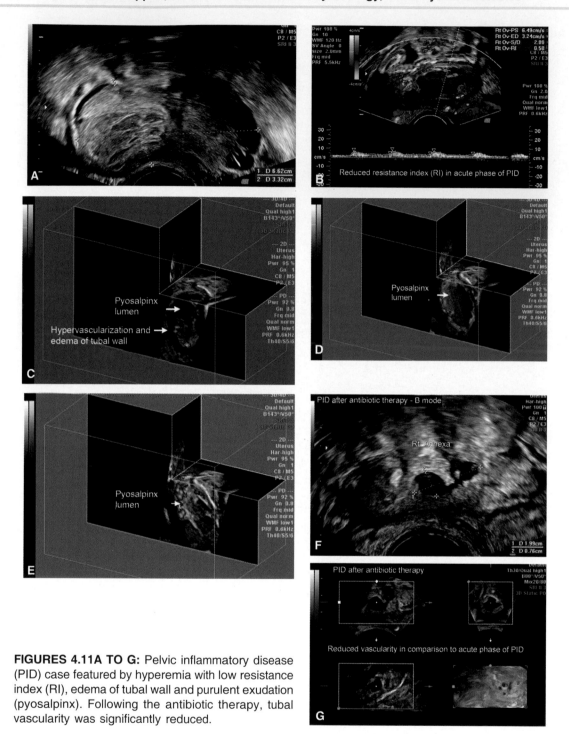

FIGURES 4.11A TO G: Pelvic inflammatory disease (PID) case featured by hyperemia with low resistance index (RI), edema of tubal wall and purulent exudation (pyosalpinx). Following the antibiotic therapy, tubal vascularity was significantly reduced.

and color Doppler ultrasound (Figures 4.12, 4.13, 4.14A to E, 4.15A to C and 4.16A to H).

Note pericystic hyperemia and fibrin strands on 3D PD and "niche" mode. Laparoscopy with coagulation of the rupture site and lavage were performed.

Our group has reported on a significant reduction in the rate of false-positive findings between 2D transvaginal and color Doppler ultrasound and combined 3D static and power Doppler ultrasound: 76.92% vs 91.67%.[76] The most illustrative is the case of a serous cystadenocarcinoma in a 38-year-old patient, measuring only 3 cm, missed by 2D transvaginal color Doppler, but successfully identified by a combined use of 3D static and power Doppler imaging. Transvaginal sonography did not demonstrate a small

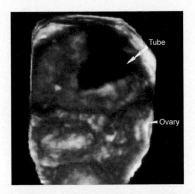

FIGURE 4.12: Three-dimensional view of a dilated tube in a patient with hydrosalpinx. Ipsilateral ovary, containing follicles, is clearly visualized close to the affected tube. This is an illustrative example of how surface rendering defines spatial relations of a tubal lesion with a nearby ovary.

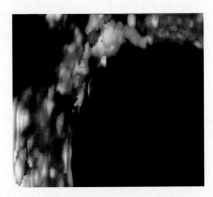

FIGURE 4.13: Three-dimensional power Doppler ultrasound demonstrated regularly separated vessels at the periphery of a fluid filled dilated tube in a patient with pelvic inflammatory disease.

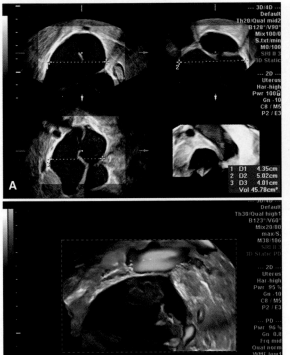

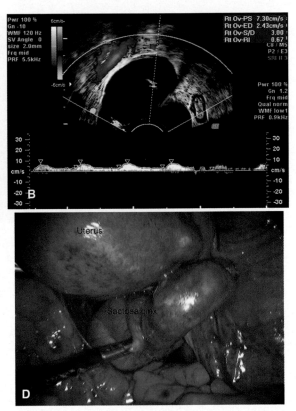

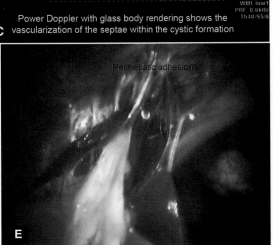

FIGURES 4.14A TO E: End-result of insufficient PID management: hydrosalpinx resembling a multicystic adnexal mass with vascularized septae. Laparoscopy reveals hydrosalpinx and perihepatic adhesions due to Chlamydia infection.

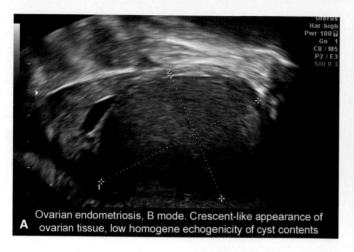

A Ovarian endometriosis, B mode. Crescent-like appearance of ovarian tissue, low homogene echogenicity of cyst contents

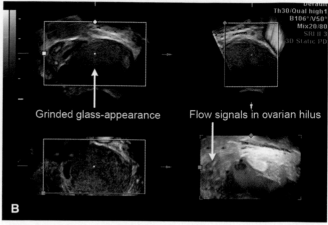

B Grinded glass-appearance   Flow signals in ovarian hilus

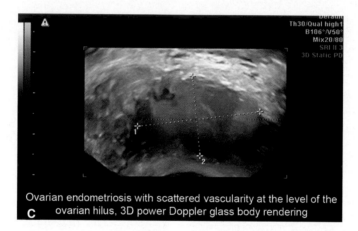

C Ovarian endometriosis with scattered vascularity at the level of the ovarian hilus, 3D power Doppler glass body rendering

FIGURES 4.15 A TO C: Ovarian endometriosis with scattered vascularity in the hilus area, "grinded glass" like low echogenicity of the intracystic fluid and "crescent" appearance of the remaining ovarian tissue.

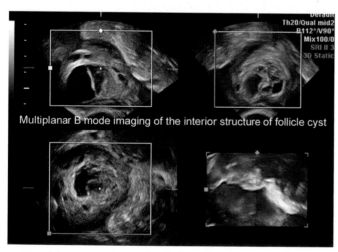

Multiplanar B mode imaging of the interior structure of follicle cyst

FIGURE 4.16A

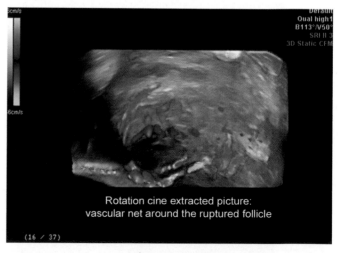

Rotation cine extracted picture: vascular net around the ruptured follicle

FIGURE 4.16B

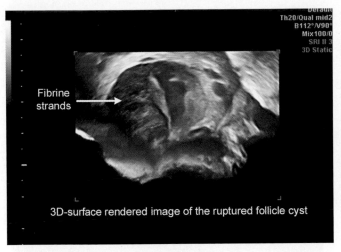

FIGURE 4.16C

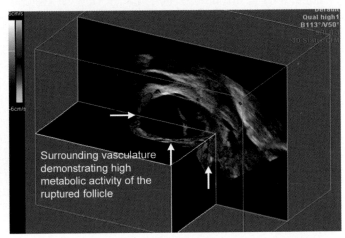

FIGURE 4.16D

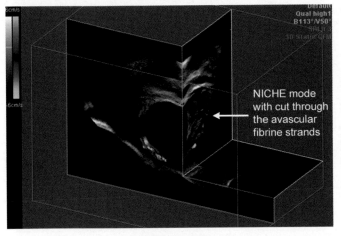

FIGURE 4.16E

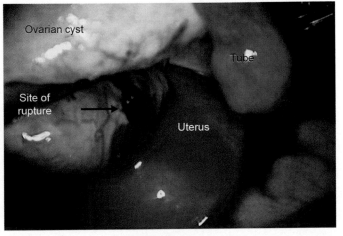

FIGURE 4.16F

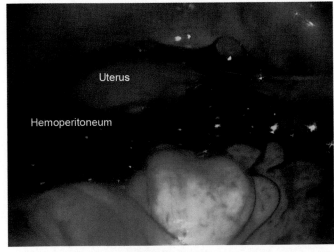

FIGURE 4.16G

FIGURE 4.16H

FIGURES 4.16A TO H: Ruptured hemorrhagic cyst with massive hemoperitoneum (0.9 L).

papillary projection (less than 5 mm in maximum diameter) extending into the cystic wall. Although pulsed Doppler waveform analysis demonstrated peripheral vascularity, resistance index values were above the cut-off value proposed for the diagnosis of ovarian malignancy and measured 0.46. Three-dimensional ultrasound clearly depicted papillary protrusions and power Doppler enabled detection of tiny irregular vessels within the papillary protrusion.

Three-dimensional power Doppler ultrasound allows the clinician to visualize the many overlapping vessels easily and quickly and assess their relationship to other vessels or surrounding tissues.[77] The implementation of the 3D display enables visualization of the pelvic structures in three dimensions interactively, rather than having to assemble the sectional images mentally. The 3D power Doppler systems improve our understanding of the tumoral vascularity and speed up the entire diagnostic process.[78]

While 2D color Doppler was useful in detecting vascularized structures, 3D power Doppler is superior for study of the vascular morphology. Evaluation of the blood vessels anatomy represents another approach to tumor diagnosis, which is extensively evaluated during the last decade.

Using 3D color and power Doppler ultrasound, Crade has described a "tissue block" technique. Several volumes of a certain region of interest (ROI) within the adnexal mass, containing vascular patterns picked up by color or power Doppler ultrasound were stored and rendered without the physical presence of a patient. Volumes were analyzed using software features like "magic cut", tomographic ultrasound imaging (TUI) and "niche" mode. The following vascularization criteria assessed by 3D power Doppler ultrasound are suggestive of malignancy:

1. Loss of tree-like branching of vessels.
2. Sacculation of arteries and veins.
3. Focal narrowing of the arteries.
4. Internal shifts in velocity within the arterial lumen.
5. "Beach ball" finding of increased and disorganized peripheral flow, surrounding the surface of a malignant lesion, thus forming a ball-like power Doppler image of vascular signals.
6. Increased flow to a center of a solid region.
7. Crowding of the vascularity.
8. "Start and stop" arteries, showing arteries that stop abruptly within the tumor, without developing the tree-like branching how it would be normally seen in a benign mass.[79]

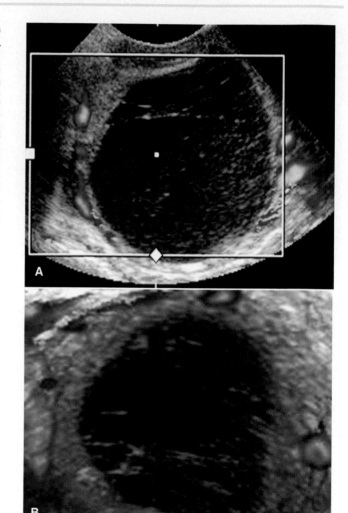

FIGURES 4.17A AND B: Two and three-dimensional power Doppler scan of an ovarian cyst. Note regular walls of the cyst and echogenic content suggestive of a benign lesion. Corpus luteum cyst was found at the time of laparoscopy. Note single vessel arrangement is clearly displayed at the periphery of the cystic lesion.

There is a distinct impression that the distribution and branching pattern of blood vessels, supplying a fast-growing tumor differ from those in a normal blood supply to normal organs. This means that blood vessel distribution seems to carry additional information that is missed in the present diagnostic approaches.

In 2000, we published a study, in which we presented results of 3D power Doppler imaging in interactive analysis of the ovarian tumors microcirculation anatomy.[80]

Benign adnexal lesions were characterized by single vessel arrangement which is clearly displayed at the periphery of the cystic lesion (Figures 4.17A and B).

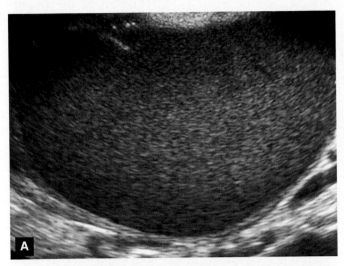
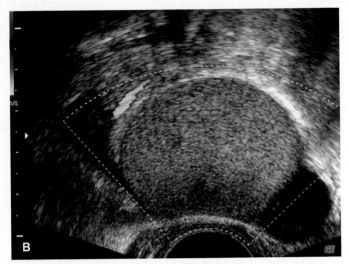

FIGURES 4.18A AND B: Two-dimensional B mode and color Doppler scan of an ovarian endometrioma. Note homogeneous high-level internal echoes typical of a chocolate paste fluid.

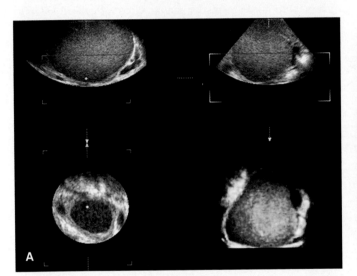
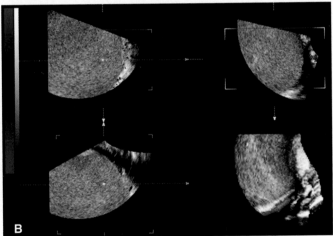

FIGURES 4.19A AND B: Three-dimensional B mode and power Doppler image of ovarian endometrioma. Note regularly separated peripheral vessel at the level of the ovarian hilus. This flow pattern is typical of ovarian endometrioma.

The most common ovarian lesion in premenopausal patients was ovarian endometrioma (26 of 58) (Figures 4.18A and B and 4.19A and B) and dermoid cysts (19 of 58), whereas the most common ovarian tumor during the postmenopausal period was serous cystadenoma (22 of 28). In ovarian endometrioma, vessels were usually straight with regularly branching pattern. Typically, endometrioma vascularity originates from a hilar vessel and runs along the surface of the tumor. Similar vascular anatomy is detected in dermoid cysts.

From nine cases of malignant ovarian tumors, the most common ovarian malignancy was serous cystadenocarcinoma detected in six postmenopausal patients (5 of 28), one perimenopausal (1 of 4) and one premenopausal patient (1 of 58). Mucinous cystadenocarcinoma was diagnosed in two postmenopausal patients (2 of 28). Three-dimensional power Doppler ultrasound accurately detected characteristic structural abnormalities of the malignant tumor vessels, such as microaneurysms, arteriovenous shunts, tumor lakes, disproportional calibration, elongation, coiling and dichotomous branching (Figures 4.20 and 4.21).

Another feature of adnexal tumor vascularity is the presence of the randomly dispersed vessels within the tumoral stroma and periphery. The course of the main tumor vessel is usually irregular with more complicated branching. The diameters of these vessels were felt to be more

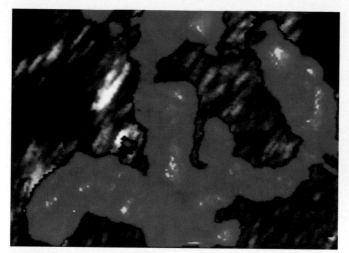

FIGURE 4.20: Malignant tumor neovascularization is characterized by arteriovenous shunts, stenosis and blind-ending lakes. All these features can be assessed using 3D power Doppler imaging.

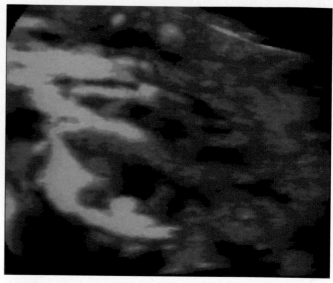

FIGURE 4.21: Three-dimensional power Doppler can of a malignant tumor neovascularization. Note the typical vascular features of adnexal malignancy: three generations of the vessels, areas of stenosis, microaneurysms and tumor lakes.

"uneven" and "thorn-like". Our pioneering study demonstrated that qualitative analysis of the tumor vascularity architecture by 3D power Doppler increased morphological 3D ultrasound assessment, reaching the sensitivity and specificity of 100 and 98.76% respectively.

FURTHER POSSIBILITIES IN THE EVALUATION OF TUMOR ANGIOGENESIS

Our group made efforts in describing branching pattern of the tumoral microvasculature. The branching pattern is the result of some principle mathematical laws that act repeatedly, so that they branch out in similar ways at different scale factors. Such objects that are self-similar at different scales are called fractals. A "fractal" is a shape that yields detail forever, no matter how far one zooms in. It is best compared to the trunk of a tree sprouting branches, which in turn split off into smaller branches which themselves yield twigs again. If the underlying rule changes, the branching pattern must change too. We postulate that blood vessel trees are an example of fractal geometry (Figure 4.22).[81]

The normal blood vessel trees (arteries and veins) form branched structures with ever-smaller branches and diameters. The underlying proposition of our hypothesis is that there is a change in fractal dimension when the branching becomes unregulated by abnormal processes, i.e. when the ordered growth is replaced by disordered growth.

Currently, the application of 3D power Doppler in the evaluation of neoplasms is mainly quantitative or

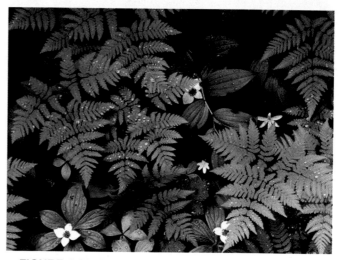

FIGURE 4.22: Fern leaf as example for fractal geometry.

semiquantitative (for example, in detecting whether the vascularity is present or not). Further development of the technology and the introduction of 3D quantification of blood flow, called the 3D color histogram, may improve our ability to differentiate between benign and malignant tumors and predict tumor prognosis.[82-84] The 3D color histogram measures the color percentage and flow amplitudes in the volume of interest. The histogram enables the vascularization and blood flow within a tissue block to be quantified, in contrast to 2D color histograms in which only single planes can be investigated.

Pairleitner et al. reported on the use of cube method for measurement of blood flow and vascularization in 3D perspective.[83] The vascularization index (VI) represents the vessels in the tissue and is important for situation of both high and low vascularization. The flow index (FI), a mean color value, is important for characterizing high flow intensities (presumably tumors). The vascularization flow index (VFI) is a combination of VI and FI and identifies the extremes between low vascularization and low blood flow on one side and high vascularization and high blood flow on the other. Although both VI and FI showed excellent reproducibility, VFI did not achieve accurate estimation between two observations, which may lead to unreliable measurement. It is expected that VI and FI may become good predictors for tumor neovascularization that can replace qualitative or semiquantitative 3D power Doppler evaluation.[84]

More recently, Kudla and Alcazar analyzed 3D vascularization indices (VI, FI and VFI) in evaluation of the advanced, metastatic and early stage ovarian tumors. In an attempt to standardize this new technique, they suggested standard settings of power Doppler gain control to avoid interpretation errors caused by extensive color "leaking": for Voluson 730 Expert (Beta 05 version, RIC 5-9 H TVS probe), which they were using, they recommended PRF = 0.6 kHz and gain 0.8.[85]

Intravenous contrast agents for ultrasound studies are commercially available.[86,87] With the utilization of ultrasound contrast agents perfusion imaging of the tumors has become less subjective. Contrast enhanced ultrasound imaging is of particular importance in cases of "slow flow, low flow and no flow." One of the most exciting areas is the use of 3D power Doppler enhanced imaging of pelvic circulation and may assist in better visualization of the vessel's continuity (in three orthogonal projections) and branching (3D vascular reconstruction). Higher detection rate of small vessels after injection of contrast agents may allow application of the mathematical models assessing 3D vascular chaos and fractals.[73]

Our group reported on the use of contrast enhanced 3D power Doppler sonography for the differentiation of adnexal lesions.[88] We found that contrast enhanced, 3D power Doppler sonography provided better visualization of the tumoral vascularity in morphologically suspicious adnexal lesions than that obtained with noncontrast 3D power Doppler sonography (Figures 4.23A to C, 4.24 and 4.25).

With respect to differential diagnosis between malignant and benign ovarian lesions, contrast enhanced, 3D power

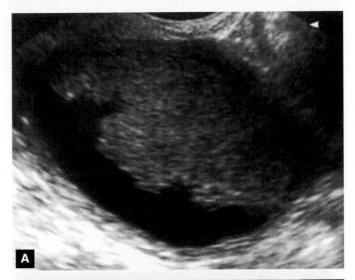

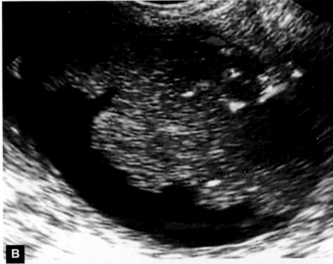

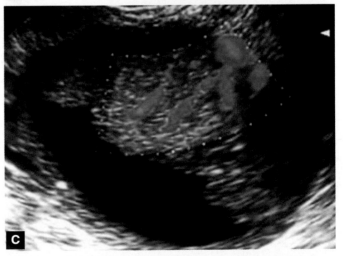

FIGURES 4.23A TO C: Two-dimensional B mode, color Doppler and power Doppler scan of a complex adnexal mass. Penetrating pattern of the tumor vasculature is suggestive of ovarian malignancy.

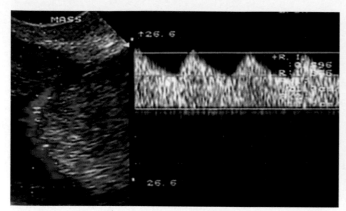

FIGURE 4.24: Pulsed Doppler waveform analysis of intratumor neovascularization demonstrates low vascular impedance blood flow signals, typical of ovarian malignancy.

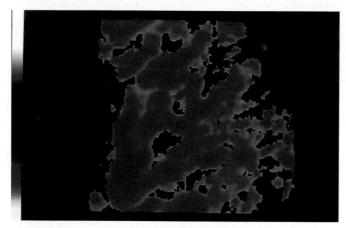

FIGURE 4.25: Enhanced 3D power Doppler ultrasound of ovarian carcinoma. More than four generations of penetrating intratumor vessels with irregular course and numerous shunts were visualized.

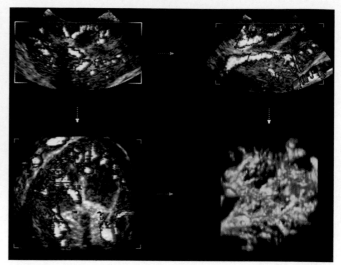

FIGURE 4.26: Simultaneous rendering of all three orthogonal sectional planes, demonstrating a vasculature of a nonpalpable postmenopausal ovary after instillation of the echo-enhancing contrast. Note the 3D view of the tumor microcirculation on the lower right figure.

ZAGREB EXPERIENCE

The question which ultrasound technique and diagnostic criteria provide the best adnexal lesion characterization has not been answered sufficiently. However, successful adnexal mass pattern recognition obviously also depends on the performance of the sonographer.[89]

Sokalska et al, performed the first multicenter study evaluating the ability of ultrasound examiners to make a specific diagnosis of an adnexal mass, using subjective gray scale and Doppler ultrasound findings criteria (pattern recognition).[90] More recently, Alcazar et al., examined 173 patients (medium age 52.4 years) with adnexal masses (117 malignant and 56 benign adnexal lesions). After logistic regression analysis only central blood flow in solid tumor areas and presence of ascites were identified as independent predictors of adnexal malignancy. Both features correlated with adnexal malignancy in 98.6% of patients. The absence of both sonographic features was detected in 82.1% of benign tumors.[91]

Our study[92] summarized a four years experience in classifying an ultrasound examination as suggestive or indicative for adnexal and endometrial malignancy. Subjects for this investigation were 292 patients who were evaluated using five complementary methods in the preoperative sonographic assessment (from January 1997 to September 2000). The inclusion criteria were clinical and/or ultrasound diagnosis of a pelvic mass and/or postmenopausal bleeding.

Doppler sonography reached diagnostic sensitivity and specificity of 100% and 93.9% respectively. The positive and negative predictive values of this method were 85.7% and 100% respectively. Therefore, the diagnostic efficiency was improved with the use of sonographic contrast agent from 86.7 to 95.6%.

Furthermore, our results show that the pattern of irregularly branching penetrating vessels in suspicious adnexal lesions demonstrated by 3D power Doppler ultrasound with or without contrast enhancement is an important feature that should be considered for prediction of the likelihood of malignancy. If used together with 3D morphologic ultrasound assessment, enhanced 3D power Doppler imaging may precisely discriminate benign from malignant adnexal lesions (Figure 4.26).

Adnexal and/or endometrial morphology and thickness/volume by 2D transvaginal and 3D ultrasound, as well as blood flow analysis by transvaginal color and pulsed Doppler and 3D power Doppler examination were performed in all the examined patients. Two hundred and fifty-one patient with adnexal masses and 41 patients with endometrial lesions were evaluated in respect of gray scale ultrasonography, adnexal/endometrial volume measurement and vascularity assessment. There were 30 histologically confirmed malignant adnexal masses and 221 benign adnexal lesions. Furthermore, histopathology revealed 9 cases of endometrial carcinoma and 32 benign endometrial lesions (18 cases of endometrial hyperplasia, 8 cases of endometrial polyps and 6 patients with atrophic or normal endometrium). Morphologic assessment by 3D ultrasound yielded additional information in 58% of adnexal lesions, especially considering small papillary projections (< 3 mm), thick septa within the inner surface of wall structure and relationship with surrounding structures in comparison with 2D ultrasound (Tables 4.3 and 4.4).

Furthermore, this modality was superior to 2D ultrasound in accurate depiction and diagnosis of two cases of fallopian tube carcinoma, by detecting intraluminal papillary projections and pseudosepta. Three-dimensional ultrasound enabled precise detection of tubal pathology in

TABLE 4.3: Two-dimensional sonographic and color Doppler criteria for the diagnosis of adnexal malignancy

Volume	< 10 cm³	0
	> 10 cm³	2
Cyst wall thickness/structure	smooth < 3 mm	0
	smooth > 3 mm	1
	papillarities < 3 mm	1
	papillarities > 3 mm	2
Septa	no septa	0
	thin septa < 3 mm	1
	thick septa > 3 mm	2
Solid parts	solid area < 1 cm	1
	solid area > 1 cm	2
Echogenicity	sonolucency/low level echo	0
	mixed/high level echo	2
Tumoral blood flow	RI > 0.42	0
	RI ≤ 0.42	2

Total score = sum of individual scores. Cut-off score greater or equal of 4 for morphology index and greater or equal to 6 for combined (morphology and vascular) index was associated with a high risk of adnexal malignancy

TABLE 4.4: Three-dimensional sonographic and power Doppler criteria for the diagnosis of adnexal malignancy

Volume	< 10 cm³	0
	> 10 cm³	2
Cyst wall thickness/structure	smooth < 3 mm	0
	smooth > 3 mm	1
	papillarities < 3 mm	1
	papillarities > 3 mm	2
Septa	no septa	0
	thin septa < 3 mm	1
	thick septa > 3 mm	2
Solid parts	solid area < 1 cm	1
	solid area > 1 cm	2
Echogenicity	sonolucency/low level echo	0
	mixed/high level echo	2
Relationship with surrounding structures	normal	0
	disturbed	1
Vessels' architecture	linear	0
	chaotic	2
Branching pattern	simple	0
	complex	2

Total score = sum of individual scores. Cut-off score greater or equal to 5 for morphology index and greater or equal to 7 for combined index was associated with high risk of adnexal malignancy

TABLE 4.5: Sensitivity, specificity, positive (PPV), and negative predictive values (NPV) of 2D US and 3D US in the detection of adnexal malignancy

Technique	Sensitivity %	Specificity %	PPV %	NPV %
2D US	80	95	71	97
3D US	87	96	74	98

both cases by simultaneous observation of the neighboring structures: uterus and ipsilateral ovary. With respect to differential diagnosis between malignant and benign adnexal lesions, better morphological assessment by 3D ultrasound slightly improved sensitivity, specificity, positive and negative predictive value in comparison with 2D sonography morphology indexing (Figures 4.27 and 4.28) (Table 4.5).

The application of 3D power Doppler significantly improved results of morphology indexing. Combined morphology and vascular index analysis revealed only one false positive (retroperitoneal fibromatosis) and one false

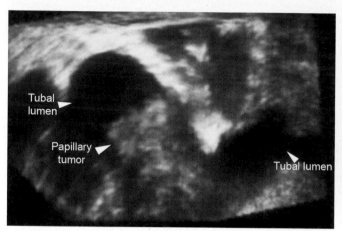

FIGURE 4.27: Three-dimensional ultrasound of a complex adnexal mass in a patient presenting with abnormal genital tract bleeding and pelvic pain. Surface view demonstrates tubular structure with papillary protrusion. The morphology was suggestive of fallopian tube malignancy, which was confirmed by histology.

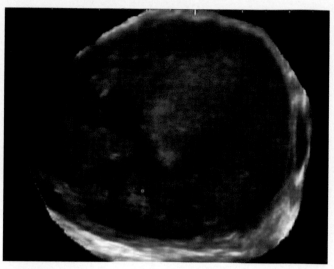

FIGURE 4.29: Complex ovarian tumor as seen by 3D ultrasound. Surface view revealed irregular wall proliferations suggestive of ovarian malignancy.

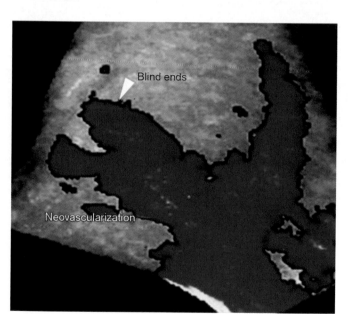

FIGURE 4.28: The same patient as in Figure 4.27 evaluated by 3D power Doppler ultrasound. The volume was rotated in all three dimensions, allowing visualization of the tumor vessels with an irregular course and branching.

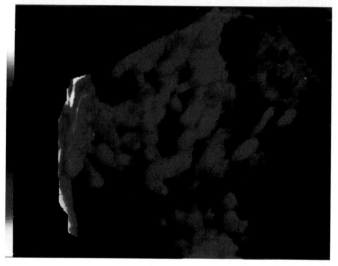

FIGURE 4.30: Three-dimensional power Doppler ultrasound of the malignant tumor vessels with the solid part. Note their irregular course and branching.

negative finding (serous cystadenocarcinoma). Demonstration of the chaotic, randomly dispersed vessels with irregular branching was suggestive of adnexal malignancy. Other structural abnormalities of the malignant tumor vessels were microaneurysms, arteriovenous shunts, tumor lakes, disproportional calibration, coiling and dichotomous branching (Figures 4.29 and 4.30).

It seems to us that 3D power Doppler ultrasound has brought us a little closer to better understanding of angiogenesis and neovascularization. Qualitative analysis of the tumor vascularity architecture, when added to morphological parameters, is clinically pertinent, reaching a sensitivity and specificity of 97% and 99% respectively (Table 4.6).

Contrast enhanced 3D power Doppler, performed in 89 patients with complex adnexal masses, improved sensitivity (100%), but regarding the criterion "highly suspicious pattern of tumor vasculature", two false-positive cases (ovarian fibroma, and fibromatosis retroperitonealis) were diagnosed. In one postmenopausal patient, with a normal size ovary (10.1 cm^3), and a solid area of 0.9 cm, 3D

TABLE 4.6: Sensitivity, specificity, positive (PPV), and negative predictive values (NPV) of 2D US/ TVCD, 3D US/3D PD and contrast enhanced 3D PD in detection of adnexal malignancy

Technique	Sensitivity %	Specificity %	PPV %	NPV %
2D US/TVCD	89	98	86	99
3D US/3D PD	97	99	97	99
Enhanced 3D PD	100	99	93	100

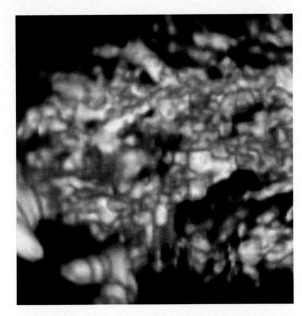

FIGURE 4.31: Three-dimensional power Doppler scan of a stage I ovarian carcinoma in a postmenopausal patient. Randomly dispersed vessels within irregular branching were the only finding, indicating ovarian malignancy what was confirmed at the time of surgery.

power Doppler revealed highly suspicious vascular pattern and the combined score for this ultrasound modality was 7, highly predictive of ovarian malignancy. Later, this case was classified as IA stage of ovarian malignancy (Figure 4.31).

Prior to entering this study, we examined 84 healthy premenopausal patients during early proliferative phase of menstrual cycle and 63 postmenopausal patients without adnexal or uterine lesions in order to estimate values of ovarian volume. All the examined patients had no history of use of oral contraception, ovary-stimulating drugs and/ or hormonal replacement therapy. In premenopausal patients, the mean ovarian volume obtained by 2D ultrasound was 5.8 ± 0.06 cm^3 and in the postmenopausal group 2.6 ± 0.03 cm^3. Ovarian volume obtained by automatic volume measurement with 3D ultrasound in premenopausal patients was 5.8 ± 0.03 cm^3, while in postmenopausal patients, the mean volume was 2.6 ± 0.01 cm^3. No differences between the volumes of the right and the left ovary were found in pre- and postmenopausal patients using both methods. Similarly, no difference was obtained in terms of ovarian volume measurement by 2D and 3D ultrasound. The overall ovarian volume of the various neoplasms obtained in this study for each age group was significantly above the normal ovarian volume (except one case of a normal sized ovary). Furthermore statistical difference in mean ovarian volume was obtained for benign versus malignant ovarian masses (109 cm^3 vs 274 cm^3) (Table 4.7).

This may suggest, the greater the size of ovarian tumor, the higher the risk of ovarian malignancy and in this light ovarian volume measurements may assist in the diagnosis of ovarian neoplasms.

TABLE 4.7: Ovarian volume obtained by automatic volume measurement by three-dimensional ultrasound

	Mean ovarian volume (cm³) ± SD
Premenopausal patients	5.8 ± 0.03
Postmenopausal patients	2.6 ± 0.01
Benign ovarian masses	109
Malignant ovarian masses	274

FUTURE CHALLENGES

Today, most traditional cancer treatments involve some combination of surgery, chemotherapy and radiation. All of these treatment options target the tumor cells directly. In contrast, selectively targeting endothelial cells, the building blocks of blood vessels, could directly inhibit the capillary support system that enables a tumor to grow. The widely held view is that these antiangiogenic therapies should destroy the tumor vasculature, thereby depriving the tumor of oxygen and nutrients.

The dependence of tumor growth on new blood vessel formation makes angiogenesis inhibition a promising treatment option for malignant disease. Encouraging results came out using monoclonal anti-VEGF antibodies or small molecule VEGF inhibitors in different cancer types.

Various additional VEGF-based and non-VEGF-based antiangiogenic therapies will be evaluated in phase II and

III studies over the coming years, which will provide more clarity regarding their potential clinical utility.

The recognition of angiogenesis and the potential for antiangiogenic therapies represents a dramatic paradigm shift in medicine and in the evolution of cancer treatment. Boehm and colleagues have shown that three different mouse tumors, treated with repeated cycles of a newly discovered angiogenesis inhibitor called endostatin, have regressed, did not become drug resistant and after a characteristic number of treatment cycles became dormant.[93] Such a treatment strategy could help circumvent many of the problems associated with current chemotherapeutic regimens, such as acquired drug resistance, attributable to tumor cell genetic instability or intrinsic resistance due to poor penetration of certain drugs into the tumor parenchyma. The results of cyclic endostatin therapy strongly suggests that drugs targeting angiogenesis and the tumor vasculature could become a major new weapon for effectively treating and indeed preventing human cancer. As with any other new treatment procedure, there are a number of important questions for the future. Indeed, a pure angiogencsis inhibitor would be expected to block new vessel growth, leaving quiescent blood vessels intact. Such an inhibitor should stop neovascularization in a tumor and should effect a static and dormant state. The neoplasm should neither grow nor regress, but should continue to be fed by its established vessels, remaining in a meta-state of proliferation balanced apoptosis.[94] Jain presented a different hypothesis on antiangiogenic drug efficacy, stating that there is emerging evidence to support that certain antiangiogenic agents can also transiently "normalize" the abnormal structure and function of tumor vasculature to make it more efficient for oxygen and drug delivery. Drugs that induce vascular normalization can alleviate hypoxia and increase the efficacy of conventional therapies, if both are carefully scheduled.[95]

Another important question rises: Are there tissue-specific differences in the vasculature and consequently in tumor vessel anatomy that affect a tumor's susceptibility to inhibition/disruption? Could 3D power Doppler help in answering these questions? This question is undoubtedly a challenge for all ultrasonographers.

CONCLUSION

Color and pulsed Doppler sonography enables visualization of the pelvic mass vascularity and provides information regarding tumor angiogenesis and/or neovascularization. This information better reflects angiogenic intensity of a mass, rather than indicating its nature. Clearly, initial attempts to classify ovarian tumors solely on the basis of their impedance to blood flow have been too simplistic.

The results reported in the literature on 3D color/power Doppler are indeed provocative and, not surprisingly, raise many new questions about the regulation of tumor angiogenesis, the density of tumor vessels, and difference between vessels' architecture in benign and malignant growths. Three-dimensional power Doppler depiction of tumor angiogenesis has many clinical implications. Improved detection and classification of tumor architecture may lead to improved diagnostic accuracy and early detection of ovarian and endometrial cancers, and consequently, reduction of false-positive findings and unnecessary invasive procedures. Undoubtedly, technological development and further improvement of real time 3D ultrasound imaging will contribute to a more objective evaluation of the adnexal tumor morphology and vascularity, which may result in a significant reduction of the morbidity and mortality, from gynecologic malignancy.

REFERENCES

1. Koonings PP, Campbell K, Mishell DR, et al. Relative frequency of primary ovarian neoplasms: A 10-year review. Obstet Gynecol 1989;74(6):921-6.
2. Kinkel K, Hricak H, Lu Y, et al. US characterization of ovarian masses: A meta-analysis. Radiology 2000;217:803-11.
3. Guerriero S, Alcazar JL, Coccia ME, et al. Complex pelvic mass as a target of evaluation of vessel distribution by color Doppler sonography for the diagnosis of adnexal malignancies: Results of a multicenter European study. Journal Ultrasound Med 2002; 21(10):1105-11.
4. Warren BA. The vascular morphology of tumors. In: Peterson HI (Ed). Tumor Blood Circulation: Angiogenesis, vascular morphology and blood flow of experimental human tumors. Boca Raton, Florida: CRC Press 1979;1-47.
5. Coman DR, Sheldon WF. The Significance of Hyperemia Around Tumor Implants. Am J Pathol 1946;22(4):821-31.
6. Algire GH, Chalkley HW, Lagallais FY, et al. Vascular reactions of mice to wounds and to normal and neoplastic transplants. J Natl Cancer Inst 1945;6:73-85.
7. Folkman J, Long DM, Becker FF. Growth and metastasis of tumor in organ culture. Cancer 1963;16:453-67.
8. Folkman J, Cole P, Zimmerman S. Tumor behavior in isolated perfused organs: In vitro growth and metastases of biopsy material in rabbit thyroid and canine intestinal segment. Ann Surg 1966;164:491-502.
9. Folkman J, Merler E, Abernathy C, et al. Isolation of a tumor factor responsible for angiogenesis. J Exp Med 1971;133(2): 275-88.

10. Klagsbrun M, D'Amore PA. Regulators of angiogenesis. Annu Rev Physiol 1991;53:217-39.

11. Folkman J. What is the evidence that tumors are angiogenesis dependent? J Natl Cancer Inst 1990;82(1):4-6.

12. Auerbach R. Angiogenesis-inducing factors: A review. In: Pick E (Ed). Limphokines, London: Academic Press 1981;4:69-88.

13. Rak JW, St Croix BD, Kerbel RS. Consequences of angiogenesis for tumor progression, metastasis and cancer therapy. Anticancer Drugs 1995;6(1):3-18.

14. Plate KH. From angiogenesis to lymphangiogenesis. Nature Med 2001;7(2):151-2.

15. Skobe M, Rockwell P, Goldstein N, et al. Halting angiogenesis suppresses carcinoma cell invasion. Nat Med 1997;3(11):1222-7.

16. Gasparini G, Weidner N, Maluta S, et al. Intratumoral microvessel density and p53 protein: Correlation with metastasis in head-and-neck squamous-cell carcinoma. Int J Cancer 1993; 55(5):739-44.

17. Gasparini G, Weidner N, Bevilacqua P, et al. Tumor microvessel density, p53 expression, tumor size and peritumoral lymphatic vessel invasion are relevant prognostic markers in node-negative breast carcinoma. J Clin Oncol 1994;12(3):454-66.

18. Weidner N. Tumor angiogenesis: Review of current applications in tumor prognostication. Semin Diagn Pathol 1993;10:302-13.

19. Folkman J, Klagsburn M. Angiogenic factors. Science 1987; 235(4787):442-7.

20. Dvorak HF, Brown LF, Detmar M, et al. Vascular permeability factor/vascular endothelial growth factor, microvascular hyperpermeability and angiogenesis. Am J Pathol 1995; 146(5):1029-39.

21. Plate KH, Breier G, Weich HA, et al. Vascular endothelial growth factor is a potential tumor angiogenesis factor in human gliomas in vivo. Nature 1992;359(6398):845-8.

22. Kim KJ, Li B, Winer J, et al. Inhibition of vascular endothelial growth factor-induced angiogenesis suppresses tumor growth in vivo. Nature 1993;362(6423):841-4.

23. Lu JJ, Stanczyk FZ, Zeng W. Expression of VEGF in ovarian epithelial tumors. J Soc Gynecol Invest 2001; 8(1)(Suppl):766.

24. Pugh CW, Ratcliffe PJ. Regulation of angiogenesis by hypoxia: Role of the HIF system. Nat Med 2003;9(6):677-84.

25. Vincent KA, Shyu KG, Luo Y, et al. Angiogenesis is induced in a rabbit model of hindlimb ischemia by naked DNA encoding an HIF-1 alpha/VP16 hybrid transcription factor. Circulation 2000;102(18):2255-61.

26. Samani AA, Yakar S, LeRoith D, et al. The role of the IGF system in cancer growth and metastasis: Overview and recent insights. Endocr Rev 2007;28(1):20-47.

27. Folkman J, Long DM, Becker FF. Growth and metastasis of tumor in organ culture. Cancer 1963;16:453-67.

28. Guilino PM. Extracellular compartments of solid tumors. In: Becker J (Ed). Cancer. New York: Plenum Press 1975:327

29. Jain RK. Determination of tumor blood flow: A review. Cancer Res.988;48:2641-6.

30. Kurjak A, Kupesic S, Breyer B. The assessment of ovarian tumor angiogenesis by three-dimensional power Doppler. In: Kurjak A (Ed). Three-dimensional power Doppler in obstetrics & gynecology. The Parthenon Publishing Group;2000.

31. Jain RK, Ward-Harley K. Tumor blood flow characterization, modifications and role in hyperthermia. Trans Sonics Ultrasonics 1984;31:504-9.

32. Vaupel P, Kallinowski F, Okunieff P. Blood flow oxygen and nutrient supply, and metabolic microenvironment of human tumors: A review. Cancer Res 1989;49(23):6449-65.

33. Dvorak HF, Brown LF, Detmar M, et al. Vascular permeability factor/vascular endothelial growth factor, microvascular hyperpermeability, and angiogenesis. Am J Pathol 1995; 146(5):1029-39.

34. Eliceiri BP, Paul R, Schwartzberg PL, et al. Selective requirement for Src kinases during VEGF-induced angiogenesis and vascular permeability. Mol Cell 1999;4(6):915-24.

35. Fleischer AC. Sonographic depiction of tumor vascularity and flow: From in vivo models to clinical applications. J Ultrasound Med 2000;19:55-61.

36. Hanahan D, Folkman J. Parameters and emerging mechanisms of the angiogenetic switch during tumorigenesis. Cell 1996; 86:353-4.

37. Kurjak A, Kupesic S, Ilijas M, et al. Preoperative diagnosis of primary fallopian tube carcinoma. Gynecol Oncol 1998;68:29-34.

38. Kurjak A, Jukic S, Kupesic S, et al. A combined Doppler and morphopathological study of ovarian tumors. Eur J Obstet Gynecol Reprod Biol 1997;71(2):147-50.

39. Emoto M, Iwasaki H, Mimura K, et al. Differences in the angiogenesis of benign and malignant ovarian tumors, demonstrated by analyses of color Doppler ultrasound, immunohistochemistry and microvessel density. Cancer 1997; 80(5):899-907.

40. Suren A, Osmers R, Kuhn W. 3D Color Power Angio TM imaging: A new method to assess intracervical vascularization in benign and pathological conditions. Ultrasound Obstet Gynecol 1998;2:133-8.

41. Kurjak A, Kupesic S. Three-dimensional ultrasound and power Doppler in assessment of uterine and ovarian angiogenesis: A prospective study. Croat Med J 1999;40(3):413-20.

42. Bourne TH, Campbell S, Steers CV, et al. Transvaginal color flow imaging: A possible new screening technique for ovarian cancer. BMJ 1989;299(6712):1367-70.

43. Kurjak A, Zalud I, Jurkovic D, et al. Transvaginal color Doppler of the assessment of pelvic circulation. Acta Obstet Gynecol Scand 1989;68(2):131-5.

44. Fleisher AC, Rodgers WH, Rao BJ, et al. Assessment of ovarian tumor vascularity with transvaginal color Doppler sonography. J Ultrasound Med 1991;10(10):563-8.

45. Kurjak A, Zalud I, Alfirevic Z. Evaluation of adnexal masses with transvaginal color ultrasound. J Ultrasound Med 1991; 10(6):295-7.

46. Weiner Z, Thaler I, Beck D, et al. Differentiating malignant from benign ovarian tumors with transvaginal color flow imaging. Obstet Gynecol 1992;79(2):159-62.

47. Kurjak A, Schulman H, Sosic A, et al. Transvaginal ultrasound, color flow and Doppler waveform of the postmenopausal adnexal mass. Obstet Gynecol 1992;80(6):917-21.

48. Hamper UM, Sheth S, Abbas FM, et al. Transvaginal color Doppler sonography of adnexal masses: Differences in blood flow impedance in benign and malignant lesions. AJR Am J Roentgenol 1993;160(6):1225-8.

49. Carter J, Saltzman A, Hartenbach E, et al. Flow characteristics in benign and malignant gynecologic tumors using transvaginal color flow Doppler. Obstet Gynecol 1994;83(1):125-30.

50. Hata K, Kata T, Kitao M. Intratumoral peak systolic velocity as a new possible predictor for detection of adnexal malignancy. Am J Obstet Gynecol 1995;172(5):1496-500.

51. Kurjak A, Jukic S, Kupesic S, et al. A combined Doppler and morphopathological study of ovarian tumors. Eur J Obstet Gynecol Reprod Biol 1997;71(2):147-50.

52. Levine D, Feldstein VA, Babcook CJ, et al. Sonography of ovarian masses: Poor sensitivity of resistive index for identifying malignant lesions. AJR Am J Roentgenol 1994;162(6):1355-9.

53. Kurjak A, Kupesic S. Transvaginal color Doppler and pelvic tumor angiogenesis: Lessons learned and future challenges. Ultrasound Obstet Gynecol 1995;6:145-59.

54. Kurjak A, Shalan H, Kupesic S, et al. Transvaginal color Doppler sonography in the assessment of pelvic tumor vascularity. Ultrasound Obstet Gynecol 1993;3:137-54.

55. Brown DL, Frates MC, Laing FC, et al. Ovarian masses: Can benign and malignant lesions be differentiated with color and pulsed Doppler US? Radiology 1994;190(2):333-6.

56. Stein SM, Laifer-Narin S, Johnson MB, et al. Differentiation of benign and malignant adnexal masses: Relative value of gray-scale, color Doppler and spectral Doppler sonography. Am J Roentgenol 1995;164:381-6.

57. Fleischer AC, Cullinan JA, Peery CV, et al. Early detection of ovarian carcinoma with transvaginal color Doppler ultrasonography. Am J Obstet Gynecol 1996;174:101-6.

58. Rubin JM, Bude RO, Carson PL, et al. Power Doppler US: A potentially useful alternative to mean frequency-based color Doppler US. Radiology 1994;190(3):853-6.

59. Rubin JM, Adler RS, Fowlkes JB, et al. Fractional moving blood volume: Estimation with power Doppler US. Radiology 1995;197(1):183-90.

60. Winsberg F. Power Doppler sonography. J Ultrasound Med 1996;15(2):164.

61. Papadimitriou A, Kalogirou D, Antoniou G, et al. Power Doppler ultrasound: A potential useful alternative in diagnosing pelvic pathological conditions. Clin Exp Obstet Gynecol 1996; 23(4):229-32.

62. Burns PN. Harmonic imaging with ultrasound contrast agents. Clin Radiol 1996;1:50-5.

63. Meyerovitz CB, Fleischer AC, Pickens DR, et al. Quantification of tumor vascularity and flow with amplitude color Doppler sonography in an experimental mode: Preliminary results. J Ultrasound Med 1996;15(12):827-33.

64. Fleischer AC, Wojcicki WE, Donnely EF, et al. Quantified color Doppler sonography of tumor vascularity in an animal model. J Ultrasound Med 1999;18(8):547-51.

65. Bonilla-Musoles F, Raga F, Osborne NG. Three-dimensional ultrasound evaluation of ovarian masses. Gynecol Oncol 1995; 59(1):129-35.

66. Merz E. Three-dimensional transvaginal ultrasound in gynecological diagnosis. Ultrasound Obstet Gynecol 1999; 14(2):81-6.

67. Geomini PM, Coppus SF, Kluivers KB, et al. Is three-dimensional ultrasonography of additional value in the assessment of adnexal masses? Gynecol Oncol 2007; 106(1):153-9.

68. Mansour GM, El-Lamie I, El-Sayed H, et al. Adnexal mass vascularity assessed by three-dimensional power Doppler: Does it add to the risk of malignancy index in prediction of ovarian malignancy?: Four hundred-case study. Int J Gynecol Cancer 2009;19(5):867-72.

69. Chase DM, Crade M, Basu T, et al. Preoperative diagnosis of ovarian malignancy: Preliminary results of the use of three-dimensional vascular ultrasound. Int J Gynecol Cancer 2009; 19(3):354-60.

70. Chan L, Lin WM, Uerpairojkit B, et al. Evaluation of adnexal masses using three-dimensional ultrasonographic technology: Preliminary report. J Ultrasound Med 1997;16(5):349-54.

71. Weber G, Merz E, Bahlmann F, et al. Ultrasound assessment of ovarian tumors— comparison between transvaginal 3D technique and conventional 2-dimensional vaginal ultrasonography. Ultraschall Med 1997;18(1):26-30.

72. Riccabona M, Nelson TR, Pretorius DH. Three-dimensional ultrasound: Accuracy of distance and volume measurements. Ultrasound Obstet Gynecol 1996;7(6):429-34.

73. Weber G, Merz E, Bahlman F. Three-dimensional sonography of cystic ovarian tumors. In: Merz E (Ed). 3D ultrasonography and gynecology. Philadelphia: Lippincott Williams & Wilkins; 1998.

74. Kurjak A, Kupesic S. Ovarian lesions assessed by three-dimensional ultrasound and power Doppler. In: Kurjak A, Kupesic S (Eds). Clinical application of 3D sonography. The Parthenon Publishing Group; 2000.

75. Kurjak A, Kupesic S, Jacobs I. Preoperative diagnosis of the primary Fallopian tube carcinoma by three-dimensional static and power Doppler sonography. Ultrasound Obstet Gynecol 2000;15(3):246-51.

76. Kurjak A, Kupesic S, Anic T, et al. Three-dimensional ultrasound and power Doppler improve the diagnosis of ovarian lesions. Gynecol Oncol 2000;76(1):28-32.

77. Downey DB, Fenster A. Vascular imaging with a three-dimensional power Doppler system. Am J Roentgenol 1995; 165(3):665-8.

78. Kurjak A, Kupesic S, Breyer B, et al. The assessment of ovarian tumor angiogenesis: what does three-dimensional power Doppler add? Ultrasound Obstet Gynecol 1998;12(2):136-46.

79. Crade M. Tissue block ultrasound and ovarian cancer-a pictorial presentation of findings. Donald School Journal of Ultrasound in Obstetrics and Gynecology 2009;3(1):41-7.

80. Kurjak A, Kupesic S, Sparac V, et al. Three-dimensional ultrasonographic and power Doppler characterization of ovarian lesions. Ultrasound Obstet Gynecol 2000;16(4):365-71.

81. Breyer B, Kurjak A. Tumor vascularization Doppler measurements and chaos: what to do? Ultrasound Obstet Gynecol 1995;5(3):209-10.

82. Fleischer AC, Pairleitner H. Transvaginal Doppler assesses ovarian flow. Diag Imag 1998;9:47.

83. Fleischer AC, Pairleitner H. 3D transvaginal color Doppler sonography: current and potential applications. Med Imag Int 1999;9:10-13.

84. Pairleitner H, Steiner H, Hasenoehrl G, et al. Three-dimensional power Doppler sonography: Imaging and quantifying blood flow and vascularization. Ultrasound Obstet Gynecol 1999; 14(2):139-43.

85. Kudla M, Alcazar JL. 3D PD imaging of ovarian pathology-Advantages and limitation of the method: How can we standardize the results? Donald School Journal of Ultrasound in Obstetrics and Gynecology 2009;3(1):48-54.

86. Ophir J, Parker KJ. Contrast agents in diagnostic ultrasound. Ultrasound Med Biol 1989;15(4):319-33.

87. Goldberg BB, Merton AD, Forsberg F, et al. Color amplitude imaging: preliminary result using vascular sonographic contrast agents. J Ultrasound Med 1996;15(2):127-34.

88. Kupesic S, Kurjak A. Contrast enhanced three-dimensional power Doppler sonography for the differentiation of adnexal masses. Obstet Gynecol 2000;96(3):452-8.

89. Van Holsbeke C, Daemen A, Yazbek J, et al. Ultrasound methods to distinguish between malignant and benign adnexal masses in the hands of examiners with different levels of experience. Ultrasound Obstet Gynecol 2009;34(4):454-61.

90. Sokalska A, Timmerman D, Testa AC, et al. Diagnostic accuracy of transvaginal ultrasound examination for assigning a specific diagnosis to adnexal masses. Ultrasound Obstet Gynecol 2009; 34(4):462-70.

91. Alcazar JL, Royo P, Pineda L, et al. Which parameters could be useful for predicting malignancy in solid adnexal masses? Donald School Journal of Ultrasound in Obstetrics and Gynecology 2009;3(1):1-5.

92. Kurjak A, Kupesic S, Sparac V, et al. Preoperative evaluation of pelvic tumors by Doppler and three-dimensional sonography. J Ultrasound Med 2001;20(8):829-40.

93. Boehm T, Folkman J, Browder T, et al. Antiangiogenic therapy of experimental cancer does not induce acquired drug resistance. Nature 1997;390(6658):404-7.

94. Holmgren L, O'Reilly MS, Folkman J. Dormancy of micro-metastases: balanced proliferation and apoptosis in the presence of angiogenesis suppression. Nat Med 1995;1(2):149-53.

95. Jain RK. Normalization of tumor vasculature: an emerging concept in antiangiogenic therapy. Science 2005;307(5706):58-62.

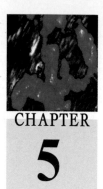

A Kurjak, U Honemeyer, S Kupesic Plavsic

CHAPTER 5

Ovarian Cancer Screening by 3D and 3D Power Doppler Ultrasound

WHY TO SCREEN FOR OVARIAN CANCER?

In developed countries more women die annually from ovarian cancer than from all other gynecologic malignancies combined. For example, in the United States approximately 22,000 new cases are diagnosed each year, and 15,000 of these women will die of the disease,[1] making it the seventh leading cause of cancer-related deaths in women.[2] In 2008, there were 21,650 cases reported, which resulted in the deaths of 15,520 women in the United States.[3]

Symptoms usually do not become apparent until the tumor compresses or invades adjacent structures, ascites develops or metastases become clinically evident. However, studies surveying ovarian cancer patients demonstrate that over 95% of epithelial ovarian cancer (EOC) patients had abdominal complaints for many months before their diagnosis.[4] The fact that the ovaries are free floating within the pelvic cavity and difficult to palpate is an obstacle to early diagnosis, especially in peri- and postmenopausal women, the group with the highest incidence of the disease. Seventy percent of patients are not diagnosed with the disease until the cancer has metastasized beyond the ovaries and is at stage III or IV.[5]

Patients with stage III or IV have a five-year survival rate of only 20 to 30%, compared with the five-year survival of over 90% in patients with stage IA ovarian cancer, when disease is confined to the ovary.[6] Given the burden of suffering associated with the development of ovarian cancer and the clear survival gradient related to the stage of disease at diagnosis,[7] there has always been much enthusiasm for the development of effective screening methods/assays for the early detection of epithelial ovarian cancer.

There are several different types of ovarian cancer depending upon the cell type of origin. Epithelial cell ovarian cancer (EOC) constitutes 90% of ovarian cancers, while gonadalstromal (6% occurrence) and germ cell (4% occurrence) tumors make-up the rest of the incidence of ovarian cancer patients.[8]

The stages (I-IV) of ovarian cancer are determined by the extent of metastasis. Stage I of EOC is confined to the ovaries, while stage II involves other pelvic structures. In stage III, the disease has spread beyond the pelvis into the upper abdominal cavity or into the draining nodal beds. Stage IV is defined as disease outside of the peritoneal cavity and often includes parenchymal liver lesions or malignant pleural effusions. Patients with stage I disease most commonly undergo bilateral oophorectomy, hysterectomy and surgical staging, including peritoneal biopsies, omentectomy, and pelvic and aortic lymph node dissection. In young patients, with localized disease who wish to preserve fertility, only the affected ovary may be removed and hysterectomy may not be required.[9]

Each cancer type typically *metastasizes* to different areas in the body. This phenomenon is called the "seed vs. soil" hypothesis, which was first observed by Stephen Paget in 1889.[10]

The "seed vs. soil" observation applies to ovarian cancer because the most common sites of metastasis are within the peritoneal cavity. This is explained by the fact that mesothelial cells that express "mesothelin" line the walls of the peritoneal cavity, as well as the organs within it. Gubbels, et al. have shown that MUC16 (CA-125), present on the surface of cancer cells, binds readily to mesothelin.[11] The peritoneal dissemination of metastasis is facilitated by the clockwise flow of the peritoneal fluid (PF).

DIFFICULTIES IN OVARIAN CANCER SCREENING

The ability to detect early-stage epithelial ovarian cancer by a simple test has long been desired, yet never achieved. Several aspects of ovarian cancer have led to the frustrations that have been encountered in attempts to screen for the disease.[12]

The time required for localized disease to progress to dissemination depends on the tumor type; therefore, the appropriate interval at which to pursue screening is at this point chosen arbitrarily. Other impediments to screening relate to the low prevalence of ovarian cancer in the general population. Therefore, a screening method should have a specificity of 99.6% to achieve a positive predictive value of 10% (i.e. to limit the number of unnecessary surgical procedures to 10 for each case of cancer detected).[13] Specificity lower than this is unacceptable for general population screening, although it may be acceptable for women with positive family history of breast or ovarian cancer.

As ovarian cancer of epithelial cell origin (EOC) is the most common type, screening methods have to take into account the specific morphological and biochemical characteristics of this tumor group. The majority of EOC cases are sporadic in nature and occur in women with no known predisposing factors. Thus, in the general population, the overall risk of EOC is low (2 to 5%). Only a small percentage (5 to 10%) of EOC patients has a genetic predisposition for the disease. Ninety percent of these patients are carriers of mutated breast cancer 1 (BRCA1) and/or breast cancer 2 (BRCA2) genes, which are also implicated in hereditary breast cancer. These genes normally act as tumor suppressors and regulate cellular proliferation and DNA repair by maintaining chromosomal integrity. Mutations in these genes render the proteins unable to perform their intended functions. The lifetime risk of ovarian cancer for patients with BRCA1 mutations is 20 to 60% and the risk for BRCA2 mutation carriers is 10 to 35%.[1,14]

The normal ovarian surface epithelium (OSE) covers the surface of the ovary. OSE is a monolayered squamous-to-cuboidal epithelium, which functions to shuttle molecules in and out of the peritoneal cavity, as well as participates in the rupture and repair that accompanies every ovulation.[15] The OSE derives from the embryonic celomic epithelial cells, which are a part of the mesoderm. The fallopian tube, uterus and endocervix are derived from the Mullerian duct, which is an invagination of the celomic epithelium. It is hypothesized that OSE cells retain the ability to differentiate into four major histological subtypes, which could explain the distinct histological EOC subtypes. There are four common subtypes of ovarian cancer of epithelial cell origin (EOC), including serous (fallopian tube-like), endometrioid (endometrium-like), mucinous (endocervical-like) and clear cell carcinoma (mesonephros-like).[2,15]

The differentiation of OSE cells from cuboidal epithelial cells to a mesenchymal phenotype that is characteristic of Mullerian duct-derived tissue is called "epithelial-mesenchymal transition (EMT)." The occurrence of EMT serves the purpose to aid cells in movement during embryo tissue generation, tissue regeneration after wounding, and obviously plays a role in the development of cancer.[16] OSE cells normally undergo EMT to heal the wound that forms following ovulation.

OSE cells express low levels of the mucin MUC16 (CA-125). Mullerian-duct derived tissues express high levels of MUC16 (CA-125), as do ovarian tumors.[17] MUC16 (CA-125) over-expression in ovarian tumors is an important marker for progression and regression of EOC.

The expression of markers that are associated with those of Mullerian-duct derived tissue are found in ovarian inclusion cysts. Inclusion cysts are known to be the site of many neoplasms. The OSE lining in inclusion cysts expresses high levels of EOC markers MUC16 (CA-125) and CA19-9. The hypothesis that epithelial ovarian cancer may derive from inclusion cysts is based upon the "incessant ovulation theory," first proposed by Fathalla in 1971.[18]

Higher ovulatory activity is associated with an increased accumulation of inclusion cysts and invaginations of the OSE, which provide a hospitable environment for tumor cell growth.[19]

This theory is supported by epidemiological data demonstrating that women who have been on oral contraceptives or who have been pregnant and/or breastfeeding, have a decreased risk of ovarian cancer.

High gonadotropin levels typical for ovulation and menopause and known to induce changes of OSE, and "oxidants," causing DNA-alterations in the OSE at the site of ovulation, lay the foundations for two more hypotheses regarding the origin of OEC – origin, however, both are linked to the incessant ovulation theory.[19,20]

Dubeau in 1999 first proposed the hypothesis that the fimbrae of the fallopian tubes, which are in close contact with the surface of the ovary during oocyte collection, and sometimes adhere to the surface of the ovary due to inflammation, are a prime site for the development of metaplasia.[21]

ATTEMPTS TO SCREEN—SOME LESSONS LEARNED

During the last 15 years, large prospective studies of screening for ovarian cancer have been performed.[22] Two distinct strategies have emerged, one based on ultrasound as the primary test and the other involving the serum tumor marker CA-125 screening with ultrasound as the secondary test (multimodal screening). Tables 5.1 and 5.2 summarize the prospective ovarian cancer screening studies in general population.[23-38] If we exclude those which used transabdominal ultrasound, an abandoned screening strategy due to unacceptably high rate of false positive results, several important lessons could be learned.

As seen on the Tables 5.1 and 5.2, the data suggest that sequential multimodal screening has greater specificity and positive predictive value compared to strategies based on transvaginal ultrasound alone. For each case of ovarian cancer, five women underwent surgery in the multimodal studies compared to 24 women in the studies using ultrasound alone. However, transvaginal ultrasound as a first line test may offer higher sensitivity for early stage disease given that 23/37 (62.2%) cancers detected using ultrasound alone were stage I, compared to 8/19 (42.1%) cancers detected by the multimodal strategy. An ultrasound-based strategy may have a greater impact on ovarian cancer mortality, albeit at higher price in the terms of surgical intervention for false positive results.

Tables 5.1 and 5.2 address the most relevant studies published until 2003. Our own ovarian cancer screening trial, which started in January 2001, is described at the end of this chapter. The developments that followed since 2003 are best summarized in reference to the screening tests, target populations and newly published trials. The possible role of 3D ultrasound technology, especially 3D power Doppler imaging in early and accurate detection of ovarian malignancy will be discussed as well.

SCREENING TESTS

Screening for ovarian cancer is based on strategies using serum tumor markers or transvaginal ultrasound images of the ovaries or a combination of both.

Serum Tumor Markers

In epithelial ovarian cancer, a number of tumor markers have been identified. Serum CA-125 continues to be the tumor marker most extensively used in ovarian cancer screening.[39] CA-125 itself is a repeating peptide epitope on the large molecular weight mucin, MUC16.[40]

This mucin is expressed at low levels by normal ovarian surface epithelium and is over-expressed by EOC tumor cells.[41]

Tumor cells secrete mucin (MUC16) into the peritoneal fluid (PF) and from the abdominal cavity this mucin leaks into the blood stream and can then be detected via the CA-125 serum assay.

Although CA-125 is elevated (> 35 U/ml) in more than 80% of patients with epithelial ovarian cancer, it is only in 25% sensitive for early stage disease.[42] Indeed, its value as an initial screening tool is limited, since picking up stage III disease at an earlier time may not alter the outcome. To improve the efficacy of CA-125 as a screening tool, an algorithm incorporating age, rate of change of CA-125 and absolute levels to calculate an individual's risk of ovarian cancer has been described.[43] This increases the sensitivity of CA-125 in comparison with a single cutoff value, because women with normal, but rising levels are identified as being at increased-risk. This approach was an integral part of the multimodal screening strategy adopted in the St Bartholomew's Hospital randomized control trial, published in the year 2000.[44]

Because CA-125 levels are elevated in less than half of the cases in early-stage ovarian cancers, underscoring the lack of sensitivity to diagnose curable disease, CA-125 appears not suitable to be used as a screening test, but mainly as a measure of disease progression, regression and the predictor of recurrence during treatment for EOC.

Another limitation of serum CA-125 represents that it is not specific for ovarian carcinoma because it can be elevated in many benign conditions, such as endometriosis, uterine fibroids, pelvic inflammatory disease, ascites or pleural effusion.[45] It is now known that the CA-125 antigen carries two major antigenic domains classified as A (the domain binding monoclonal antibody OC-125) and B (the domain binding monoclonal antibody M11). New generation assays, combining monoclonal antibodies to the two distinct regions of the molecule, have been shown to have improved specificity for the detection of early ovarian cancer.[46]

Lysophosphatidic acid (LPA), a bioactive phospholipide with mitogenic and growth factor-like activities,[47] is a tumor marker, which was considered promising in ovarian cancer screening. In a small pilot series plasma LPA levels were elevated in 9 out of 10 patients with stage I ovarian cancer, 24 of 24 patients with stage II, III and IV ovarian cancer and all 14 patients with recurrent ovarian cancer.[48]

Ovarian Cancer Screening by 3D and 3D Power Doppler Ultrasound

TABLE 5.1: Prospective ovarian cancer screening studies using ultrasound as the primary test in the general population

Study	Inclusion criteria	Screening strategy	No. screened	No. of invasive epithelial ovarian cancers detected[a]	No. of positive screens	No. of positive screens/cancer detected[b]
ULTRASOUND (US) APPROACH						
GRAY SCALE US (LEVEL 1 SCREEN), than repeat GRAY SCALE US (LEVEL 2 SCREEN)						
van Nagell et al.[7]	Age > 50 years and postmenopausal or > 30 with positive family history	TVS annual screens mean 4 screens/women	14469	11 (6) 5 stage I	180	16,4
Hayashi et al.[8]	Age > 50 years	TVS	23451	3 (3)	258	c
Tabor et al.[9]	Aged 46-65 years	TVS	435	0	9	–
Campbell et al.[10]	Age > 45 years or with positive family history (4%)	TAS 3 screens at 18 monthly intervals	5479	2 (3) 2 stage I	326	163
Goswamy et al.[11]	Age 39-78 years postmenopausal	TAS	1084	1 1 stage I	not precised	–
GRAY SCALE US and CDI (LEVEL 1 SCREEN)						
Vuento et al.[12]	Aged 56-61 years	TVS and CDI	1364	(1)	5	–
Kurjak et al.[13]	Aged 40-71 years	TVS and CDI	5013	4 4 stage I	38	9,5
Schulman et al.[14]	Age > 40 years or > 30 with positive family history	TVS and CDI	2117	1	18	18
GRAY SCALE US (LEVEL 1 SCREEN) and other tests (LEVEL 2 SCREEN)						
Sato et al.[15]	Age > 30 years	TVS then tumor markers if TVS +, CT and MRI if all previous +	51550	16 (6) 12 stage I	324	20,3
Parkes et al.[16]	Aged 50-64 years	TVS then CDI if TVS +	2953	1 1 stage I	15	15
Holbert et al.[17]	Postmenopausal aged 30-89 years	TVS then CA-125 if TVS +	478	1 1 stage I	33[d]	–
TOTAL[e]				37 (16) 23 stage I	880	23,8

TAS = transabdominal ultrasound; TVS = transvaginal ultrasound; CDI = Color Doppler imaging
[a]The borderline/granulosa tumors detected are shown in parentheses.
[b]Only invasive epithelial ovarian cancers included.
[c]Only 95 women consented to surgery and there are no follow-up details on the remaining.
[d]Only 11 of these women underwent surgery.
[e]Studies used TAS are excluded.

TABLE 5.2: Prospective ovarian cancer screening studies using serum CA-125 as the primary test in the general population

Study	Inclusion criteria	Screening strategy	No. screened	No. of invasive epithelial ovarian cancers detected[a]	No. of positive screens	No. of positive screens/cancer detected
CA-125 ONLY						
Einhorn et al.[18]	Age > 40 years	Serum CA-125	5550	6 2 stage I	175	29,2
MULTIMODAL APPROACH						
CA-125 (LEVEL 1 SCREEN), then GRAY SCALE US (LEVEL 2 SCREEN)						
Jacobs et al.[19]	Age > 45 years Postmenopausal	RCT Serum CA-125 TAS/TVS, if CA-125 3 annual screens	10958	6 3 stage I	29	4,8
Jacobs et al.[20]	Age > 45 years Postmenopausal	Serum CA-125 TAS, if CA-125	22000	11 4 stage I	41	3,7
Adonakis et al.[21]	Age > 45 years	Serum CA-125 TVS, if CA-125	2000	1 (1) 1 stage I	15	15
Grover et al.[22]	Age > 40 years or with positive family history (3%)	Serum CA-125 TAS/TVS, if CA-125 3 screens	2550	1	16	16
TOTAL[a]				19 (1) 8 stage I	101	5,3

RCT = randomized controlled trial
[a]Only multimodal approach studies included.

Among a subset of patients with ovarian cancer, only 28 out of 47 had elevated CA-125 levels, including 2 of 9 patients with stage I disease. Larger studies on the use of LPA in primary screening in combination with other procedures, such as transvaginal ultrasound are required.[49]

Moore, et al. reported on the use of multiple novel tumor biomarkers for the detection of ovarian carcinoma in patients with a pelvic mass. Serum and urine samples were obtained preoperatively from women undergoing surgery for an adnexal mass. The samples were analyzed for the levels of CA-125, SMRP, HE4, CA72-4, activin, inhibin, osteopontin, epidermal growth factor (EGFR) and ERBB2 (Her2) were compared with the final pathology results. Two hundred and fifty-nine patients with adnexal masses were enrolled. Of these, 233 patients were eligible for analysis: 67 invasive epithelial ovarian cancers and 166 benign ovarian tumors. In the analysis, HE4 had the highest sensitivity for detecting ovarian cancer as a single tumor marker, especially for stage I disease.

Combined CA-125 and HE4 were a more accurate predictor of malignancy than either alone.[50]

Recently, Anderson et al. published a nested case-control study, assessing the *lead time* of several potential ovarian cancer biomarkers: CA-125, human epididymis protein 4 (HE4), mesothelin, B7-H4, decoy receptor 3 (DcR3) and spondin-2. Except for CA-125, their behavior in the prediagnostic period had not been evaluated. As per their results, smoothed mean concentrations of CA-125, HE4 and mesothelin (but not of B7-H4, DcR3 and spondin-2) began to increase (visually) in cancer patients relative to control subjects approximately three years before diagnosis, but reached detectable elevations only within the final year before the diagnosis of ovarian malignancy. The authors concluded that serum concentrations of CA-125, HE4 and mesothelin may provide the evidence of ovarian cancer three years before clinical diagnosis, but the likely lead time associated with these markers appears to be less than one year.[51]

Transvaginal Ultrasound

Transvaginal ultrasound is used in the most screening strategies either as the sole screening modality or as a secondary test after primary screening with serum CA-125 (multimodal screening). As data regarding outcome accumulate with long-term follow-up of the participants of the early screening trials, it has been possible to define further risk of ovarian cancer associated with various ultrasound findings.

Particular results of the largest ultrasound-based ovarian cancer screening project from the University of Kentucky might have a definitive impact on the design of the future of ovarian cancer screening in general population.[52] Van Nagell, et al. established that unilocular ovarian cysts less than 10 cm in diameter, found in 256 out of 7705 (3.3%) asymptomatic women aged more than 50 years, were associated with a minimal risk for ovarian cancer because there were no cases of ovarian carcinoma during a five-year follow-up period.[53] In contrast, 7 out of the 250 women in the same study with complex cystic ovarian tumors, including wall abnormalities or solid areas, had ovarian carcinoma suggesting that these morphologic appearances are associated with a significant risk for ovarian malignancy.

In many screening algorithms, volume cut-offs are used in addition to morphology characteristics to identify women for intensive surveillance. Based on the data of 58,673 observations of ovarian volume, the authors concluded that the upper limit of normality for ovarian volume is 20 cm^3 in premenopausal women and 10 cm^3 in postmenopausal women.[54] Such data are very valuable in determining optimal strategies for operative intervention.

More recently, Kurman, et al. suggested another approach for the early detection of ovarian cancer focusing on low volume rather than low stage of the disease, in order to intercept the more aggressive tumors like high-grade serous carcinoma, malignant mixed mesodermal tumors (carcinosarcomas) and undifferentiated carcinomas, which account for the majority of ovarian cancers. According to this research group, a more rational approach for early detection of ovarian cancer is to focus on a low-ovarian-volume neoplasms, rather than low stage of disease.[55]

Postmenopausal women from general population with an elevated serum CA-125 level but normal ovarian morphology on ultrasound were found to have a cumulative risk of ovarian cancer during a median follow-up of 6.8 years, of 0.15%, which was similar to 0.22% of the entire population of 22,000 women.[56] In contrast, those with an elevated serum CA-125 level and abnormal ovarian morphology on ultrasound had a significantly increased cumulative risk of 24%. Using ovarian morphology to interpret pelvic ultrasound images has been shown to increase the sensitivity, and using a morphology, scoring index for complex ovarian tumors may improve the positive predictive value of a multimodal screening strategy.[57]

In a recent Korean study, 202 patients undergoing surgery for ovarian tumors were reviewed retrospectively from September 2000 to July 2006. In all patients, the morphology index (MI) score and serum CA-125 level were measured preoperatively.

The association of the final pathologic diagnosis with the MI score and serum CA-125 level was evaluated. The sonographic MI system was an accurate and simple method to differentiate a malignant from a benign ovarian tumor. The accuracy of the sonographic MI system improved when the serum CA-125 level was considered and ovarian teratomas were excluded.[58]

Ovarian cancer screening in general population in the United Kingdom (UKCTOCS) during the period between 2001 and 2005 has included 202,638 postmenopausal women aged 50-74 years.

Control group consisted of 101,359 women who were randomly assigned to no treatment. Fifty thousand six hundred and forty (50,640) women had annual CA-125 screening (using a risk of ovarian cancer algorithm) with transvaginal ultrasound scan as a second-line test (multimodal screening [MMS]). Fifty thousand six hundred and thirty-nine (50,639) women underwent annual screening with transvaginal ultrasound (USS) alone in a 2:1:1 ratio using a computer generated random number algorithm. In the interpretation of the results the authors considered the sensitivity of the MMS and USS screening strategies as encouraging. Specificity was higher in the MMS than in the USS group, resulting in lower rates of repeat testing and surgery. This in part reflects the high prevalence of benign adnexal abnormalities and more frequent detection of borderline tumors in the USS group. The prevalence screen could establish that the screening strategies are feasible. The results of ongoing screening are awaited so that the effect of screening on mortality can be determined.[59]

The first prospective randomized report of a multimodal ovarian cancer screening originates from a Japanese research group: Asymptomatic postmenopausal women were randomly assigned between 1985 and 1999 to either an intervention group (n = 41.688) or a control group (n = 40,799) in a ratio of 1:1, with follow-up of mean 9.2 years, in Shizuoka district, Japan. The original intention was to offer women in the intervention group annual screens by gynecological examination (sequential pelvic ultrasound [US] and serum CA-125 test). Women with abnormal US findings and/or elevated CA-125 values were referred for surgical investigation by a gynecological oncologist. The proportion of stage I ovarian cancer was higher in the screened group (63%) than in the control group (38%), which did not reach statistical significance (P = 0.2285).[60]

TARGET POPULATIONS

Participants for ovarian cancer screening trials are recruited from general and high-risk populations on the basis of the risk factors for the disease.

GENERAL POPULATION

Age and Menopausal Status

The majority of ovarian cancers occur in the general population, and postmenopausal patients. According to the International Federation of Gynecology and Obstetrics (FIGO) report,[6] ovarian cancer was most common among women during early postmenopause, at average age of 54 years. Law et al[61] used national statistics to determine the number of years of life lost through deaths from a particular cancer at each age. They concluded that screening would be the most effective (i.e. associated with the largest number of years of life saved per person screened), if done five years before the loss of life peak. Since, in ovarian cancer, the peak occurs during the age range from 55 years to 59 years, the authors have proposed that screening should start at 50 years.

High-risk Population

Family History and/or Genetic Predisposition

Approximately 5 to 10% of ovarian cancers are inherited. Mutations in BRCA1 and BRCA2 genes account for about 75% of families with a history of highly penetrant dominantly inherited breast or ovarian cancer. Recent estimates of the lifetime risk for ovarian cancer in women harboring a BRCA1 mutation are 40 to 60%.[62] Various studies have put forward schemes for stratifying women into different categories of risk for breast and ovarian cancer by virtue of a family history, genetic predisposition, or both. Pharoah et al[63] reviewed the relevance of family history in defining the target population for familial ovarian cancer screening and proposed the adoption of a unified management strategy based on eligibility criteria from UK National Familial Ovarian Cancer Screening Study (Table 5.3). A survey by Vasen et al.[64] of the European Familial Breast Cancer Collaborative Group suggested that the following high-risk populations were offered ovarian cancer screening: BRCA1 and BRCA2 mutation carriers; members of breast/ovarian cancer families and in some centers, members of "breast cancer only" families with an early onset of breast cancer.

TABLE 5.3: Eligibility criteria for the UKCCCR National Familial Ovarian Cancer Screening Study[39]

An eligible woman must be over 25 years of age and a first degree relative of an affected member of an "at risk" family. At risk families are defined by the following criteria:

1. Two or more first degree relatives[a] with ovarian cancer.

2. One first degree relative with ovarian cancer and one first degree relative with breast cancer diagnosed under 50 years of age.

3. One first degree relative with ovarian cancer and two first or second degree relatives[b] with breast cancer diagnosed under 60 years of age.

4. An affected individual with one of the known ovarian cancer predisposing genes.

5. Three first degree relatives with colorectal cancer with at least one diagnosed before the age of 50 years and at least one first degree relative with ovarian cancer.

[a] A first degree female relative is mother, sister or daughter.
[b] A second degree female relative is grandmother, grand-daughter, aunt or niece.

OVARIAN CANCER SCREENING TRIALS

Clinical trials of ovarian cancer screening have involved strategies using ultrasound alone and a multimodal approach with CA-125 as a primary test and ultrasound as a secondary test. Prospective studies have involved both the general and high-risk populations.

General Population

Ultrasound Screening

In the evaluation of data from the 2000 University of Kentucky trial, the results of annual transvaginal ultrasound screening performed on 14,469 asymptomatic women aged 50 years or more and women aged 25 years or more with a family history of ovarian cancer were reported.[23] Hundred and eighty patients with persisting transvaginal abnormalities were subjected to a surgical intervention. Seventeen primary ovarian cancers were detected of which 11 were epithelial ovarian cancers (EOC), three were granulosa cell tumors and three were borderline tumors. Of the EOC, 5 were stage I, 3 were stage II and 3 were stage III. In this study, transvaginal ultrasound (TV US) as a screening modality was associated with sensitivity of 81%, specificity of 98.9%, positive predictive value of 9.4% and negative predictive value of 99.97% for the detection of all primary ovarian cancers. The survival of patients with EOC in the annually screened population was 92.9% at 2 years and 83.6% at 5 years.

What is encouraging about these results is that annual TV US screening appeared to achieve the primary goal of earlier detection of the disease, which translates into a reduction in mortality associated with ovarian carcinoma. On the other hand, data from this study suggested that in certain cases, length of time required for ovarian cancer to progress from a localized sonographically detectable tumor to widespread regional disease is quite short. In four patients in the false-negative group, disease progression from sonographically normal ovaries to stage II or III ovarian cancer occurred in less than 12 months. Authors stated that for future screening algorithms, a screening interval of six months should be taken into consideration. In 2000, the Japanese ovarian cancer screening trial was published: 51,550 women aged 30 years or more attending for annual cervical screening underwent TV US screening for ovarian cancer.[31] Three hundred twenty four women with masses of more than 60 mm in diameter or with a mixed echo pattern or persistently raised tumor markers underwent laparotomy. Twenty two primary ovarian tumors and two metastatic tumors were detected. Of the 22 primary tumors, 16 were EOCs, four were borderline malignancies and two were germ cell tumors. 11 (68.7%) of the EOCs were stage I, with tumor markers positive in 5 (45.4%) of the 11 cases. The positive predictive value of the screening strategy was 4.9%; in other words 20 operations were undertaken for each detected case of ovarian cancer. As no follow-up data were reported on any of the trial participants, it is difficult to assess the sensitivity of the screening strategy. Before the onset of the screening, the authors noted that only 29.7% out of 35 cancers diagnosed in the department, were stage I, while after the trial was initiated, 58.8% of 85 ovarian cancers treated were stage I.

Multimodal Screening

One of the most active groups in screening for ovarian malignancy lead by Jacobs, reported the results of the first completed randomized trial of ovarian cancer screening.[35] This study, which was published in 1999, randomized asymptomatic postmenopausal women aged 45 years or older to no screening (n = 10.977) or to annual multimodal screening for 3 years (n = 10.958). In the screening group, 29 women with elevated CA-125 values and abnormal ultrasound findings were referred for surgical investigation. All six ovarian cancers detected were EOCs, three were stage I and three were stage III. Using this algorithm, the authors found a high positive predictive value of 20.7% and were encouraged by a longer median survival (72.9 months) in patients with ovarian cancer in the screened group when compared to the control group (41.8 months). The mortality rates, however, were not significantly different between the groups. The authors concluded that the results do not justify general population ovarian cancer screening but do support the need for a larger randomized trial that is powered to assess the impact of screening on mortality.

The Kentucky Ovarian Cancer screening trial confirmed that screening can detect ovarian cancer at an earlier stage than it is normally detected without screening. It also established the fact that the combination of serum CA-125 with transvaginal sonography (TVS) is probably more effective than TVS alone. The study design suggested that if the ultrasound was abnormal, a repeated TVS in four weeks was performed. If the repeated ultrasound was abnormal, CA-125 blood test and morphology indexing (MI) of the ovarian mass were performed. To improve accuracy in differentiating a benign ovarian tumor from ovarian cancer, MI was used to identify certain patterns that are associated with benign or noncancerous tumors. If the patient's CA-125 was normal and the morphology index indicated a benign tumor, the patient was not considered for surgery and was followed periodically with ultrasound.[65]

Both the Kentucky trial and the trial from the United Kingdom (UKCTOCS) detected ovarian cancer at a significantly earlier stage than when women did not have screening. The University of Kentucky Ovarian Cancer Screening Program is an ongoing trial, results from this trial were published in 2007 in the journal Cancer. Of women whose ovarian cancer was detected by screening, 82% had Stage I or II disease compared to 30% of women in the unscreened population. Without screening, about 70% of women presented with stage III or IV disease. This is important to note because only 30% of women with advanced ovarian cancer will be alive in five years after the treatment and two-thirds of them will still have disease that cannot be cured. The ultimate cure rate for a woman with advanced ovarian cancer is only about 10%. Therefore, something needs to be done to increase early detection.

High-risk Population

For women with a known germ line BRCA1, 2 mutation or with a family history suggesting a significant possibility of a genetic predisposition to ovarian cancer, the appropriate screening strategy remains undefined. In several studies, most authors advocate screening using TVUS and serum CA-125 in patients who elect to delay or decline prophylactic oophorectomy. However, there is no consensus concerning the appropriate interval for screening.

Karlan et al, reported the results of an ovarian cancer screening program launched in 1991, involving 1,261 women aged over 35 years with a family history of ovarian, breast, colon or endometrial carcinoma or a personal history of breast cancer.[66] Screening with TVUS, color Doppler imaging and CA-125 was initially performed biannually until 1995 and annually thereafter. Two tumors of low malignant potential, at stage one, EOC and seven cases of primary peritoneal serous papillary carcinoma were diagnosed. Ultrasound abnormalities triggered surgical exploration in all the three cases of the ovarian disease. In two out of seven cases, elevated levels of CA-125 were the harbinger of peritoneal serous papillary carcinoma, in two patients abnormal ultrasound findings prompted diagnosis and three developed interval cancers 5, 6 and 16 months after screening. At least three of the patients with primary peritoneal cancer carried mutations of the BRCA1 gene.

Multifocal peritoneal serous papillary carcinoma may be a phenotypic variant of familial ovarian cancer and screening strategies for these women cannot rely on ultrasound and CA-125 testing to detect an early disease.

OVARIAN CANCER—THE ROLE OF 3D ULTRASOUND AND 3D POWER DOPPLER IMAGING

Improvements in ultrasound technology, such as 3D volume acquisition and 3D power Doppler imaging may have clinical utility in a more reliable identification of an abnormal ovarian vascularity and vessels architecture. 3D volume acquisition allows for the careful evaluation of the internal surfaces of cyst walls for excrescences otherwise not appreciated by 2D ultrasound.[67,68] While the addition of 3D power Doppler provides a new tool for measuring the quality of ovarian tumor angiogenesis,[69] improving accurate diagnosis of ovarian malignancies,[70] its clinical value for the early detection of ovarian carcinoma has yet to be determined.

What Does 3D Ultrasound Add?

In the pioneer work, Bonilla-Musoles et al. [67] tried to determine whether 3D ultrasound may offer advantages over 2D ultrasound as a screening tool for the evaluation of ovarian lesions. Seventy-six women with ovarian masses first detected with 2D ultrasound were then evaluated with 3D ultrasound. The 3D sonographic criteria, used for diagnosing ovarian malignancy were based on the morphologic scoring system for 2D transvaginal ultrasound examinations proposed by different authors.[71-74] A score greater than 4 was suggestive of a malignant ovarian mass.[74] The images were dissected in the three perpendicular planes and the areas indicative of malignancy, as suggested by 2D ultrasonography, were determined to be either negative or positive and confirmatory. Five lesions observed on 2D ultrasound were suspected to be malignant. 3D sonography identified four of these lesions as malignant. The remaining one suspected to be malignant on 2D ultrasound was diagnosed as endometriosis with 3D sonography. One additional ovarian carcinoma was diagnosed by 3D scanning. Two of the malignant lesions were FIGO stage IA. The other tumors were FIGO stages IC, IIC, and IIIB, respectively. Authors stated that observation of papillary projections (especially those less than 3 mm), characteristics of cystic walls, and the extent of capsular infiltration was superior with 3D ultrasound in comparison to conventional 2D sonographic measurements, as was the calculation of the ovarian tumor volume. They also pointed out that eventually 3D ultrasound imaging will allow diagnosis of ovarian malignancy at an earlier stage than it is possible with currently established diagnostic techniques.

Advantages of 3D Power Doppler Imaging

There are two potential advantages of this new imaging modality: more accurate visualization of the ovarian tumor neovascularization and more effective detection of stage I disease.

More Accurate Visualization of Ovarian Tumor Neovascularization

In order to determine whether three-dimensional power Doppler can improve the ability to differentiate benign from malignant ovarian masses, Kurjak et al[75] performed transvaginal color Doppler and 3D power Doppler analysis on 120 patients with ovarian lesions. As a result, in each of 11 ovarian malignancies, preoperative diagnosis by 3D power Doppler was confirmed by histopathology. Transvaginal color Doppler missed one case of serous cystadenocarcinoma, while three benign lesions (dermoid cyst, ovarian fibroma and ovarian cystadenofibroma) where considered false positive. In a case of cystadenofibroma, 3D power Doppler findings were falsely positive. Authors emphasized that irregular and randomly dispersed vessels with complex branching, depicted by 3D power Doppler imaging, were indicative for ovarian malignancy. Such qualitative analysis of the tumor vascularity architecture had

a sensitivity, specificity and positive predictive value (PPV) of 100, 99.08 and 91.67% in the detection of ovarian malignancy, respectively. In a study published by Cohen et al,[76] 71 women with a known complex pelvic mass were referred for a preoperative ultrasound evaluation with both two-dimensional grayscale and 3D power Doppler ultrasound. All the women underwent surgical exploration and 14 had ovarian cancer. Two-dimensional gray scale ultrasound identified 40 masses as suspicious for cancer, including all 14 malignancies, yielding a sensitivity, specificity and PPV of 100, 54 and 35% respectively. However, evaluation with 3D power Doppler identified only 28 cases as suspicious, including all cancers, resulting in a sensitivity, specificity and PPV of 100, 75 and 50%, respectively. Even though all malignancies were correctly identified by both 2D and 3D imaging, the specificity was significantly improved with the addition of 3D power Doppler. This improved diagnostic accuracy may promote improved patient care by separating complex benign masses from ovarian cancer, and by facilitating the appropriate and timely physician's referral.

Despite the inability of currently available screening algorithms to achieve the desired positive predictive value (PPV) of 10, there may be an advantage in producing a stage migration to lower stages at the time of diagnosis, thereby resulting in improved survival. Equally important recent studies have demonstrated that women who have their initial surgery performed by gynecologic oncologists and women who have their surgeries at centers experienced in the treatment of ovarian cancer have higher survival rates. A cost-effectiveness analysis conducted by Bristow et al. revealed that the strategy of expert center referral had an overall cost per patient of $50.652 and had an effectiveness of 5.12 quality-adjusted life years (QALYs). The strategy of referral to a less experienced center carried an overall cost of $39,957 and had an effectiveness of 2.33 QALYs. The expert center strategy was associated with an additional 2.78 QALYs at an incremental cost of $10,695 but was more cost-effective, with a cost-effective ratio of $9,893 per QALY compared with $17,149 per QALY for the less experienced center referral strategy.[77]

Kupesic and Kurjak reported on the use of contrast-enhanced, 3D power Doppler ultrasound in the differentiation of benign and malignant adnexal lesions.[78] A total of 45 patients with complex adnexal lesions of uncertain malignancy at transvaginal B mode and/or color Doppler ultrasound were prospectively evaluated with 3D power Doppler before and after the injection of the contrast agent. There were 12 cases of ovarian malignancy and 33 benign adnexal lesions. Of 12 ovarian cancers, seven (58.3%) showed vascular distribution suggestive of malignancy at nonenhanced 3D power Doppler imaging. After injection of the contrast agent, a penetrating vascular pattern and/or a mixed penetrating and peripheral pattern were detected in all the cases of ovarian malignancy. One cystadeno-fibroma demonstrated penetrating vessels at initial scan, whereas two benign lesions (fibroma and cystadenofibroma) were misdiagnosed as malignant with contrast-enhanced 3D power Doppler. The use of a contrast agent with 3D power Doppler showed diagnostic efficiency (95.6%) that was superior to that of nonenhanced 3D power Doppler ultrasound. The authors concluded that contrast-enhanced 3D power Doppler imaging might more precisely discriminate benign from malignant complex adnexal masses.

Methods for "vascular sampling" by 3D power Doppler angiography in solid and cystic-solid adnexal masses were described by Alcazar and Prka in 2009, in a study which analyzed the difference in reproducibility of 3D-PD vascular sampling between manual and 5 cm sphere sampling. 3D power Doppler angiography has been proposed as a method of predicting malignancy in adnexal masses. This new technique allows the objective assessment of tumor vascularization by means of power Doppler signals. The rationale of the technique is based on the fact that malignant ovarian tumors have a higher microvascular density than do benign tumors. Vascularity Index (VI) is thought to reflect vascular density, flow index (FI) is thought to reflect blood flow in those vessels.[79]

"Vascular Sampling" – a term created by Alcazar – is based on the manual outlining of a solid tumor area using the VOCAL software (GE Medical Systems) to measure the tumor neovascularization. Both manual and 5 cm sphere sampling by 3D-PD angiography data sets were proved to be reproducible.[80]

As previously stated, ultrasound screening may be more effective when a morphology indexing system is used. This may be of value, especially for less experienced sonographers. Ameye et al. conducted a multicenter study with 1,573 patients forming four subgroups of adnexal masses to improve pattern recognition: 1 unilocular cyst, 2 multilocular cyst, 3 tumor with at least one solid component but no papillation and 4 tumor with papillation. In each subgroup, the associated likelihood of malignancy was calculated, using all the possible combinations of the variables ranging from demographic characteristics, grayscale findings, blood flow indices, tumor marker CA-125, family history of breast or/and ovarian cancer, to color score (no flow, minimal flow, moderate, strong flow). The authors concluded that the subgroup system with likelihood calculation may improve the characterization of ovarian tumors by nonexperts in gynecological sonography.[81]

Detection of Stage I Disease

Preliminary results of Zagreb group showed that 3D power Doppler ultrasound can enhance and facilitate morphological and functional evaluation of an early stage ovarian cancer.[82] A five-year retrospective analysis was performed on the data from 43 referred patients with suspected stage I ovarian cancer subsequently confirmed by histopathologist. All the patients were preoperatively evaluated by four complementary sonographic methods: 2D transvaginal grayscale, 2D transvaginal color Doppler, 3D ultrasound and 3D power Doppler, during the week prior to surgery. Our results clearly demonstrated the significant impact of 3D power Doppler imaging on the accurate detection of stage I ovarian cancer. By using a combined 3D morphology and vascular score indexing, the diagnostic accuracy of preoperative sonographic assessment has reached 97.7% (Table 5.4). These findings justify the implementation of 3D ultrasound with power Doppler facilities in ovarian cancer screening programs, especially as a secondary screening tool.

ZAGREB OVARIAN CANCER SCREENING TRIAL

Following the first attempt to screen for ovarian cancer by transvaginal color Doppler ultrasound[29] Zagreb group has initiated ovarian cancer screening trial using 2D transvaginal US, 2D transvaginal color Doppler, 3D US and 3D power Doppler ultrasound.

Subjects and Methods

During a five-year period, approximately 10,000 asymptomatic postmenopausal women with a positive family history of ovarian and/or breast cancer in at least one primary or secondary relative were offered to participate in the trial. The screening algorithm is illustrated in Figure 5.1.

Primary screening included annual transvaginal ultrasound (TV US) and transvaginal color Doppler (TV CD) examination/scoring according to the existing sonographic and color Doppler criteria.[83] Women with an abnormal first level screen underwent a repeat TV US and TV CD sonogram depending on morphologic appearance: In the case of simple ovarian cyst after 4-6 weeks, while if complex ovarian cyst persisted, within two weeks. In patients with a persistently abnormal screen, secondary

TABLE 5.4: Diagnostic accuracy of four different techniques (2D transvaginal US, 2D transvaginal color Doppler, 3D US, and 3D power Doppler) in preoperative sonographic assessment of 43 patients with suspected stage I ovarian cancer[53]

Technique	Preoperatively	
	No. of detected cancers (%)	No. of missed cancers (%)
2D US	30 (69,8)	13 (30,2)
Combined 2D US and Doppler score	37 (86,0)	6 (14,0)
3D US	32 (74,4)	11 (25,6)
3D PD US	41 (95,3)	2 (4,7)
Combined 3D US and Doppler score	42 (97,7)	1 (2,3)

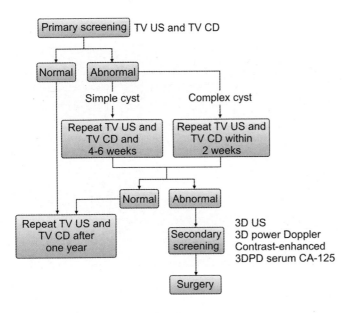

FIGURE 5.1: Screening algorithm of the Zagreb ovarian cancer screening trial.

screening will be considered necessary, including 3D, 3D power Doppler and contrast-enhanced 3D power Doppler ultrasound evaluation, with a serum CA-125 determination. For an examination/scoring of the 3D US data, previously established 3D sonographic and power Doppler criteria were used.[83] In the case of an abnormal second level screen, surgical removal of the tumor and pathological examination were performed.

Illustrative Case No. 1—More Accurate Diagnosis of Ovarian Cancer

In an asymptomatic, 51-year-old postmenopausal patient, complex ovarian tumor suspicious of an early stage ovarian cancer was detected. Family history was positive, because her aunt and uncle (mother's brother) died from colorectal cancer. In the first step, transvaginal gray scale ultrasound

was performed, which revealed a complex cystic-solid tumor of the left ovary, measuring 4.5 cm in the largest diameter, with detection of several high-level echo foci within the solid component of the lesion (Figure 5.2). According to the sonographic criterias, morphology score of 6 (volume > 10 cm³, solid area > 1 cm and mixed/high-level echo pattern) finding was suggestive of ovarian malignancy. Another step in our primary screening represented transvaginal color Doppler analysis of intratumoral blood flow within the solid part of the tumor. It revealed RI of 0.36 (Figure 5.3A) to 0.40 (Figure 5.3B) as the lowest values.

According to color Doppler criteria for ovarian malignancy, these findings were indicative for a malignant ovarian lesion. Three-dimensional ultrasound scan, as a part of the secondary screening process, clearly depicted a hyperechoic area within the solid part of a complex ovarian

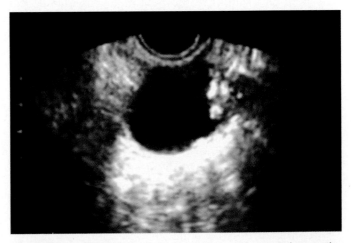

FIGURE 5.2: Transvaginal ultrasound scan of a complex cystic-solid ovarian tumor in a 51-year-old postmenopausal patient. Note several high-level echo foci within the solid component of the lesion.

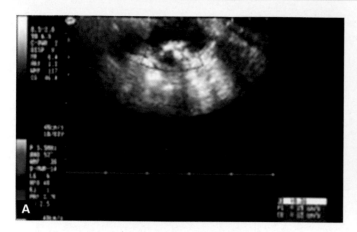
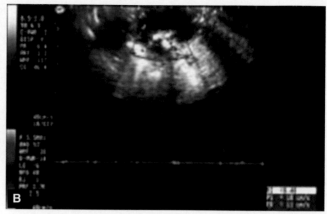

FIGURES 5.3A AND B: Further analysis of tumoral blood flow within the solid part of the tumor using transvaginal color Doppler ultrasound revealed RI of 0.36 to 0.40, suggestive of ovarian malignancy.

tumor (Figure 5.4). 3D ultrasound didn't add any significant morphological findings in comparison to 2D transvaginal gray scale US, besides more precise volume calculation.

However, the vascular pattern obtained by 3D power Doppler imaging revealed single-vessel arrangement and regularly separated vessels within the solid part of the tumor (Figure 5.5), indicative of a benign ovarian lesion. 3D US combined index score of 6, and regular course of the peripheral vessels was suggestive of a benign ovarian lesion, despite complex ovarian morphology. Also, CA-125 serum level of 10.5 U/ml was within the normal ranges. Unilateral adnexectomy was performed via laparotomy and "ex tempore" biopsy of the left ovary reported a benign cystic teratoma. This surgical procedure was considered adequate and the final histopathological analysis has confirmed the previous finding.

From this case, we can learn the following facts, which may help us to improve the multimodal ovarian cancer screening:

1. False-positive findings on transvaginal color Doppler analysis tend to involve non-neoplastic lesions that contain dilated vessels (due to underlying inflammatory process or necrosis).
2. The addition of 3D power Doppler (to study tumor vessels architecture) as a secondary screening tool may significantly improve the specificity of this screening test. This imaging modality might accurately discriminate benign from malignant complex ovarian lesions on the basis of qualitative analysis of tumoral microcirculation.
3. Improved diagnostic accuracy may improve patient care in terms of different surgical approaches to benign vs. malignant ovarian tumors (laparoscopy vs. laparotomy),[84] therefore, facilitating appropriate physician's referral.

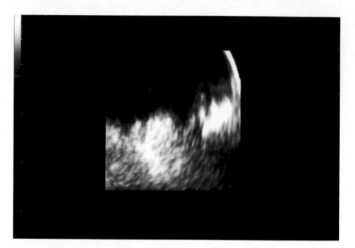

FIGURE 5.4: The same patient as in Figures 5.2 and 5.3 Three-dimensional ultrasound scan of a hyperechoic areas within the solid part of a complex ovarian tumor.

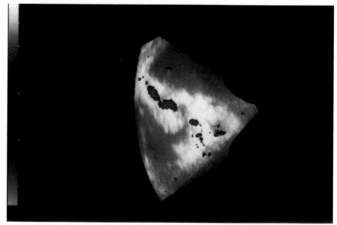

FIGURE 5.5: Transvaginal 3D power Doppler imaging of the same patient revealed single-vessel arrangement and regularly separated vessels within the solid part of the tumor, indicative of a benign ovarian lesion. Histopathology revealed benign cystic teratoma.

Illustrative Case No. 2—The Detection of Stage I Disease

Here we present an illustrative case of successfully detected stage IA ovarian cancer in an asymptomatic, 57-year-old postmenopausal patient with positive family history of breast cancer (mother and mother's sister). Besides regular mammography and gynecological check-ups, patient decided to perform gynecological ultrasound in an outpatient clinic for the first time in her life.

Transvaginal gray scale sonography, performed by her primary care gynecologist, revealed a complex cystic-solid tumor of the right ovary, measuring 8 cm in diameter, with detectable papillary protrusions and thick, irregular septations (Figure 5.6).

Regarding ovarian morphology indicative for malignancy, she was immediately directed to a tertiary center for further ultrasound evaluation. Previous TVUS finding was confirmed and morphology score of 8 was highly suspicious of ovarian malignancy. Another step represented transvaginal color Doppler analysis of the tumoral blood flow, which revealed RI of 0.40 as the lowest value (Figure 5.7). According to color Doppler criteria, this finding was indicative for a malignant ovarian lesion.

The vascular pattern obtained by further analysis with 3D power Doppler imaging clearly depicted disorganized, randomly dispersed vessels with irregular branching in the papilla (Figure 5.8) and solid parts (Figure 5.9) of the tumor, strongly associated with ovarian malignancy.

As a result, 3D US combined index score of 12, using data on tumor vessels architecture enabled us to make a correct preoperative sonographic diagnosis of an early stage ovarian cancer. On the other hand, CA-125 serum level of 16.3 U/ml was within the normal range, giving a false negative impression of a benign ovarian tumor. Standard oncological surgical procedure was performed and histopathology reported stage IA endometroid adenocarcinoma of the ovary.

Illustrative Case No. 3—The Detection of Stage I Disease

A 51-year-old patient was admitted to emergency room because of the lower back pain, lasting five weeks. Patient had normal menstrual bleeding and no children. Ultrasound showed a complex ovarian cyst on the right side, and she was referred to the primary care gynecologist. Vaginal examination revealed a hard mass in the right small pelvis. Transvaginal ultrasound demonstrated a complex ovarian cyst on the right side, with intracystic fluid of low echogenecity, and intracystic proliferations, which was not

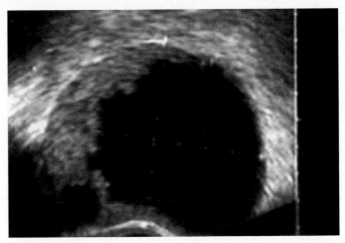

FIGURE 5.6: Complex ovarian tumor in a 57-year-old post-menopausal patient, with noticeable solid component protruding into the cystic cavity. Note thick, irregular septa on the basis of the lesion.

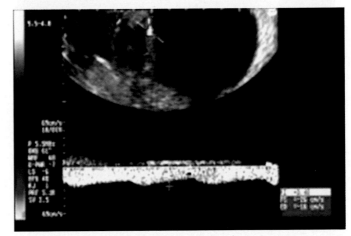

FIGURE 5.7: Further analysis of the tumoral blood flow with transvaginal color Doppler ultrasound in the same patient revealed RI of 0.40 as the lowest value. According to 2D color Doppler criteria, this finding was indicative of ovarian malignancy.

visualized on transabdominal ultrasound (Figure 5.10) measuring 7 × 9.2 cm, with a volume 256 ccm (Figure 5.11).

On 3D color and power Doppler ultrasound vascularization of the papillary intracystic projections, demonstrated irregular branching and evidence of stenosis, microaneurysms and lacunae (Figure 5.12). Pulsed wave Doppler showed a continuous flow of venous type (Figure 5.13). Using combined 3D morphology and vascular score indexing, these sonographic findings were highly suspicious of ovarian malignoma (Figures 5.14A to E). Serum levels of CA-125 were not elevated. MRI did not show any signs of regional or systemic metastasis. The patient was

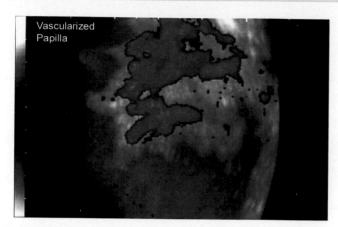

Vascularized Papilla

FIGURE 5.8: The same patient as in Figures 5.6 and 5.7. 3D power Doppler imaging added important information on tumor microcirculation architecture. Numerous randomly dispersed vessels are shown within the papilla, indicating malignant nature of the ovarian tumor.

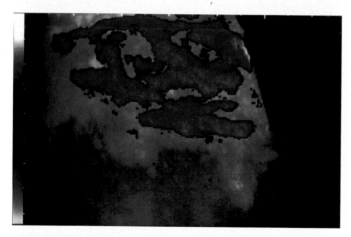

FIGURE 5.9: Further 3D power Doppler analysis in the same patient revealed typical signs of malignant neovascularization within the solid part of the lesion, characterized by irregular course of the tumoral vessels and complicated branching. Histopathological finding was stage IA ovarian endometroid adenocarcinoma.

scheduled for laparoscopy/laparotomy with frozen section. Laparoscopy showed an immobile cystic ovarian tumor with smooth surface, of which only 1/5 was visible (Figure 5.15). Under these circumstances, conversion to laparotomy was continued using midline incision. An immobile right ovarian tumor was released after spilling-free removal of the intracystic fluid (Figure 5.14E). Frozen section diagnosed ovarian adenocarcinoma. Preliminary diagnosis was followed by staging and hysterectomy, left adnectomy, omentectomy, and paraaortic and iliac lymphadenectomy. The final histological diagnosis was clear cell carcinoma, staging pT1a. Focal endometriosis was found in both ovaries and the right fallopian tube (Figures 5.16A to C).

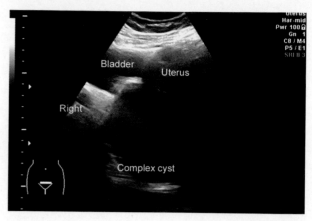

Bladder   Uterus

Right

Complex cyst

FIGURE 5.10: Ovarian carcinoma IA transabdominal ultrasound. The adnexal mass was not obtained due to shadowing and limited penetration/depth.

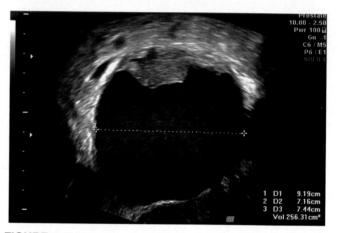

1	D1	9.19cm
2	D2	7.16cm
3	D3	7.44cm
		Vol 256.31cm³

FIGURE 5.11: Transvaginal sonogram of ovarian cancer IA by B-mode. Note echogenic fluid and papillary intracystic projections. Sonographic finding was suggestive of ovarian carcinoma.

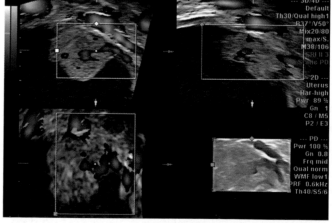

FIGURE 5.12: Ovarian carcinoma IA by 3D power Doppler. Three-dimensional power Doppler ultrasound demonstrated randomly dispersed vascular signals within the papillary protrusion.

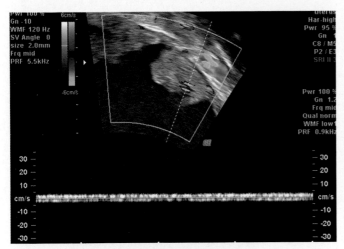

FIGURE 5.13: Color Doppler and pulsed Doppler waveform analysis of ovarian carcinoma stage IA. Note continuous low-resistance flow within the tumoral papilla.

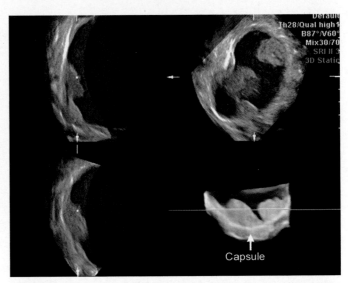

FIGURE 5.14B: 3D surface rendering and "magic cut" through the basis of the papillary lesion. These modalities improve depiction of infiltrative lesions.

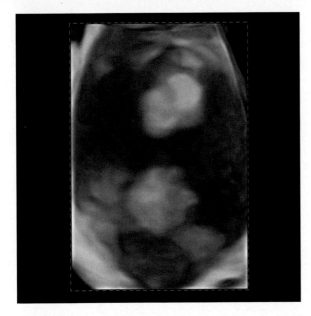

FIGURE 5.14A: 3D surface rendering of the same patient.

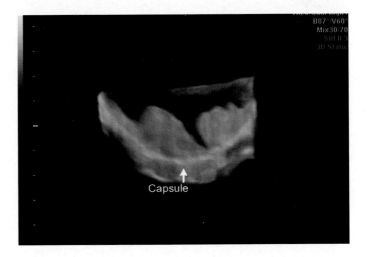

FIGURE 5.14C: 3D surface rendering with "magic cut" through the papillae demonstrates continuity of the ovarian capsule. Note an echogenic band showing no interruptions. With tomographic ultrasound imaging (TUI), a systematic macroscopic evaluation of the capsule could be obtained.

The surprisingly good staging result, looking at a tumor volume of 256 ccm, demands additional explanation. Kurman et al. suggested a new model dividing ovarian cancer patients into two groups designated as type I and type II. Type I tumors are slow growing tumors, generally confined to the ovary at diagnosis, which develop from the well-established precursor lesions so-called borderline tumors. Type I tumors include low-grade micropapillary serous carcinoma, mucinous, endometrioid and clear cell carcinomas. They are genetically stable and are characterized by mutations in a number of different genes, including KRAS, BRAF, PTEN and beta-catenin.[55] Type II tumors are rapidly growing, highly aggressive neoplasms that lack well-defined precursor lesions; most are advanced stage at, or soon after, their inception. These include high-grade serous carcinoma, malignant mixed mesodermal tumors (carcinosarcomas) and undifferentiated carcinomas. Type II tumors are characterized by mutation of TP53 and a high level of genetic instability. Screening tests that focus on stage I disease may detect low-grade type I.[55]

For several decades, endometriosis has been suspected of playing a role in the etiology of ovarian cancer.

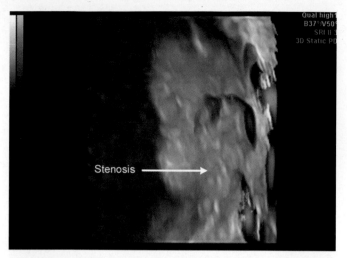

FIGURE 5.14D: Power Doppler in glass body rendering of the tumor papilla. Prominent changes of the vascular caliber and depiction of stenosis and lacunae due to abnormal chaotic tumor angiogenesis are suggestive of ovarian malignancy.

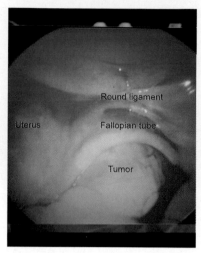

FIGURE 5.15: Ovarian carcinoma IA, laparoscopy: The tumor is incarcerated in the right small pelvis, immobile due to endometriotic adhesions.

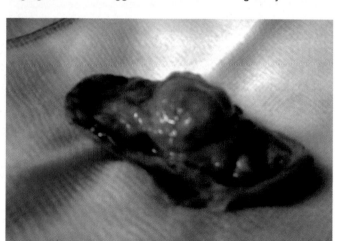

FIGURE 5.14.E: Macroscopic specimen of ovarian carcinoma IA. Correlate the macroscopic and ultrasound findings.

atypical endometriosis in a spatial and chronological association with ovarian cancer. Finally, molecular studies have detected common alterations in endometriosis and ovarian cancer. These data suggest that some tumors, especially endometrioid and clear-cell carcinomas, can arise from endometriosis. Moreover, endometriosis-associated ovarian cancer represents a distinct clinical entity, with a more favorable biological behavior, given a lower-stage distribution and better survival rate than nonendometriosis-associated ovarian cancer.[85]

Epidemiological evidence from large-cohort studies confirms endometriosis as an independent risk factor for ovarian cancer. Further circumstantial evidence for this link was found in the common risk factors for ovarian cancer and endometriosis. These risk factors influence retrograde menstruation and endometriosis in the same positive or negative way. Based on the data from the literature, the prevalence of endometriosis in epithelial ovarian cancer has been calculated to be 4.5, 1.4, 35.9 and 19% for serous, mucinous, clear-cell and endometrioid ovarian carcinoma, respectively.[85] The risk of malignant transformation in ovarian endometriosis was calculated at 2.5% but this might be an underestimation. In addition, some authors described

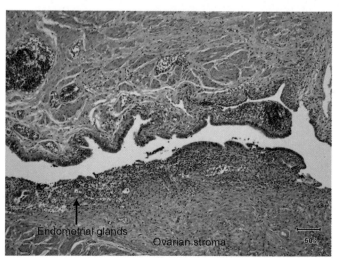

FIGURE 5.16A: Ovarian IA clear cell carcinoma, histology: Endometrial glands, embedded in ovarian stroma (*Courtesy:* Dr Hala Abdelaziz).

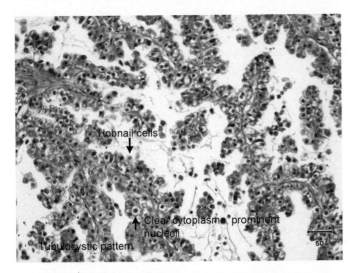

FIGURE 5.16B: Ovarian carcinoma IA. Note tubulocystic pattern of the tumor, tubuli lined by hobnail cells with clear cytoplasma and prominent nucleoli (*Courtesy:* Dr Hala Abdelaziz).

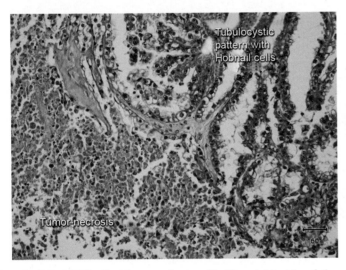

FIGURE 5.16C: Ovarian carcinoma IA. The right side of the image demonstrates tubulopapillary pattern with Hobnail cells, while on the left side there is an area of tumor-necrosis (*Courtesy:* Dr Hala Abdelaziz).

Illustrative Case No. 4—The Detection of Stage III Disease

A 48-year-old patient with lower abdominal discomfort and bloating for three months, came to a primary care gynecologist for her annual examination. She had hypertension and diabetes mellitus type 2, for which she took metformine. Her obstetrical history was significant for two normal vaginal deliveries. One of her sisters suffered from breast cancer. The patient had a normal gynecological check-up result one year before by a gynecologist, but no

ultrasound has been performed on that occasion. Recently, she noticed irregular menstruation.

Ultrasound showed bilateral complex adnexal masses, measuring 7 cm in mean diameter. Color Doppler demonstrated randomly dispersed vessels within the echogenic portion of the lesion (Figures 5.17 and 5.18).

Preoperative CA-125 measured 1404 IU per ml. At the time of laparotomy metastases were detected in the omentum and paraaortal lymph nodes. Cytology of the peritoneal fluid (PF) was positive for cancer cells. Final diagnosis was stage III bilateral high-grade serous-papillary carcinoma, moderately differentiated.

Based on these examples it can be concluded that:

1. 3D power Doppler qualitative analysis of tumor angiogenesis allows accurate detection of the earliest appearance of ovarian malignancy, i.e. stage IA ovarian cancer.

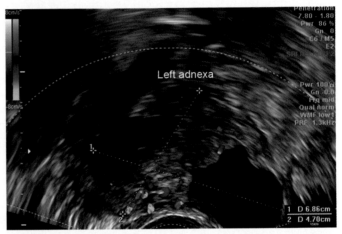

FIGURE 5.17: Bilateral ovarian carcinoma stage III/IV. Note randomly dispersed flow in the solid part of the cystic-solid mass.

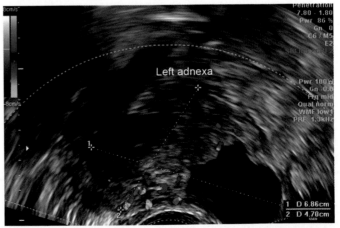

FIGURE 5.18: Bilateral ovarian carcinoma stage III/IV. Bizarre contour of the solid component is typical of ovarian malignancy.

2. 3D ultrasound technology may be utilized in clinical and university hospital settings as a secondary screening tool.

3. As published by Holbert, and noted in the cases above, routine screening for ovarian cancer by standard 2D ultrasound modalities, in terms of primary screening, is a valuable addition to the yearly pelvic examination in outpatient clinics and private gynecology office settings.

Aims

Application of 3D ultrasound imaging with power Doppler facilities in patients with positive standard ultrasound tests represents an innovation compared with previous ovarian cancer screening trials. It has been demonstrated that a secondary screening-based on morphologic and vascular parameters assessed by 3D ultrasound, 3D power Doppler and contrast-enhanced 3D power Doppler may improve early detection of ovarian cancer and accuracy of ultrasound screening strategy in high-risk population.

CONCLUSION

Evaluation of the ovarian cancer screening trials leads to the conclusion that a routine screening of a high-risk population appears to be advantageous. In high-risk groups, fewer women need to be screened for each case detected, prevalence of the disease is markedly higher and the ratio of false positives to true positives is lower.

Because most of the ovarian cancers occur during postmenopause, there has been a growing interest for screening asymptomatic postmenopausal women. Two main strategies, multimodal and ultrasound-based screening have emerged, both with some limitations for implementation in a routine screening practice. For the first one, the great challenge is to improve the sensitivity of serum CA-125 as a primary screening tool. The risk assessment by means of ovarian cancer algorithm (ROCA), an exponential model using data from several prior scans and testing for an exponential rise in the value of the marker, is likely to improve the sensitivity of CA-125 as the first line screening test. More promising ovarian tumor markers appear on the horizon.

Color Doppler's role in the detection of ovarian carcinoma is based on the fact that malignant tumors are characterized by neovascularization and formation of new blood vessels with a poorly developed "muscular media." The blood flow in these vessels is marked by low vascular impedance. Initial 3D power Doppler ultrasound studies with volume and histogram analysis have demonstrated increased specificity and positive predictive value (PPV)

in ovarian cancer detection. Three-dimensional power Doppler (3D-PD) clearly depicts disorganized, randomly dispersed vessels with irregular branching, the features that are typical of ovarian malignancy.[86] Therefore, researchers from the field of ultrasound hope that the problem of low PPV of 2D ultrasound studies may be solved by introducing enhanced and nonenhanced 3D ultrasound technology, used as a secondary screening procedure.

REFERENCES

1. Greenlee RT, Murray T, Bolden S, et al. Cancer statistics, 2000. CA Cancer J Clin 2000;50(1):7-33.
2. Gubbels JA, Claussen N, Kapur AK, et al. The detection, treatment, and biology of epithelial ovarian cancer. J Ovarian Res 2010;3:8.
3. Jemal A, Siegel R, Ward E, et al. Cancer statistics, 2008. CA Cancer J Clin 2008;58:71-96.
4. Lowe KA, Andersen MR, Urban N, et al. The temporal stability of the Symptom Index among women at high-risk for ovarian cancer. Gynecol Oncol 2009;114(2):225-30.
5. Permuth-Wey J, Sellers T. Epidemiology of ovarian cancer. Methods Mol Biol 2009;472:413-37.
6. Heintz APM, Odicino F, Maisonneuve P, et al. Carcinoma of the ovary. In: 24th Volume of the FIGO Annual Report on the Results of Treatment in Gynecological Cancer. J Epidemiol Biostat 2001;6(1):107-38.
7. Kirwan JM, Tincello DG, Herod JJ, et al. Effect of delays in primary care referral on survival of women with epithelial ovarian cancer: Retrospective audit. BMJ 2002;324 (7330): 148-51.
8. Holschneider CH, Berek JS. Ovarian cancer: Epidemiology, biology, and prognostic factors. Semin Surg Oncol 2000; 19(1):3-10.
9. Hoskins WJ, Perez CA, Young RC. Principles and Practice of Gynecologic Oncology. Philadelphia: Lippincott-Raven Publishers 1997.
10. Paget S. The distribution of secondary growths in cancer of the breast. Cancer Metastasis Rev 1989;8(2):98-101.
11. Gubbels JA, Belisle J, Onda M, et al. Mesothelin-MUC16 binding is a high-affinity, N-glycan dependent interaction that facilitates peritoneal metastasis of ovarian tumors. Mol Cancer 2006;5(1):50.
12. Paley PJ. Screening for the major malignancies affecting women: Current guidelines. Am J Obstet Gynecol 2001; 184(5):1021-30.
13. Urban N. Screening for ovarian cancer. We now need a definitive randomised trial. BMJ 1999;319(7221):1317-8.
14. Antoniou A, Pharoah PD, Narod S, et al. Average risks of breast and ovarian cancer associated with BRCA1 or BRCA2 mutations detected in case Series unselected for family history: A combined analysis of 22 studies. Am J Hum Genet 2003; 72(5):1117-30
15. Auersperg N, Wong AS, Choi KC, et al. Ovarian surface epithelium: Biology, endocrinology, and pathology. Endocr Rev. 2001;22:255-88.

16. Ahmed N, Thompson EW, Quinn MA. Epithelial-mesenchymal interconversions in normal ovarian surface epithelium and ovarian carcinomas: An exception to the norm. J Cell Physiol 2007;213:581-8.

17. Neunteufel W, Breitenecker G. Tissue expression of CA-125 in benign and malignant lesions of ovary and fallopian tube: A comparison with CA 19-9 and CEA. Gynecol Oncol 1989; 32:297-302.

18. Fathalla MF. Incessant ovulation—A factor in ovarian neoplasia? Lancet 1971;2(7716):163.

19. Ozols RF, Bookman MA, Connolly DC, et al. Focus on epithelial ovarian cancer. Cancer Cell 2004;5(1):19-24.

20. Murdoch WJ, Townsend RS, McDonnel AC. Ovulation-induced DNA damage in ovarian surface epithelial cells of ewes: Prospective regulatory mechanisms of repair/survival and apoptosis. Biol Reprod 2001;65:1417-24.

21. Dubeau L. The cell of origin of ovarian epithelial tumors and the ovarian surface epithelium dogma: Does the emperor have no clothes? Gynecol Oncol 1999;72:437-42.

22. Bell R, Petticrew M, Sheldon T. The performance of screening tests for ovarian cancer: results of a systematic review. Br J Obstet Gynecol 1998;105(11):1136-47.

23. Van Nagell JR, DePriest PD, Reedy MB, et al. The efficacy of transvaginal sonographic screening in asymptomatic women at risk for ovarian cancer. Gynecol Oncol 2000;77(3):350-6.

24. Hayashi H, Yaginuma Y, Kitamura S, et al. Bilateral oophorectomy in asymptomatic women over 50 years old selected by ovarian cancer screening. Gynecol Obstet Invest 1999;47(1):58-64.

25. Tabor A, Jensen FR, Bock JE, et al. Feasibility study of a randomised trial of ovarian cancer screening. J Med Screen 1994;1(4):215-9.

26. Campbell S, Bhan V, Royston P, et al. Transabdominal ultrasound screening fo early ovarian cancer. BMJ 1989; 299(6712):1363-7.

27. Goswamy RK, Campbell S, Whitehead MI. Screening for ovarian cancer. Clin Obstet Gynecol 1983;10(3):621-43.

28. Vuento MH, Pirhonen JP, Makinen JI, et al. Evaluation of ovarian findings in asymptomatic postmenopausal women with color Doppler ultrasound. Cancer 1995;76(7):1214-8.

29. Kurjak A, Shalan H, Kupesic S, et al. An attempt to screen asymptomatic women for ovarian and endometrial cancer with transvaginal color and pulsed Doppler sonography. J Ultrasound Med 1994;13(4):295-301.

30. Schulman H, Conway C, Zalud I, et al. Prevalence in a volunteer population of pelvic cancer detected with transvaginal ultrasound and color flow Doppler. Ultrasound Obstet Gynecol 1994;4(5):414-20.

31. Sato S, Yokoyama Y, Sakamoto T, et al. Usefulness of mass screening for ovarian carcinoma using transvaginal ultrasonography. Cancer 2000;89(3):582-8.

32. Parkes CA, Smith D, Wald NJ, et al. Feasibility study of a randomised trial of ovarian cancer screening among the general population. J Med Screen 1994;1(4):209-14.

33. Holbert TR. Screening transvaginal ultrasonography of postmenopausal women in a private office setting. Am J Obstet Gynecol 1994;170:1699-1704.

34. Einhorn N, Sjovall P, Knapp RC, et al. Prospective evaluation of serum CA-125 levels for early detection of ovarian cancer. Obstet Gynecol 1992;80(1):14-8.

35. Jacobs IJ, Skates SJ, MacDonald N, et al. Screening for ovarian cancer: A pilot randomised controlled trial. Lancet 1999; 353(9160):1207-10.

36. Jacobs IJ, Skates SJ, Davies AP, et al. Risk of diagnosis of ovarian cancer after raised serum CA-125 concentration: A prospective cohort study. BMJ 1996;313(7069):1355-8.

37. Adonakis GL, Paraskevaidis E, Tsiga S, et al. A combined approach for the early detection of ovarian cancer in asymptomatic women. Eur J Obstet Gynecol Reprod Biol 1996; 65(2):221-5.

38. Grover S, Quinn MA, Weidman P, et al. Screening for ovarian cancer using serum CA-125 and vaginal examination: Report on 2550 females. Int J Gynecol Cancer 1995;5:291-5.

39. Meyer T, Rustin GJ. Role of tumour markers in monitoring epithelial ovarian cancer. Br J Cancer 2000;82(9):1535-8.

40. Yin BW, Dnistrian A, Lloyd KO. Ovarian cancer antigen CA-125 is encoded by the MUC16 mucin gene. Int J Cancer. 2002; 98:737-40.

41. Niloff JM, Knapp RC, Schaetzl E, et al. CA-125 antigen levels in obstetric and gynecologic patients. Obstet Gynecol 1984; 64:703-7.

42. Bohm-Velez M, Mendelson E, Bree R, et al. Ovarian cancer screening. American College of Radiology. ACR Appropriateness Criteria. Radiology. 2000; 215 (Suppl):861-71.

43. Skates SJ, Xu FJ, Yu YH, et al. Toward an optimal algorithm for ovarian cancer screening with longitudinal tumor markers. Cancer 1995;76(10 Suppl):2004-10.

44. Menon U, Jacobs IJ. Ovarian cancer screening in the general population. Ultrasound Obstet Gynecol 2000;15:350-3.

45. Buamah P. Benign conditions associated with raised serum CA-125 concentration. J Surg Oncol 2000;75(4):264-5.

46. Verheijen RH, von Mensdorff-Pouilly S, van Kamp GJ, et al. CA-125: Fundamental and clinical aspects. Semin Cancer Biol 1999;9:117-24.

47. Fang X, Gaudette D, Furui T, et al. Lysophos-pholipid growth factors in the initiation, progression, metastases and management of ovarian cancer. Ann N Y Acad Sci 2000; 905:188-208.

48. Xu Y, Shen Z, Wiper D, et al. Lysophosphatidic acid as a potential biomarker for ovarian and other gynecologic cancers. JAMA 1998;280(8):719-23.

49. Roberts JA. Searching for a biomarker for ovarian cancer. JAMA 1998;280(8):739.

50. Moore RG, Brown AK, Miller MC, et al. The use of multiple novel tumor biomarkers for the detection of ovarian carcinoma in patients with a pelvic mass. Gynecol Oncol 2008; 108(2):402-8.

51. Anderson GL, McIntosh M, Wu L, et al. Assessing lead time of selected ovarian cancer biomarkers: A nested case-control study. J Natl Cancer Inst 2010;102(1):26-38.

52. Fishman DA, Cohen LS. Is transvaginal ultrasound effective for screening asymptomatic women for the detection of early-stage epithelial ovarian carcinoma? Gynecol Oncol 2000; 77(3):347-9.

53. Bailey CL, Ueland FR, Land GL, et al. The malignant potential of small cystic ovarian tumors in postmenopausal women. Gynecol Oncol 1998;69(1):3-7.

54. Pavlik EJ, DePriest PD, Gallion HH, et al. Ovarian volume related to age. Gynecol Oncol 2000;77(3):410-2.

55. Kurman RJ, Visvanathan K, Roden R, et al. Early detection and treatment of ovarian cancer: Shifting from early stage to minimal volume of disease based on a new model of carcinogenesis. Am J Obstet Gynecol 2008;198(4):351-6.

56. Menon U, Talaat A, Jeyarajah AR, et al. Ultrasound assessment of ovarian cancer risk in postmenopausal women with CA125 elevation. Br J Cancer 1999;80:1644-7.

57. Menon U, Talaat A, Rosenthal AN, et al. Performance of ultrasound as a second line test to serum CA125 in ovarian cancer screening. BJOG 2000;107:165-9.

58. Jeoung HY, Choi HS, Lim YS, et al. The efficacy of sonographic morphology indexing and serum CA-125 for preoperative differentiation of malignant from benign ovarian tumors in patients after operation with ovarian tumors. J Gynecol Oncol 2008;19(4):229-35.

59. Menon U, Gentry-Maharaj A, Hallett R, et al. Sensitivity and specificity of multimodal and ultrasound screening for ovarian cancer, and stage distribution of detected cancers: Results of the prevalence screen of the UK Collaborative Trial of Ovarian Cancer Screening (UKCTOCS). Lancet Oncol 2009; 10(4):327-40.

60. Kobayashi H, Yamada Y, Sado T, et al. A randomized study of screening for ovarian cancer: A multicenter study in Japan. Int J Gynecol Cancer. 2008; 18(3):414-20.

61. Law MR, Morris JK, Wald NJ. The importance of age in screening for cancer. J Med Screen 1999;6(1):16-20.

62. Boyd J. Molecular genetics of hereditary ovarian cancer. Oncology (Williston Park) 1998;12(3):399-406.

63. Pharoah PD, Stratton JF, Mackay J. Screening for breast and ovarian cancer: The relevance of family history. Br Med Bull. 1998; 54(4):823-38.

64. Vasen HF, Haites NE, Evans DG, et al. Current policies for surveillance and management in women at risk of breast and ovarian cancer: A survey among 16 European family cancer clinics. European Familial Breast Cancer Collaborative Group. Eur J Cancer 1998;34(12):1922-6.

65. Van Nagell JR, DePriest PD, Ueland FR, et al. Ovarian cancer screening with annual transvaginal sonography: Findings of 25,000 women screened Cancer 2007;109(9):1887-96.

66. Karlan BY, Baldwin RL, Lopez-Luevanos E, et al. Peritoneal serous papillary carcinoma, a phenotypic variant of familial ovarian cancer: Implications for ovarian cancer screening. Am J Obstet Gynecol. 1999; 180:917-28.

67. Bonilla-Musoles F, Raga F, Osborne NG. Three-dimensional ultrasound evaluation of ovarian masses. Gynecol Oncol. 1995; 59(1):129-35.

68. Chan L, Lin WM, Verpairojkit B, et al. Evaluation of adnexal masses using three-dimensional ultrasonographic technology: Preliminary report. J Ultrasound Med 1997;16(5):349-54.

69. Kurjak A, Kupesic S, Breyer B, et al. The assessment of ovarian tumor angiogenesis: what does three-dimensional power Doppler add? Ultrasound Obstet Gynecol. 1998; 12(2):136-46.

70. Kurjak A, Kupesic S, Sparac V, et al. Three-dimensional ultrasonographic and power Doppler characterization of ovarian lesions. Ultrasound Obstet Gynecol 2000;16(4):365-71.

71. Sassone MA, Timor-Tritsch IE, Artner A, et al. Transvaginal sonographic characterization of ovarian disease: Evaluation of a new scoring system to predict ovarian malignancy. Obstet Gynecol 1991;78(1):70-6.

72. Lerner JP, Timor-Tritsch IE, Federman A, et al. Transvaginal ultrasonographic characterization of ovarian masses with an improved, weighted scoring system. Am J Obstet Gynecol 1994;170(1):81-5.

73. DePriest PD, Shenson D, Fried A, et al. A morphology index based on sonographic findings in ovarian cancer. Gynecol Oncol 1993;51(1):7-11.

74. Kurjak A, Predanic M. New scoring system for prediction of ovarian malignancy based on transvaginal color Doppler sonography. J Ultrasound Med 1992;11(12):631-8.

75. Kurjak A, Kupesic S, Anic T, et al. Three-dimensional ultrasound and power Doppler improve the diagnosis of ovarian lesions. Gynecol Oncol 2000;76(1):28-32.

76. Cohen LS, Escobar PF, Scharm C, et al. Three-dimensional power Doppler ultrasound improves the diagnostic accuracy for ovarian cancer prediction. Gynecol Oncol 2001;82(1):40-8.

77. Bristow RE, Santillan A, Diaz-Montez TP. Centralization of care for patients with advanced-stage ovarian cancer: A cost-effectiveness analysis. Cancer 2007;109(8):1513-22.

78. Kupesic S, Kurjak A. Contrast-enhanced three-dimensional power Doppler sonography for the differentiation of adnexal masses. Obstet Gynecol 2000;96(3):452-8.

79. Alcazar JL, Prka M. Evaluation of two different methods for vascular sampling by three–dimensional power Doppler angiography in solid and cystic-solid masses. Ultrasound Obstet Gynecol 2009;33(3):349-54.

80. Alcazar JL, Merce LT, Garcia Manero M. Three-dimensional power Doppler sampling: A new method for predicting ovarian cancer in vascularised complex adnexal masses. J Ultrasound Med 2005;24:689-96.

81. Ameye L, Valentin L, Testa AC, et al. A scoring system to differentiate malignant from benign masses in specific ultrasound-based subgroups of adnexal tumors. Ultrasound Obstet Gynecol 2009;33(1):92-101.

82. Kurjak A, Kupesic S, Sparac V, et al. The detection of stage I ovarian cancer by three-dimensional sonography and power Doppler. Gynecol Oncol 2003;90(2):258-64.

83. Kurjak A, Kupesic S, Sparac V, et al. Preoperative evaluation of pelvic tumors by Doppler and three-dimensional sonography. J Ultrasound Med 2001;20:829-40.

84. Mettler L. The cystic adnexal mass: patient selection, surgical techniques and long-term follow-up. Curr Opin Obstet Gynecol 2001;13(4):389-97.

85. Van Gorp T, Amant F, Neven P, et al. Endometriosis and the development of malignant tumours of the pelvis. A review of literature. Best Pract Res Clin Obstet Gynaecol 2004; 18(2):349-71.

86. Kurjak A, Prka M, Arenas JB. Screening for ovarian cancer by different modes of transvaginal sonography. In: Kurjak A, Bajo Arenas J (Eds).Textbook of Transvaginal Sonography, New Delhi: Jaypee Brothers 2005;465-78.

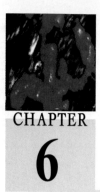

S Kupesic Plavsic, A Kurjak, K Baston

CHAPTER

6

Ovarian Endometriosis

INTRODUCTION

Endometriosis is defined as the presence of endometrial tissue in an abnormal anatomical location. Endometrial tissue may implant itself in the myometrium, leading to the formation of adenomyosis. The myometrium may respond to this intrusion with muscular overgrowth and a nodule called an adenomyoma may be formed consisting of an island of endometrial tissue circumscribed within the myometrium.[1]

Endometriosis was first described by Daniel Shroen in 1690. Later, WW Russel in 1899 raised interest in the hemorrhagic cyst of the ovary, describing a case of a woman of reproductive age who had "the right ovary enveloped in adhesions of the posterior face of the broad ligament." Microscopic examination showed "areas, which were an exact prototype of normal uterine mucous membrane."[2] It took more than 20 years before the endometrial tissue was recognized as a cause of the hemorrhagic cyst by Sampson,[3] and the cyst was later called endometrioma. Sampson observed similarity between the peritoneal implants and ectopic endometrium and formulated the hypothesis that peritoneal endometriosis originates by a mechanism of menstrual regurgitation and implantation. Progress in laparoscopy has led to an increased recognition of endometriosis as this method is a gold standard for early diagnosis and accurate staging of this disease.

Endometriosis is a unique disease characterized by its invasive but non-neoplastic growth pattern, the presence of endometrium at ectopic sites and the evidence of hormonal responsiveness with menstrual cyclicity.[4] However, the dissemination of viable endometrial cells can occur by routes other than transplantation and regurgitation and in some cases can only be explained by the metaplasia

theory.[5] Although endometriosis is a common benign gynecologic condition, there is still much to learn about its etiology and pathogenesis.

SYMPTOMS

Chronic pelvic pain, dysmenorrhea, deep dyspareunia and infertility are the main symptoms of pelvic endometriosis. Mahmood et al.[6] and Fedele et al.[7] reported that deep dyspareunia and chronic pelvic pain affect one-third of the patients with endometriosis. Later investigation demonstrated the lack of correlation between the stage of the disease as determined by revised American Fertility Society classification and the prevalence and severity of the symptoms. Koninckx et al. found a strong correlation between the sites of focal tenderness on examination and the presence of the implants on the uterosacral ligaments and cul-de-sac.[8] The psychological status of the woman can influence the perception of pain and sometimes it is difficult to recognize whether the psychological disturbance proceeds or aggravates the pain or if it results from the chronic exposure to it.[9]

ENDOMETRIOSIS IN INFERTILE PATIENTS

Endometriosis is an extremely common disease and unsuspected endometriosis accounts for approximately 15% of infertility.[10] Many asymptomatic women are found to have endometriosis and some of them are reported to have severe disease discovered after the incidental detection of an ovarian mass or during laparoscopy for infertility. The classic symptom of endometriosis is pelvic pain associated with menstruation (or during the immediate premenstrual phase).[11]

Suspicion is heightened when the infertile patient complains of dysmenorrhea and dyspareunia. Pelvic adhesions, ovarian dysfunction, altered prostaglandin secretion and peritoneal fluid macrophages are implicated as possible pathophysiological mechanisms.[12] Sonography is accurate in determining the type (cystic, mixed or solid), shape and location of endometriosis.[13] Ovarian cystic lesions, which constitute about 30 to 62% of endometriosis cases are seen as irregular cysts with some evidence of septation. The sonographic appearance in the mixed type is compatible with pelvic inflammatory disease of an infectious cause, while a solid pattern may even suggest ovarian malignancy. Sometimes it is difficult to differentiate a "chocolate cyst" from a hemorrhagic ovarian cyst or corpus luteum cyst. Fibrinolysis of the hemolytic content of a hemorrhagic ovarian cyst may change its pattern.[14]

Endometriomas usually remain constant as nonechogenic cysts with a semisolid content of a "parenchymatous" texture representing "chocolate" paste-like fluid within a cyst.[10] The most common sites of their deposition are the ovaries. Endometriomas may mimic developing follicles or functional cysts. Sometimes endometriomas increase in size during ovulation induction and mimic developing follicles. The experienced ultrasonographer may distinguish them accurately on the basis of low-level echoes, irregular shape, persistence during several cycles, and observation of their behavior. Transvaginal sonography can be used for monitoring the regression of these collections under hormonal therapy.

Many years ago Scott and Te Linde[15] presented the sites of endometriosis detected in a series of 516 cases. They showed the ovaries to be the most common site followed by pelvic peritoneum. Another study, including 182 infertile women demonstrated that the ovaries were the primary site of endometriosis in 54.9% of patients, followed by a posterior broad ligament (35.2%), the anterior or posterior pouch of Douglas (each 34%) and uterosacral ligaments (28%).[16]

Common physical findings associated with endometriosis also include the fixation of the pelvic structures secondary to adhesions. In many patients, the uterus is retroverted.[17] Nodularity and tenderness of the uterosacral ligaments are noted in one-third of patients with endometriosis.[18] The condition has aroused much interest and controversy in recent years with regard to its accurate diagnosis, infertility association and proper treatment. Even with the recent ongoing achievements in operative endoscopy, clinicians are still faced with a problem of correct diagnosis, both in the sense of missing this pathology and of treating a luteinic cyst instead of an endometrioma.[19,20] Therefore, any diagnostic technique that could differentiate accurately and reliably between hemorrhagic luteinic cyst, cystadenoma, dermoid cyst, ovarian malignancy and endometrioma would be a useful additional tool for the better management of this enigmatic disease.

ULTRASOUND DIAGNOSIS

Ovarian endometrioma presents different sonographic patterns, such as purely cystic, cystic with few septations or minimal debris, complex mass and largely solid lesions. There were several papers about the role of transabdominal sonography in the diagnosis of endometriosis.[13,21-23] Typically, an ovarian endometrioma was described as a cystic mass that is entirely or predominantly echogenic.[22,23] In other reports[21,24] endometrioma was characterized as a complex mass. In a transvaginal study by Kupfer et al.,[20] 82% of 32 surgically proved endometriomas showed the presence of a homogeneous hyperechoic "carpet" of low level echoes (Figure 6.1). Introduction of transvaginal color Doppler ultrasound increased the potential for *in vivo* characterization of adnexal masses, particularly in the differentiation between benign and malignant conditions.[25] The addition of color Doppler capabilities to transvaginal transducers can detect vascularity within an ovarian endometrioma.[26] Endometriotic cysts are supported by already existing vessels within the ovarian hilus showing moderate vascular impedance (Figure 6.2). If present, inflammatory changes may show alteration in perfusion that is characterized by marked reduction in blood flow resistance. This finding may be wrongly interpreted as ovarian malignancy.[27,28]

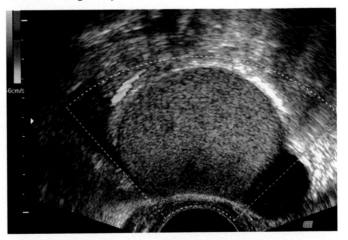

FIGURE 6.1: Transvaginal color Doppler scan of an ovarian endometrioma. Note the homogeneous "carpet-like" echoes of the cystic lesion and peripheral blood flow signals.

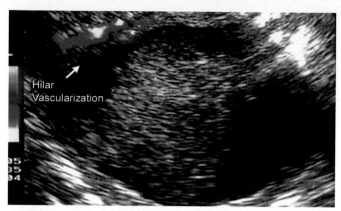

FIGURE 6.2: Transvaginal color Doppler scan of an ovarian endometriotic cyst. Note the homogeneous high-level internal echoes and prominent vascularization at the level of the ovarian hilus.

TABLE 6.1: Scoring system for endometriosis based on transvaginal color and pulsed Doppler sonography

	Score
Reproductive age	2
Chronic pain (premenstrual or menstrual)	1
Infertility	1
B-mode	
Position (medially, retrouterine)	2
Bilaterality	1
Serial sonography positive	2
Thick walls	2
Homogeneous echogenicity	2
Clear demarcation from the ovary	1
Transvaginal color Doppler	
Vascularization	2
Pericystic/hilar location	2
Regularly separated vessels	2
Existence of notching	1
RI < 0.40 (menstrual phase)	2
RI = 0.41 to 0.60 (late follicular/corpus luteum phase)	2
CA-125 (> 35 IU/ml)	2

With permission from the reference 29.

Kurjak and Kupesic[29] were the first who reported on the combined use of transvaginal color Doppler and CA-125 levels in patients with ovarian endometrioma. A new noninvasive scoring system (Table 6.1), using clinical signs and symptoms, CA-125 levels, sonographic findings, and transvaginal color and pulsed Doppler parameters, was developed and used for preoperative recognition of ovarian endometriosis. The authors performed a five-year prospective study in patients undergoing laparotomy and laparoscopy. The study group consisted of 544 women with clinically suspected adnexal masses who were undergoing laparotomy and 112 patients who were undergoing laparoscopy. In the second group, management of ovarian mass and additionally, lysis of adhesions in infertile patients were the indications for diagnostic and/or operative laparoscopy. The mean age of the patients enrolled in this study was 46 years. Ovarian endometriosis was proven histologically in 103 patients. The average age of the patients with ovarian endometriosis was 31 years (range 19 to 45 years).[29]

The scoring system, using age, clinical signs and symptoms (pelvic pain associated with menstruation and presentation of infertility), CA-125 levels, sonographic findings and transvaginal color and pulsed Doppler parameters, was created in an effort to improve sensitivity and specificity in the diagnosis of ovarian endometriosis.

Patients were sonographically examined at least twice, when they were admitted to the hospital, as well as the day before the intervention. Patients with mild endometriosis and peritoneal implants were excluded from the analysis because no role can be expected from pelvic sonography in the minimal or mild endometriosis detection. B-mode was used to evaluate location, appearance and width of the ovarian lesions. The morphological scoring system analyzed internal borders of the cyst, quality of the cyst, fluid echogenicity, position and existence of the adnexal mass bilaterality. The sonographic criteria for the diagnosis of endometriosis were thick walls, regular margins and homogeneous low echogenicity of the fluid. The presence of the cyst was confirmed at least twice in different cycles before surgery (the interval between the first and second ultrasound ranged from 42 to 84 days). In 427 patients, serial ultrasound examinations were performed.

The part of the scoring system, dedicated to color Doppler evaluation has been derived from vascular location, type of vascularization and vascular quality. The vascular location typical for endometrioma is pericystic, at the level of ovarian hilus. The type of vascularization represents regularly separated pericystic vessels or scattered hilar vessels with low-to-moderate vascular resistance.

The threshold value for discrimination between ovarian endometriosis and other ovarian lesions was a value of 20 for the combined scoring system. The histopathological diagnosis was considered definitive in all cases.

Ovarian endometriomas appeared as thick-walled cystic structures, containing marked internal echoes in 86 patients, multilocular cysts in 7 patients and a solid-cystic appearance in 10 patients. The median diameter of the endometrioma was 55.3 mm. Although, at times the internal pattern represented a predominantly solid appearance, some acoustic enhancement was always demonstrated. In such cases, ballotement through the abdominal wall caused movements of the echoes, confirming the liquid mass. Most of the ovarian endometriomas were positioned medially or retrouterine. A well-demarcated separation between the endometrioma and the normal adjacent ovarian stroma was detected ultrasonically and proven surgically in 43.7% of cases.

Endometrioma was confused morphologically for an acute hemorrhagic cyst in seven patients, which is not surprising because of the similar blood content. In seven patients with hemorrhagic cysts, sonography indicated endometriomas. Acute onset of the symptoms in these patients was suggestive of the hemorrhage, whereas a history of chronic pain was associated with endometriosis. In follow-up, endometriomas remained constant both in size and internal echo pattern, whereas all the hemorrhagic cysts resolved or decreased in size during the one or two ensuing cycles. Seven more false-negative cases were observed: the sonographic reports indicated five cystic teratomas and two ovarian cystadenomas.

Five false-negative cases by morphologic scoring system alone were caused by cystic teratomas in patients with partly solid appearance of endometriosis. In three patients surrounding scarification process was obvious. These structures were confused for high amplitude reflectors with acoustic shadowing typical for dermoid cysts. Two patients with ovoid, huge multilocular endometriomas were interpreted incorrectly as mucinous cystadenomas. Sonographic evaluation, whether alone or in combination with tumor markers, did not determine the exact nature of the lesion with acceptable accuracy. In one patient with ovarian cystadenocarcinoma, the septations, papillary projections and solid areas were absent. Pelvic sonography demonstrated a small unilocular cyst of 28 mm with a smooth cystic wall, containing homogeneous fluid of low echogenicity. Eight more false-positive cases were observed: the morphological scoring system indicated endometriomas in six patients with homogeneous dermoid cysts and two with cystadenomas.

Therefore, the sensitivity of vaginal sonographic characterization of ovarian endometrioma was 83.9%. Specificity and positive predictive values of this scoring system were 97.1% and 82.0%, respectively. The negative predictive value of transvaginal sonography was 97.5%.[29]

COMBINED STUDIES BY DOPPLER ULTRASOUND AND CA-125 VALUES

Even though a combination of transvaginal ultrasonography and color Doppler flow imaging may identify ovarian endometriosis with great reliability, measurement of CA-125 levels seems to enhance sensitivity of the new scoring system. CA-125 is a cell surface antigen expressed on certain cells derived from embryonic coelomic epithelium. Its measurement may aid in the diagnosis and clinical follow-up of patients with ovarian carcinoma.[30]

Elevation of CA-125 levels has been noted in patients with other benign conditions of the pelvis, such as endometriosis, myoma, adenomyosis, acute pelvic inflammatory disease and ovarian cysts.[31] The mechanism by which the elevated serum concentration of CA-125 occurs in women with endometriosis has not been clarified yet. Mc Bean and Brumstead[32] showed that the endometrium of women with advanced endometriosis represents a potential source of elevated serum levels of CA-125. Disruptions of normal barriers between the tissue and intravascular space could explain increased amounts of this antigen. A majority of studies measuring CA-125 values in patients with endometriosis have demonstrated elevation of serum CA-125 levels during menses.[33] Elevation, specifically during menses, may result from a retrograde flow and increased peritoneal inflammation, which is more pronounced than in women without disease.

It was demonstrated that screening tests based on the relationship of multiple CA-125 levels throughout the menstrual cycle are more sensitive for the detection of endometriosis than tests based on a single CA-125 level.[31] When CA-125 analysis was performed in 14 false-negatives by morphological score,[29] an increased CA-125 value was detected in nine patients. Color and pulsed Doppler showed vascularization typical for endometrioma in 13 patients: regularly separated or scattered vessels at the level of ovarian hilus with a RI between 0.40 and 0.56. The existence of notching was noticed in 10 of 14 false negatives. When serum CA-125 levels were analyzed in 16 false-positives, 14 normal results were found.[29] Color and pulsed Doppler analysis showed typical luteal blood flow in six hemorrhagic cysts. Five dermoid cysts showed no areas of vascularity, whereas two cystadenomas had a RI > 0.50. The morphological score indicated endometrioma in a patient with endometrioid cystadenocarcinoma (stage Ia). Color Doppler demonstrated massive diastolic flow and RI of 0.38, suggestive of ovarian malignancy.[29]

In 13 of 14 patients with a false-negative diagnosis by B-mode, color Doppler was decisive in definitive diagnosis when used in combined assessment for ovarian endometriosis.[29] Endometrioma supplying vessels were identified in 91 patients. The most prominent vascular area in these cystic structures was at the level of the ovarian hilus. The resistance index values measured from this location were usually greater than 0.45. Blood flow indices varied between low (RI = 0.36 to 0.40) in 5.83%, intermediate (RI = 0.41 to 0.50) in 41.75% (Figure 6.3), and high (RI = 0.51 to 0.60) in the remaining 40.77%. The total absence of blood flow was noticed in 11.65% patients. In 11 patients with inflammatory changes surrounding the endometrioma, color Doppler showed intermediate RI values (0.41 to 0.50). Moderate elevation of serum CA-125 has been observed in 63.11% of patients suffering from endometriosis. The sensitivity and specificity of preoperative CA-125 levels, using a cut-off of >35 IU/ml, were 63.10% and 83.28%, respectively, whereas positive and negative predictive values were 36.93% and 93.57%, respectively.[29]

In 104 patients, the combined scoring system resulted in suspicion for an endometrioma. A vascularized homogeneous cystic teratoma and hemorrhagic cyst caused the false-positive results. Elevated serum CA-125 levels (40 IU/ml for cystic teratoma and 42 IU/ml for hemorrhagic cyst) were seen. In both cases, color Doppler demonstrated an intermediate RI in the tumoral vessels: in the first case, within the small bulge on the lateral cystic wall (RI = 0.48) and in the second case, at the edge of inner wall of the ovarian cyst (RI = 0.45). Both ovarian tumors had a total score value of 21. One false-negative result was observed when the combined noninvasive scoring system for endometriosis indicated a corpus luteum cyst. The serum CA-125 level in this case was 28 IU/ml, whereas color Doppler had not revealed any area of angiogenesis. Sensitivity of the combined scoring system was 99.04%. Specificity and positive predictive values were 99.64% and 98.10%, respectively. The negative predictive value of the new scoring system was 99.82%.[29]

Of 103 patients, 45 were diagnosed correctly as having bilateral endometrioma. No malignancy was observed in the group of patients in which the combined score was suggestive of endometriosis.

Alcazar et al.[34] performed a similar study trying to assess the diagnostic accuracy of transvaginal sonography alone and combined with color flow velocity imaging in differentiating ovarian endometrioma from other non-endometriotic masses. Twenty-seven (32.9%) of the 82 masses were proven to be ovarian endometriomas. Morphological assessment correctly diagnosed 24 (88.9%)

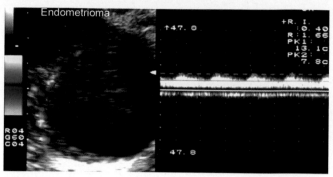

FIGURE 6.3: Pulsed Doppler analysis (right) shows low-resistance flow (RI = 0.40) when there is a hemorrhage in the menstrual phase of the cycle.

of 27 endometriomas. A typical flow pattern (pericystic flow at the level of the ovarian hilus) was present in 90.5% of endometriomas. CA-125 levels in patients with endometrioma (45.6 ± 6.3 U/ml; mean ± SEM) were significantly higher than in patients with nonendometriotic masses (26.5 ± 5.5 U/mL). The sensitivity, specificity, and positive and negative predictive values of transvaginal ultrasonography alone and combined with color velocity imaging and pulsed Doppler were 88.9%, 91%, 84.2% and 94.5%, and 76.2%, 88.9%, 82.4% and 82.4%, respectively. For CA-125 levels, using a cut-off ≥ 35 U/ml, these figures were 79.3%, 84.6%, 79.3% and 84.6%, respectively. The authors concluded that the use of color velocity imaging and pulsed Doppler does not improve the diagnostic accuracy of transvaginal ultrasound in the diagnosis of ovarian endometrioma. However, they did not perform serial ultrasound examination, vascular resistance was not related to the phase of the menstrual cycle and CA-125 levels were evaluated separately.

Aleem et al.[35] reported on the specific vascular pattern of ovarian endometrioma. Peripheral endometrioma vessels had the mean RI and PI of .59 ± 0.02 (range from 0.5 to 0.74), and 0.95 ± 0.1 (range from 0.59 to 1.59), respectively. There were no significant differences between the flow indices for ovarian endometrioma and other benign cystic lesions. Scattered hilar vascularity helps to differentiate them from other lesions of dense vascular distribution, such as corpora lutea or ovarian neoplasms. Guerriero et al[36] used the same method, transvaginal color Doppler imaging for the detection of ovarian endometrioma. They found color Doppler evaluation more accurate in the diagnosis of ovarian endometriomas than B-mode sonography. According to the logistic regression equation obtained, the probability of the presence of endometrioma varied between a minimum of 1.4% for patients with no risk factors to a maximum of 95.6% for patients with two risk factors.[36]

There were several multicentric studies on the successful use of transvaginal color and pulsed Doppler in the early detection of ovarian malignancy.[25,37,38] The most common cause of false-positive results in screening for ovarian carcinoma in premenopausal patients was ovarian endometrioma. It seems that a new scoring system for reliable detection of endometriomas can potentially reduce the number of false positives in screening programs for ovarian malignancy.[29]

At laparoscopy or laparotomy, most of the typical endometriotic lesions are surrounded by a substantial amount of blood vessels. According to the transplantation theory of Sampson,[3] viable endometrial cells that reach the peritoneal cavity by a retrograde menstruation could implant and form an endometriotic lesion. Further progression of the lesion depends on different factors, which include the hormonal, immunologic and vascular environment. Oosterlynck et al.[39] investigated the presence of angiogenic factors in the peritoneal fluid of women with endometriosis. They found that increased angiogenetic activity could be important for further outgrowth and progression of these ectopic endometrial implants. It seems that the extent of fibrosis and the presence of local hemorrhage correlate with hormonal responsiveness of these implants. The collagen layer may alter the vascularity and the diffusion of the nutrients and oxygen into the endometrioma.[40] It is possible that toxic factors within the lesion or increased pressure caused by accumulation of chocolate fluid alter the vascularity and result in impaired response to cyclic endogenous hormones.

Color Doppler ultrasound is a method of choice for noninvasive assessment of blood flow patterns in patients with ovarian endometriosis. Low impedance/high diastolic flow (RI = 0.36 to 0.40) is present during the menstrual phase of a cycle.[29] The existence of notch in such cases indicates persistence of an initial resistance from the muscular lining of pre-existing arterioles and is suggestive for benign tumors.[41] Therefore, to distinguish this condition from ovarian malignancy, a careful study of ovarian endometrioma vascularity during the late follicular phase or early luteal phase is recommended. Serial color and pulsed Doppler evaluation is useful in indeterminant cases.[29]

It is postulated that the effect of medical treatment is highly dependent on the arrival of metabolically active products via an intact blood supply. Based on our experience, varying vascularity between lesions may determine the efficacy of therapy.[29] Medical treatment of ovarian endometriomas with fibrotic plaques is never successful.[42] Intraperitoneal injection of GnRH analogs could be used successfully in patients with optimal vascular pattern. The scarification process surrounding the implants modifies the vascularization, which is possible to detect by transvaginal color Doppler. Treatment for avascular lesions must therefore be surgical removal.

A recent study of Alcazar et al.[43] correlated ovarian endometrioma vascularization with the presence of pelvic pain. Peak systolic velocity (PSV, cm/s) and pulsatility index (PI) were assessed by transvaginal color Doppler ultrasonography and CA-125 plasma concentrations were retrospectively analyzed in 74 patients who had undergone surgery for cystic ovarian endometriosis. Fifty-two patients were asymptomatic (group A) and 22 presented with pelvic pain (group B). Blood flow was found in 66.1% and 88.5% of endometriomas in groups A and B, respectively. Pulsatility index was significantly lower and CA-125 concentrations were significantly higher in group B. The authors concluded that vascularization of ovarian endometriomas in patients presenting with pelvic pain is higher than in asymptomatic patients.[43]

OVARIAN ENDOMETRIOMA ASSESSED BY 3D ULTRASOUND

Three-dimensional ultrasound is a new and emerging technology that provides additional information for the evaluation of ovarian tumors. Multiplanar and volume-rendering display combined with the ability to rotate volume data into standard orientations are essential components of the current and future success of 3D ultrasound. The surface-rendering mode allows exploration of the outer wall surface of the tumor, while combined angiographic and rendering mode allows simultaneous analysis of the morphology, texture, and vascularization.

On 3D ultrasound scan, ovarian endometrioma presents with homogeneous high-level internal echoes, some blood clots within the "chocolate" paste-like fluid and regular echogenicities at the periphery, indicative of scarification (Figure 6.4).

More recently, Guerriero et al.[44] reported that ultrasound is able to detect or exclude the presence of adhesions in patients with ultrasonographic suspicion of endometriosis. Presence of fixation of the ovary to the uterus was considered characteristic of the presence of ovarian adhesions. The probability of pelvic adhesions was 74%, and was increased to 96% when fixation of at least one ovary to the uterus was present and fell to 27% when this ultrasonographic finding was absent.[44] Alcazar et al.[45] found that 3D ultrasound assessment of mean gray value

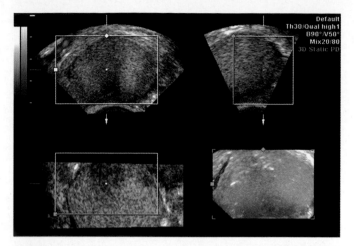

FIGURE 6.4: Three-dimensional power Doppler ultrasound of ovarian endometrioma. "Chocolate" paste-like fluid is typical for ovarian endometrioma. Note regular course of the peripheral vessels. Hyperechogenicities at the periphery are suggestive of fibrotic changes.

(MGV) may help to differentiate endometrioma from other unilocular cysts in premenopausal women because the cyst content MGV was significantly higher in endometriotic cysts. Three-dimensional sonography may also be helpful in the assessment of patients with deep and infiltrating endometriosis. Tomographic ultrasound imaging could be particularly useful for evaluation of the extension of endometriotic nodules in the rectovaginal septum, estimation of the depth of infiltration, and assessment of the relationship with the rectosigmoid junction or ureter.[46]

Three-dimensional ultrasound allows detection of the surface of the endometrioma, visualization of the preserved ovarian tissue, and assessment of the relationship with neighbouring pelvic structures. Power Doppler of ovarian endometrioma provides visualization of the scattered vascularity at the level of the ovarian hilus and detection of the regularly separated peripheral vessels. Both vascular features are typical of an ovarian endometrioma and are easily depicted by 3D power Doppler. Meticulous investigation of the ovarian lesions by 3D ultrasound reduces false-positive findings and is especially useful for the evaluation of complex ovarian lesions, such as ovarian endometriotic cysts, ovarian dermoids, fibromas and corpus luteum cysts, which may often give a wrong impression of malignancy when evaluated by conventional transvaginal sonography and color Doppler ultrasound.[47]

CONCLUSION

Transvaginal color Doppler is a promising noninvasive method for the detection of ovarian endometriosis.[29,33,35,36]

It is hoped that combined scoring systems that use both transvaginal ultrasound color flow imaging and CA-125 assessment can stand in place of laparoscopy in obvious cases. Furthermore, study of the vascularity seems to be an efficient guideline for the management of patients suffering from endometriosis.[29] Reliable blood flow analysis of the endometriotic implant has the overwhelming advantage, after which the effective treatment can be instituted. The success of medical treatment is dependent upon delivering metabolically active products via the blood supply to the endometrioma. Surrounding inflammation and scarification processes may alter the delivery of the medication. Therefore, in avascular lesions, surgical therapy should be recommended.[29]

Transvaginal color Doppler is a method of choice for the analysis of the regional blood flow in patients with adnexal masses and is complementary to laparoscopy. More recent introduction of 3D power Doppler may provide additional help in the evaluation of the ovarian endometrioma vascularization and decision making about the best treatment options available for infertile patients suffering from endometriosis. Further studies are needed to determine whether 3D ultrasound has improved clinicians' accuracy in differentiating between malignant and benign ovarian lesions, especially by reducing the false-positive findings in patients with benign conditions that may mimic ovarian malignancy.

REFERENCES

1. Flowers CE, Wilborn WH. New observation in the physiology of menstruation. Obstet Gynecol 1978;51:16-24.
2. Russel WW. Aberrant portions of the Müllerian duct found in an ovary. Johns Hopkins Hosp Bull 1899;10:8-10.
3. Sampson JA. Perforating hemorrhagic (chocolate) cysts of the ovary. Arch Surg 1921;3:245-323.
4. Ridley JH. The histogenesis of endometriosis: a review of facts and fancies. Obstet Gynecol Survey 1968;23:1-25.
5. Donnez J, Nisolle M, Casanas-Roux, et al. Endometriosis: pathogenesis and pathophysiology. In: Shaw RW (Ed). Endometriosis. Lancashire: Parthenon Publishing 1989;11-29.
6. Mahmood TA, Templeton AA, Thomson L, et al. Menstrual symptoms in women with pelvic endometriosis. Br J Obstet Gynecol 1991;98(6):558-63.
7. Fedele L, Bianchi S, Bocciolone L, Pain symptoms associated with endometriosis. Obstet Gynecol 1992;76:767-9.
8. Koninckx PR, Muyldermans M, Maloman P, et al. CA-125 concentrations in ovarian 'chocolate' cyst fluid can differentiate an endometriotic cyst from a cystic corpus luteum. Hum Reprod 1992;7(9):1314-7.
9. Brosens I. Endometriosis. In: Brosens I, Wamsteker K (Eds). Diagnostic imaging and endoscopy in gynecology. London: WB Saunders Co Ltd 1997;228-43.

10. Hill ML. Infertility and reproductive assistance. In: Nyberg DA, Hill LM, Bohm-Valez M, et al. (Eds). Transvaginal ultrasound. St. Louis: Mosby Year Book 1992;43-6.

11. Barlow DH, Kennedy. Endometriosis: clinical presentation and diagnosis. In: Shaw RW (Ed). Endometriosis. Lancashire: Parthenon Publishing 1989;1-10.

12. Doddy MC, Gibbons WE, Buttram VC. Linear regression analysis of ultrasound growth series: evidence for an abnormality of follicular growth in endometriosis patients. Fertil Steril 1988;49(1):47-51.

13. Friedman H, Vogelzang RL, Mendelson EB, et al. Endometriosis detection by ultrasound with laparoscopic correlation. Radiology 1985;157(1):217-20.

14. Kupesic S, Kurjak A, Stilinovic K. The assessment of female infertility. In: Kurjak A (Ed). An Atlas of Transvaginal Color Doppler. London: Parthenon Publishing 1994;171-97.

15. Scott RB, Te Linde RW. External endometriosis: the scourge of the private patient. Ann Surg 1950;131:706-9.

16. Jenkins S, Olive DL, Haney AF. Endometriosis: pathogenic implications of anatomic distribution. Obstet Gynecol 1986;67(3):335-8.

17. Dodson MG. Infertility. In: Dodson MG (Ed). Transvaginal ultrasound. New York: Churchill Livingstone 1995;157-62.

18. Speroff L, Glass RH, Kass NG. Endometriosis and infertility. In: Speroff L, Glass RH, Kase NG (Eds). Clinical Gynecologic Endocrinology and Infertility, 4th Edition. Baltimore: Williams & Wilkins 1989;853-71.

19. Brosens IA. Classification of endometriosis revisited. Lancet 1993;341(8845):630.

20. Kupfer MC, Schwimer RS, Lebovic J. Transvaginal sonographic appearance of endometriomata: spectrum of findings. J Ultrasound Med. 1992; 11:129-32.

21. Sandler MA, Karo JJ. The spectrum of ultrasonic findings in endometriosis. Radiology 1978;127(1):229-31.

22. Coleman BG, Arger PH, Mulhern CB. Endometriosis: clinical and ultrasonic correlation. AJR Am J Roentgenol 1979; 132(5):747-9.

23. Athey A, Diment DD. The spectrum of sonographic findings in endometriosis. J Ultrasound Med 1989;8(9):487-91.

24. Goldman SM, Minkin SI. Diagnosing endometriosis with ultrasound: accuracy and specificity. J Reprod Med 1980; 25(4):178-82.

25. Kurjak A, Shalan H, Kupesic S, et al. Transvaginal color Doppler sonography in the assessment of pelvic tumor vascularity. Ultrasound Obstet Gynecol 1993;3(2):137-54.

26. Kurjak A, Jurkovic D, Alfirevic Z. Transvaginal color Doppler imaging. J Clin Ultrasound 1990;18(4):227-34.

27. Kurjak A, Zalud I, Alfirevic Z, et al. Evaluation of adnexal masses with transvaginal color ultrasound. J Ultrasound Med 1991;10(6):295-7.

28. Kurjak A, Schulman H, Sosic A, et al. Transvaginal ultrasound, color flow and Doppler waveform analysis of the postmenopausal adnexal mass. Obstet Gynecol 1992;80:917-21.

29. Kurjak A, Kupesic S. Scoring system for prediction of ovarian endometriosis based on transvaginal color and pulsed Doppler sonography. Fertil Steril 1994;62(1):81-8.

30. Bast RC, Klug TL, St John E. A radioimmunoassay using monoclonal antibody to monitor the course of epithelial ovarian cancer. N Engl J Med 1983;309(15):883-7.

31. O'Shaughnessy A, Check JH, Nowroozi K, et al. CA-125 levels measured in different phases of the menstrual cycle in screening for endometriosis. Obstet Gynecol 1993;81(1):99-103.

32. McBean JH, Brumstead JR. In vitro CA-125 secretion by endometrium from women with advaced endometriosis. Fertil Steril 1993;59(1):89-92.

33. Jager W, Meier C, Wildt L, et al. CA-125 serum concentrations during the menstrual cycle. Fertil Steril 1988;50:223-7.

34. Alcazar JL, Laparte C, Jurado M, et al. The role of transvaginal ultrasonography combined with color velocity imaging and pulsed Doppler in the diagnosis of endometrioma. Fertil Steril 1997;67:487-91.

35. Aleem F, Pennisi J, Zeitoum K, et al. The role of color Doppler in diagnosis of endometriomas. Ultrasound Obstet Gynecol 1995;5:51-4.

36. Guerriero S, Ajossa S, Mais V, et al. The diagnosis of endometriomas using colour Doppler energy imaging. Hum Reprod 1998;13(6):1691-5

37. Campbell S, Bourne TH, Reynolds K, et al. Role of color Doppler in an ultrasound based screening programme. In: Sharp F, Mason WP, Creasman W (Eds). Ovarian cancer. Biology, diagnosis and management. London: Chapman and Hall Medical 1992;237-47.

38. Kurjak A, Predanic M. New scoring system for prediction of ovarian malignancy based on transvaginal color Doppler sonography. J Ultrasound Med 1992;11(12):631-8.

39. Oosterlynck DJ, Meuleman C, Sobis H, et al. Angiogenic activity of peritoneal fluid from women with endometriosis. Fertil Steril 1993;59(4):778-82.

40. Metzger DA, Szpk CA, Haney AF. Histologic features associated with hormonal responsiveness of ectopic endometrium. Fertil Steril 1993;59(1):83-8.

41. Fleischer AC. Color Doppler sonography of benign and malignant pelvic masses: the spectrum of findings. In: Kurjak A, Fleischer AC (Eds). Doppler Ultrasound in Gynecology. Lancshire, London: Parthenon Publishing 1998;27-37.

42. Malinak LR, Wheeler JM. Combination medical-surgical therapy for endometriosis. In: Shaw RE (Ed). Endometriosis. Lancshire, London: Parthenon Publishing 1990;85-91.

43. Alcazar JL. Transvaginal colour Doppler in patients with ovarian endometriomas and pelvic pain. Hum Reprod 2001;16(12): 2672-5.

44. Guerriero S, Ajossa S, Garau N, et al. Diagnosis of pelvic adhesions in patients with endometrioma: the role of transvaginal ultrasonography. Fertil Steril 2010 in press.

45. Alcazar JL, Leon M, Galvan R, et al. Assessment of cyst content using mean gray value for discriminating endometrioma from other unilocular cysts in premenopausal women. Ultrasound Obstet Gynecol 2010;35(2):228-32.

46. Guerriero S, Alcazar JL, Ajossa S, et al. Three-dimensional sonographic characteristics of deep endometriosis. J Ultrasound Med 2009;28(8):1061-6.

47. Kurjak A., Kupesic S, Anic T, et al. Three-dimensional ultrasound and power Doppler improve the diagnosis of ovarian lesions. Gynecol Oncol 2000;76(1):28-32.

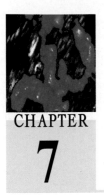

S Kupesic Plavsic, A Kurjak, K Baston

CHAPTER 7

Pelvic Inflammatory Disease

Pelvic inflammatory disease (PID) is defined as inflammation of the uterus, fallopian tubes and ovaries, caused by the ascending spread of microorganisms (unrelated to pregnancy or surgery) from the vagina or cervix. This serious complication of sexually transmitted bacterial infection can lead to infertility, ectopic pregnancy and chronic pelvic pain. It is estimated that in the USA, 10 to 15% of women of reproductive age have had at least one episode of PID. Each year almost 1,000,000 new cases develop.[1] About 30% of infertility and 50% of ectopic pregnancies are attributed to PID.[1] Every year about 50,000 surgeries are performed for PID as a primary indication. Nearly 40,000 ectopic pregnancies each year are attributed to PID and only 50% of these women will become pregnant again.[2,3] It has been reported that pregnancies, following PID, have an increased incidence of an adverse outcome.[4]

Sexually active adolescents are at the greatest risk for PID. Other risk factors include multiple sex partners, a high number of sex partners throughout life, use of an intrauterine device (IUD), untreated infected male sex partner(s), history of previous PID and frequent vaginal douching. PID causes significant morbidity for the following three major reasons:
1. Women fail to be hospitalized when appropriate.
2. Many women receive inadequate or inappropriate antibiotic therapy.
3. The male sex partner is not treated or is treated inadequately.

TRANSVAGINAL ULTRASOUND AND COLOR DOPPLER ASSESSMENT OF PID

Although early acute PID may not have detectable signs, there is a characteristic sequence in which findings appear on transvaginal sonogram. Early on, the sonographic findings may be entirely normal, except for fluid collection in the uterine cavity or in the pelvis. Fluid in the uterine cavity may be the only sign of endometritis. As the infection progresses, an increased number of changes occur in the pelvic organs with characteristic sonographic features. Visualization of the fallopian tubes greatly improves the accuracy of the diagnosis. If there is significant fluid accumulation in the pelvis, the fallopian tubes are readily visualized thus, proving the diagnosis of PID. Hyperemia, swelling and tortuosity of the fallopian tubes, together with purulent exudate from the tubal lumen and serosal surface of the tubes are the main characteristics of acute PID. In this phase of the disease, the tubal walls are thick and incomplete septations are seen. Low-level echogenic fluid, representing purulent exudate, may also be seen within the thickened tube. Sometimes fluid levels are noted during ultrasound examination. Table 7.1 presents an algorithm for diagnosis of the pelvic inflammatory disease using clinical signs, ultrasound and color Doppler findings.

The typical sonographic image of salpingitis, with evidence of tubal wall thickening and central hyperechoic mucosa with or without low-level echo-filled lumen, should not be confused with a sonographic image of appendicitis.

During the early phase of PID, blood vessels within the tubal wall are easily identified by color Doppler ultrasound. The ovaries are enlarged, globular and usually contain multiple cystic structures, representing the infected follicles (Figure 7.1). The margins may be indistinct due to the accompanying perio-ophoritis.

Since an inflammatory process in the pelvis may affect ovarian blood flow, many studies have been undertaken to assess blood flow changes during the course of PID.[1] Ovarian blood flow changes due to its proximity to the

TABLE 7.1: Diagnostic algorithm for diagnosis of the PID patients

Diagnosis	Clinical signs	Ultrasound findings	Color Doppler findings
Acute salpingitis	• Low abdominal tenderness/pelvic pain • Increased or normal body temperature • Lab findings: ESR ↑, WBC count ↑	• Tubes filled with inflammatory secretion • Tubular-shaped tubes	• Low-to-moderate resistance index (RI = 0.53 ± 0.09)
Tubo-ovarian abscess	• Low abdominal and pelvic pain • High-fever • Lab findings: ESR ↑, WBC count ↑	• Multilocular or unilocular fluid filled structure • In case of gas producing bacteria infection, air bubbles are visualized within the fluid	• Low vascular resistance signals (RI = 0.40 ± 0.08) obtained from septa or periphery of the complex adnexal mass
Chronic salpingitis	• Mild or absent symptomatology • Infertility	• "Cogwheel sign" • Distended tubes with incomplete septa • Hyperechogenic "knots" visualized every few millimeters in a transverse section	• High vascular resistance (RI = 0.71 ± 0.09) • Absence of the diastolic flow indicates irreversible scarification

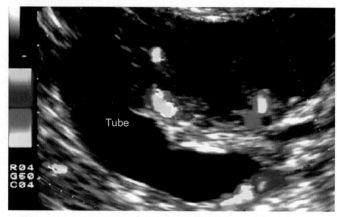

FIGURE 7.1: Transvaginal ultrasound of a complex adnexal mass, containing a sausage like structure (dilated tube) and enlarged ovary with indistinct border and fluid-filled cystic cavities. Color Doppler reveals abundant vascular signals.

tube, which is the primary focus of infection. In addition, because of its anatomical location, the ovary shares a significant part of its blood supply with the ipsilateral tube.

Our team evaluated the role of transvaginal color Doppler in the assessment of pelvic inflammatory disease.[5] One hundred and two patients were evaluated and among these, 10 were IUD-users. Uterine findings indicated ongoing inflammation in 72 (70.6%) patients. The findings included mild-to-moderate uterine enlargement, increased endometrial thickness (>12 mm) and altered echogenicity of the endometrium. The presence of endometrial fluid was associated with acute endometritis in 17 (16.7%) patients. Increased endometrial vascularity (RI = 0.50 ± 0.005) was the only uterine abnormality demonstrated in 49 (68%) patients. Sixty-six of 102 (64.7%) patients had unilateral

adnexal pathology and six of them had undergone previous contralateral salpingo-oophorectomy. The remaining 36 (35.3%) patients had bilateral adnexal pathology detected on B mode transvaginal ultrasound. Adnexal findings included enlarged ovaries, adnexal tubular anechoic structures or complex adnexal masses. All the sonographic findings were confirmed by laparoscopy. Anechoic fluid within the tube was visualized in 16 patients with hydrosalpinx. The appearance of internal echoes in the deflated tubal lumen suggested pyosalpinx and was demonstrated in six patients. A complex adnexal mass with the septations and irregular external margins, scattered internal echoes and fluid debris levels was present in 74 (72.5%) patients with tubo-ovarian abscess. As it may resemble a variety of benign and malignant adnexal conditions (tubal abortion, hematosalpinx and ovarian tumors), evaluation of clinical, biochemical, morphologic and Doppler findings enabled correct diagnosis.

Color signals were obtained from the septa or external margins in 56 (75.7%) patients presenting with complex adnexal masses. Tubal arteries were identified in 12 (54.6%) patients with tubular tubal appearance. Extensive inflammation, suppuration and subsequent adhesion formation may aggravate the identification of the tube and the ovary. Additionally, the formation of adhesions leads to a significant loss of motion and "sliding organ sign" (in the absence of adhesions and in response to the pressure by transvaginal probe, the pelvic organs move freely, while in patients with adhesions the organs move together). In 31 (41.9%) patients presenting with complex adnexal mass, the ovary could clearly be delineated from the remaining complex mass. On the contrary, the ipsilateral ovary was demonstrated in all 22 patients (100%) presenting with tubular anechoic adnexal structure. Therefore, ovarian morphology was recognized in 59 patients (55.9%), while the ipsilateral ovarian flow was altered in 50 (84.7%) of them. Free fluid in the cul-de-sac was demonstrated in 39 (38.2%) patients.

After that the patients were divided into the two groups according to their clinical presentation and histopathologic finding (acute vs. chronic), a significant difference in the tubal artery and ovarian parenchymal blood flow was observed between the groups. In the early phase of PID, ovarian parenchymal blood flow was characterized by low-to-moderate resistance to blood flow (RI = 0.53 ± 0.09) (Figure 7.2). In the chronic stage, RI was increased (RI = 0.71 ± 0.09) ($p < 0.05$) (Figure 7.3). When comparing the two subgroups presenting in the chronic stage (chronic pelvic pain and infertility cases suspected of tubal etiology), no significant difference was observed. These values of ovarian blood flow correlated with histopathologic findings. The findings obtained during the acute stage demonstrated rapidly changing patterns.[5] The ongoing vasodilatation mediated by local products of inflammation caused a decrease in RI, while the subsequent edema of the ovarian parenchyma caused an increase in the RI. As the ovarian capsule may vary in its rigidity, the intraovarian pressure was different from case to case. Adhesions and encapsulation of the ovaries affected the intensity of the intraovarian blood flow and was reflected in variable values of RI. Furthermore, fluid collection within the tubes has influenced the blood flow characteristics by compressing the vessel walls. As the process advanced, the proliferation of the fibroblasts and scar tissue formation caused the reduction of the tubal blood flow, which was demonstrated by a progressive increase in RI. Very similar results were reported by other authors.[1,6-8]

Tinkanen and Kujansu[6] examined ten patients with tubo-ovarian infectious complex. Doppler velocity waveforms were quantitated by the resistance index (RI) and pulsatility index (PI). A low-resistance blood flow was found at the margin of the infectious complex. Moderate vascular impedance (RI of 0.50) was detected in six patients during the acute or subacute phase of infection. The severity of the infection as determined by C-reactive protein values was inversely correlated to RI and PI.

Another interesting study correlated the infectious parameters (sedimentation, leukocyte count, C-reactive protein) and vascular parameters (RI and PI) during the course of PID.[9] Transvaginal color Doppler ultrasound was

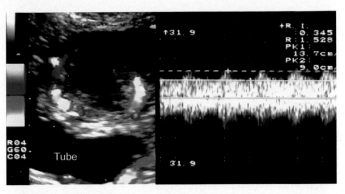

FIGURE 7.2: In the same patient as in Figure 7.1, pulsed Doppler wave form analysis shows low-vascular resistance (RI = 0.35) indicative of acute pelvic inflammatory disease.

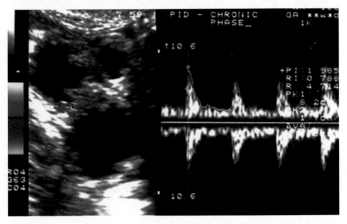

FIGURE 7.3: Moderate to high-resistance blood flow signals (RI = 0.79) are depicted from the walls of the fallopian tube in a patient suffering from infertility.

performed on days 1, 7 and 30 of the diagnosis of PID. It was demonstrated that as the infection subsided, the changes in vascular flow returned to normal values prior to the infectious parameters. Therefore, the authors of this study suggested that color Doppler ultrasound may be used to assess the regression of the infection, because Doppler parameters had better accuracy than the acute phase reactants.

Quillin and Siegel[7] used color Doppler to scan an adolescent population with ovarian masses associated with pain. They confirmed that low-resistance blood flow may be detected in various conditions, such as PID, hemorrhagic cyst and ovarian endometriosis. Therefore, Doppler parameters should always be used in the context of patient's history and clinical findings.

Tepper and coworkers[8] assessed the role of Doppler in predicting the response to antibiotic treatment in patients with PID. They analyzed 24 patients with the diagnosis of PID. Twelve patients responded favorably to the antibiotic treatment (the conservative treatment group), while the other patients showed no clinical improvement and underwent surgery (surgical treatment group). The mean resistance index in the conservative treatment group was significantly higher (0.60 ± 0.15) than in the surgical treatment group (0.52 ± 0.08, p < 0.05). The authors concluded that the decrease of the fallopian tube artery resistance index due to hyperemia and inflammation correlates well with the severity of PID.[9]

TUBO-OVARIAN ABSCESS

Tubo-ovarian abscess has variable sonographic presentations, but the underlying common appearance includes a complex cystic and solid structure, which often does not allow for distinct identification of the tube and the ovary. Tubo-ovarian abscesses may be seen in either the acute or chronic phase of the PID, although they are considered to be the hallmark of a severe acute PID episode. The continuous spillage of purulent material from the tube reaches the ovarian surface and neighboring structures (bowel and omentum). The end result is formation of an adnexal conglomerate with a complex sonographic appearance. The initial impression is that of a solid mass, but the acoustic enhancement and absence of blood flow confirm the presence of dense fluid. In patients with tubo-ovarian complex, the anatomy of the tube and the ovaries is not recognized.[10]

Tubo-ovarian abscess is demonstrated as a multilocular or unilocular large fluid-filled structure occupying the adnexa or cul-de-sac. Sometimes the two adnexa may show slightly different images as if they are out of phase. The reason for this finding is that one side was affected first, and inflammatory changes were spread later on to the other side. If gas producing bacteria are present, the image usually shows highly echogenic speckles within the abscess. As the disease advances, the tubo-ovarian abscess loses its anatomical borders and is ill-defined on transvaginal scan.

CHRONIC PID

This condition can develop either as a consequence of an acute, symptomatic infection or as a consequence of a silent asymptomatic disease in patients without any clinical evidence of salpingitis. Taipale et al.[11] have prospectively evaluated 86 patients with PID. Three months following PID, 6% of the patients exhibited a hydrosalpinx for the first time. This finding encourages clinicians to perform transvaginal ultrasound three months after the onset of the symptoms of PID.[11] The exudate from the fallopian tubes

during the acute stage of PID causes a strong peritoneal reaction. Many inflammatory cells migrate towards the affected site and start a cascade of events, resulting in the formation of pelvic adhesions and hydrosalpinx, the hallmark of chronic PID. Hydrosalpinx is formed when the fimbrial part of the tube is closed due to pelvic adhesions, resulting in accumulation of tubal mucus.

In a study of 42 women with suspected PID, Toth and coworkers[1] performed color Doppler ultrasound examination prior to diagnostic laparoscopy. Fourteen patients had negative findings, while the remaining 28 women had PID with some degree of permanent tissue damage (PID residual syndrome). The intraovarian resistance was increased in all but two patients, as indicated by a higher pulsatility index (PI) with a range of 0.9-2.8. The PI in the controls ranged between 0.4 and 1.1. The absence of significant difference in Doppler parameters may be explained by the fact that no acute PID cases were included in this study.[1]

In another observation of six patients with primary infertility, four had laparoscopically proven permanent tubal damage caused by infection ("silent PID"). They all had PI > 1.52. In the cases of acute PID, the authors found that the ovarian resistance indices varied between non-detectable and high-resistance values.[1]

Sonographic appearance of hydrosalpinx differs depending on the stage of the disease. During the acute phase, the tubal wall is thick and tender to the probe touch, while in the chronic phase, hydrosalpinx shows thin and nontender walls[10]. Chronic hydrosalpinx is usually discovered accidentally on a routine transvaginal scan or during an infertility procedure. The patients are often unaware of their pelvic pathology but can recall an episode of pelvic pain or overt pelvic inflammation. Sometimes, fibrotic remnants of endosalpingeal tissue form strings. When viewed on cross-sectional examination, these tubes resemble a cogwheel, and thus "the cogwheel sign" is considered to be an ultrasound marker of hydrosalpinx.[12] When viewed longitudinally, these fibrous strings look like knots tied every few millimeters along the tubal wall, mimicking a "beads on a string" appearance, another ultrasound sign of hydrosalpinx (Figure 7.4).[13]

Hydrosalpinx can occasionally be mistaken for a parovarian cyst, although it is usually easily recognized by its tubular shape, folded configuration and short linear echoes protruding into the lumen. A fluid filled tube is easily differentiated from the bowel loops by the lack of peristalsis. Sometimes, a tubular anechoic structure can confuse the ultrasonographer. Color Doppler imaging is of

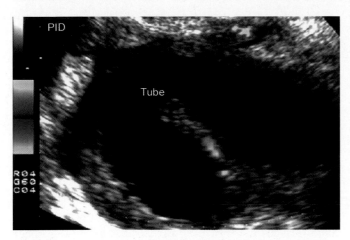

FIGURE 7.4: Complex adnexal mass with thick vascularized pseudosepta. The scarring process causes alteration of the blood flow.

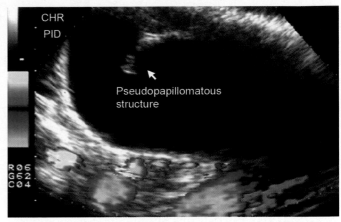

FIGURE 7.5: Color Doppler image of the avascular pseudopapillomatous structure protruding into the tubal lumen. This finding suggests chronic pelvic inflammatory disease.

great help in these cases and usually solves the diagnostic problem. The absence of blood flow on color Doppler helps to differentiate hydrosalpinx from a large blood vessel.

Color Doppler studies showed that in most cases hydrosalpinx is characterized by the lack of blood flow on color Doppler imaging.[13,14] The ovarian parenchymal blood flow is almost invariably decreased, while the ovarian volume is normal or increased.

Since blood flow indices assessed by color Doppler ultrasound change with the progression of the disease and introduction of the antibiotic treatment, it is recommended to use this method for diagnosis and follow-up of the patients with PID. Our data indicate that in patients with successful antibiotic treatment (36 (48.65%) patients) adnexal blood flow indices return to normal values.[5]

Color Doppler ultrasound is also very useful in differentiating hydrosalpinx from the dilated veins in patients suffering from pelvic congestion syndrome or pyosalpinx from hematosalpinx in patients with ectopic pregnancy.

As the inflammation may mimic a wide variety of findings and sometimes may even suggest malignancy, serial assessment by transvaginal color Doppler ultrasound is recommended. Serial examination demonstrates morphologic changes, as well as variation in blood flow intensity according to the stage of the PID. Doppler studies may be particularly useful in the assessment of the patients with chronic stage of PID who present with complex adnexal masses, thick and incomplete septations and pseudopapillomatous lesion, which may morphologically suggest ovarian or tubal malignancy (Figure 7.5). The absence of blood flow and/or high vascular resistance,

typical for this stage, helps to differentiate chronic PID from the adnexal malignancy (Figure 7.6). During the acute stage of PID, low vascular resistance is associated with typical clinical and laboratory findings (high sedimentation rate, C-reactive protein, etc.). Serial B mode and color Doppler ultrasound examinations reveal the morphological and hemodynamic changes that correlate with the pathophysiology of the pelvic inflammatory process.

In patients with tubo-ovarian abscess, abscess drainage under transvaginal sonographic guidance can hasten the recovery process and improve the efficacy of the antibiotic therapy.[15,16] Addition of the color Doppler imaging facilitates visualization of the large pelvic vessels and thereby may reduce the complication rate of the drainage procedure. Careful clinical examination, ultrasound

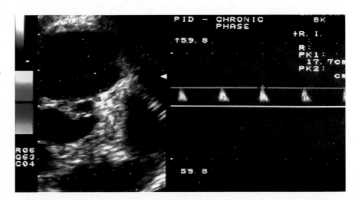

FIGURE 7.6: Complex adnexal mass with thick vascularized septa (left). The area resembles ovarian tissue undergoing extensive scarring. Absent diastolic flow (RI = 1.0) (right) is detected in the ovary of the women with laparoscopically proven chronic salpingitis.

evaluation and blood tests are required before performing the procedure to avoid the propagation of infection.

Initial results by Kupesic et al.[5] and Tinkanen et al.[6] were confirmed by other authors.[17,18] Using color Doppler ultrasound Zalel et al.[17] evaluated 25 patients with adnexal masses. Significantly higher-resistance index values were obtained at the periphery of hydrosalpinx (0.75 ± 0.04), than from the tubo-ovarian abscess (0.44 ± 0.04; P < 0.0001).[17]

It has been demonstrated that transvaginal power Doppler sonography may assist in the diagnosis of PID.[18] Molander et al.[18] evaluated 30 patients with clinically suspected acute PID. Laparoscopy confirmed the diagnosis of PID in 20 (67%) patients. Specific ultrasound findings, such as wall thickness > 5 mm, cogwheel sign, incomplete septa and the presence of fluid in the cul-de-sac discriminated women with acute PID form the patients with hydrosalpinx. Power Doppler ultrasound revealed hyperemia in all the patients presenting with acute PID, but in only two women with hydrosalpinx. Pulsatility indices were significantly lower in the acute PID group than in the control group (0.84 ± 0.04 vs 1.50 ± 0.10; P < 0.01).[18] According to these data, power Doppler was 100% sensitive and 80% specific in the diagnosis of PID, reaching the overall accuracy of 93%. Application of B mode and color/power Doppler ultrasound assists in the clinical diagnosis of PID and allows simple classification of the severity of the disease.

Evaluation of tubal patency is the next step in patients with a history of previous PID, infertility, or ectopic pregnancy. Hysterosalpingosonography with isotonic saline or positive contrast media seems to be the method of choice in a variety of clinical cases. For more information concerning this technique, the interested reader is referred to the chapter on "Hystero-Contrast-Salpingography".

THREE-DIMENSIONAL ULTRASOUND

Three-dimensional (3D) ultrasound and multiplanar view may help in the spatial delineation of inflammatory conglomerates. Any scanned volume can be rotated in all dimensions and thus it is possible to observe the borders of tissues and organs. By conventional B-mode ultrasound, hydrosalpinx can sometimes be mistaken for a multilocular cyst, but when 3D ultrasound is applied, the true spatial position of the ovary and the tube are clearly visible. By using 3D volume sections it is possible to visualize the tortuous structure and contiguous spread of hydrosalpinx[19] (Figure 7.7). Three-dimensional ultrasound enables the three perpendicular planes to be visualized simultaneously.

By moving the cursor, the sonographer "sees through" the slices of the hydrosalpinx. Another useful mode is the so-called niche mode that enables the "cut-into" view of a certain tissue. With the use of this mode we can demonstrate the spatial anatomic orientation of hydrosalpinx, and at the same time visualize the lumen. Furthermore, incomplete septations and pseudopapillomatous structures within the tubal lumen can be better assessed. The surface of the papillary protrusions can be thoroughly scanned by surface mode and its subtype "X-ray mode".[19] When applying this mode, the spaces that appeared anechoic on the conventional ultrasound scan are even darker, while the echoic tissues are shown lighter, so that the whole image gains more sharpness and contrast.

Inflammatory conglomerates pose a significant diagnostic problem to the ultrasonographer. Inflammatory conglomerates may form a tubo-ovarian abscess or remain encapsulated by two sheets of the peritoneum in the retrouterine space.[19] Because of increased echogenicity and low vascular resistance assessed by color Doppler ultrasound, these structures can be mistaken for a malignant lesion.

Halperin et al.[20] have studied 173 patients (42 women with clinical and sonographic evidence of tubo-ovarian abscess and 121 patients with PID) to define the predictors discriminating between the patients with tubo-ovarian abscess and those with non-tubo-ovarian abscess PID on the day of admission to the hospital. It seems that

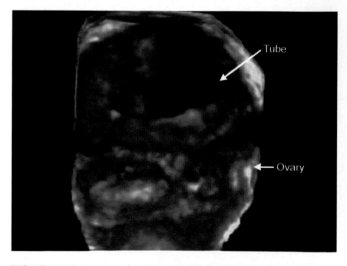

FIGURE 7.7: A case of a distended fallopian tube in an infertile patient. The ovary containing a preovulatory follicle is clearly separated from the occluded tube. This is an illustrative example of how surface rendering defines spatial relations of a tubal lesion with a nearby ovary.

parameters obtained by transvaginal ultrasound can be used as predictor of tubo-ovarian abscess and prolonged hospital stay.

Assessment of the vascularity by 3D power Doppler ultrasound and 3D color histogram may further improve our understanding of the hemodynamic changes during the course of PID. The vascularity index (VI) measures the number of color voxels in the cube, representing the vessels in the tissue. The flow index (FI), a mean color value of all blood flow or induced flow intensities, represents the intensity of flow at the time of 3D sweep. These indices assist in quantification of the blood flow and may differentiate the phases of the inflammatory process. The changes caused by vasodilatation or those influenced by a scar tissue formation can be better understood and more objectively evaluated.

CONCLUSION

B mode, color Doppler and 3D ultrasound are useful tools in the diagnosis and follow-up of the patients with PID. These modalities help to differentiate between the dilated vessels and fluid filled tubes and may assist in the diagnosis of tubo-ovarian abscess. Measurement of the intra-ovarian and tubal arterial blood flow reveals rapidly changing patterns of pelvic inflammatory disease. Low vascular impedance blood flow signals are obtained during the acute phase of PID. An increased resistance to blood flow during the chronic phase is most likely related to extensive scarring. This condition of reduced perfusion may have long-term effects on the endocrine function of the ovary.

The introduction of 3D ultrasound technology enables better spatial delineation of the inflammatory conglomerates. It was demonstrated that this modality reduces the rate of false negative findings obtained by conventional B-mode ultrasound (for example, patients with hydrosalpinx whose adnexal finding was mistaken for a multilocular ovarian cyst). Calculation of 3D color histogram indices may improve a clinician's ability to distinguish the phase of the inflammatory process.

REFERENCES

1. Toth M, Chervenak FA. Infection as the cause of infertility. In: Kupesic S and De Ziegler D (Eds). Ultrasound and Infertility. London: Parthenon Publishing 1999;205-14.
2. Cates W, Wasserheit JN. Genital chlamydial infections: Epidemiology and reproductive sequelae. Am J Obstet Gynecol 1991;164:1771-81.
3. Sweet RL, Blankfort-Doyle M, Robbie MO, et al. The occurrence of chlamydial and gonococcal salpingitis during the menstrual cycle. JAMA 1986;255(15):2062-4.
4. Westrom L. Incidence, prevalence, and trends of acute pelvic inflammatory disease and its consequences in industrialized countries. Am J Obstet Gynecol 1980;138:880-92.
5. Kupesic S, Kurjak A, Pasalic L, et al. The value of transvaginal color Doppler in the assessment of pelvic inflammatory disease. Ultrasound Med Biol 1995;21(6):733-8.
6. Tinkannen H, Kujansuu E. Doppler ultrasound findings in tubo-ovarian infectious complex. J Clin Ultrasound 1993;21(3):175-8.
7. Quillin SS, Siegel MJ. Transabdominal color Doppler ultrasonography of the painful adolescent ovary. J Ultrasound Med 1994;13(7):549-55.
8. Tepper R, Aviram R, Cohen N, et al. Doppler flow characteristics in patients with pelvic inflammatory disease: Responders versus nonresponders to therapy. J Clinical Ultrasound 1998;26(5):247-9.
9. Alatas C, Aksoy E, Akarsu C, et al. Hemodynamic assessment in pelvic inflammatory disease by transvaginal color Doppler ultrasonography. Eur J Obstet Gynecol Reprod Biol 1996;70(1):75-8.
10. Timor-Tritsch IE. Adnexal Masses. In: Goldstein SR and Timor-Tritsch IE (Eds). Ultrasound in Gynecology. Churchill Livingstone Inc 1995;103-14.
11. Taipale P, Tarjanne H, Ylostalo P. Transvaginal sonography in suspected pelvic inflammatory disease. Ultrasound Obstet Gynecol 1995;6(6):430-4.
12. Timor-Tritsch IE, Rottem S, Lewitt N. The fallopian tube. In: Timor-Tritsch IE, Rottem S (Eds). Transvaginal Sonography, 2nd edn. New York: Chapman and Hall 1991;131-44.
13. Hata K, Makihara K, Hata T, et al. Transvaginal color Doppler imaging for hemodynamic assessment of reproductive tract tumors. Int J Gynaecol Obstet 1991;36(4):301-8.
14. Fleischer AC, Rogers WH, Rao BK, et al. Transvaginal color Doppler sonography of ovarian masses with pathological correlation. Ultrasound Obstet Gynecol 1991;1(4):275-8.
15. Teisala K, Heinonen PK, Punnonen R. Transvaginal ultrasound in the diagnosis and treatment of tubo-ovarian abscess. Br J Obstet Gynaecol 1990;97(2):178-80.
16. Kuligowska E, Keller E, Ferrucci JT. Treatment of pelvic abscesses: Value of one-step sonographically guided transrectal needle aspiration and lavage. AJR Am Journal of Roentgenol 1995;164(1):201-6.
17. Zalel Y, Soriano D, Lipitz S, et al. Contribution of color Doppler flow to the ultrasonographic diagnosis of tubal abnormalities. J Ultrasound Med 2000;19(9):645-9.
18. Molander P, Sjoberg J, Paavonen J, et al. Transvaginal power Doppler findings in laparoscopically proven acute pelvic inflammatory disease. Ultrasound Obstet Gynecol 2001;17(3):233-8.
19. Kurjak A, Kupesic S, Zodan T. Three-dimensional ultrasound and the Fallopian tube. In: Kurjak A, Kupesic S (Eds). Clinical application of 3D sonography. London, New York: Parthenon Publishing Group 2000;43-54.
20. Halperin R, Svirsky R, Vaknin Z, et al. Predictors of tubo-ovarian abscess in acute pelvic inflammatory disease. J Reprod Med 2008;53:40-4.

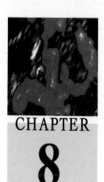

CHAPTER

8

Endoscopic Surgery in Gynecology

*V Sparac, A Kurjak, I Bekavac,
S Kupesic Plavsic*

INTRODUCTION

During the last two decades endoscopic surgery has played very important role in the process of development of gynecologic surgery. Endoscopy has oriented gynecologic care toward minimally invasive treatment that preserves forms while restoring function. This approach permits diagnoses and treatments that were previously unavailable except by massive compromise of body integrity.

There are many obvious advantages of endoscopic surgery over classical approach (Table 8.1).

With regard to enhanced surgical benefits and decreased morbidity, endoscopy may in many cases be viewed as a preferable option to laparotomy. Generally, the choice of an endoscopic route means a shorter recovery period, outpatient management and decreased costs.[1] Furthermore, early ambulation in endoscopy leads to fewer respiratory and thromboembolic complications. The typical gynecologic patient undergoing operative endoscopy will most probably return to work in several days. A similar procedure by laparotomy means about four weeks of convalescence. The endoscopic procedure permits the modern woman to minimize the disruption to her life from gynecologic disease.

Modern endoscopic surgery is known for about one hundred years, although first attempt to illuminate inside the body can be find since the era of Hippocrates.[2] During the last two decades, endoscopy has passed transformation from mainly diagnostic procedure to therapeutic surgical technique, which is capable to treat the most of the benign gynecological diseases and some of the malignant lesions.

Endoscopic procedures in gynecology are divided into two main categories: laparoscopy and hysteroscopy (Table 8.2). Common characteristic of these two techniques is indirect visual control through the optic system with

TABLE 8.1: Advantages of endoscopic approach vs laparotomy

* Shorter time of operation
* Better visualization (magnification up to 10×)
* Better precision of procedure (less traumatic for surrounding tissues)
* Reduction of pain
* Reduction of morbidity and medication
* Faster recovery and working ability
* Reduction of scars on abdominal wall
* Reduction of treatment expenses

integrated light and camera source. Approach is different; hysteroscopy uses a physiological openings: vagina, cervix and uterine cavity (Figure 8.1), while laparoscopy demands minimal incisions in abdominal wall (Figure 8.2); Instruments are also different: hysteroscope, laparoscopic telescope, scissors, graspers, etc.

LAPAROSCOPY

The roles of diagnostic and operative laparoscopy are still interfering in modern gynecology, but tendency to implement operative procedure is more and more obvious in all kinds of gynecological pathologies.[3]

There is a huge variety of the instruments and technologic advancements in endoscopic surgery over the last decade. The current array of instruments including powerful insufflators, light sources and new generation cameras have overcome the majority of technical problems, which were limitative factors in early period of laparoscopy, allowing transformation of endoscopy from diagnostic to operative procedure.

TABLE 8.2: Endoscopic procedures in gynecology

Laparoscopy	Hysteroscopy
Ovarian cystectomy	Resection of submucosal myoma
Adnexectomy	Removal of uterine polyps
Salpingectomy	Incision of uterine septa
Oophorectomy	Removal of retained IUD
Lysis of adhesions	Lysis of intrauterine synechia
Tubal reconstruction	Endometrial ablation
Treatment of ectopic pregnancy	
Treatment of endometriosis	
Sterilization	
Myomectomy	
Hysterectomy	
Presacral neurectomy	
Uterosacral nerve interruption	
Retroperitoneal dissection	

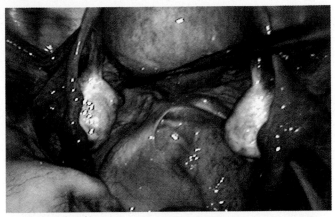

FIGURE 8.2: Laparoscopic view of the female pelvis and pelvic organs.

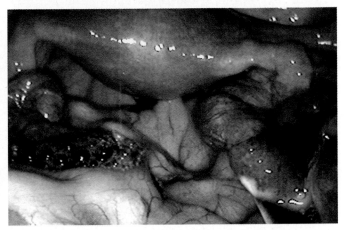

FIGURE 8.3: Diagnostic laparoscopy in an infertile patient. Normal fallopian tube patency is detected following contrast injection.

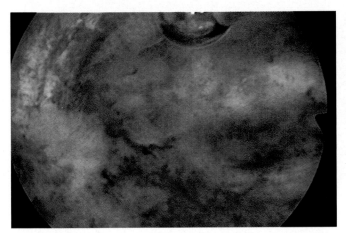

FIGURE 8.1: Uterine cavity view through the diagnostic hysteroscope.

Diagnostic laparoscopy plays an important role in the detection of acute and/or unclear clinical status in gynecology (for example, evaluation of a patient presenting with chronic pain without pathological substrate) (Table 8.3). Today, all the emergency departments include diagnostic laparoscopy as a standard procedure for the evaluation of the patients with unclear diagnosis (Figure 8.3).

TABLE 8.3: Indications for diagnostic laparoscopy

Abdominal and pelvic pain
Suspect adnexitis
Infertility
Congenital anomalies
Endometriosis
"Second look" after the previous therapy of:
– Malignant disease
– Endometriosis

If necessary during the same act it is possible to transform a diagnostic procedure into the operative and cure the patient at the same time.

Operative laparoscopy has become a golden standard for the treatment of the benign tumors and tumor-like changes, as well as for the management of infertility (Table 8.4).

Treatment of malignant gynecologic diseases by laparoscopy is still controversial. Obviously, the most experienced surgeons are capable to perform lymphadenectomy during the laparoscopic procedure, but the real cost-benefit of these procedures has to be analyzed. A paucity of prospective, randomized studies prevents a definitive answer, which technique, laparoscopy or laparotomy is superior for the efficient treatment of an oncologic female patient.

Recent development of robotics contributed to better visualization and precision of the most demanding

TABLE 8.4: Indications for operative laparoscopy

Benign ovarian tumors (cystic and solid)
Ectopic pregnancy
Sterilization
Periadnexal adhesions
Ampular tubal occlusion
Endometriosis
Drilling of polycystic ovaries
Myomectomy
Laparoscopic (LH) or laparoscopic assisted vaginal hysterectomy (LAVH)
Chronic pelvic pain (uterosacral nerve ablation/presacral neurectomy)

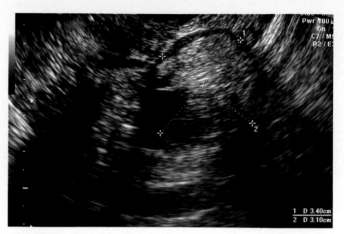

FIGURE 8.4: Transvaginal ultrasound scan of a dermoid cyst. Note the complex hyper and hypoechogenic intratumoral content.

minimally invasive procedures.[4] Even more, robotic remote control operation allows the application of real telemedicine, what literally means executing surgical procedure with the remoteness of thousands of miles between the surgeon and the patient.

Contraindications for laparoscopy are few and are divided in absolute and relative ones (Table 8.5).

Intra-abdominal bleeding is not contraindication per se for laparoscopy, especially, if the surgeon is skillful and has a potent suction/irrigation system. However, in hemodynamically instable patients, increase of intra-abdominal pressure and continuation of bleeding during the suction of blood may be fatal.

Previous abdominal surgery is not contraindication for laparoscopic procedure, but every patient has to be reevaluated according to the type of previous operation, abdominal wall scar and risk of bowel adhesion formation.[5]

Pregnancy is a relative contraindication because gravid uterus becomes too large for successful exposure of the adnexa and the risk of laceration of the uterus with trocars is increasing with ongoing weeks of pregnancy.

Properly performed "preoperative assessment" is necessary to achieve all the advantages of minimal invasive surgery. Ultrasound as a noninvasive technique has proved itself as one of the most important procedures in diagnostic process.

According to their ultrasound characteristics, the ovarian tumors are divided into cystic, cystic-solid, solid-cystic and solid tumors. Each of these characteristics has relative specificity in differentiation of the ovarian lesion and should be valued within the framework of other clinic findings.

Transvaginal ultrasound is capable to differentiate cystic from solid masses and categorize cystic masses by visualization of internal morphological characteristics (Figure 8.4). These morphological characteristics according to the ultrasonic pattern are further categorized in septations, loculations, solid lesions, papillae, daughter cysts and liquid phase. A statistically significant correlation is found between the ovarian malignancy and presence of the sonographic ovarian lesions, such as papillae, solid components ($p < 0.001$) and thick septa ($p < 0.003$).[6]

Further improvement has been made with the introduction of color and pulsed Doppler ultrasound. Arrangement of pre-existing blood vessels inside and around the tumor(s), type of branching of tumoral microcirculation and analysis of Doppler patterns are parameters, which are developed for this method with the purpose to better differentiate benign from malignant neoplasms (Figure 8.5). Sensitivity and specificity of sonographic evaluation are increased by adding the information on the lowest vascular resistance index (RI) or pulsatility index (PI) to morphological analysis of the ovarian lesion.

Doppler characteristics of benign ovarian tumors are pre-existing vascularization with one or two afferent vessels, regular branching (arborization) of the arteries and arterioles, resistance index (RI) over 0.42 and pulsatility index (PI) over 1.00.

Vascularization of malignant ovarian masses is characterized with blood flow with RI of 0.42 at the base

TABLE 8.5: Contraindications for laparoscopic procedure

Absolute	Relative
Massive intra-abdominal bleeding	Excessive obesity
Hemodynamic shock	Large abdominal tumors
Acute ileus	Pregnancy (> 16 weeks)
Extensive intra-abdominal adhesions	
Decompensate cardiorespiratory disease	

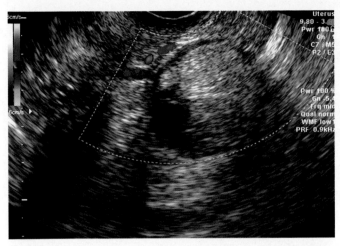

FIGURE 8.5: Color Doppler analysis of the cystic tumor from Figure 8.4. Note the lack of any intratumoral vascularization, typical for dermoid cyst.

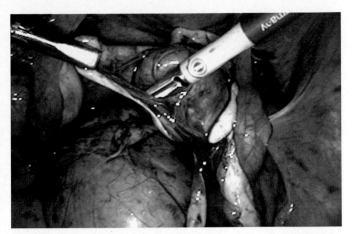

FIGURE 8.6: Cautious extirpation of intact ovarian cysts from the right ovary.

of the papillae, within the septa and/or in the solid part of an ovarian mass.

Cystic structures in the adnexal region necessarily may not belong to the ovary itself. Paraovarian cysts, peritoneal inclusion cysts, occluded tubes and other tubo-ovarian tumors may be visualized separately from the ovary, which may help to distinguish them from the ovarian tumors.

Three-dimensional (3D) ultrasound is a new technology that provides additional information for the evaluation of gynecological tumors. Recent technological advances, such as 3D power Doppler may aid in early identification of abnormal vascularity and architecture. While 2D color Doppler ultrasound is useful in detecting the pre-existing vessels and neovascular signals, 3D power Doppler ultrasound is an excellent tool for the evaluation of the vascular morphology. The addition of 3D power Doppler provides a new tool for measuring the quality of the ovarian tumor vascularity. Thus, this modality may assess the ovarian tumor microcirculation anatomy and speed up the entire patient management process.[4]

LAPAROSCOPY OF ADNEXAL LESIONS

Ovarian Cysts and Solid Tumors

Laparoscopic treatment of ovarian cystic tumors is a well established routine procedure, and, indeed, we live and practice during the endoscopic era, meaning that reservation about the practical use of this technique is not any more actuelle.[8] The fact that incidental rupture of undetected stage I ovarian carcinoma is changing the stage from Ia to

Ic was the prime argument against laparoscopic treatment of ovarian cysts.[9] Factors predictive for relapse of the ovarian cancer are grade, dense adherence and large volume ascites, whereas cyst rupture, capsula penetration, bilaterality and tumor size do not seem to be predictive for recurrence.[9] According to these results cyst rupture does not disseminate the disease or worsen the prognosis. Of course, concerns about the failure to diagnose ovarian cancer preoperatively and during the procedure has the highest priority in planning the surgical procedure. Detailed preoperative evaluation, including assessment of tumor markers, is a diagnostic imperative.[10]

During the laparoscopic procedure, it is important to visually detect suspicious locations on the cystic walls or intracystic growths. The suspicious structures should be sent for emergency histopathological analysis so called "frozen section." With this kind of the approach, we can maximally reduce the risk of the incompetent treatment of a malignant disease. If the proper preoperative evaluation is done (bimanual check-up, tumor markers, transvaginal sonography with color Doppler and more recently three-dimensional power Doppler ultrasound), and surgical procedure is properly conducted (Figure 8.6), the risk of malignant ovarian neoplasms is estimated to less than 1%.[11,12] However, all intact tumors should be extracted by an endo-bag, which prevents unintentional spillage of a liquid content.

Procedure with solid tumors and cystic-solid tumors (for example, fibromas and dermoid cysts) should follow the same protocol, but extraction of the solid tumors in toto may be problematic without the morcellation. In these cases, it is recommended to use leiomyoma morcellating device.

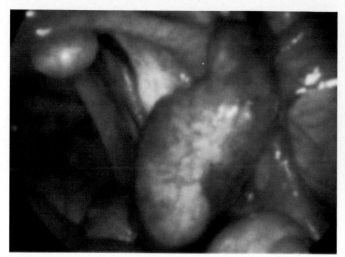

FIGURE 8.7: Ectopic pregnancy in the ampular region of the fallopian tube.

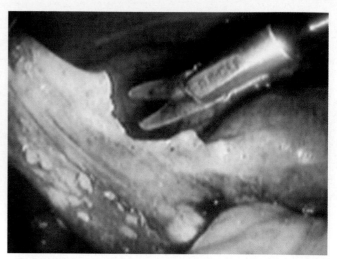

FIGURE 8.8: Detachment of the isthmic portion of the fallopian tube.

Ectopic Pregnancy

Laparoscopy has become a "golden standard" procedure for the treatment of the ectopic pregnancy (Figure 8.7). Laparoscopic procedure leads to short hospitalization, fast recovery, reduction of morbidity and costs and high fertility rates following linear salpingostomy.[9,10] However, surgical success depends on the experience of the surgeon. Following conservative laparoscopic treatment of ectopic pregnancy Bruhat et al, reported 67% intrauterine pregnancy rate and 12% recurrence ectopic pregnancy rate.[15] This compares favorably with the rates of intrauterine pregnancy after laparotomy with salpingectomy (54%), microsurgery (53%) and conservative treatment (64%).[15]

Lundorff et al., studied the risk of postoperative adhesion formation following salpingotomy. They randomized 105 patients with ectopic pregnancy for laparotomy or laparoscopic treatment. In 73 cases, they performed "second look" laparoscopy and found significantly more adhesion formation on the ipsilateral side in patients treated by laparotomy than by laparoscopy.[16] However, there was no statistically significant difference in tubal patency between these two groups.

Sterilization

Since mid-60s of the last century, sterilization was the first widely accepted surgical application of laparoscopy. It is very simple, safe and cost-effective procedure based on bipolar coagulation of the fallopian tubes in their isthmic region, with incision of a coagulated part to ensure the interruption of tubal integrity (Figure 8.8). Sterilization may be performed mechanically using one of the numerous types of endoclips that are available on the market today.

Salpingo-ovariolysis and Neosalpingostomy

Several studies proved laparoscopic adhesiolysis to be superior classic microsurgery. After laparoscopic treatment de novo adhesion formation is significantly reduced and less dense.[17] In review of the literature, slightly higher, but not statistically significant pregnancy rates were reported following laparoscopy.[18] Moderate increase of pregnancy rates together with decrease of the morbidity and risk of adhesion formation make laparoscopic adhesiolysis the technique of choice.

Degree of tubal damage is the most important independent prognostic factor for the rate of intrauterine pregnancy. Results of laparoscopic corrective treatment of tubal obstruction are comparable to the results of microsurgery.[19,20] A review of literature demonstrates higher, but statistically insignificant pregnancy rates after laparoscopy. However severe cases should be directed immediately to *in vitro* fertilization procedures (Figure 8.9).

Endometriosis

Resection of the endometriotic cysts and vaporization of the endometriotic nodules is the most common indication for operative laparoscopy according to the American Association of Gynecological Laparoscopists (AAGL).[8] Laparoscopy is an optimal technique for the diagnosis and treatment of all the stages of endometriosis (Figure 8.10). Combination of mechanical tools (graspers and scissors)

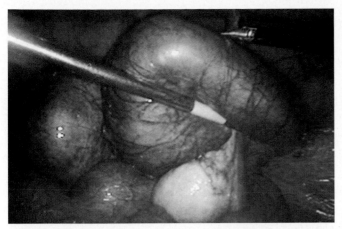

FIGURE 8.9: Severe case of sactosalpinx in a patient with the history of perforated appendix.

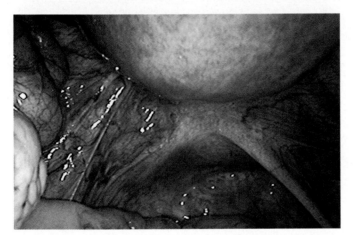

FIGURE 8.10: Subtle brownish lesions and white scars of pelvic endometriosis. Note the exaggerated vascular pattern of pelvic blood vessels as a result of endometriotic process.

allows surgeon to excise the "chocolate-like" cystic structures (Figure 8.11), and by applying different vaporization power sources (monopolar and bipolar coagulation, CO_2 laser or "harmonic knife") which destroy small lesions that can not be excised. Advantage of the laparoscopic treatment of the mild and/or moderate endometriosis is equal, or even more effective than medical treatment. Patient can plan pregnancy from the very first next cycle and does not have to wait for six months.

However, laparoscopic treatment of advanced deep infiltrating endometriosis can be technically demanding, and requires knowledge, training, skill, experience and in complicated cases of bowel and rectovaginal septum endometriosis, collaboration with abdominal surgeon. Deep infiltrating endometriosis is form of endometriotic process

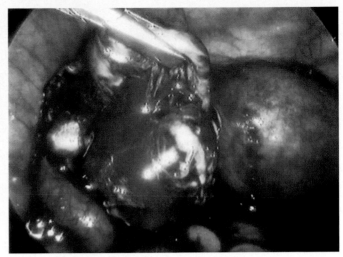

FIGURE 8.11: Chocolate-like fluid content of endometriotic cyst.

that penetrates >5 mm under the peritoneal surface. At last but not the least, well trained, motivated assistant and sophisticated equipment are very important for the success of this type of endoscopic surgery.

Needless to say, accurate preoperative diagnosis (application of transvaginal color Doppler, CA-125 and careful bimanual palpation) are of the highest priority in planning the laparoscopic procedure and follow-up of the patients with endometriosis.[21]

Polycystic Ovaries (PCO)

Polycystic ovaries are very common sonographic finding, usually combined with infertility problems. Depending on the patient's symptoms and preferences, management includes medical treatment, induction of ovulation, ovarian monopolar cautery or laser evaporization are treatment options.[22]

Advantages of the medical treatment are noninvasiveness, correction of associated problems (beneficial cosmetic effects) and possibility of multiple applications. Patients, who do not react properly to medical stimulation, may be directed to laparoscopy. There are few concerns about laparoscopic treatment of PCO patients. One should be aware that it has a temporary effect; approximately six months after the procedure patient reaches an ovulatory cycles again. Second is the risk of periovarian adhesion formation. However, it seems that deep multiple monopolar cautery incisions or laser evaporization tends to form less adhesions than ovarian wedge resection.

Conclusion

Although laparoscopy has certain technical limitations and is operator dependent, this technique has become an important part of modern gynecologic surgery. Laparoscopic surgery is sometimes time consuming, but in properly selected cases, it is not only an attractive alternative to traditional laparotomy, but has become a "golden standard" for the treatment of adnexal lesions.

In the future, we can expect miniaturization of laparoscopes and further improvement of the tools that will bring even more elegance in surgical practice and potentially broaden the indications. In this light, performance of more accurate sonographic preoperative analysis is more than welcome.

LAPAROSCOPIC MYOMECTOMY

With prevalence of about 25%, myomas are the most frequent benign genital tumors. They develop from the smooth muscle cells and may be located in any part of uterus. According to their number and location, myoma may cause a variety of symptoms. Irregular bleeding, abdominal pain and infertility are the most frequent symptoms. Preoperative assessment (bimanual examination, transvaginal ultrasound with color Doppler or 3D ultrasound) plays a crucial role in decision making, regarding the surgical approach.

Laparoscopic procedure is mostly reserved for subserosal and intramural fibroids, but even larger submucosal fibroids (larger than 5 cm), may be scheduled for this type of surgery. In case of multiple myomas, dilemma between laparoscopy and laparotomy depends on number, size and location of the fibroids, as well as on surgeon's experience.

Although number and size of fibroids suitable to be laparoscopically treated are still matter of controversies, solitary myoma larger than 12 cm or more than three fibroids larger than 5-6 cm in diameters, justify laparotomy.

Technique of laparoscopic procedure differs according to the location of fibroid. Pedunculated myomas can be easily electrocoagulated at the pedicle level or pedicle can be strangulated by an endoscopic loop. Subserosal myomas with wider basis can be coagulated and excised from the basis or surpassed by an endoloop. During the excision and coagulation of a fibroid, loop is gradually tightened around the basis.

Intramural fibroids are much more demanding. An incision is made on the thinnest serosal layer over the myoma. Once the myoma is reached, it is extracted by

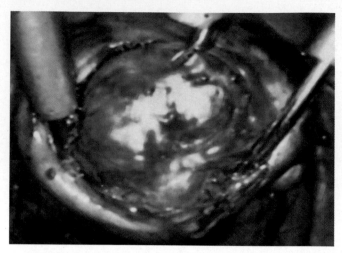

FIGURE 8.12: Extraction of the intramural myoma after incision of the fibroid's capsule.

pulling the myoma with a screw instrument and pushing the myometrial edges with graspers (Figure 8.12). Suction-irrigation instrument is often used as a blunt probe for easier dissection process. Larger blood vessels are coagulated and dissection proceeds until the complete extraction of myoma. Deep intramural defects after the extraction are approximated by intra- or extracorporeal knots.

Finally, myomas are removed from the abdominal cavity with some of the available electrically driven myomorcellators. The other possibilities include extraction through the posterior colpotomy or intra-abdominal cutting in smaller chunks and extraction with a grasper through the one of the abdominal wall incisions.

LAPAROSCOPIC HYSTERECTOMY

After the cesarean section hysterectomy is at this moment, the most frequent surgical procedure performed in women. Hysterectomy by laparotomy is performed since 19th century, while vaginal route was introduced in the beginning of 20th century. In 1988, Harry Reich described the first laparoscopic hysterectomy (LH).[23] Since then thanks to the development of a new instrumentation and increase of endoscopic knowledge, it became a standard surgical procedure.

Indications for LH are more or less the same as for laparotomy, but LH should not be a substitute for the surgeries that are carried via vagina. Laparoscopic approach to hysterectomy has the same advantages as other laparoscopic procedures. In experienced hands, it shortens the hospitalization time and reduces patients' morbidity and mortality.

According to the level at which surgery is performed, the laparoscopic hysterectomy may be divided into the:

- *Laparoscopic supracervical hysterectomy (LSH):* In which uterine corpus is laparoscopically detached, while the cervix is preserved. This surgery is performed in cases with absence of cervical pathology. Pros for this approach are preservation of the pelvic floor with preservation of bladder and rectal positions, while cons is the possibility of cervical cancer development.

- *Laparoscopic-assisted vaginal hysterectomy (LAVH):* It considers laparoscopic ligation of the vascular and detachment of the ligamentous structures above the uterine vessels. Remaining surgical procedure is performed vaginally.

- *Total laparoscopic hysterectomy (TLH):* It is performed completely via a laparoscopic route. This includes laparoscopic closure of the vaginal cuff.

There are a wide variety of approaches for laparoscopic hysterectomy that go beyond the extensity of this chapter. However, each laparoscopic technique demands a skillful and experienced endoscopic surgeon.

LAPAROSCOPY IN GYNECOLOGIC ONCOLOGY

The first role of laparoscopy in treatment of an oncologic patient was a lymph node, sampling as a part of surgical staging. Numerous studies reported a good correlation between extent of the disease according to FIGO classification and patient's prognosis.[24-31] Enabling maximal reliability with minimal of intraoperative aggressiveness surgical staging by laparoscopy became superior when compared to conservative clinical approach. When lymphadenectomy performed by laparotomy was correlated with laparoscopic approach, there was a significant difference in terms of intra- and perioperative morbidity.

In gynecologic patient, the primary metastases of endometrial, cervical and ovarian carcinoma are located in the lymph nodes from the pelvic floor to the abdominal aorta. Since the Dargent's first description of laparoscopic lymphadenectomy in 1989, laparoscopic approach was proved as a reliable diagnostic and therapeutic method. However, laparoscopy has to be critically observed in oncology, according to the possibility of tumor cell spillage and port-site metastasis, although these complications are known from the open surgery as well.[24,25]

The laparoscopic oncologic procedure seems to be safe and feasible option, with significantly lower short- and long-term complication rates than laparotomy, but has a considerable learning curve for the surgeon.

Endometrial Carcinoma

Endometrial carcinoma was the first indication where oncologic laparoscopic surgery proved itself as a valuable treatment method. As the forth most common malignant disease, it affects women mostly after the age of 50. Due to very early symptoms of irregular bleeding, about 80% of cases are diagnosed at stage I, with an excellent five-year survival of 85 to 90%.[24] Although abdominal hysterectomy with bilateral adnexectomy and lymphadenectomy used to be the gold standard for the surgical treatment of endometrial carcinoma, today many patients with stage I adenocarcinoma undergo laparoscopic surgery. After the thorough inspection of all the intra-abdominal organs and peritoneal surfaces, the procedure begins with coagulation of the fallopian tubes at the isthmic level. Extrafascially extirpated uterus with adnexa is then removed via vagina, while pelvic lymphadenectomy and para-aortic lymphadenectomy, if necessary, are completed at the end of the procedure. Alternative route is laparoscopically assisted surgical staging procedure (LASS), described for the first time by Childers and Surwit.[26] Hysterectomy is accomplished by the vaginal route with combination of laparoscopically removed lymph nodes and peritoneal washings.

Staging of the endometrial carcinoma includes assessment of the iliac (common, external, internal) and obturator lymph nodes. If the para-aortic lymph nodes are to be removed, upper border is the line of the inferior mesenteric artery.

Cervical Carcinoma

Cervical carcinoma is the second most frequent solid tumor in women under 35 years of age. Traditionally, Wertheim's radical hysterectomy was used in early stages of disease. Laparoscopic lymphadenectomy or lymph node sampling may be combined with laparoscopically assisted vaginal radical hysterectomy for patients with stages IA-IIA (Coelio-Schauta) as an alternative to classic abdominal approach.[27] Although the main portion of the laparoscopic procedure is oriented toward pelvic lymphadenectomy, radical hysterectomy may also be accomplished by laparoscopic route.

Another similar procedure is radical trachelectomy, where transvaginal amputation of the cervix and surrounding tissues is combined with laparoscopic staging of pelvic lymph nodes. Although named radical trachelectomy, the main purpose is to preserve the uterine corpus and patient's future fertility.[28] It seems that procedure of radical trachelectomy is sufficiently reliable and has similar relapse rate as radical hysterectomy.[29] However, the surgical staging (including laparoscopy) in the advanced cases of cervical carcinoma is still the matter of controversial discussions.[30]

Ovarian Carcinoma

Laparoscopy is the standard procedure for the clarification of undefined ovarian masses but treatment of ovarian carcinoma is still under the evaluation in specialized centers and clear recommendations have not been made yet. Although laparoscopy in early stages of epithelial ovarian cancer is feasible and laparoscopic comprehensive surgical staging is a valuable alternative treatment to laparotomy, there are still many questions regarding the laparoscopic treatment of advanced stages of the ovarian malignancy.

Laparoscopic procedure for surgical treatment of ovarian carcinoma is mainly indicated in two groups of patients. First group consists of patients in early stages of the disease. In these cases, complete surgical procedure may be successfully accomplished with laparoscopy. It includes aspiration of free fluid, usually bilateral adnexectomy with hysterectomy, intraperitoneal excision of all suspicious areas, omentectomy with sampling of the para-aortic and pelvic lymph nodes. This includes iliac (common, external, internal), obturator and para-aortic lymph nodes under the level of renal arteries. Second group consists of patients with previously advanced stage of ovarian malignancy, who were already treated by chemotherapy and surgery. Purpose of second-look operations in this population is to follow the effect of the therapy and eventually detect early forms of intra- or retroperitoneal metastases. Surgical procedure includes the aspiration of abdominal free fluid and thorough inspection, with possible excision of intraperitoneal structures and lymph nodes suggestive of a disease spread.

However, laparoscopy may be an induction factor for tumor spread in patients with ovarian cancer, especially for dissemination of port-site metastasis. Fortunately, recent results do not show a dramatic impact of abdominal wall metastasis on a long-term outcome.[31]

HYSTEROSCOPY

Although the first attempts to illuminate the uterine cavity began during the course of 19th century (Bozzini 1806, Pantaleoni 1869) nothing important has changed until the late 80s of the past century, when rapid technological development allowed the miniaturization of diagnostic and therapeutic instruments. Awareness about the increasing

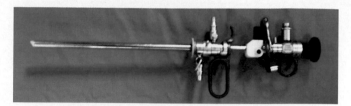

FIGURE 8.13: 8.5 mm hysteroresectoscope.

number of the uterine abnormalities and infertility problems was the main driving force for the development of diagnostic and therapeutic hysteroscopic procedures.

One of the main advantages of hysteroscopy over the other techniques of minimally invasive approach is in the use of natural openings (vagina, cervical channel, uterine cavity). This means avoidance of surgical cuttings of the abdominal wall or peripheral pelvic organs. Result of hysteroscopic surgery is express recovery within 24 hours with and literally normal working ability.

Fixed instrumentation is mainly identical to laparoscopic ones. It consists of a moveable trolley (tower) with monitor, light source (cold fountain light), endoscopic camera, monopolar/bipolar electric generator and pressure delivery system (endoscopic pump). Main difference is in the hand-hold part of the instrumentation. Hysteroscope per se is a pistol like instrument with integrated optical rod lens system, bipolar/monopolar electrode, working channel for mechanical instrument and a channel for circulation of the fluid distension media (Figure 8.13).

Hysteroscopic procedures are divided into the two main groups:
- Diagnostic hysteroscopy, and
- Operative hysteroscopy.

Overall, indications for diagnostic and operative hysteroscopy are the same (Table 8.6).

TABLE 8.6: Indications for diagnostic/operative hysteroscopy

- Uterine bleeding disorders
- Congenital uterine anomalies
- Intrauterine adhesions
- Idiopathic infertility
- Submucosal leiomyomas
- Endometrial and intracervical polyps
- Adenomyosis
- Endometrial hyperplasia
- Endometrial cancer
- Intrauterine foreign bodies (for example dislocated IUD)

Of course, hysteroscopy is still an invasive procedure, so there are few contraindications for it (Table 8.7).

TABLE 8.7: Contraindications for diagnostic/operative hysteroscopy

Absolute
- Pelvic inflammatory disease (PID)
- Pregnancy

Relative
- Severe uterine bleeding
- Positive cervical smears/acute cervicitis

Intrauterine bleeding is one of the main hysteroscopic indications but severe uterine hemorrhage can be a relative contraindication due to obscured visualization.

DIAGNOSTIC HYSTEROSCOPY

Although many physicians who are familiar with transvaginal ultrasound are relatively indifferent towards hysteroscopy, its clinical importance has increased during the course of last two decades. On the other hand, not many endoscopic surgeons are highly skilled in the ultrasound examination procedures. That results in necessity to directly visualize the problem, which has to be cured. This was the main promoting factor for further development of diagnostic hysteroscopy.

There are some pros and cons for this method. Skillful sonographer is capable to detect almost any kind of intrauterine pathology with the sensitivity of 95%.[32] In combination with hysterosonography or three-dimensional saline infusion sonography (3D SIS) sensitivity rises up to 98%.[32,33] But there are still some limitations of these noninvasive techniques. First, ultrasound cannot detect some minor, but clinically important endometrial changes, such as strawberry-like pattern of the endometrium in patients with chronic endometrial inflammation or some other causes of endometrial bleeding (Figure 8.14). Inspection of the endometrium with special attention at vascular pattern can reliably distinguish normal (functional/atrophic) from the pathologic mucosa.

"Uterine bleeding disorders" are the most frequent reason for visit to gynecologist. Routine examination includes pelvic exam and transvaginal ultrasound. Other cases with abnormal uterine bleeding (with exemption of dysfunctional uterine bleeding) require further evaluation. Fortunately, hysteroscopy has replaced D and C procedure, which used to be a golden standard for many years. The main advantages of hysteroscopy are minimal invasiveness and high sensitivity.[34]

The main reasons for abnormal uterine bleeding are:
- Submucosal myomas
- Endometrial and intracervical polyps

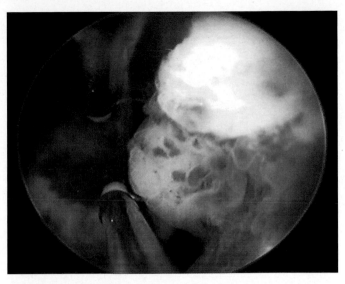

FIGURE 8.14: Strawberry-like pattern of the endometrium in a case of chronic inflammation.

- Residual placental tissue
- Atrophic endometrium
- Endometrial hyperplasia
- Endometrial cancer

Submucosal leiomyomas and polyps are elaborated in the part on operative hysteroscopy.

Detection of residual placental tissue, following the termination of pregnancy, is one of the possible applications of diagnostic/operative hysteroscopy.[35] Residual tissue is usually located in the cornual regions as a fringed-like structure and may be easily differentiated from the normal pale endometrial tissue by its brownish-violet color.

Atrophic mucosa is a physiologic state of postmenopausal endometrium and may cause postmenopausal bleeding. Lack of hormone stimulation makes the epithelial layer of the mucosa and superficial blood vessels much thinner. In combination with the lose of glandular mucosal elements, it causes uterine bleeding in up to 48% of postmenopausal women and represents the most common reason of postmenopausal bleeding.[36] Hysteroscopic image is typical: pale, very thin (usually not more than 1 mm thick) endometrium and underneath blood vessels. Due to its very high fragility, distension of the uterine cavity during hysteroscopy may cause small petechial bleedings (Figure 8.15).

Different types of endometrial hyperplasia give full spectrum of hysteroscopic findings. Hysteroscopically, it is impossible to differentiate them, so the biopsy is necessary to divide the low-risk hyperplasia from high-risk

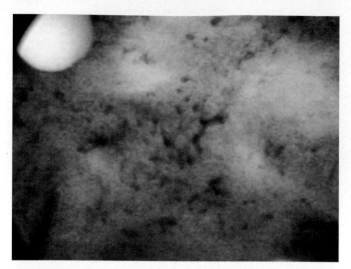

FIGURE 8.15: Petechial bleeding from atrophic endometrium.

hyperplasia. According to the established risk for endometrial carcinoma, endometrial hyperplasia without cellular atypia is a low-risk pathology (less than 2% will undergo malignant alteration), while those with cellular atypia alter in 23% of patients and are considered a high-risk atypia.[37]

Hysteroscopically, low-risk hyperplasia has some mutual characteristics:
- Increase of mucosal thickness,
- Inhomogeneous mucosal growth,
- Increased vascular pattern,
- Polypoid structures,
- Cystic irregularly located glandular elements, and
- Necrotic regions.

Whenever some of these characteristics are located, visually directed biopsy is mandatory. High-risk hyperplasia shows complex pathological vascular patterns, such as irregular course, altered arborization and cork-screw image of the vessels.

Endometrial cancer is sometimes hardly distinguishable from the benign endometrial lesions. Macroscopic characteristics of endometrial carcinoma are numerous fringe-like structures with many necrotic regions and bleeding from the irregular vessels. In early phase of the disease changes are usually located in the cornual regions.

The main advantage of diagnostic hysteroscopy is its capability of directing the endometrial sampling leading to improved precision than blind procedure of D and C. Fractioned curettage may overlook early stages of the endometrial carcinoma, smaller myomas and paradoxically larger endometrial polyps.[38]

During the work-up of infertility cases, traditional method for evaluation of the uterine cavity and tubal patency was X-ray hysterosalpingography (HSG). More recently diagnostic hysteroscopy became an alternative to HSG for detection of the uterine abnormalities. On X-ray, HSG uterine anomalies and intracavitary lesions are visualized as filling defects, what leads to a relatively high percentage (8 to 35%) of false (positive/negative) results.[39,40] However, hysteroscopy is not capable of analyzing the tubal status, so these two methods remain complementary in infertility work-up.

Sometimes foreign bodies may be "lost" within the uterine cavity. Mainly those are intrauterine devices (IUD) with too short, retroverted or broken thread. In such cases hysteroscopy may aid in directing the extraction by a mechanical grasper.

Thanks to newly developed miniature diagnostic hysteroscopes of only 3 mm, hysteroscopy has become a routine procedure in office setting. These hysteroscopes have a continuous flow circulation of saline solution and many minor surgical procedures (polypectomy, septal incision or lysis of intrauterine adhesions) can be resolved by mechanical or bipolar working elements. The size and shape of the hysteroscope is merited that patient requires no anesthesia.[41]

In conclusion, transvaginal ultrasound and diagnostic hysteroscopy are complementary methods and should be used together with purpose to reach better sensitivity and specificity of diagnostic process.

OPERATIVE HYSTEROSCOPY

Indications and contraindications for operative hysteroscopy are identical to the diagnostic ones. It should not be neglected that operative hysteroscopy, although minimally invasive has all operative and anesthesiologic risks as other procedures, so preoperative work-up and firm indication are mandatory.

Hysteroscopic Myomectomy and Polypectomy

Myomas are by far the most common benign pelvic tumors. It is estimated that fibroids can be present in up to 40% of women older than 40 years of age. Symptoms more often depend upon the location, then to the size and number of the fibroids. Although they can be located in all of the uterine layers, submucosal myomas are of the special interest for hysteroscopists. They cause a wide range of symptoms that represent indications for hysteroscopic myomectomy (Table 8.8).

TABLE 8.8: Indications for hysteroscopic myomectomy

- Hypermenorrhea
- Menorrhagia
- Metrorrhagia
- Infertility

Protrusion of myoma in the uterine cavity mostly provokes different types of abnormal bleeding (Figure 8.16). Incidence in infertility population is almost doubled in correlation with control group.[42] The mechanism of infertility and pregnancy loss for submucosal fibroids remains uncertain.

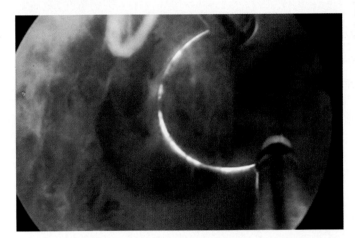

FIGURE 8.16: Submucosal leiomyoma type I before the resection procedure.

European Society of Hysteroscopy (ESH) classifies fibroids according to the level of their protrusion in the uterine cavity (Table 8.9).

TABLE 8.9: Classification of submucosal fibroids according to ESH

- **Type 0:** Fibroid is located completely in the uterine cavity, attached to the wall with tiny pedicle or very narrow basis.
- **Type 1:** Fibroid is located in the uterine cavity with more than 50% of its own volume (angle between the fibroid and uterine wall is less than 90°).
- **Type 2:** Fibroid is located in the uterine cavity with less than 50% of its own volume (angle between the fibroid and uterine wall is more than 90°).

While the submucosal myomas type 0 can be successfully resected even by a less experienced surgeon, type 2 demands large experience and meticulous preoperative assessment (precise sonographic analysis of the fibroid site, with special respect to the thickness of the underlying muscle layer). Minimal thickness of underlying muscle should be between 5-7 mm[43] (Figure 8.17).

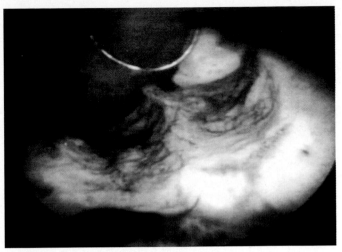

FIGURE 8.17: Intracavitary submucosal leiomyoma (type 0) during resection procedure.

One of the most important maneuvers during the resection procedure is periodic reduction of intrauterine pressure. Changes of the intrauterine pressure force the uterus to contract and result is further protrusion of the fibroid to the uterine cavity. With this hydromassage maneuver, surgeon avoids deep intramural resection and significantly reduces the perforation risk.

Maximal size of the fibroids suitable for resection is not precisely established. Hysteroscopic resection is a viable option for fibroids, measuring less that 5 centimeters but very important information is on the position of the myoma.[43] If it is located at easily approachable position, even fibroids measuring 6 centimeters may be removed by hysteroscopy. Fibroids located at the anterior and posterior uterine wall are the easiest for resection, while those located at side walls and fundal region are more complicated. The most complicated location is the cornual region due to thin wall and limited space for resection.

Efficiency of hysteroscopic myomectomy is in scale between 74-90% for bleeding disorders and 70%, respectively for infertility cases.[42,44,45]

Hysteroscopic polypectomy has almost the same principles as myomectomy, but the procedure is much easier (Figure 8.18). Working element is also the loop, but the mechanical pressure is usually enough to separate the polypoid tissue from the underlying endometrium (Figure 8.19). This is particularly important in infertility cases where introduction of electrical loop in myometrial layer could promote the formation of intrauterine adhesions. Endometrial polyps can also be resected by mechanical

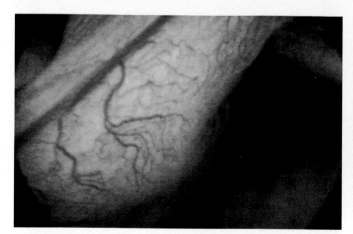

FIGURE 8.18: Endometrial polyp with regular vascular arborization pattern.

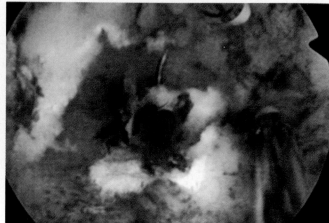

FIGURE 8.20: Incision of intrauterine adhesions in the right uterine horn.

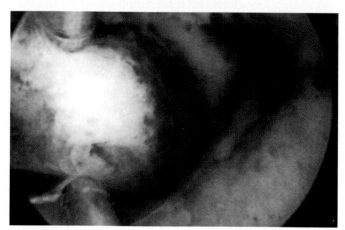

FIGURE 8.19: Mechanical pressure of the loop at the base of the pedicle of the polyp during hysteroscopic polypectomy.

hysteroscopic scissors or graspers introduced through the working channel.

Hysteroscopic Adhesiolysis

Asherman's syndrome is the formation of intrauterine adhesions or synechia with consequent hypo- or amenorrhea, dysmenorrhea and/or infertility. In some cases, obliteration of the isthmic region or internal cervical os results in hematometra and painful labor-like contractions.

Etiologically, destruction of the endometrial basal layer is responsible for the formation of the adhesions. Functional layer is fully renewable and is not prone to scarring process.

Adhesions may be caused by pyogenic endometritis or more often, vigorous curettage. Hysteroscopic myomectomy is also one of the independent risk factors. Although some studies report prevalence of up to 30% for post-operative adhesions after deeper myomectomies, it seems

that newly developed bipolar hysteroscopes significantly lower those numbers to about 7.5%.[46]

Other possible causative factors are manual removal of the placenta, operative correction of Müllerian malformations and uterine tuberculosis. Diagnosis is mainly made with transvaginal ultrasound examination or diagnostic hysteroscopy. Ultrasound usually depicts inhomogeneous endometrium at longitudinal section. Periovulatory period is the best time for examination due to proliferation and triple line appearance of the endometrium. Visualization of hyperechogenic or inhomogeneous inclusions within the hypoechoic layers of the endometrium is suggestive of fibrotic adhesions.

Tender adhesions may be easily resected during the diagnostic procedure, while rigid adhesions require operative hysteroscopy. The procedure is usually completed by scissors or mono/bipolar needle electrodes (Figure 8.20). YAG laser is another treatment option in experienced hands, but due to its expensiveness, it is not available in all endoscopic units.

In the most complicated cases, simultaneous laparoscopy is advisable to prevent perforation and bowel injury (bowels are removed away from the uterus). Reproductive outcome depends on the extent of the adhesions and volume of the reformed endometrial cavity.

Hysteroscopic Endometrial Ablation

Although development of levonorgestrel-releasing intrauterine system (LNG-IUS) during the last fifteen years has reduced the clinical significance of this procedure, prominent uterine bleeding is still an indication for endometrial ablation.[47]

After the exclusion of uterine malignancy, abnormal uterine bleeding cases are usually directed to conservative hormonal treatment. In cases with no response to conservative treatment, physician has to decide between endometrial destruction techniques and hysterectomy. Hysteroscopic endometrial ablation is one of the endometrial destruction techniques, together with radioblation, hot water and electricity. The main idea of hysteroscopic endometrial ablation is to destroy complete functional and underlying basal layer of the endometrium. Often it means a destruction of the superficial myometrial layer. However, not all the patients are suitable for this procedure. The most important demand is the absence of any premalignant or malignant mucosal changes. Contraindications are listed in Table 8.10.

Surgical techniques are different and the most utilized one is the excision of the endometrial tissue by a loop. Due to a reduced space, roller-ball electrode is a preferred method to destroy the endometrium in the cornual regions. The same outcome has been reported by the use of touch or non-touch laser.

TABLE 8.10: Contraindications for endometrial ablation

- Histologically verified premalignant/malignant changes
- Uterine cavity larger than 12 cm
- Adenomyosis
- Significantly distorted uterus due to fibroid changes
- Fertility preservation
- Other gynecological problems that require radical operative treatment

Although procedure often results with sterility, endometrial ablation is not considered a sterilization technique, so it is advisable to perform a simultaneous laparoscopic sterilization, with purpose to avoid undesired pregnancy.

Congenital Uterine Anomalies

Although congenital uterine anomalies show a wide variety of anatomical findings, the septate uterus is the most interesting one. There are the two main reasons for it: first, the highest incidence rate (8-10 times more often then bicornuate or duplex uterus) and second, this anomaly is easily correctible by hysteroscopy.[48] Congenital uterine anomalies are commonly associated with infertility problems. Septate uterus is associated with increased risk of miscarriages, preterm deliveries, anomalies of fetal position, intrauterine growth retardation and primary infertility problems. The mechanism of obstetric complications is not clearly understood because the uterine septum is not built from avascular fibrotic tissue.

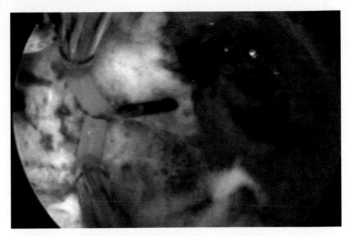

FIGURE 8.21: Well vascularized underlaying structure of the uterine septum during incision procedure.

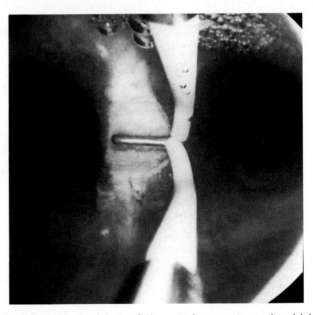

FIGURE 8.22: Incision of the uterine septum should be performed in a midline, with a needle electrode pointing towards the tubal ostia.

Histologically uterine septum is formed from well vascularized myometrial tissue and hypothetically, such a uterus may develop irregular and intense contractions that may result in pregnancy loss (Figure 8.21).[32,49,50]

Preoperative ultrasound assessment is an important tool to differentiate between the septate and bicornuate uterus. Bicornuate uterus is not hysteroscopically correctible anomaly and misdiagnosed cases may result in uterine perforation.

Operative procedure itself considers incision of the septal protrusion in midline between the anterior and posterior uterine wall (Figure 8.22). If the shape of the fundal region is convex or planar on preoperative 2D or 3D ultrasound, incision is extended until the level of tubal ostia. Incision may be performed mechanically by scissors with electrical needle electrode (monopolar/bipolar) or with laser. In demanding cases with a concave form of uterine fundus (less than 1 cm), it is recommended to perform a simultaneous laparoscopy.

REFERENCES

1. Azziz R, Steinkampf MP, Murphy A. Postoperative recuperation: relation to the extent of endoscopic surgery. Fertil Steril 1989;51(6):1061-4.
2. Robinson V. Preface. In: Leonardo R (Ed). History of gynecology. New York: Forben Press 1944.
3. Candiani GB, Vercellini P, Fedele L, et al. Conservative surgical treatment for severe endometriosis in infertile women: Are we making progress? Obstet Gynecol Surv 1991;46(7):490-8.
4. Lambaudie E, Houvenaeghel G, Walz J, et al. Robot-assisted laparoscopy in gynecologic oncology. Surg Endosc 2008;22(12):2743-7.
5. Audebert AJM. The role of microlaparoscopy for safer wall entry: incidence of umbilical adhesions according to past surgical history. Gynaecological Endoscopy 1999;8(6):363-7.
6. Rottem S, Levit N, Thaler I, et al. Classification of ovarian lesions by high-frequency transvaginal sonography. J Clin Ultrasound 1990;18(4):359-63.
7. Kurjak A, Sparac V, Kupesic S, et al. Three-dimensional ultrasound and three-dimensional power Doppler in the assessment of adnexal masses. Ultrasound Rev Obstet Gynecol 2001;1:167-83.
8. Peterson HB, Hulka JF, Phillips JM. American Association of Gynecologic Laparoscopists 1988 membership survey on operative laparoscopy. J Reprod Med 1990;35(6):587-9.
9. Dembo AJ, Davy M, Stenwig AE, et al. Prognostic factors in patient with stage I epithelial ovarian cancer. Obstet Gynecol 1990;75:263.
10. Kurjak A, Kupesic S, Sparac V, et al. Preoperative evaluation of pelvic tumors by Doppler and three-dimensional ultrasonography. J Ultrasound Med 2001;20(8):829-40.
11. Audabert AJM. Ovarian surgery: Why expect more problems from laparoscopy than from laparotomy? Gynaecological Endoscopy 1995;4:1-2.
12. Nezhat F, Nezhat C, Welander CE, et al. Four ovarian cancers diagnosed during laparoscopic management of 1011 women with adnexal masses. Am J Obstet Gynecol 1992;167(3):790-6.
13. Vermesh M, Lilva PD, Rosen GF, et al. Management of unruptured ectopic gestation by linear salpingostomy: a prospective randomized clinical trial of laparoscopy vs. laparotomy. Obstet Gynecol 1988;73:889.
14. Ghosh S, Mann C, Khan K, et al. Laparoscopic management of ectopic pregnancy. Semin Laparosc Surg 1999;6(2):68-72.
15. Bruhat MA, Mage G, Chapron C, et al. Present day endoscopic surgery in gynecology. Eur J Obstet Gynecol Reprod Biol 1991;41(1):4-13.
16. Lundroff P, Hahlin M, Sjoblom P, et al. Persistent trophoblast after conservative treatment of tubal pregnancy: Prediction and detection. Obstet Gynecol 1991;77(1):129-33.
17. Operative Laparoscopy Study Group. Postoperative adhesion development after operative laparoscopy: Evaluation at early second look procedures. Fertil Steril 1991;55:700-4.
18. Prapas Y, Prapas N, Papanicolaou A, et al. Laparoscopic tubal surgery. A retrospective comparative study of open microsurgery vs. laparoscopic surgery. Acta Eur Fertil 1995;26(2):81-3.
19. Tourgeman DE, Bhaumik M, Cooke GC, et al. Pregnancy rates following fimbriectomy reversal via neosalpingostomy: A 10-year retrospective analysis. Fertil Steril 2001;76(5):1041-4.
20. Milingos SD, Kallipolitis GK, Loutradis DC, et al. Laparoscopic treatment of hydrosalpinx: Factors affecting pregnancy rate. J am Assoc Gynecol Laparosc 2000;7(3):355-61.
21. Kurjak A, Kupesic S. Scoring system for prediction of ovarian endometriosis based on color and pulsed Doppler sonography. Fertil Steril 1994;62(1):81-8.
22. Liguori G, Tolino A, Moccia G, et al. Laparoscopic ovarian treatment in infertile patients with polycystic ovarian syndrome (PCOS): Endocrine changes and clinical outcome. Gynecol Endocrinol 1996;10(4):257-64.
23. Reich H, DeCaprio J, McGlynn F. Laparoscopic hysterectomy. J Gynecol Surg 1989;5:213-6.
24. Sanjuan A, Hernandez S, Pahisa J, et al. Port-site metastasis after laparoscopic surgery for endometrial carcinoma: Two case reports. Gynecol Oncol 2005;96:539-42.
25. Chen CC, Straughn JM, Kilgore LC. Early abdominal incision reccurence in a patient with stage I adenocarcinoma of endometrium. Obstet Gynecol 2004;104:1170-2.
26. Childers JM, Surwit EA. Combined laparoscopic and vaginal surgery for the management of two cases of stage I endometrial cancer. Gynecol Oncol 1992;45(1):468-71.
27. Schneider A, Possover M, Kamprath S, et al. Laparoscopy-assisted radical vaginal hysterectomy modified according to Schauta-Stockel. Obstet Gynecol 1996;88:1057-60.
28. Kim JH, Park JY, Kim DY, et al. Fertility-sparing laparoscopic radical trachelectomy for young women with early stage cervical cancer. BJOG 2010;117(3):340-7.
29. Burnett AF. Radical trachelectomy with laparoscopic lymphadenectomy: Review of oncologic and obstetrical outcomes. Curr Opin Obstet Gynecol 2006;18(1):8-13.
30. Ulrich U. Laparoscopic staging in advanced cervical cancer: the pros and cons of an oncological concept. Gynecol Surg 2005;2:151-4.
31. Heitz F, Ognjenovic D, Harter P, et al. Abdominal wall metastases in patients with ovarian cancer after laparoscopic surgery: incidence, risk factors, and complications. Int J Gynecol Cancer 201;20(1):41-6.
32. Kupesic S, Kurjak A. Septate uterus: detection and prediction of obstetrical complication by different forms of ultrasonography. J Ultrasound Med 1998;17:631-6.

33. R Salim, C Lee, A Davies, et al. A comparative study of three-dimensional saline infusion sonohysterography and diagnostic hysteroscopy for the classification of submucosal fibroids. Human Reprod 2005;20(1):2537.

34. Karageyim Karsidag AY, Buyukbayrak EE, Kars B, et al. Transvaginal sonography, onohysterography and hysteroscopy for investigation of focal intrauterine lesions in women with recurrent postmenopausal bleeding after dilatation & curettage. Arch Gynecol Obstet 2010;281(4):637-43.

35. Cohen SB, Kalter-Ferber A, Weisz BS, et al. Hysteroscopy may be the method of choice for managment of residual trophoblastic tisue. J Am Assoc Gynecol Laparoscop 2001;8(2):199-202.

36. Cacciatire B, Ramsay T, Lehtovirta P, et al. Transvaginal sonography and hysteroscopy in postmenopausal bleeding. Acta Obstet Gynecol Scand 1994;73(5):413-6.

37. Iliæ-ForkoJ, Babiæ D. Korpus Uterusa. In: Jukiæ S (Ed). Patologija •enskog spolnog sustava. Zagreb:AGM, 1995;107-44.

38. Brooks PG, Serden SP. Hysteroscopic findings after unsuccesful dilatation and curettage for abnormal uterine bleeding. Am J Obstet Gynecol 1988;158:1354-7.

39. Wang CW, Lee CL, Lai YM, et al. Comparison of hysterosal-pingography and hysteroscopy in female infertility. J Am Assoc Gynecol Laparosc 1996;3(4):581-4.

40. Brown SE, Coddington CC, Schnorr J, et al. Evaluation of outpatient hysteroscopy, saline infusion hysterosonography and hysterosalpingography in infertile women: a prospective randomized study. Fertil Steril 2000;74(5):1029-34.

41. Betocchi S, Ceci O, Nappi L, et al. Operative office hysteroscopy without anesthesia: analysis of 4863 cases performed with mechanical instruments. J Am Assoc Gynecol Laparosc 2004;11(1):59-61.

42. Giatras K, Berkeley AS, Noyes N, et al. Fertility after hysteroscopic myomectomy of submucosal myomas. J Am Assoc Gynecol Laparosc 1999;6(2):155-8.

43. Yang JH, Lin BL. Changes in myometrial thickness during hysteroscopic resection of deeply invasive submucosal myomas. J Am Assoc Gynecol Laparosc 2001;8(4):501-5.

44. Fernandez H, Kadoch O, Capella-Allouc S, et al. Hysteroscopic resection of submucosal myomas: long term results. Ann Chir 2001;126(1):58-64.

45. Wamsteker K, Emanuel MH, de Kruif JH. Transcervical hysteroscopic resection of submucosal fibroids for abnormal uterine bleeding: results regarding the degree of intramural extension. Obstet Gynecol 1993;82(5):736-40.

46. Touboul C, Fernandez H, Deffieux X, et al. Uterine synechiae after bipolar hysteroscopic resection of submucosal myomas in patients with infertility. Fertil Steril 2009;92:1690-3.

47. Kaunitz AM, Meredith S, Inki P, et al. Levonorgestrel-releasing intrauterine system and endometrial ablation in heavy menstrual bleeding: a systematic review and meta-analysis. Obstet Gynecol 2009;113(5):1104-16.

48. Portuondo J, Camara MM, Echanojauregui AD, et al. Müllerian abnormalities in fertile women and recurrent aborters. J Reprod Med 1986;31(7):616-9.

49. Dabirashrafi H, Bahadori M, Mohammad K, et al. Septate uterus: New idea on the histological features of the septum in the abnormal uterus. Am J Obstet Gynecol 1995;172:105-7.

50. Sparac V, Kupesic S, Ilijas M, et al. Histologic architecture and vascularization of hysteroscopically excised intrauterine septa. J Am Assoc Gynecol Laparosc 2001;8(1):111-6.

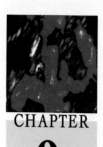

S Kupesic Plavsic, A Kurjak, N Zafar

CHAPTER 9

Color Doppler and Three-Dimensional Ultrasound Imaging in Infertility

Infertility is defined as a failure to conceive a desired pregnancy after 12 months of unprotected intercourse and it affects almost 10% of couples. With recent technological development and proper use of medically assisted reproduction techniques, one half of these couples will become pregnant. More than any other new method, ultrasound has made significant improvements in the modern management of female infertility. Transvaginal sonography provides the reproductive endocrinologist with a tool that cannot only evaluate normal and stimulated ovarian cycles, but may also assist in follicle aspiration and subsequent transfer of the embryo. The addition of color Doppler capabilities to the transvaginal probes permits the visualization of small intraovarian and endometrial vessels, allowing depiction of normal and abnormal physiologic changes in the ovary and uterus. It may help in the prediction of ovulation and detection of certain ovulatory disorders and diagnosis of the luteal phase defects. In patients with ovulation induction, Doppler investigation of the ovarian blood flow may improve early detection of ovarian hyperstimulation syndrome. Initial impressions concerning the usefulness of blood flow studies in infertile patients have been confirmed by numerous studies during the last two decades. This chapter reviews the role of ultrasound in the assessment of ovarian, uterine and tubal causes of infertility and discusses the current and future role of color Doppler and three-dimensional (3D) ultrasound in the field of reproductive endocrinology.

UTERINE CAUSES OF INFERTILITY

The uterine cavity should provide an environment for successful sperm migration from the cervix to the fallopian tube. The normality of the mucosal lining, glandular secretion and vascularity are necessary to support implantation and placentation. Uterine anomalies, polyps, submucosal fibroids, neoplasia, infections and intrauterine scar tissue may lead to a poor reproductive performance. Attempts have been made to correlate the sonographic parameters (such as thickness and reflectivity) and endometrial receptivity.

Uterine Perfusion in Infertile Patients

Transvaginal color and pulsed Doppler sonography has been established as an additional tool in the management of infertile patients. In anovulatory cycles, a continuous increase of the uterine artery resistance index, RI has been detected[1, 2] (Figure 9.1). Moreover, in some infertile patients, an end-diastolic flow is absent.[3] Some Doppler studies indicate that the absent diastolic flow might be associated with infertility and a poor reproductive performance. Therefore, the uterine artery blood flow could potentially be used to predict a hostile uterine environment prior to embryo transfer (Figure 9.2). Steer et al.[4] calculated the probability of pregnancy by using the pulsatility index, (PI) values obtained from the uterine artery on the day of embryo transfer. With the use of these measurements, the highest probability of becoming pregnant was obtained in patients whose uterine artery PI values were bellow 3.0. Statistical analysis confirmed that mean uterine artery PI of more than 3.0 on the day of embryo transfer can predict up to 35% of pregnancy failures.[4] Tsai et al.[5] evaluated the prognostic value of uterine perfusion on the day of human chorionic gonadotropin (hCG) administration in patients who were undergoing intrauterine insemination. They evaluated the ascending branch of the uterine artery pulsatility index on the day of administration of hCG and

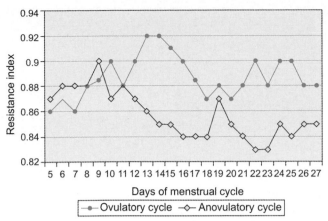

FIGURE 9.1: Changes in the uterine artery blood flow in ovulatory and anovulatory cycles.

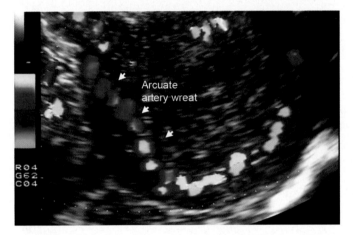

FIGURE 9.2: Uterine circulation demonstrated by color Doppler ultrasound. The uterine artery is demonstrated lateral to the cervix at the level of the cervicocorporeal junction. The arcuate arteries are visualized in the outer third of the myometrium. Radial arteries are demonstrated within the myometrial portion of the uterus (From reference 1, with permission).

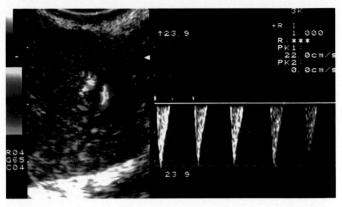

FIGURE 9.3: Absent diastolic flow of the uterine artery may be associated with infertility or poor reproductive performance.

compared the uterine artery vascular resistance to the outcome of intrauterine insemination. No pregnancy occurred when the pulsatility index of the ascending branch of the uterine arteries was more than 3 (Figure 9.3). The fecundity rate was 18% when the PI was less than 2 and was 19.8% when the PI was between 2 and 3. Their data suggest that the measurement of uterine perfusion on the day of hCG administration may have a predictive value regarding fecundity in patients undergoing intrauterine insemination. In infertile women, uterine artery PI measured during the midluteal phase of natural cycles, correlates inversely with endometrial thickness,[6] suggesting a direct effect of uterine perfusion on the endometrial growth.[7] Furthermore, pulsatility index correlates directly with the age of the patients,[3] suggesting a detrimental effect of age on uterine perfusion. Cacciatore et al.[8] did not find any correlation between the uterine artery PI measured on the day of embryo transfer (ET) and endometrial thickness or the age of the patients. These findings may be explained by the fact that all the patients evaluated in this study had controlled ovarian hyperstimulation and elevation of estradiol (E2) levels that reduce the difference between the individuals.

Increased uterine artery impedance was also reported among the infertile patients diagnosed with endometriosis.[6] Women with a history of endometriosis have significantly higher pulsatility and resistance index values than patients with other causes of infertility, even after hormonal stimulation. This evidence, although gained in different settings, seem to suggest an adverse effect of endometriosis on uterine perfusion. This could be another way in which endometriosis may compromise a woman's fertility potential. Whether this is due to mechanical effects on the pelvic vessels as a result of adhesions or is mediated by the production of agents with vasoactive properties, remains to be explained.

Endometrial Thickness, Endometrial Volume and Vascularity

The question on correlation between endometrial thickness and the likelihood of conception, in the context of assisted conception, remains a contentious issue. However, a very thin endometrium (below 7 mm) seems to be accepted as a reliable sign of suboptimal implantation potential. In a review of 2,665 assisted conception cycles from 25 reports, eight reports have demonstrated a statistically significant difference in the mean endometrial thickness of conception and nonconception cycles, while 17 reports found no significant difference.[9] They concluded that results from various trials are conflicting and that insufficient data exist describing a linear correlation between endometrial thickness and the probability of conception. The main advantage of measuring endometrial thickness is its high negative predictive value in patients with minimal endometrial thickness. Early transvaginal studies reported absence of pregnancies in donor insemination cycles where the endometrium thickness did not reach at least 6 mm.[10] Similarly, in a group of oocyte recipients, no pregnancies were reported in women who had an endometrial thickness of less than 5 mm, whereas several pregnancies occurred in patients with an endometrium thinner than 7.5 mm.[11] In IVF cycle's minimal endometrial thickness of 7 mm was reported to be compatible with pregnancy.[12]

Endometrial pattern is defined as the relative echogenicity of the endometrium and the adjacent myometrium as demonstrated on a longitudinal ultrasound scan. In a prospective study, Serafini et al.[13] found that a multilayered endometrial pattern on the day of hCG administration was more predictive of implantation than any other ultrasound parameter. Sher et al.[14] demonstrated that a nonmultilayered echo pattern was commonly visualized in patients with advanced reproductive age and uterine abnormalities. In the literature, of 13 studies evaluating the value of endometrial pattern in predicting pregnancy, only four failed to confirm its predictive value.[9] The endometrial pattern does not appear to be influenced by the type of ovarian stimulation and it is of prognostic value for both fresh IVF and frozen embryo transfer cycles.

Subendometrial blood flow is another parameter to be analyzed in patients undergoing medically assisted reproduction.[15] Endometrial thickness, endometrial morphology, presence or absence of the subendometrial or intraendometrial color flow, degree of intraendometrial vascular penetration and subendometrial blood flow velocimetry on the day of hCG administration were assessed in 96 patients undergoing IVF/ET (Figure 9.4). The overall pregnancy rate was 32.3% (31/96) and there was no significant difference between the pregnant and nonpregnant groups with regard to endometrial thickness, subendometrial peak systolic blood flow velocity (V_{max}) or subendometrial pulsatility index (PI). The pregnancy rates based on endometrial morphology was not significantly

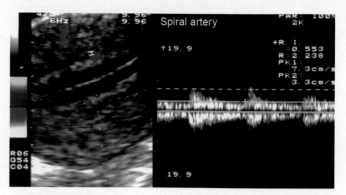

FIGURE 9.4: Blood flow velocity waveforms of the spiral arteries during the follicular phase. Note a triple-line endometrium (left) and moderate resistance index (RI = 0.55) (right) obtained from the spiral arteries.

different, being 17.6% (3/17), 33.3% (2/6) and 35.6% (26/73) for types A (hyperechoic), B (isoechoic) and C (triple-line) endometrium, respectively. In eight (8.3%) patients, subendometrial color flow and intraendometrial vascularization was not detected. Absence of blood flow was associated with failure of implantation (p < 0.05). The pregnancy rates related to the zones of vascular penetration into the subendometrial and endometrial regions were: 26.7% (4/15) for Zone 1 (subendometrial zone), 36.4% (16/44) for Zone 2 (outer hyperechogenic zone) and 37.9% (11/29) for Zone 3 (inner hypoechogenic zone) and were not significantly different.

Endometrial thickness obtained by two-dimensional (2D) sonography is considered the most important parameter of endometrial growth. However, this parameter does not include the total volume of the endometrium. Retarded endometrial development may be associated with primary infertility, and, therefore, endometrial volume assessment by 3D ultrasound maybe a clinically relevant parameter. The ability to quantify the volume of the endometrium using 3D ultrasound may help to correlate the cycle outcome using this as a quantitative parameter, rather than endometrial thickness, which is prone to greater subjective variation in measurement.[16] By stepping through the volume in the multiplanar mode, the outer border of the endometrium is traced and the volume calculation is performed. High accuracy and low inter- and intraobserver variability of this method have already been described.[17,18] The endometrium shows a good contrast to the surrounding myometrial tissue and therefore, in most cases endometrial volume estimation may be precisely performed.

Measurements could be reproduced in longitudinal and transverse viewing planes. Other sources of measuring error may derive from the low contrast of the caudal end of the endometrium and the uterus. Endometrial fluid may also increase measuring error because the fluid volume may be too small to be accurately measured by 3D ultrasound. Lee et al.[19] were the first to demonstrate volume estimation of the endometrium by 3D ultrasound. Using the same method Kyei-Mensah et al.[20] assessed the reliability of 3D ultrasound of endometrial volume measurements on twenty patients undergoing ovarian stimulation. Endometrial volumes obtained on the day of hCG administration demonstrated the intraobserver and interobserver coefficient of variation of 8% and 11%, respectively. Reproducibility within and between the investigators was also expressed as the Intra CC and Inter CC. The coefficients describe the proportion of variation in a measurement, which is caused by true biological subject differences. For a single measurement of endometrial volume, the Intra CC was 0.90 and the Inter CC was 0.82. These results clearly demonstrate that 3D ultrasound volume measurements are highly reliable, with a small measure of error. However, higher interobserver differences were noticed for localization of the internal os and endometrial margins, which may explain greater interobserver variability for the endometrial than for the ovarian volume assessment. Since 3D ultrasound is applied in the same manner as 2D vaginal ultrasound it does not cause additional patients' discomfort. Quantification of the endometrial volume by 3D ultrasound in combination with blood flow studies may be the best way to predict the pregnancy rates in patients undergoing medically assisted reproduction.

Kupesic et al.[21] investigated the usefulness of transvaginal color Doppler and 3D power Doppler ultrasonography for the assessment of endometrial receptivity in patients undergoing IVF/ET procedures. Endometrial thickness and volume, endometrial morphology and subendometrial perfusion were evaluated on the day of embryo transfer. Neither the volume, nor the thickness of the endometrium on the day of embryo transfer had a predictive value for conception during *in vitro* fertilization cycles. Patients who became pregnant were characterized by a significantly lower resistance index (0.53 ± 0.04 versus 0.64 ± 0.04), obtained from the subendometrial vessels by transvaginal color Doppler ultrasonography and a significantly higher flow index (13.2 ± 2.2 versus 11.9 ± 2.4), as measured by a 3D power Doppler histogram. No difference was found in the predictive value of scoring systems analyzing endometrial thickness and volume, endometrial morphology and subendometrial perfusion by color Doppler and 3D power Doppler ultrasonography. However, a high degree of endometrial perfusion illustrated by both techniques on the day of embryo transfer may indicate a more favorable endometrial milieu for successful implantation.

Congenital Anomalies

Congenital uterine malformations are variable in frequency and are usually estimated to represent 3% to 4%, although less than half have clinical symptoms.[22-24] The respective frequency of symptomatic malformations is dominated by a septate uterus.[24,25] During the first trimester of pregnancy, the risk of spontaneous abortion in this group is between 28% and 45%, while during the second trimester the frequency of late spontaneous abortions is approximately 5%.[24] Premature deliveries, abnormal fetal presentations, irregular uterine activity and dystocia at delivery are likely to prevail in cases of a septate uterus.[26] Poor vascularization of the septum was proposed as a potential cause of miscarriages.[25] Electron microscopy study by Fedele et al.[27] indicated a decrease in the sensitivity of the endometrium, covering the septa of the malformed uteri to the preovulatory changes. This could play a role in the pathogenesis of primary infertility in patients with a septate uterus.

It is clear that unfavorable obstetric prognosis can be transformed by surgical correction of the intrauterine septum. Hysteroscopic treatment was currently proposed as the procedure of choice for the management of uterine anomalies. This simple and effective treatment has an obvious advantage that the uterus is not weakened by a myometrial scar. Cararach et al.[28] and Goldenberg et al.[29] reported 75% and 88.7% pregnancy rates after operative hysteroscopy. The clear, simplicity and effectiveness of hysteroscopic metroplasty have placed the clinician into a need for an early and correct diagnosis of uterine anomalies. When used as a screening test for the detection of congenital uterine anomalies, the transvaginal ultrasound has a sensitivity of almost 100%.[30,31] However, a clear distinction between the different types of abnormalities is impossible and operator dependent.[32,33]

X-ray hysterosalpingography (X-ray HSG) is an invasive test, which requires the use of contrast medium and exposure to radiation. Although HSG provides a good outline of the uterine cavity, the visualization of minor anomalies and clear distinction between different types of

TABLE 9.1: Sensitivity, specificity, positive (PPV) and negative predictive (NPV) values of various imaging modalities for the diagnosis of a septate uterus in 420 patients with a history of infertility and recurrent abortions

Imaging modality	Sensitivity (%)	Specificity (%)	PPV (%)	NPV(%)
Transvaginal sonography	95.21	92.21	95.86	91.03
Transvaginal color Doppler	99.29	97.93	98.03	98.61
Hysterosonography	98.18	100.00	100.00	95.45
Three dimensional ultrasound	98.38	100.00	100.00	96.00

From reference 40, with permission

fusion and resorption disorders is sometimes impossible. Hysterosonography, with the application of transvaginal ultrasound after distension of the uterine cavity by instillation of saline solution was introduced over twenty years ago.[34] This simple and minimally invasive approach allows anatomical imaging of the endometrium and myometrium, accurate depiction of the septate uterus and even the measurement of the thickness and height of the septum.[35] Although some reports have indicated a high diagnostic accuracy of magnetic resonance imaging[36,37] in the diagnosis of congenital uterine anomalies, this technique is rarely, routinely used for this indication. More recently, 3D ultrasound has shown a high diagnostic accuracy in detection of uterine anomalies[38] suggesting that invasive procedures, such as CO_2 diagnostic hysteroscopy are not needed in patients scheduled for a corrective surgery.[39]

Kupesic and Kurjak attempted to evaluate the combined use of transvaginal ultrasound, transvaginal color and pulsed Doppler sonography, hysterosonography and 3D ultrasound in the preoperative diagnosis of a septate uterus.[40]

A total of 420 infertile patients undergoing operative hysteroscopy were included in this study. With the use of B-mode transvaginal sonography, the morphology of uterus was carefully explored with emphasis on the endometrial lining in both sagittal and transverse sections. The septum was visualized in a transverse plane, based on detection of the two endometrial echoes in the upper portion of the uterine cavity. Once an experienced sonographer completed B-mode examination, another skilled operator who was unaware of the previous finding performed a transvaginal color Doppler examination.

Color and pulsed Doppler were superimposed to visualize intraseptal and myometrial vascularity. Flow velocity waveforms were obtained from all the interrogated vessels. For each recording, at least five waveform signals of good quality were obtained. During each procedure, the resistance index (RI) was automatically calculated. The RI was calculated from the maximum frequency envelope using the formula: peak systolic velocity minus end-diastolic velocity divided by a peak systolic velocity. Instillation of isotonic saline (hysterosonography) was carried out on a gynecological examination table. Transverse and sagittal sections were carefully explored, and the septum was visualized as an echogenic portion separating the uterine cavity into two parts. Eighty-six women undergoing hysteroscopy were examined by 3D ultrasound. When these patients were evaluated on 3D ultrasound, three perpendicular planes of the uterus were simultaneously displayed on the screen, allowing a detailed analysis of the uterine morphology. Frontal reformatted sections were particularly useful for detection of the uterine abnormalities.

Table 9.1 summarizes the sensitivity, specificity, positive and negative predictive values of transvaginal sonography, transvaginal color and pulsed Doppler ultrasound, hysterosalpingography and 3D ultrasound for the diagnosis of a septate uterus. The sensitivity of the transvaginal sonography in the diagnosis of septate uteri was 95.21%. The transvaginal color and pulsed Doppler enabled the diagnosis of a septate uterus in 276 cases, reaching the sensitivity of 99.29%. In one patient with an endometrial polyp and one with intrauterine synechiae, the septate uterus was not correctly diagnosed. Therefore, the reliability of color and pulsed Doppler examination was reduced when other intracavitary structures, such as an endometrial polyp or a submucosal leiomyoma were present.

Color and pulsed Doppler studies of the septal area revealed vascularity in 198 (71.22%) patients. The RI values obtained from the septum ranged from 0.68 to 1.0 (mean RI = 0.84 ± 0.16) (Figures 9.5A and B). Hysterosonography reached 100% specificity and positive predictive value. In one patient with extensive intrauterine synechiae, hysterosonography did not detect an intrauterine septum. The sensitivity and specificity of a 3D ultrasound was 98.38% and 100%, respectively. One false-negative result was reported in a patient with a fundal fibroid distorting the uterine cavity. Interestingly, in our study, a septate uterus

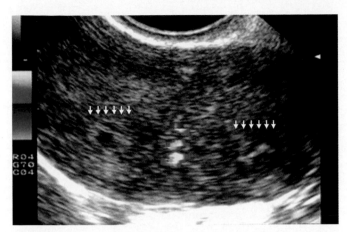

FIGURE 9.5A: Septate uterus demonstrated by color Doppler imaging. Vascularity within the septal area indicated that septum is built from myometrial tissue.

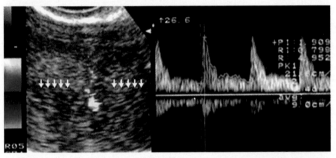

FIGURE 9.5B: The same patient as in Figure 9.5A. Pulsed Doppler waveform analysis (right) reveals moderate to high vascular resistance (RI = 0.79) of the vessels involved in the septum.

was never mistaken for a bicornuate uterus. However, in patients with a bicornuate uterus, transvaginal ultrasonography misinterpreted it as a septate uterus.

One hundred and eighty eight patients underwent X-ray HSG within 12 months prior to our study. The sensitivity of X-ray HSG in the diagnosis of septate uteri was only 26.06%. Fedele et al.[27] recently indicated that an intrauterine septum may be a cause of primary infertility. The ultrastructural morphologic alterations of the septal area were indicative of irregular differentiation and estrogenic maturation of the septal endometrial mucosa. Since the hormonal levels of the patients enrolled in this study were normal for the cycle phase, the most convincing hypothesis is that endometrial mucosa covering the septum is poorly responsive to estrogens probably due to the scanty vascularization of the septal connective tissue.

Dabirashrafi et al.[41] performed a histological study of the uterine septa from 16 patients undergoing abdominal metroplasty. Statistical analysis confirmed less connective tissue in the septum compared to the amount of muscle

tissue, which was contradictory to the classic view of the histopathologic features of the uterine septum. Less connective tissue in the septum may explain poor decidualization and placentation in the area of implantation.[35] Increased amounts of muscle tissue in the septum may lead to an abortion by higher and uncoordinated contractility of these muscles. In our study, we also found no correlation between the septal height and thickness and the occurrence of obstetrical complications ($p > 0.05$).[40] Pregnancy loss rates correlated significantly with septal vascularity. Patients with vascularized septa had a significantly higher incidence of early pregnancy failure and late pregnancy complications than those with an avascularized septa ($p < 0.05$).[40] Three-dimensional ultrasound enables planar reformatted sections through the uterus, which allows a precise evaluation of the fundal indentation and the length of the uterine septum (Figures 9.6 and 9.7). Based on our experience, 3D ultrasound may give a wrong impression of an arcuate uterus in patients with a fundal location of a leiomyoma. In these cases, the uterine cavity has a concave shape, while the fundal indentation is shallower. Shadowing caused by the uterine fibroids, irregular endometrial lining and decreased volume of the uterine cavity (in cases of intrauterine adhesions) are obvious limitations of 3D ultrasound. More recently 3D power Doppler was used to detect vascularization of the uterine septa in a combined angio and gray rendering mode. This approach allows simultaneous analysis of the septal morphology, texture and vascularization.

Balen et al.[42] described a technique for the 3D reconstruction of the uterine cavity using a positive contrast medium (Echovist). The main problem encountered with Echovist was an acoustic shadowing artifact owing to its highly reflective properties. An alternative approach is 3D

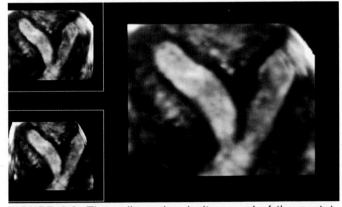

FIGURE 9.6: Three-dimensional ultrasound of the septate uterus. Note complete division of the uterine cavity and planar shape of the uterine fundus.

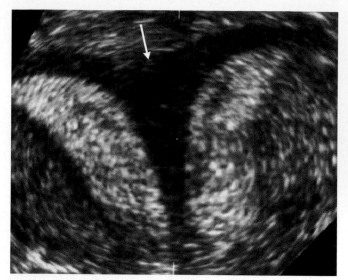

FIGURE 9.7: Frontal reformatted section of a bicornuate uterus. Note complete division of the uterine cavity and concave shape of the uterine fundus. Since the fundal cleft is more than 1 cm, this uterine anomaly is defined as a bicornuate uterus. The finding was confirmed at the time of the hysterolaparoscopic procedure.

saline contrast hysterosonography. This also offers a comprehensive image of the uterine cavity and the surrounding myometrium and gives access to planes unobtainable by conventional 2D ultrasound examination.[43] Further research is required to document whether contrast instillation contributes to a better diagnosis of the uterine cavity pathology when compared to unenhanced frontal reformatted section analysis.

Kupesic et al.[44] studied the incidence of surgically correctable uterine abnormalities (congenital uterine anomalies, submucous leiomyoma, endometrial polyps and intrauterine synechiae) in the infertile population, attending a tertiary infertility clinic. All the infertile patients enrolled in the study were evaluated by 3D ultrasound. Another objective was to assess pregnancy rates before and after operative hysteroscopy in patients affected by uterine causes of infertility. The prevalence of uterine abnormalities in our study was 7.9%.[44] The most common uterine abnormality accounting for 77.1% of the uterine causes of infertility was the septate uterus.[44] Out of 310 patients who were followed-up, 225 (72.6%) patients achieved pregnancy after hysteroscopic metroplasty for an intrauterine septum.

Endometrial Polyps

Endometrial polyp is the anatomic defect that is implicated in the etiology of a recurrent pregnancy loss and infertility. Polyps appear as a focal thickening of the endometrium.

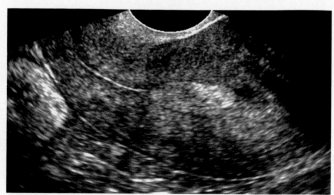

FIGURE 9.8: Transvaginal ultrasound scan of a focal endometrial thickening. The endometrial polyp was confirmed by hysteroscopy.

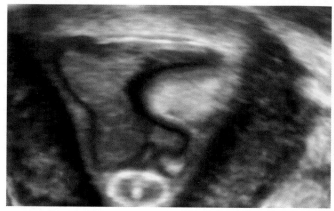

FIGURE 9.9: Saline infusion sonography by three-dimensional ultrasound demonstrates an endometrial polyp.

Using sonohysterography, an intracavitary polyp is seen surrounded by anechoic fluid. If ultrasound examination is performed during the follicular phase, the use of a distending medium is not necessary to detect an abnormal endometrial thickening (Figure 9.8). However, during the periovulatory and secretory phase, polyps are better visualized when outlined by intracavitary fluid. Using transvaginal color and pulsed Doppler, minor arteries supplying the growth of an endometrial polyp can be visualized. Three-dimensional ultrasound allows a detailed analysis of the uterine cavity in frontal reformatted sections, which enables clear demarcation of the endometrial polyp (Figure 9.9).

Submucosal Leiomyomas

The diagnosis of a submucosal leiomyoma is based on the distortion of the uterine contour, uterine enlargement and textural changes. Leiomyomas have a varying amount of smooth muscle and connective tissue, such that these benign tumors have a variety of sonographic features. Sonographic texture ranges from hypoechoic to echogenic, depending on the amount of smooth muscle and connective tissue. Central ischemia, which is a consequence of tumor enlargement and inadequate blood supply, is usually followed by various stages of degeneration. The most common cause of calcification within the uterus is calcific degeneration within the fibroid. Other types of degeneration include cystic, myxomatous and hyaline degeneration. Sometimes, because of the variety of appearances, submucosal leiomyomas may be mistaken for endometrial polyps, endometrial carcinoma, blood or mucus. The uterine environment of patients with a submucosal leiomyoma may not be conducive to the nidation of a fertilized ovum and the blood supply might be inadequate. Leiomyomas grow centripetally as proliferations of smooth muscle cells and fibrous connective tissue, creating a pseudocapsule of compressed muscle fibers. Therefore, color Doppler demonstrates most of the myometrial blood vessels at its periphery (Figure 9.10). Presence of blood vessels in the central portion of the leiomyomas is usually correlated with necrotic, degenerative and inflammatory changes. These vessels display lower RI values than peripherally located vessels and sometimes can be misinterpreted for malignant neovascular pulsed Doppler signals.[45] Vascular impedance to blood flow in the myometrial supplying vessels depends not only on the size, but location within the uterus. A significant difference is shown in blood flow characteristics of the leiomyoma supplying vessels between entirely subserosal versus intramural and submucosal leiomyomas. Lower impedance value for subserosal leiomyomas can be explained by the fact that these leiomyomas are supplied with blood vessels through a contact area with loose connective tissue. Therefore, these vessels are usually dilated with very low vascular impedance to blood flow. On the other hand, submucosal and intramural leiomyomas are supplied by blood vessels with higher vascular impedance. High basal tonus of the myometrial tissue surrounding the intramural or submucosal leiomyomas increases the vascular impedance in the leiomyoma vessels. Transvaginal color Doppler evaluation of 101 patients with palpable uterine fibroids and 60 healthy volunteers analyzed the mean resistance index from the myometrial vessels.[45] The mean RI value in the leiomyoma vessels was 0.54 and the mean PI value was 0.89. The histopathologic finding was a benign uterine tumor in all the cases, even when RI was very low. Lowered resistance indices were present in

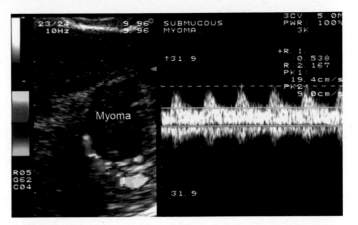

FIGURE 9.10: Transvaginal color Doppler scan of the uterus with submucosal leiomyoma. Waveform analysis (right) indicates moderate resistance of the tumor blood flow (RI = 0.54).

cases with necrosis and secondary degenerative and inflammatory changes within the fibroid. Increased blood flow velocity and decreased RI (mean RI = 0.74) in both uterine arteries occurred in patients with uterine fibroids.[45]

Adenomyosis

Adenomyosis is characterized by the in-growing of the endometrium into the myometrium and is usually asymptomatic, but may present with uterine bleeding, pain and infertility. Patients with adenomyosis have a diffusely enlarged uterus with a heterogeneous myometrium, streaky lines with posterior shadowing and/or multiple small cysts within the myometrium.[46] Disordered echogenicity of the middle and distal layers of the myometrium is present in some severe cases. Reported sensitivity and specificity of transvaginal ultrasound in detection of this benign entity is 86% and 50%, respectively.[46] Color Doppler may reveal increased vascularity mainly characterized by moderate vascular resistance.

Endometritis

Chronic endometritis is characterized with an increased echogenicity, thickness and vascularity of the endometrium. The most common cause of a chronic endometrial infection in the past was *Mycobacterium tuberculosis*. During the activation of an infection, pregnancy often terminates ectopically or as an abortion. The transvaginal sonographic findings may include calcified pelvic lymph nodes or smaller irregular calcifications in the adnexa and deformity of the endometrial cavity suggestive of adhesions in the absence of a history of prior curettage or abortion. In the acute stage of endometritis low to moderate impedance blood flow signals are easily obtained at the periphery of the endometrium. On the contrary, in chronic cases with irreversible tissue damage, blood flow is usually absent. Transvaginal sonography allows a better elucidation of the abnormal endometrial morphology, after which appropriate cultures should be taken and broad-spectrum antibiotic therapy administered. In order to prevent the development of intrauterine adhesions (especially following D&C procedures) administration of conjugated estrogen for one to two months is recommended. This therapy allows regeneration of a healthy endometrium, which is paralleled by a sharp increase in end-diastolic velocities of the spiral arteries at the time of color flow and pulsed Doppler analysis.

Asherman's Syndrome

Destruction of the endometrium may result in scarring and development of the bands of the scar tissue or synechiae, within the uterine cavity. This destruction may occur as a result of a vigorous curettage of the uterus following an abortion or more often, after curettage of an advanced pregnancy. Tuberculosis may also cause uterine synechiae, but only in rare cases. This may result in the formation of adhesive bands of different size with a subsequent partial or total obliteration of the endometrial cavity. Amenorrhea or hypomenorrhea are typical clinical patterns. Patients with endometrial adhesions, such as Asherman's syndrome, may have a distorted endometrial pattern with areas that have no visualized endometrium, mixed with areas that have a normal endometrial appearance. Adhesions are observed as endometrial irregularities or hyperechoic bridges within the endometrial cavity. Schlaff and Hurst[47] analyzed seven amenorrhoic patients with severe Asherman's syndrome. Transvaginal sonography demonstrated a well-developed endometrial stripe in three of the seven women, while the remaining four patients had virtually no endometrium seen. Excluding the lower uterine segment, patients with an endometrium visualized on a transvaginal ultrasound that were found to have adhesions, had a resumption of normal menses and normalization of the cavity following hysteroscopy. Women with a minimal endometrium had no cavity identified and derived no benefit from hysteroscopic surgery. The endometrial pattern on transvaginal sonography is highly predictive of both surgical and clinical outcome of the patients with severe Asherman's syndrome characterized by a complete obstruction of the cavity at hysterosalpingogram.

Intrauterine synechiae do not present with increased vascularity on color Doppler examination. In patients with preserved menstrual function adhesions are better visualized either during menstruation when the intracavitary fluid outlines them or following hysterosonography. When a 3D ultrasound of the uterus visualizes a uterus with synechiae, it also demonstrates a significant reduction of the endometrial cavity volume in all reformatted sections.

OVARIAN CAUSES OF INFERTILITY

Transvaginal sonography is considered the most reliable method for monitoring the follicular growth. It enables the accurate prediction of ovulation and detection of ovulation abnormalities.

The success of IVF treatment is dependent on the ability of the ovary to respond to controlled stimulation by gonadotropins and to develop a reasonable number of mature follicles and oocytes, simultaneously. Failure to respond is associated with cancellation of the cycle or poor outcome of the treatment. Prior prediction of the likelihood of optimal ovarian response is therefore essential in identifying the patients who are most likely to benefit from an IVF treatment. Zaidi et al.[48] were the first to show that there was a relationship between ovarian stromal blood flow velocity and ovarian follicular response. They measured the ovarian stromal PSV in the early follicular phase and showed that poor responders had low ovarian blood flow PSV. Increased ovarian stromal blood flow velocity was detected in polycystic ovaries, in combination with a relatively unchanged impedance to blood flow. This may reflect increased intraovarian perfusion and thus a greater delivery of gonadotropins to the granulosa-thecal cell complex, with a resultant greater number of follicles being produced. This mechanism may help to explain why patients with polycystic ovaries tend to respond excessively to the administration of gonadotropins and may possibly explain their increased risk of ovarian hyperstimulation syndrome.

Documentation of ovarian stromal vascularity at the initial baseline scan is important and may provide useful information for assisted reproduction techniques. Measurement of the ovarian stromal blood flow in the early follicular phase may be related to subsequent ovarian responsiveness in IVF treatment.[48] This is particularly useful since the ability to predict ovarian response to stimulation by exogenous gonadotropins is still central for success in any IVF program. Most centers still determine the dose of gonadotropins used for the first attempt based on the chronological age of the patient, with adjustments being made in subsequent attempts depending on their initial response. Unfortunately, the ovarian age (capacity of the ovary to produce fertilizable oocytes) and chronological age are not always synchronous, leading to a degree of unpredictability in the number of developing follicles and collected oocytes. Certainly, if an inadequate dose of gonadotropins is used there may be a relatively poor response, which reduces the number of the oocytes retrieved, whereas if an excessive dose is used, there may be an increased risk of ovarian hyperstimulation syndrome (Figures 9.11A and B).

Engman et al.[49] speculated that the ovarian stromal blood flow velocity after 2-3 weeks of pituitary suppression is a true representative of a baseline ovarian blood flow, because the ovaries are in a quiescent state. The primordial follicles in the ovary have no independent capillary networks, lying simply among the vessels of the stroma and therefore, depend on their proximity to the stromal vessels for the delivery of nutrients and hormones. The subsequent growth of primary follicles leads to the acquisition of a vascular sheath through the process of angiogenesis. The administration of a GnRH agonist suppresses follicular activity and consequently the ovaries become inactive. Ovarian stromal blood flow at this time might be at its lowest and may truly reflect the baseline ovarian blood flow. Therefore, ovarian stromal blood flow velocity after pituitary suppression may be predictive of ovarian responsiveness and the outcome of IVF treatment. One might speculate that by improving the ovarian stromal blood flow velocity, the delivery of gonadotropins to the follicles will be improved, resulting in higher number and quality of the mature oocytes with higher implantation rates.

The accuracy of diagnosis and monitoring of infertility treatments, such as ovulation induction has increased greatly because of the availability of sophisticated ultrasound technology and equipment.[20] Accurate follicular assessment is essential for a safe and effective infertility treatment. In IVF-ET cycles, follicles with a mean follicular diameter of 12 to 24 mm are associated with optimal rates of oocyte recovery, fertilization and cleavage.[50] This corresponds to follicular volumes of between 3 mL and 7 mL. In the hands of experienced operators, ultrasound alone suffices for cycle monitoring, with no necessity of additional hormonal estimations.[51-53] The basic structural information provided by conventional scans in the longitudinal and transverse planes now can be augmented by 3D ultrasound evaluation, which provides an additional

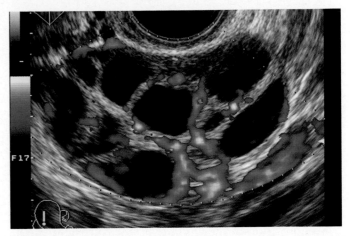

FIGURE 9.11A: Power Doppler ultrasound of enlarged and hyperstimulated ovary. Power Doppler demonstrates dilated perifollicular vessels.

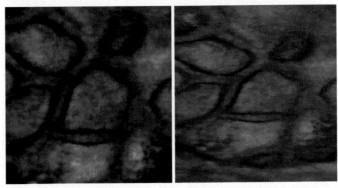

FIGURE 9.11B: Three-dimensional ultrasound of an enlarged and hyperstimulated ovary.

view of the coronal or C-plane, which is parallel to the transducer face.[20] The computer-generated scan is displayed in three perpendicular planes. Translation or rotation can be carried out in one plane, while maintaining the perpendicular orientation of all three so that serial translation results in an ultrasound tomogram from which volumetric data are captured.[54] Kyei-Mensah et al[20], evaluated the accuracy of 3D ultrasound measurement of the follicular volume and standard ultrasound techniques by comparing the volume of individual follicles estimated by both methods with the corresponding follicular aspirates. The volume of follicular fluid aspirated was compared with the corresponding volume of the follicle measured by 3D ultrasound and conventional 2D ultrasound volume measurement calculated by using the formula $0.52 \times (D_1 \times D_2 \times D_3)$. The limits of agreement and 95% confidence intervals were calculated and systematic biases between the methods were analyzed. The limits of agreement between the volume of follicular aspirate and follicular volume determined by ultrasound were +0.96 to –0.43 mL for 3D measurements and +3.47 to –2.42 mL for 2D measurements. High accuracy of 3D measurement of follicular volume is clearly demonstrated in this study by the limits of agreement, which are within 1 mL of the true volume. These limits encompass 95% of the volume measurements. On the other hand, the 2D method produced limits of agreement that were up to 3.5 mL above or 2.5 mL below the true volume. The shape and number of the follicles influence the reliability of the standard 2D ultrasound technique of follicular volume measurement. Measurement of the follicular diameter may be difficult when its shape is distorted because of compression by adjacent follicles. Penzias et al.[55] showed that mean follicular diameter accurately predicted volume in round and polygonal follicles, but not in ellipsoid ones. Round follicles were most prevalent in patients with the fewest follicles. Patients selected for this study have produced fewer follicles than normal and therefore, represent the group in which the conventional technique was likely to be most accurate. Kyei-Mensah[20] found that 3D assessment of the follicular volume produced a more accurate reflection of the true volume. This is because 3D measurement is not affected by the follicular shape since the changing contours are outlined serially to obtain the specific volume measurement. The disparity in accuracy between 3D assessment of the follicular volume and conventional 2D ultrasound is likely to increase significantly, if there is a florid multifollicular ovarian response, because the conventional formula is less precise with ellipsoid follicles, which are likely to predominate in these cases. One limitation of 3D volume assessment is that follicles with a mean diameter of <10 mm cannot be assessed accurately because the limits of agreement are too wide in this range.

It has been reported that 3D ultrasound may be useful for distinction of the ovarian cysts from the ovarian follicles.[56] Since both the ovarian cysts and follicles demonstrate an elevation of the serum estradiol levels, it is difficult to distinguish these two entities by E2 assay alone. For the purpose of the prospective observational study, the authors evaluated 50 IVF patients after ovulation induction. Three-dimensional ultrasound was used to search for the presence of cumuli in follicles greater than 15 mm. Only cumuli demonstrable in all three planes by multiplanar imaging predicted mature oocytes recovery.

Follicles without visualization of the cumulus in all three planes were not likely to contain mature fertilizable oocytes.

Lass et al.[57] tested the hypothesis that small ovaries measured on transvaginal sonography are associated with a poor response to ovulation induction by human menopausal gonadotropin (hMG) for in vitro fertilization (IVF). A total of 140 infertile patients with morphologically normal ovaries undergoing IVF was studied and represented. The mean ovarian volume of each patient was measured on transvaginal sonography before the start of ovulation induction. Subsequent routine IVF management was conducted without prior knowledge of the results of transvaginal sonography. The mean ovarian volume was 6.3 cm^3 (range 0.5 – 18.9, SD = 3.1). Seventeen patients with small ovaries measuring less than 3 cm^3 represented group A. Both groups were of similar age (mean 35.8 versus 34.4 years). Early basal FSH concentrations were increased in group A (9.5 versus 7.0 mIU/ml, P = 0.025). The cycle was abandoned before planned oocyte recovery in nine patients (52.8%) from group A and in 11 patients (8.9%) from group B because of poor response to ovulation induction. Oyesanya et al.[58] measured the total ovarian volume before the administration of hCG in 42 women undergoing treatment for infertility by in vitro fertilization. Seven women who subsequently developed moderate or severe ovarian hyperstimulation syndrome (OHSS) (n = 7; group 1) were compared with 35 matched controls (five matched controls per case; n = 35; group 2) of similar age, number of follicles and duration of infertility who underwent follicular stimulation, oocyte recovery, in vitro fertilization and embryo transfer during the same period but did not develop moderate or severe OHSS. The mean age, duration of infertility and total number of follicles were similar, but the mean total ovarian volume was significantly higher in the group of women who developed moderate or severe OHSS compared with controls (271.00 ± 87.00 versus 157.30 ± 54.20 ml).

Kupesic and Kurjak[59] designed a study to evaluate whether the ovarian antral follicle number, ovarian volume, stromal area and ovarian stromal blood flow are predictive of ovarian response and in vitro fertilization (IVF) outcome. Total ovarian antral follicle number, total ovarian volume, total stromal area and mean flow index (FI) of the ovarian stromal blood flow were determined by 3D and power Doppler ultrasound after pituitary suppression. Pretreatment 3D ultrasound ovarian measurements were compared with subsequent ovulation induction parameters (peak estradiol on hCG administration day and number of the oocytes) and for the cycle outcome (fertilization and pregnancy rates). The total number of antral follicles achieved the best predictive value for a favorable IVF outcome, followed by ovarian stromal FI, total ovarian stromal area and total ovarian volume.

Kupesic et al.[60] evaluated whether ovarian antral follicle number, ovarian volume and ovarian stromal blood flow changed with a women's age and if they are predictive of ovarian response and in vitro fertilization (IVF) outcome. Total ovarian antral follicle number, ovarian volume and mean flow index (FI) of the ovarian stromal blood flow were determined by 3D and power Doppler ultrasound after pituitary suppression. Patients were separated into the three groups based upon age and in each group the median values of 3D ultrasound parameters (total ovarian antral follicle number, total ovarian volume and mean ovarian stromal vascularity) were measured and presented. Pretreatment 3D ultrasound ovarian measurements were compared with a subsequent ovulation induction parameter (number of the oocytes) and a cycle outcome (fertilization and pregnancy rates). Increasing age was associated with poor ovarian response, smaller ovarian volume, lower antral follicle count and poor stromal vascularity.

Clearly, there is a place for 3D ultrasound in the assessment of the ovaries prior to ovulation induction and with medically assisted reproduction.

POLYCYSTIC OVARIAN SYNDROME

Polycystic ovarian syndrome (PCOS) is one of the causes of anovulation and amenorrhea. In its classic form, it is characterized by infertility, oligo- and amenorrhea, hirsutism, acne or seborrhea and obesity. In 1986, Adams et al. defined the criteria for ultrasonographic diagnosis of polycystic ovaries: multiple (n > 10), small (2-8 mm) peripheral cysts around a dense core of stroma in enlarged ($\geq$ 8 ml) ovaries.[61] However, ovaries, which are normal in volume may also be polycystic, as demonstrated by histological and biochemical studies. Anatomic structure of the ovaries can be adequately assessed by transabdominal approach in about 42% of cases. Underlying causes are obesity, limited resolution of low-frequency transducers, full bladder distorting pelvic anatomy and bowel loops, covering the adjacent ovary. High frequency transvaginal probes avoid the need for a full bladder and bypass the problems of attenuation and artifacts associated with obesity. Furthermore, transvaginal ultrasonography has the advantage of improved resolution, better visualization of the pelvic organs and greater acceptance among patients.

The number of follicles necessary to establish the diagnosis of polycystic ovaries by ultrasonography has been reported, varies between five and fifteen. In many reports, the highest number of atretic follicles obtained in normal control patients was 10 per ovary, so it was conventionally established that in polycystic ovaries, the number of atretic follicles per ovary would be at least ten ($\geq$ 10) . Matsunaga and colleagues identified two types of polycystic ovaries on the basis of ultrasonographic follicular distribution; the peripheral cystic pattern (PCP) and the general cystic pattern (GCP).[62] In the PCP, small cysts are distributed in the subcapsular region of the ovary, whereas in the GCP they are scattered through the entire ovarian parenchyma. Recently, Takahashi and colleagues showed that these two different ovarian morphologies reflect histopathologic differences and that the PCP and GCP appearances reflect specific endocrine PCOS patterns.[63]

Another parameter considered in the diagnosis of polycystic ovaries is the ovarian volume. However, the wide volume overlap between normal and PCOS patients suggests that the discriminative capacity of ovarian volume alone is not sufficient for ultrasound diagnosis of PCOS.[64] The role of a hyperechogenic ovarian stroma has been emphasized, but appraisal of the ovarian stroma echodensity,[65] although comparable with computerized quantification,[66] is absolutely subjective and may be differently interpreted by the operator.

Color Doppler studies of the patients with polycystic ovarian syndrome have demonstrated that ovarian vascularization changes occur at the level of the intraovarian arteries (Figure 9.12). Although intraovarian arteries are usually not seen before day 8 to 10 of the 28-day cycle,[67] Battaglia detected distinct arteries with characteristic low vascular impedance as early as day 3 to 5 of the 28-day cycle.[68] This blood flow pattern was associated with typical PCOS hormonal parameters and was inversely correlated with the LH/FSH ratio. Tonic hypersecretion of LH during the follicular phase of the menstrual cycle occurs in PCOS and is associated with theca cells and stromal hyperplasia with consequent androgen overproduction.[68] Elevated LH levels may be responsible for increased stromal vascularization by different mechanisms that may act individually or in a cumulative way, such as neoangiogenesis, catecholaminergic stimulation, and leukocyte and cytokine activation. In the same study, the PCOS patients showed higher uterine pulsatility index (PI) values than non-hirsute normally menstruating women. This finding was correlated with androstenedione levels,

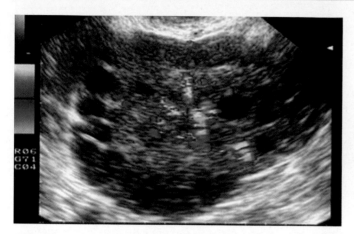

FIGURE 9.12: Color Doppler image of a polycystic ovary. Small cystic structures are crowded together and stand out from the enlarged ovarian stroma. Stromal vessels are easily visualized by color Doppler imaging.

confirming a possible direct androgen vasoconstrictive effect due to activation of specific receptors in the arterial vessel walls, and collagen and elastin deposition in smooth muscle cells. The above condition, by reducing the uterine perfusion, has been theorized as the cause that prevents blastocyst implantation, and increases the incidence of miscarriages in PCOS patients. Zaidi[69] and Aleem[70] have obtained similar results and confirmed that the Doppler analysis of stromal arteries in PCOS may be useful to improve the diagnosis and provide further information about the pathophysiology and evolution of the PCOS. Doppler evaluation showed that PCP patients, in comparison with GCP patients, present significantly lower resistance index (RI) values at the level of the ovarian stromal arteries and that in 22% of GCP patients, the intraovarian vessels are not recognized.[71] In addition, the GCP appearance of the ovary is more common in the early phase of the disease[62, 63] during the peripubertal period. Thus, the ovarian morphology may evolve from a normal multicystic to a polycystic PCP pattern, passing through an ovarian GCP aspect. Clearly, PCOS is a progressive syndrome and ultrasound plays an important role in follow-up of these patients. Comparisons of oligo- and amenorrheic PCOS patients have clearly demonstrated that amenorrheic patients are older and present with higher PI values in uterine arteries and with lower RI values in intraovarian vessels than oligomenorrheic patients.[72] This finding is associated with a higher plasma LH and androstenedione levels and with a more elevated LH/FSH ratio.

Furthermore, significantly higher ovarian volumes and subcapsular small-sized follicles are observed in amenorrheic PCOS patients. This data shows that as the number of ovarian microcysts increases, ovarian volume increases and Doppler indices worsen, the clinical and endocrine abnormalities become more remarkable and the menstrual disturbances become more severe.[71] It has also been demonstrated that obese PCOS women show higher PI uterine artery values than lean patients.[73] These findings are associated with higher hematocrit values, hyperinsulinemia, higher triglyceride levels and lower high-density lipid (HDL) concentrations.

In overweight patients, hyperinsulinemia is usually demonstrated together with increased uterine artery vascular resistance, obesity, lipid abnormalities and cardiovascular disease.[73, 74] Assuming that PCOS patients are at increased risk for cardiovascular disease, it is possible to affirm that obesity may further increase the risk. Unopposed estrogen stimulation, obesity and chronic anovulation are important contributing factors for endometrial carcinoma.

Recent advances in 3D ultrasound have made accurate noninvasive assessment of the pelvic organs feasible. The ability to visualize the oblique or coronal plane allows for accurate volume measurements, especially of irregularly shaped objects.[17, 20] Due to an accurate track of the individual variations in structure during the measurement process, measurements are considered reliable and highly reproducible.[16]

Wu et al.[75] studied 44 patients with PCOS who presented with a history of irregular menstrual periods. The diagnosis of PCOS was based on the clinical symptoms (e.g. menstrual problems, obesity, acne, hirsutism), endocrinologic data (reversed serum LH/FSH ratio) and ultrasonographic features (increased ovarian stroma and volume, subcapsular cysts and thickened capsule). Another 22 women with regular ovulatory cycles were recruited as normal controls. There was no statistically significant difference in age (range, 17-35 years) between the patient groups. Three-dimensional ultrasonography was performed to store and document the ovarian volumes for detailed ultrasound evaluation. Three perpendicular planes of both ovaries were rotated to obtain the largest dimensions and ovarian volumes were measured using the trapezoid formula. The ovaries of the patients with PCOS were larger in size, area and volume than the ovaries of normal controls. The mean ovarian volumes of PCOS patients (three dimensions; mean SD) were 11.3 ± 3.5 cm^3 compared to 5.5 ± 1.4 cm^3 in the normal controls (P < 0.0001). The volumes of the right ovary were 12.2 ± 4.7 cm^3 and 5.3 ± 2.0 cm^3 and volumes of the left ovary were 10.5 ± 3.6 cm^3

and 5.7 ± 1.6 cm^3 in the PCOS and normal groups, respectively. In patients with PCOS, the right ovary demonstrated a larger volume than the left ovary ($P < 0.0001$); however, the left ovary was significantly larger than the right one in the normal controls ($P < 0.0001$). The ovaries in PCOS were increased in size, stroma and volume ($P < 0.0001$) compared with the ovaries in a control group. Cut-off values for ovarian area, stroma and volume in PCOS were 5.2 cm^2 (sensitivity 93%, specificity 91%), 4.6 cm^2 (sensitivity 91%, specificity 86%) and 6.6 cm^3 (sensitivity 91%, specificity 91%), respectively. The stroma, total ovarian areas and volume detected by careful rotation and outlining of the longitudinal ovarian cut were increased in 84% (37 of 44), 89% (39 of 44) and 80% (35 of 44) of the patients with PCOS, in comparison with normal controls. The total ovarian area was highly correlated with the stromal area ($r^2 = 0.66$).

Undoubtedly, 3D ultrasonography facilitates noninvasive retrospective evaluation and volume calculation. The examination time is short and does not increase the patient's discomfort. Three maximal dimensions of the ovaries can be measured easily once the digital volume is documented from either transvaginal or transabdominal 3D ultrasonography. In addition, superior volume determination is obtained from the 3D images. The volume measurement in 3D ultrasonography is accurate and highly reproducible. The volume of follicles may be precisely determined and the volume of the ovary from 3-D sonography correlates better with a direct measurement of the surgical specimen than the ovarian volume assessed by 2D ultrasonography.[20] The ability of reconstruction increases the diagnostic potential for PCOS. The ovaries in PCOS are usually enlarged bilaterally, but may be of normal size (up to 20% in our study). The stromal area in PCOS is hypertrophic and provides yet another subjective ultrasonographic criterion that could differentiate PCOS from the multifollicular ovary. Multifollicular ovaries demonstrate normal or slightly increased size, but an increased number of follicles are noted without an increased amount of the ovarian stroma. Using the computerized quantification measurement, PCOS patients demonstrate an increased total ovarian area of > 5.5 cm^2 that highly correlate with an increased ovarian stroma at a strict longitudinal ovarian section.[66]

Three-dimensional ultrasonography allows precise measurement of the ovarian stroma, which is obtained after subtracting the sum area of the ovarian follicles from the total ovarian area. Also, 3D ultrasound obtains a more accurate volume data by outlining the contour of the ovary, which is more accurate than the traditional 2D ultrasonographic calculation, using the ellipsoid formula (height × width × thickness × 0.523).

Hence, 3D ultrasonography can complement 2D ultrasonography for the diagnosis of PCOS. It allows excellent spatial evaluation of the polycystic ovaries, measurement of the ovarian volume and assessment of the follicular and stromal areas. Apart from the morphological and volume assessment of the ovaries, Doppler evaluation of the hemodynamic parameters may be added to the traditional endocrinologic and ultrasonographic parameters clinically used for diagnosis and evaluation of the patients with PCOS.

Patients with PCOS undergoing ovulation induction for IVF are more likely to develop a greater number of follicles and generate more oocytes compared with women who have normal ovaries even though they require less gonadotropin stimulation.[76] These patients develop more follicles of all sizes, in particular small- and medium-sized follicles and are at greater risk of ovarian hyperstimulation syndrome (OHSS).[77] This suggests that patients with PCOS are more sensitive to gonadotropin stimulation. The exact mechanism is unknown, although it is possible that the increased ovarian stromal blood flow velocity, in combination with a relatively unchanged impedance to blood flow, may reflect increased intraovarian perfusion leading to a greater delivery of gonadotropins to the granulosa cells of the developing follicles. PCOS patients have significantly increased blood flow velocity within the ovarian stroma, detected by transvaginal color Doppler ultrasound, which may explain the excessive ovarian response when they are administered gonadotropins. Increased stromal blood flow velocity on color, power and pulsed Doppler ultrasound may be an additional marker in the diagnosis of PCOS. It seems that the evaluation of the ovarian stromal vascularity by 3D power Doppler may further increase our knowledge about this enigmatic syndrome.

Luteinized Unruptured Follicle Syndrome

Luteinized unruptured follicle (LUF) syndrome is characterized by regular menses and presumptive ovulation, suggested by a cyclic hormonal profile, similar to that seen in normal ovulatory women, but without release of the oocyte. Although LUF was first diagnosed at laparoscopy by the absence of an ovulation signs and demonstration of the lower concentrations of estradiol and progesterone in peritoneal fluid compared with normal ovulatory cycles, diagnosis is most commonly made on ultrasound examination, due to the persistence of the ovarian follicle with progressive loss of its typical echo-free cystic appearance and accumulation of internal echogenicity. The precise etiology of LUF remains uncertain, but impairment of the mid-cycle luteinizing hormone (LH) surge, the absence of the preovulatory progesterone rise, abnormalities of prostaglandin synthesis and a primary abnormality of the oocyte has all been suggested as possible causes. There is a possible association between LUF syndrome and unexplained infertility, chronic pelvic infection and endometriosis. The estimated frequency of this syndrome is between 6% and 47%.

Kupesic et al.[78] evaluated the intraovarian resistance index, RI in 47 healthy volunteers with ovulatory cycles, 28 patients with luteal phase defect (LPD) and four patients with luteinized unruptured follicle (LUF syndrome). Ovulatory cycles were diagnosed based on daily ultrasound measurement of the mean follicular diameter, detection of follicular collapse, visualization of a solid or complex structure representing the corpus luteum and demonstration of the extraovarian signs, such as thickened endometrium and presence of free fluid in the cul-de-sac. All these findings were suggestive of ovulation. Doubtful cases (nonvisualization of the corpus luteum and/or lack of the serial measurement) were excluded from the study. LUF syndrome was documented by daily ultrasound observations and endocrinological measurement. During the period of expected ovulation, the follicle remained the same size and maintained a tense appearance. Luteinization of the unruptured follicle was seen as a progressive accumulation of the strong echoes located on its periphery. There was also evidence of progesterone increase during the luteal phase of the menstrual cycle. In the group with regular ovulatory cycles, moderate to high RI (0.56 ± 0.06) was obtained at the rim of the follicle. Significant decline of the RI occurred on the day of LH peak (RI 0.44 ± 0.04). The lowest RI values were obtained during the midluteal phase (RI 0.42 ± 0.06), with a return to higher vascular resistance of 0.50 ± 0.04 during the late luteal phase. In 15 patients, endometrial biopsy was performed and normal endometrial dating was detected. In patients with LUF syndrome, no difference in terms of intraovarian RI was obtained after the LH peak. Similar RI values were obtained during the follicular and luteal phase (0.55 ± 0.04 vs 0.54 ± 0.06). There was no difference between the sides in terms of intraovarian vascular resistance. The mean progesterone value in this group was 14.1 ± 6.2 ng/ml and normal

endometrial dating was obtained from all the patients with LUF syndrome. Similar results were reported by Merce et al.[79] who did not observe any decrease in perifollicular intraovarian resistance after the LH peak. The so called "luteal conversion" did not take place in patients with LUF syndrome, indicating that the perifollicular angiogenesis was altered in LUF, probably because of follicular failure.

An increase in the perifollicular blood flow during the periovulatory period appears to be primarily regulated by LH. Ovulatory cycles are characterized with progressive decrease of vascular resistance and increase of the blood flow velocity of the perifollicular vessels. Stable vascular impedance and decreased blood flow velocity of the peripheral follicular vessels are diagnostic Doppler parameters of LUF syndrome.[69] The reduction in perifollicular blood flow velocity has also been reported in a patient with drug-associated LUF.[80] Additional Doppler studies and biochemical research are needed to clarify the causes and consequences of LUF syndrome.

Luteal Phase Defect

The formation of the corpus luteum is an important event in reproductive cycle and one of the crucial factors in early pregnancy support. After ovulation, blood vessels of the theca layer invade the cavity of the ruptured follicle starting the formation of the corpus luteum. Small luteal cells produce more and more LH receptors and thus, amplify the production of progesterone. This chain reaction continues until the so called midluteal phase, which is characterized by peak values of blood LH, progesterone and the lowest resistance index (RI) in corpus luteum blood vessels, as proven by transvaginal color and pulsed Doppler by Kupesic et al.[81]

Consequently progesterone suppresses the secretion of gonadotropins, LH and progesterone levels decrease and RI in the vessels of the corpus luteum increases. Whether because of "intrinsic error of mechanism" or because of the interference with external factors (e.g. strenuous exercise, ovulation stimulating drugs), a condition called luteal phase defect (LPD) occurs. Various names have been assigned to this disorder, such as short luteal phase, luteal insufficiency, inadequate luteal phase, luteal defect and luteal phase deficiency (LPD). All these names describe the same condition: lack of progesterone, luteal phase of the cycle shorter than 11 days and when related to endometrium, an out-of-phase endometrium by two or more days. The new method to detect an abnormality with the corpus luteum is color Doppler ultrasound. Until recently, research in this field was carried out mainly using B mode. Glock et al.[82] investigated whether the ultrasound appearance, size or change in size of the corpus luteum during early pregnancy correlates with serum progesterone, estradiol E2 or 17-hydroxyprogesterone or were even predictive of pregnancy outcome. They hypothesized that the corpus luteum volumes during early pregnancy correlate with the serum concentration of steroids produced by the corpus luteum, the appearance of the corpus luteum may be correlated with pregnancy outcome and that a decreased volume of the corpus luteum volume may be associated with pregnancy loss. Disappointingly, the acquired data showed a lack of correlation between the corpus luteum size and steroid products, and no correlation between changes in volume and changes in steroid production during early pregnancy. However, decreasing corpus luteum volume before 8 weeks gestation was associated with increased risk of pregnancy loss. In this study, color and pulsed Doppler was used to determine a dominant ovary (containing corpus luteum). Dominant ovary showed low impedance blood flow signals with RI between 0.39 and 0.49. The contralateral ovary demonstrated significantly higher impedance to blood flow (RI from 0.69 to 1.0), characteristic of a nondominant ovary. Patient with ovarian RI of 0.74 obtained from a dominant ovary and RI of 0.79 in the nondominant ovary experienced pregnancy loss.

Kupesic at al.[81] evaluated intraovarian resistance index in 47 healthy fertile volunteers with ovulatory cycles and compared them with 28 patients with luteal phase defect (LPD) and four patients with luteinized unruptured follicle (LUF syndrome). Serial sonography allowed daily measurement of the mean follicular diameter, visualization of the follicular collapse and demarcation of the hypoechoic structure with an irregular wall, solid or complex structure representing the corpus luteum, as well as observation of the thickened endometrium and free fluid in the cul-de-sac. All of these findings were suggestive of ovulation. Doubtful cases (nonvisualization of the corpus luteum and/or lack of the serial measurements) were excluded from this study. LPD was diagnosed by measuring the progesterone levels and performing the endometrial biopsy during the midluteal phase of the menstrual cycle. Sonographic and Doppler findings were correlated to hormonal and histopathologic data.[81]

In the group with regular ovulatory cycles (n = 47), different ovarian RI values have been observed. During the stage of the follicular growth and development, moderate to high RI (mean 0.56 ± 0.06) were obtained at the rim of the follicle. Significant decline of the RI occurred on the day of the LH peak (RI 0.44 ± 0.04). The lowest RI values were obtained during the midluteal phase (RI 0.42 ± 0.06), with a return to a higher vascular resistance of 0.50 ± 0.04 during the late luteal phase. In the LPD group (n = 28) no difference was obtained in terms of intraovarian RI during the follicular phase. However, the mean RI throughout the luteal phase (RI 0.56 ± 0.04) was significantly higher when compared to the control group. Furthermore, it did not show any difference between the early, middle and late luteal phase in LPD group.[81]

In the control group, both follicular and luteal RI was significantly lower on the dominant side. However, in the LPD group no difference occurred in terms of intraovarian RI between the sides. Mean progesterone levels were significantly lower in the LPD group (6.9 ± 2.3 ng/ml) than in the controls (24.1 ± 11.4 ng/ml), while histopathology revealed delayed endometrial pattern in all the patients with LPD. There was a correlation between progesterone levels and intraovarian resistance index during the midluteal phase.[81]

"Luteal conversion" is a term describing intraovarian Doppler findings obtained during the luteal phase. Increased turbulence of the blood flow with "luteal conversion" signals are easily obtained from the ovarian stroma, have an increased intensity in the frequency spectrum, have extensive dispersion of maximum frequencies and superposition of the multiple waveforms presenting variable maximum systolic velocities, and exhibit an increased intensity of color signals occupying most of the ovary.[79] In patients with LPD, the dominant and nondominant ovaries demonstrate similar resistance index values, and there are no significant differences in intraovarian vascularity between the follicular and luteal phases of the menstrual cycle.[81]

Glock and Brumsted[83] correlated the intraovarian blood flow with the values of progesterone throughout the cycle. Mean progesterone levels were significantly lower for LPD patients than for the control group during the luteal phase. The mean resistance index in LPD patients was significantly higher compared with the control group during the follicular and luteal phase of the menstrual cycle. Although systolic and diastolic velocities were observed to be lower in LPD patients compared with normal women, these differences were not statistically different. High correlations were observed between the progesterone and resistance index of the intraovarian flow for each of the luteal time points, achieving the highest value during the midluteal phase. The conversion signals obtained from the dominant ovary had significantly lower vascular impedance than the nondominant ovary in the control group (0.50 versus 0.65). In patients with LPD conversion, the luteal signals had resistance index of 0.60 and were not statistically different from the contralateral ovary (RI of 0.66 P = 0.37). In both ovaries, in a single anovulatory subject, the resistance index values remained high (mean 0.76, range 0.70 to 0.82). This study[83] demonstrated a correlation between the resistance index of the corpus luteum blood flow and plasma progesterone in the natural cycle. The strongest correlation was obtained for the midluteal phase, the period that corresponds to the peak angiogenesis of the corpus luteum. Consistent with this finding, the authors have shown an increase in blood flow impedance during the late luteal phase, the period associated with the onset of corpus luteum regression. These findings suggest that the resistance index of the corpus luteum blood flow may be used as an index of luteal function and adjunct to plasma progesterone assay for detection of the patients with LPD.

Tinkanen[84] did not prove the hypothesis that LPD is due to a premature vascular regression of the corpus luteum, and documented no difference between the luteal blood flow in patients with a normal luteal function and those with a short luteal phase. Strigini et al.[85] observed the change of impedance during the luteal phase of FSH-treated cycles. The uterine pulsatility index during stimulated cycles, both before and after ovulation, was significantly reduced compared with spontaneous cycles. That was explained by the increase of plasma E2. Furthermore, Strigini advocates an administration of exogenous progesterone as a supplementation to FSH treated cycles, stating that the uterine pulsatility index after administration of progesterone decreased even more than in spontaneous or only with FSH treated cycles.

Our study correlating Doppler velocimetry, histological and hormonal markers[81] has documented that mean progesterone levels were significantly lower in the group with a luteal phase defect (10.2 ± 4.3 ng/ml) than in the control group (21 ± 4.2 ng/ml). The FSH/LH ratio was significantly lower in the group with a delayed endometrial pattern compared to normal subjects during the follicular and periovulatory phases (0.70 vs 1.24; 0.58 vs 0.75, respectively). There was a close correlation between estradiol levels and the mean diameter of the dominant follicle from days −5 to −1 relative to the days of sonographically observed ovulation. An increase in follicular diameter and endometrial thickness was noted for

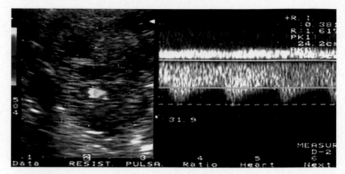

FIGURE 9.13: Transvaginal color Doppler scan of a mature corpus luteum. Pulsed Doppler waveform analysis shows high velocity and low resistance index (RI = 0.34), both indicative of a normal corpus luteum function.

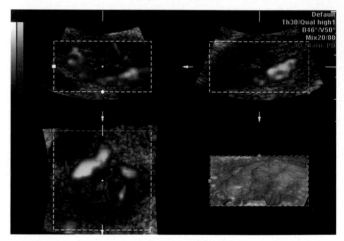

FIGURE 9.14: Three dimensional power Doppler ultrasound of corpus luteum angiogenesis.

both normal and luteal phase defect groups. Intraovarian blood flow resistance showed no difference between the groups during the proliferative phase. A significant decline of the RI occurred in the control group for the day of the LH peak (RI = 0.45 ± 0.04), with a return to the follicular phase level of 0.49 ± 0.02 during the second phase of the menstrual cycle (Figures 9.13 and 9.14). The mean intraovarian RI for the luteal phase defect group (RI = 0.58 ± 0.04) was significantly higher than in the control group throughout the luteal phase (Figure 9.15). Patients in the control group had a significantly lower RI in the dominant than in the nondominant ovary, whereas LPD patients had the almost same RI in both ovaries. Spiral arteries in the control group demonstrated mean RI of 0.53 ± 0.04 during the periovulatory phase, and RI values of 0.50 ± 0.02 and 0.51 ± 0.04 were obtained during the midluteal and late luteal phase, respectively. Higher impedance values during

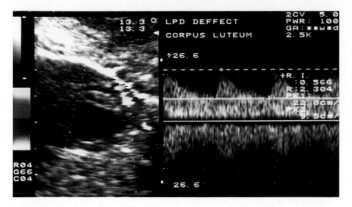

FIGURE 9.15: Intraovarian blood flow during the midluteal phase in a patient with a luteal phase defect demonstrates increased resistance index (RI = 0.56).

the periovulatory phase (RI = 0.70 ± 0.06, p < 0.001), midluteal phase (RI = 0.72 ± 0.06, p < 0.001) and late luteal phase (RI = 0.72 ± 0.04, p < 0.001) were obtained from the spiral arteries in the luteal phase defect group. A close correlation has been found between plasma estradiol levels and the mean diameter of the follicle. Patients with normal endometrial development show a similar trend of regression for uterine, radial and spiral artery impedance from the follicular to the luteal phase. In contrast, patients with a delayed endometrial pattern are characterized by increased uterine vascular resistance during the luteal phase. Since the most significant difference in terms of RI is obtained for the spiral arteries, it might be expected that endometrial blood flow changes could be used to predict the development of the endometrium and likelihood of pregnancy.

Salim et al.[86] correlated luteal blood in normal pregnancies to the flow in abnormal pregnancies. Their study proved the hypothesis that an absence of luteal flow cannot coexist with normal pregnancy. Impedance to intraovarian blood flow is significantly higher in patients with abnormal early pregnancy (missed, incomplete and threatened abortion) than in women with normal pregnancy outcome. However, this was not confirmed in patients with blighted ovum, molar and ectopic pregnancy. In these groups of patients, the luteal blood flow was almost the same as in normal pregnancy. This difference among the subgroups of an abnormal early pregnancy may be a consequence of a different natural history of the disease. Missed and incomplete abortions are manifested as failed early pregnancy with no prospects for further development. A threatened abortion is potentially a similar condition.

Whether a decreased corpus luteum blood flow is a potential cause or a consequence of the event remains unclear. Anembryonic pregnancies, molar or ectopic pregnancies are somewhat different. These pathologic conditions are usually progressive and not self-limited. This can explain why luteal vascular impedance in these women is similar to the luteal flow of the patients with a normal pregnancy outcome.

Increased intraovarian vascular resistance in patients with missed abortion may be explained by a failure of early pregnancy to develop and impaired production of human chorionic gonadotropin, which in turn could have a negative effect on luteal function. However, Alcazar et al.[87] found no statistically significant difference in intraovarian RI of the patients with threatened abortion.

TUBAL CAUSES OF INFERTILITY

The tubal mucosa responds to the hormonal changes during the menstrual cycle in order to facilitate the sperm and oocyte transport in the process of fertilization. During the luteal phase, decreased tubal secretion and more prominent ciliary activity propel the oocyte into the uterine fundus. If conception does not occur, the secretory and ciliary cells are significantly reduced in number due to withdrawal of the endocrine support.

The normal Fallopian tubes are narrow and usually not seen by transabdominal or transvaginal ultrasound unless they contain fluid within their lumina or are surrounded by fluid. The motility and transport function of the oviducts are impaired during all stages of pelvic inflammatory disease. First, in the acute phase, the tube becomes thick and edematous and a large amount of purulent exudate fills the lumen. Later on, the inflammatory process may be organized to form a tubo-ovarian abscess, which will, in most cases lead to scarring and occlusion of the tube. Chronic hydrosalpinx is the ultimate remnant of PID with a thin-walled, occluded and fluid filled tube. Infertility caused by tubal dysfunction is found in approximately 35% of patients. A history of pelvic inflammatory disease, septic abortion, intrauterine contraceptive device, ruptured appendix, tubal surgery or ectopic pregnancy should alert the physician to the possibility of tubal damage. Amorphous acellular plugs in the proximal tube have been identified in nearly 50% of women whose tubes did not opacify on hysterosalpingography. Improved pregnancy rates after uterotubal insufflation and hysterosalpingography suggests that their therapeutic effects may result from dislodgment of the Fallopian tube debris. Reversible spasm at the uterotubal junction is another cause of apparent obstruction on conventional hysterosalpingography. Evaluation of a 100 patients with a nonfilling fallopian tubes on an initial hysterosalpingogram, found that only 39 had persistent occlusion after pharmacologic manipulation and selective tubal salpingography.[88] In the remaining 61 patients, the apparent cause of tubal nonfilling was spasm and debris in 49 patients, submucosal fibroids in six, synechiae in three, salpingitis isthmica nodosa in two, and a septate uterus in one.[88]

Until a few years ago, the assessment of the uterine cavity and the Fallopian tube lumen relied on complicated, painful and invasive procedures. The major problem was how to visualize the hollow space within pelvic organs and how to describe the contours of uterine and oviduct walls. Uterine cavity distorted by a submucosal myoma or endometrial polyp may be an obstacle to implantation, while a tortuous and narrow tube with PID changes prevents fertilization.

Hysterosalpingography, using radio-opaque dye for X-ray assessment of tubal and uterine anatomy, has been the standard form of investigation for several decades. The disadvantage of this investigation is that ionizing radiation presents a risk to the oocyte. If the conception takes place in the investigation cycle, congenital fetal anomalies may occur. Furthermore, iodine-containing dyes used for X-ray hysterosalpingography may cause an allergic reaction. During the last two decades, laparoscopy has become the gold standard for the assessment of tubal status. However, it requires general anesthesia and carries the risk of anesthetic and surgical complications, such as bowel or vascular injury, false pneumoperitoneum and postoperative discomfort.

With the development of transvaginal, color Doppler and 3D ultrasound, a totally new concept of diagnostic procedures has been developed. In the chapter on hystero-contrast-salpingography, an interested reader may find relevant information about the benefits and limitations of the sonographic evaluation of tubal patency.

CONCLUSION

Introduction of the transvaginal color Doppler and 3D power Doppler ultrasound has made a significant improvement in the assessment of infertility. Ultrasound may predict ovulation, diagnose ovulatory disorders, predict ovarian reserve and detect polycystic ovaries.[89,90,91] Measurements of the endometrial thickness and evaluation of uterine perfusion may determine likelihood of pregnancy in patients undergoing medically assisted reproduction.

Absence of subendometrial and intraendometrial vascularization on the day of hCG administration is a useful predictor of failure of implantation in IVF cycles, irrespective of the ultrasound appearance of the endometrium. Studies of spiral artery perfusion represent a noninvasive assay of the uterine receptivity, which provides additional information on the pathophysiology of infertility, especially in patients with unexplained causes.[92,93,94] It was demonstrated that dynamic changes in endometrial volume and thickness between the day of embryo transfer and two weeks later may predict IVF outcome.[95] The main clinical application of ultrasound is the assessment for uterine anomalies and intrauterine pathology, especially if combined with the procedure of saline infusion into the uterine cavity.[38,40,44] In conclusion, color Doppler and 3D ultrasound are exciting research and clinical tools in hands of experienced sonographers, but their widespread clinical use still remains to be elucidated.

REFERENCES

1. Kurjak A, Kupesic-Urek S, Schulman H, et al. Transvaginal color Doppler in the assessment of ovarian and uterine blood flow in infertile women. Fertil Steril 1991;56(5):870-3.
2. Kurjak A and Kupesic-Urek S. Normal and abnormal uterine perfusion. In: Jaffe R and Warsof LS (Eds). Color Doppler Imaging in Obstetrics and Gynecology. New York: McGraw Hill 1992;255-63.
3. Goswamy RK, Silliams G, Steptoe PC. Decreased uterine perfusion—a cause of infertility. Hum Reprod 1988;3(8):955-9.
4. Steer CV, Mills CV, Campbell S. Vaginal color Doppler assessment on the day of embryo transfer (ET) accurately predicts patients in an in vitro fertilization programme with suboptimal uterine perfusion who fail to become pregnant. Ultrasound Obstet Gynaecol 1994;1:79-82.
5. Tsai YC, Chang JC, Tai MJ, et al. Relationship of uterine perfusion to outcome of intrauterine insemination. J Ultrasound Med 1996;15:633-6.
6. Steer CV, Tan SL, Mason BA, et al. Midluteal-phase vaginal color Doppler assessment of uterine artery impedance in a subfertile population. Fertil Steril 1994;61(1):53-8.
7. Kupesic S. The first three weeks assessed by transvaginal color Doppler. J Perinat Med 1996;24(4):301-17.
8. Cacciatore B, Simberg N, Fusaro P, et al. Transvaginal Doppler study of uterine artery blood flow in vitro fertilization-embryo transfer cycles. Fertil Steril 1996;66(1):130-4.
9. Freidler S, Schenker JG, Herman A. The role of ultrasonography in the evaluation of endometrial receptivity following assisted reproductive treatments: a critical review. Hum Reprod 1996;2:323-35.
10. Gonen Y, Calderon M, Direnfeld M, et al. The impact of sonographic assessment of the endometrium and meticulous

hormonal monitoring during natural cycles in patients with failed donor artificial insemination. Ultrasound Obstet Gynecol 1991;1(2):122-6.

11. Abdalla HI, Brooks AA, Johnson MR, et al. Endometrial thickness: a predictor of implantation in ovum recipients? Hum Reprod 1994;9(2):363-5.

12. Khalifa E, Brzyski RG, Oehninger S, et al. Sonographic appearance of the endometrium: the predictive value for the outcome of in vitro fertilization in stimulated cycles. Hum Reprod 1992;7(5):677-80.

13. Serafini P, Batzofin J, Nelson J, et al. Sonographic uterine predictors of pregnancy in women undergoing ovulation induction for assisted reproductive treatments. Fertil Steril 1994;62(4):815-22.

14. Sher G, Herbert C, Maassarani G, et al. Assessment of the late proliferative phase endometrium by ultrasonography in patients undergoing in vitro fertilization and embryo transfer (IVF/ET). Hum Reprod 1991;6(2):232-7.

15. Zaidi J, Campbell S, Pitroff R, et al. Endometrial thickness, morphology, vascular penetration and velocimetry in predicting implantation in an in vitro fertilization program. Ultrasound Obstet Gynecol 1995;6(3);191-8.

16. Kyei-Mensah A, Maconochie N, Zaidi J, et al. Transvaginal three-dimensional ultrasound: reproducibility of ovarian and endometrial volume measurements. Fertil Steril 1996;66(5):718-22.

17. Riccabona M, Nelson TR, Pretorius DH. Three-dimensional ultrasound: accuracy of distance and volume measurements. Ultrasound Obstet Gynecol 1996;7(6):429-34.

18. Gilja OH, Smievoll I, Thune N, et al. In vivo comparison of 3D ultrasonography and magnetic resonance imaging in volume estimation of human kidney. Ultrasound Med Biol 1995;21(1):25-32.

19. Lee A, Sator M, Kratochwil A, et al. Endometrial volume change during spontaneous menstrual cycles: volumetry by transvaginal three-dimensional ultrasound. Fertil Steril 68(5):831-5.

20. Kyei-Mensah A, Zaidi J, Pittrof R. Transvaginal three-dimensional ultrasound: accuracy of follicular volume measurements. Fertil Steril 1996;65(2):371-6.

21. Kupesic S, Bekavac I, Bjelos D, et al. Assessment of endometrial receptivity by transvaginal color Doppler and three-dimensional power Doppler ultrasonography in patients undergoing in vitro fertilization procedures. J Ultrasound Med 2001;20(2):125-134.

22. Ashton D, Amin HK, Richart RM, et al. The incidence of asymptomatic uterine anomalies in women undergoing transcervical tubal sterilization. Obstet Gynecol 1988;72(1):28-30.

23. Sorensen S. Estimated prevalence of mulerian anomalies. Acta Obstet Gynecol Scand 1988;67(5):441-5.

24. Gaucherand P, Awada A, Rudigoz RC. Obstetrical prognosis of septate uterus: a plea for treatment of the septum. Eur J Obstet Gynecol Reprod Biol 1994;54(2):109-12.

25. Fedele L, Arcaini L, Parazzini F, et al. Metroplastic hysteroscopy and fertility. Fertil Steril 1993;59:768-70.

26. Heinonen PK, Saarikoski S, Pystynen P, et al. Reproductive performance of women with uterine anomalies. An evaluation of 182 cases. Acta Obstet Gynecol Scand 1982;61:157-62.

27. Fedele L, Bianchi S, Marchini M, et al. Ultrastructural aspects of endometrium in infertile women with septate uterus. Fertil Steril 1996;65(4):750-2.

28. Cararach M, Penella J, Ubeda J. Hysteroscopic incision of the septate uterus: scissors versus resectoscope. Hum Reprod 1994;9(1):87-9.

29. Goldenberg M, Sivan E, Sharabi Z. Reproductive outcome following hysteroscopic management of intrauterine septum and adhesions. Hum Reprod 1995;10(10):2663-5.

30. Valdes C, Malini S, Malinak LR. Ultrasound evaluation of female genital tract anomalies: a review of 64 cases. Am J Obstet Gynecol 1984;149(3):285-92.

31. Nicolini U, Bellotti B, Bonazzi D, et al. Can ultrasound be used to screen uterine malformation? Fertil Steril 1987;47:89-93.

32. Reuter KL, Daly D, Cohen SM. Septate versus bicornuate uteri: errors in imaging diagnosis. Radiology 1989;172(3):749-52.

33. Randolph J, Ying Y, Maier D, et al. Comparison of real time ultrasonography, hysterosalpingography, and laparoscopy/ hysteroscopy in the evaluation of uterine abnormalities and tubal patency. Fertil Steril;1986;5:828-32.

34. Richman TS, Viscomi N, Cherney AD, et al. Fallopian tubal patency assessment by ultrasound following fluid injection. Radiology 1984;152:507-10.

35. Salle B, Sergeant P, Gaucherand P, et al. Transvaginal hysterosonographic evaluation of septate uteri: a preliminary report. Hum Reprod 1996;11(5):1004-7.

36. Marshall C, Mintz DI, Thickman D. et al. MR evaluation of uterine anomalies. Radiology 1987;148:287-9.

37. Carrington BM, Hricak M, Naruddin RN. Mullerian duct anomalies: MR evaluation. Radiology 1990;170:715-20.

38. Jurkovic D, Giepel A, Gurboeck K, et al. Three-dimensional ultrasound for the assessment of uterine anatomy and detection of congenital anomalies: a comparison with hysterosalpingography and two-dimensional sonography. Ultrasound Obstet Gynecol 1995;5(4):233-7.

39. Taylor PJ, Cumming DC. Hysteroscopy in 100 patients. Fertil Steril 1979. 31(3):301-4.

40. Kupesic S, Kurjak A. Septate uterus: detection and prediction of obstetrical complications by different forms of ultrasonography. J Ultrasound Med 1998;17(10):631-6.

41. Dabrashrafi H, Bahadori M, Mohammad K, et al. Septate uterus: New idea on the histologic features of the septum in this abnormal uterus. Am J Obstet Gynecol 1995;172:105-7.

42. Balen FG, Allen CM, Gardener JE, et al. 3-dimensional reconstruction of ultrasound images of the uterine cavity. Br J Radiol 1993;66(787):588-91.

43. Weinraub Z, Maymon R, Shulman A, et al. Three-dimensional saline contrast rendering of uterine cavity pathology. Ultrasound Obstet Gynecol 1996;8(4):277-82.

44. Kupesic S, Kurjak A, Skenderovic S, et al. Screening for uterine abnormalities by three-dimensional ultrasound improves perinatal outcome. J Preinat Med. 30(1):9-17.

45. Kurjak A, Kupesic S, Miric D. The assessment of benign uterine tumor vascularization by transvaginal color Doppler. Ultrasound Med Biol 1992;18:645-9.

46. Brosens JJ, de Souza NM, Barker FG, et al. Endovaginal ultrasonography in the diagnosis of adenomyosis uteri: identifying the predictive characteristics. Br J Obstet Gynaecol 1995;102(6):471-4.

47. Schlaff WD, Hurst BS. Preoperative sonographic measurement of endometrial pattern predicts outcome of surgical repair in patients with severe Asherman's syndrome. Fertil Steril 1995;63(2):410-3.

48. Zaidi J, Barber J, Kyei-Mensah A, et al. Relationship of ovarian stromal blood flow at baseline ultrasound to subsequent follicular response in an in vitro fertilization program. Obstet Gynecol 1996;88(5):779-84.

49. Engmann L, Sladkevicius P, Agrawal R, et al. Value of ovarian stromal blood flow velocity measurement after pituitary suppression in the prediction of ovarian responsiveness and outcome of in vitro fertilization treatment. Fertil Steril 1999;71(1):22-9.

50. Wittmaack FM, Kreger DO, Blasco L, et al. Effect of follicular size on oocyte retrieval, fertilization, cleavage and embryo quality in in vitro fertilization cycles: a 6-year data collection. Fertil Steril 1994;62(6):1205-10.

51. Golan A, Herman A, Soffer Y, et al. Ultrasonic control without hormone determination for ovulation induction in in-vitro fertilization/embryo-transfer with gonadotrophin-releasing hormone analogue and human menopausal gonadotrophin. Hum Reprod 1994. 9(9):1631-3.

52. Shoham Z, DiCarlo C, Pater A, et al. Is it possible to run a successful ovulation induction program based solely on ultrasound monitoring? The importance of endometrial measurements. Fertil Steril 1991;56(5): 836-41.

53. Tan SL. Simplification of IVF therapy. Curr Opin Obstet Gynecol 1994;6:111-4.

54. Steiner H, Staudach A, Spitzer D, et al. Three-dimensional US in obstetrics and gynaecology: technique, possibilities and limitations. Hum Reprod 1994;9(9):1773-8.

55. Penzias AS, Emmi AM, Dubey AK, et al. Ultrasound prediction of follicle volume: is the mean diameter reflective? Fertil Steril 1994;62(6):1274-6.

56. Feichtinger W. Transvaginal three-dimensional imaging for evaluation and treatment of infertility. In: Merz (Ed). 3-D Ultrasound in Obstetrics and Gynecology. Philadelphia: Lipincott Williams & Wilkins;1998;37-43.

57. Lass A, Skull J, McVeigh E, et al. Measurement of ovarian volume by transvaginal sonography before ovulation induction with human menopausal gonadotrophin for in-vitro fertilization can predict poor response. Hum Reprod 1997;12(2):294-7.

58. Oyesanya OA, Parsons JH, Collins WP, et al. Total ovarian volume before human chorionic gonadotrophin administration for ovulation induction may predict the hyperstimulation syndrome. Hum Reprod 1995;10(12):3211-12.

59. Kupesic S, Kurjak A. Predictors of IVF outcome by three-dimensional ultrasound. Hum Reprod 2002;17(4):950-5.

60. Kupesic S, Kurjak A, Bjelos D, et al. Three-dimensional ultrasonographic measurements and in vitro fertilization outcome are related to age. Fertil Steril 2003;79(1):190-7.

61. Adams J, Franks S, Polson DW, et al. Multifollicular ovaries: clinical and endocrine features and response to pulsatile gonadotropin-releasing hormone. Lancet 1985;2:1375-9.

62. Matsunaga I, Hata T, Kitao M. Ultrasonographic identification of polycystic ovary. Asia-Oceania J Obstet Gynaecol 1985;11(2):227-32.

63. Takahashi K, Ozaki T, Okada M, et al. Relationship between ultrasonography and histopathological changes in polycystic ovarian syndrome. Hum Reprod 1994;9(12):2255-8.

64. Battaglia C, Artini PG, D'Ambrogio G, et al. Uterine and ovarian blood flow measurement. Does the full bladder modify the flow resistance? Acta Obstet Gynecol Scand;1994;73(9):716-8.

65. Ardaens Y, Robert Y, Lemaitre L, et al. Polycystic ovarian disease: contribution of vaginal endosonography and reassessment of ultrasonic diagnosis. Fertil Steril 1991;55(6): 1062-8.

66. Robert Y, Dubrulle F, Gaillandre L, et al. Ultrasound assessment of ovarian stroma hypertrophy in hyperandrogenism and ovulation disorders: visual analysis versus computerized quantification. Fertil Steril 1995;64(2):307-12.

67. Merce LT, Garces D, Barco MJ, et al. Intraovarian Doppler velocimetry in ovulatory, dysovulatory and anovulatory cycles. Ultrasound Obstet Gynecol 1992;2(3):197-202.

68. Battaglia C, Artini PG, D'Ambrogio G, et al. The role of color Doppler imaging in the diagnosis of polycystic ovary syndrome. Am J Obstet Gynecol 1995;172:108-13.

69. Zaidi J, Campbell S, Pittrof R, et al. Ovarian stromal blood flow in women with polycystic ovaries—a possible new marker for diagnosis? Hum Reprod 1995;10(8):1992-6.

70. Aleem FA, Predanic M. Transvaginal color Doppler determination of the ovarian and uterine blood flow characteristics in polycystic ovary disease. Fertil Steril 1996;65(3):510-6.

71. Battaglia C, Artini PG, Salvatori M, et al. Ultrasonographic patterns of polycystic ovaries;color Doppler and hormonal correlations. Ultrasound Obstet Gynecol 1998;11:332-6.

72. Battaglia C, Artini PG, Genazzani AD, et al. Color Doppler analysis in oligo- and amenorrheic women with polycystic ovary syndrome. Gynecol Endocrinol 1997;11(2):105-10.

73. Battaglia C, Artini PG, Genazzani, AD, et al. Color Doppler analysis in lean and obese women with polycystic ovary syndrome. Ultrasound Obstet Gynecol 1996;7(5):342-6.

74. Wild RA, Van Nort JJ, Grubb B, et al. Clinical signs of androgen excess as risk factors for coronary artery disease. Fertil Steril 1990;54(2):255-9.

75. Wu MH, Tang HH, Hsu CC, et al. The role of three-dimensional ultrasonographic images in ovarian measurement. Fertil Steril 1998;69(6):1152-5.

76. MacDougall MJ, Tan SL, Balen A, et al. A controlled study comparing patients with and without polycystic ovaries undergoing in-vitro fertilization. Hum Reprod 1993;8:233-7.

77. MacDougall MJ, Tan SL, Jacobs HS, et al. In-vitro fertilization and the ovarian hyperstimulation syndrome. Hum Reprod 1992;7(5):597-600.

78. Kupesic S, Kurjak A. The assessment of normal and abnormal luteal function by transvaginal color Doppler sonography. Eur J Obstet Gynecol Reprod Biol 1997;72(1):83-7.

79. Merce LT, Garces D, De la Fuente F. Conversion lutea de la onda de velocidad de fluio ovarica: nuevo parametro ecografico de ovulacion y funcion lutea. Acta Obstet Gynecol Scand. 2:113-4.

80. Bourne TH, Reynolds K, Waterstone J, et al. Paracetamol-associated luteinized unruptured follicle syndrome: effect on intrafollicular blood flow. Ultrasound Obstet Gynecol 1991;1(6):420-5.

81. Kupesic S, Kurjak A, Vujisic S, et al. Luteal phase defect: comparison between Doppler velocimetry, histological and hormonal markers. Ultrasound Obstet Gynaecol 1997;9(2):105-12.

82. Glock JL, Blackman JA, Badger GJ, et al. Prognostic Significance of Morphologic Changales of the Corpus Luteum by Transvaginal Ultrasound in Early Pregnancy Monitoring. Obstet Gynecol 1995;85(1):37-41.

83. Glock JL, Brumsted JR. Color flow pulsed Doppler ultrasound in diagnosing luteal phase defect. Fertil Steril 1995;64:500-4.

84. Tinkanen H. The role of vascularization of the corpus luteum in the short luteal phase studied by Doppler ultrasound. Acta Obstet Gynecol Scand 1994. 73:321-3.

85. Strigini FAL, Scida PAM, Parri C, et al. Modifications in uterine and intraovarian artery impedance in cycles of treatment with exogenous gonadotropins: effects of luteal phase support. Fertil Steril 1995;64(1):76-80.

86. Salim A, •alud I, Farmakides G. Corpus luteum blood flow in normal and abnormal early pregnancy: Evaluation with transvaginal color and pulsed Doppler sonography. J Ultrasound Med 1994;13:971-5.

87. Alcazar JL, Laparte C, Lopez-Garcia G. Corpus luteum blood flow in abnormal early pregnancy. J Ultrasound Med 1996;15:645-9.

88. Lang EK. Organic vs. functional obstruction of the fallopian tubes: differentiation with prostaglandin antagonist-and B2-mediated hysterosalpingography and selective ostial salpingography. AJR 1991;157: 77-80.

89. Lam PM, Raine-Fenning N. The role of three-dimensional ultrasonography in polycystic ovary syndrome. Hum Reprod 2006;21(9):2209-15.

90. Ng E, Tang O, Chan C, et al. Ovarian stromal vascularity is not predictive of ovarian response and pregnancy. Reprod Biomed Online 2006;12(1):43-9.

91. Hendriks D, Kwee J, Mol B, et al. Ultrasonography as a tool for the prediction of outcome in IVF patients: a comparative meta-analysis of ovarian volume and antral follicle count. Fertil Steril 2007;87(4):764-75.

92. Mercé L, Barco M, Bau S, et al. Are endometrial parameters by three-dimensional ultrasound and power Doppler angiography related to in vitro fertilization/embryo transfer outcome? Fertil Steril 2008;89(1):111-7.

93. Järvelä IY, Sladkevicius P, Kelly S, et al. Evaluation of endometrial receptivity during in-vitro fertilization using three-dimensional power Doppler ultrasound. Ultrasound Obstet Gynecol 2005;26(7):765-9.

94. Ng E, Chan C, Tang O, et al. The role of endometrial and subendometrial vascularity measured by three-dimensional power Doppler ultrasound in the prediction of pregnancy during frozen-thawed embryo transfer cycles. Hum Reprod 2006;21(6):1612-7.

95. Zohav E, Bar Hava I, Meltcer S, et al. Early endometrial changes following successful implantation. 2D and 3D ultrasound study. Clin Exp Obstet Gynecol 2008;35:255-6.

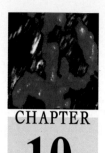

S Kupesic Plavsic
A Kurjak, N Zafar

CHAPTER

10

Color Doppler and 3D Power Doppler Hystero-Contrast-Salpingography

The number of cases of tubal sterility is on the rise. Tubal factors, such as tubal dysfunction or obstruction, account for approximately 35% of the causes of infertility.[1,2] A history of pelvic inflammatory disease, septic abortion, use of an intrauterine contraceptive device, ruptured appendix, tubal surgery or an ectopic pregnancy should alert the physician to the possibility of tubal damage. One aspect of the infertility investigation, which has changed little over the last 20 years, is the assessment of the Fallopian tube patency. Until now, the most frequently used procedures to demonstrate tubal patency have been X-ray hysterosalpingography (HSG) and chromopertubation during laparoscopy.[3]

Hysterosalpingography, using radio-opaque dye for X-ray studies to assess tubal and uterine anatomy, has been a standard form of investigation for several decades. The disadvantage of this type of investigation is that ionizing radiation has inherent risks to the oocyte, which may result in congenital malformations, especially if conception takes place during the investigation cycle. Furthermore, allergy to iodine-containing dyes is a contraindication to an X-ray HSG. Knowledge acquired from an X-ray HSG includes the following: whether or not there is opacification of the tubal lumen, demonstration of an ampullary rugal pattern and visualization of the intramural or intraluminal abnormalities of the Fallopian tube. The risk factors include pelvic inflammatory disease (PID), dye sensitivity and infection. Anesthesia is not required and procedure is carried out on an outpatient basis.

Hysteroscopy is a technique, which complements HSG. It can accurately differentiate between the endometrial polyps and submucosal leiomyomas and can subsequently be used as a treatment modality for those pathologies. The same method is useful in establishing the definitive diagnosis and the treatment of intrauterine adhesions and some congenital anomalies of the uterus. Risk factors include perforation, hemorrhage, infection and inherent risk of anesthesia.

Hysteroscopy-directed falloscopy may detect obstruction of the tubal ostium and is utilized to examine the entire length of the tubal lumen.[4] Treatment of the proximal tubal obstruction can immediately follow the diagnosis. Transcervical tubal cannulation or balloon tuboplasty performed by hysteroscopic approach are the methods of choice.[5]

Laparoscopy has been used as the gold standard for investigation of the tubal status during the last three decades, but it requires general anesthesia and carries the risk of anesthesia itself, surgical complications, such as bowel or vascular injury, hemorrhage, infection, false pneumoperitoneum and postoperative discomfort. With a Jarcho-type of cannula in the uterine cavity, one can manipulate the uterus. In addition, by instilling indigo-carmine saline, or other tinted saline, one is able to evaluate for tubal competence. By the use of laparoscopy, the operator is equally able to visualize the total pelvic anatomy and the upper abdominal cavity. It is also useful for the evaluation of ovarian diseases, genital anomalies, tubal patency and pelvic distortions.

Furthermore, laparoscopy is the gold standard for classification and staging of endometriosis of the pelvis. Another advantage of laparoscopy is that it can be used as an adjunct for assessing possible causes of pelvic pain, the extent of pelvic neoplasia, as well as for a prognostic review of previous infertility surgical procedures. It is also helpful in obtaining peritoneal washings and cultures in

TABLE 10.1: The accuracy of sonographic HSG compared to X-ray HSG

Authors (year)	Total number	Accuracy N (%)	Sensitivity (%)	Specificity (%)
Richman et al. (1984)[13]	36		100%	96%
Peters et al. (1991)[6]	27	19 (70, 37)		
Stern et al. (1992)[8]	89	72 (80, 90)		
Volpi et al. (1991)[7]	21	19 (92, 20)		

patients with a positive history of PID. With the advent of high-frequency vaginal ultrasound probes, ultrasound imaging of the pelvic organs has significantly improved. In addition, the need for bladder filling is avoided. The normal Fallopian tube is usually not seen by vaginal sonography unless some fluid surrounds it. The contrasting fluid usually includes one of the following: normal serous fluid, follicular fluid during or after ovulation, blood, ascitic fluid or products of an exudative or infectious process. If the Fallopian tube is not filled with fluid, its lumen cannot be detected. More recently, ultrasound was introduced for evaluation of the tubal patency and function. Advantages of an ultrasound guided hysterosalpingography (hystero-sono-salpingography or hystero-contrast-salpingography) include: avoidance of the ionization or idiosyncratic reaction to contrast media, noninvasiveness and increased intraprocedural active participation of the patient (increased patient's knowledge of tubal status). The results of this "real time" procedure of analyzing tubal motility may be stored, reviewed, analyzed and viewed by the infertile couple, using a DVD or video recorder. Anesthesia is not required and the procedure is completed in an office setting. The accuracy of the sonographic HSG, compared to an X-ray HSG, varies from 70.37 to 92.20%[6,7] (Table 10.1). The accuracy of a sonographic HSG compared to chromopertubation varies from 81.82[8] to 100%[9,10] (Table 10.2).

HISTORICAL DEVELOPMENT OF THE ULTRASONIC ASSESSMENT OF THE FALLOPIAN TUBE

In 1954, Rubin was the first clinician who attempted insufflation of the Fallopian tubes.[11] Sonographic evaluation of the tubes was first described by Nanini, Richman and Randolph,[12,13,14] who performed abdominal sonography following the intracervical injection of the contrast fluid. Richman was the first to report on the transabdominal sonographic evaluation of tubal patency using the ultrasonic contrast medium.[13] In his study, the accumulation of fluid in the cul-de-sac was accepted as an indicator of tubal patency. Randolph used transabdominal ultrasound for the

TABLE 10.2: The accuracy of sonographic HSG compared to chromopertubation

Authors (year)	Total number	Accuracy (%)
Allahbadia et al. (1993)[33]	27	25 (92, 59)
Tüfekci et al. (1992)[20]	38	37 (97, 37)
Peters et al. (1991)[6]	58	50 (86, 20)
Kupesic et al. (1994)[9]	47	43 (91, 48)
Stern et al. (1992)[8]	121	99 (81, 82)
Deichert et al. (1992)[10]	16	16 (100, 00)
Volpi et al (1996)[7]	29	24 (82.7)
Battaglia (1996)[31]	60	52 (86)
Raga (1996)[35]	42	39 (92)
Sladkevicius (2000)[38*]	67	-
Jeanty (2000)[30]	115	
Kiyokawa (2000)[41*]	25	

* Three-dimensional HSG

observation of the cul-de-sac after injecting 200 ml of isotonic saline through the Rubin cannula.[14] The accumulation of retrouterine fluid was accepted as a criterion for the patency of one or both tubes. In addition, tubal patency was deduced indirectly from the presence of increasing fluid in the pouch of Douglas, without differentiation of the sides. Following instillation of dextran or saline solution into the uterine cavity, it is possible to visualize lesions, such as submucous myomas and endometrial polyps, subsequently confirming their presence by hysteroscopy. While intracavitary lesions are clearly delineated by anechoic media, very small hollow cavities, such as the lumen of normal tubes, are rarely visualized using this technique.[13,15] The demonstration of small hollow cavities, such as lumen of tubes, requires visualization of the movement of fluid, which in turn requires the use of a highly echogenic medium.[16,17,18]

Deichert was the first to report on transvaginal sonographic evaluation of tubal patency, following transcervical injection of echogenic ultrasonic contrast fluid.[19] The method was called Hy-Co-Sy, which stands for transvaginal hysterosalpingo-contrast-sonography. Tüfekci has developed a simplified technique using injection of isotonic saline.[20]

Transvaginal sonosalpingography is a safe, cost-effective, noninvasive and easily repeatable method for the evaluation of the tubal status. In addition, there is no idiosyncratic reaction with contrast agents.

ULTRASOUND CONTRAST AGENTS

All media having a different echogenicity from that of the human body can be used as a contrast media. Contrast media are divided into two groups: hypoechogenic and hyperechogenic media.

Isotonic saline, ringer or dextran solutions belong to the group of hypo- or anechoic contrast media. Instillation of these media facilitates the detection of echogenic border surfaces. The main disadvantage is that it is not possible to visualize the phenomena of motion and flow.

Hyperechogenic contrast media enhance echo signals, allowing detection of the flow by both B-mode and Doppler ultrasound. Gramiak Shah[21] and Meltzer[22] found that small gas bubbles effectively reflect ultrasonic waves. This observation has lead to the development of the commercial echo contrast media containing microbubbles. Echovist and Levovist (Schering AG, Berlin) represent the suspension of microbubbles made of special galactose microparticles. Galactose microparticle granules are suspended either in galactose solution (Echovist) or in a sterile water (Levovist).[23]

Echovist (SHU 454) is an ultrasound contrast medium consisting of a suspension of monosaccharide microparticles (50% galactose, diameter 2 mm) in a 20% aqueous solution of galactose (w/v). The echogenic suspension is reconstituted immediately before the use from granules and a vehicle solution (200 mg microparticles in 1 ml of suspension).[24] This contrast medium has been licensed for gynecological intracavitary applications in 1995.

Levovist (SHU 508) are microparticle granules, which contain a very low concentration of palmitic acid and are used systemically. A few minutes before the use of these contrast agents, the granules have to be shaken vigorously for 5-10 seconds then dissolved by an appropriate volume of aqueous galactose solution (Echovist) or sterile water (Levovist). A milky suspension of galactose microparticles in a solution is thus created after disaggregation of the microparticle "snowball". The suspension of Echovist is stable for about 5 min after preparation. Due to its extended stability, Levovist may be administered up to 10 min after the suspension is created. Depending on the indication and the imaging modality (B-mode or Doppler), clinically adequate suspensions of Echovist has concentrations of 200 and 300 mg/ml. For Levovist, the maximum concentration is 400 mg/ml. The predominant limitation at concentrations lower than 200 mg/ml is decreased suspension stability. Concentrations exceeding 400 mg/ml are limited by a rapid increase of the viscosity.

After intrauterine administration and emergence of Echovist from the fimbriae into the pelvis, the galactose microparticles dissolve. This process is accelerated by warming to body temperature and dilution by the peritoneal fluid. In vitro, a rise in temperature of the Echovist suspension to 37°C leads to a complete dissolution within 30 minutes. The dissolved galactose is subsequently absorbed and metabolized.

Numerous clinical studies in the field of echocardiography, venous vascular system analysis and HSG showed no evidence of serious side effects.

Absolute contraindication for the instillation of these fluids is galactosemia (an autosomal recessive disorder, due to deficiency of galactose-1-phosphate uridyltransferase, galactose cannot be metabolized into glucose).

Administration of the ultrasound contrast via the vascular system or into the body cavities changes the acoustic properties of the body region under investigation. The acoustic parameters, which improve the tissue imaging by conventional sonographic units include backscattering, attenuation and the velocity of the sound.

TECHNIQUE OF HYSTERO-CONTRAST-SALPINGOGRAPHY

Requirements

Prior to implementing this technique, a complete history should be obtained from the patient to rule out the possibility of galactosemia. Although a rare condition, it is, in addition to acute inflammatory disease of the genital organs, the only absolute contraindications for this investigation. A gynecological and ultrasound examination prior to the procedure is necessary to define the uterine position and anomalies if present, as well as to visualize both of the adnexal regions. For legal purposes, prior to any intervention, a pregnancy test should be performed. The possibility of local or systemic infections is excluded by the clinical examination of the patient, such as absence of elevated temperature and inspection of the genital tract. The procedure should not be performed on patients with active pelvic infections. Antibiotic prophylaxis (doxycycline and metronidazole) should be used in patients with a history of pelvic inflammatory disease. Hy-Co-Sy should always be performed during the early follicular phase of the menstrual cycle, after complete cessation of menses. This avoids dispersion of the menstrual debris into the peritoneal cavity. Procedures done during this period allow absorption of the media prior to ovulation, thus, avoiding the presence of a foreign substance around the time of an imminent corpus luteum formation. This decreases any theoretic effect the media may have on tubal transport.

Patients are given a detailed description of the procedure, including the possible risks and benefits associated with it. Anesthesia is generally not required for Hy-Co-Sy and the patient can follow the course of the examination on the monitor. If Hy-Co-Sy is performed without sedation, patients occasionally report discomfort, especially if the tubes are occluded. The degree of discomfort depends on the individual response to pain. Premedication or sedation is routinely used. 5-10 mg of intravenous diazepam has been found to be beneficial, especially in anxious patients. Pain signifies the obstruction of the tubes and potential intravasation of the contrast material or tubal rupture and should not be masked by anesthesia. However, tubal spasm may occur if Hy-Co-Sy is performed without anesthesia, which may mimic a tubal occlusion. Pretreatment with atropine (0.5 mg) may prevent this complication. The parenteral administration of 1 mg glucagon may relieve the spasm and allow the flow of the contrast.

Procedure

The patient voids and is positioned supine on the gynecological table. With the patient's legs flexed, a speculum is inserted into the vagina and positioned such that the entire cervix is visualized and the os is easily accessible. The cervix and the vagina are then thoroughly scrubbed with Betadine solution. A tenaculum is placed on the anterior lip of the cervix and the cannula is gently guided into the endocervical canal. Application of the contrast medium is performed via a small and very thin uterine catheter fitted with a balloon for stabilization and occlusion of the internal cervical os. The first observation to be made is of the uterine cavity, with verification of the catheter placement. After removal of the tenaculum, the transvaginal probe is gently introduced into the posterior fornix of the vagina. The contrast (sterile saline) is then slowly injected under the control of ultrasound. Usually, no more than 2 to 5 ml of the contrast is instilled into the uterine cavity. At this stage sonographer observes the morphology of the uterus and its endometrial lining. Duplication anomalies of

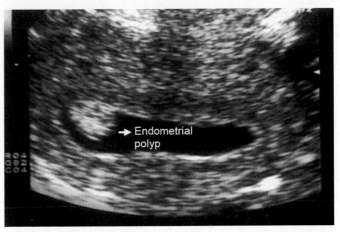

FIGURE 10.1: Transvaginal scan of the uterus demonstrating a focal area of increased echogenicity within the endometrial portion. An endometrial polyp is easily visualized after instillation of the anechoic contrast medium.

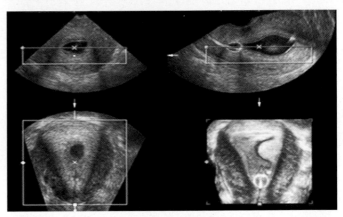

FIGURE 10.2: Three-dimensional Hy-Co-Sy demonstrating an endometrial polyp.

the uterus, existence of endometrial polyps or submucous fibroids protruding into the uterine cavity are clearly marked with anechoic contrast (Figures 10.1 and 10.2). Saline infusion sonography may be performed by 2D or 3D ultrasound.

If used by a trained physician hysterosonosalpingography allows reproducible and reliable assessment of the tubal patency without exposure to radiation. This procedure carried out in an office setting, is well tolerated, rapid and shows tubal patency to the patient in "real time". The sonographer should be aware that tubal spasm may lead to misdiagnosis of tubal occlusion and that the tubal flow may give a false impression of tubal patency in hydrosalpinx. The learning curve is very steep and at least 10 to 20 investigations are needed to acquire competency for this technique. Benefits and limitations of hysterosonosalpingography are listed in Table 10.3.

TABLE 10.3: Benefits and limitations of hysterosonosalpingography

Benefits	Limitations
• Reproducible and reliable assessment of tubal patency if used by a trained physician	• Tubal spasm may lead to misdiagnosis of tubal occlusion (spasm also seen with other methods)
• Avoids radiation exposure	• In hydrosalpinx, tubal flow may give a false impression of tubal patency
• Avoids allergic reactions	• Inability to visualize the bowel and intrapelvic pathology
• Avoids general anesthesia	• Requires a degree of technical competence
• Performed in an office setting	• 10-20 investigations needed to acquire competency for this new technique
• Rapid	
• Well tolerated: little discomfort and few adverse events	
• Demonstrates tubal patency of the patient in "real time"	

GRAY-SCALE HYSTERO-CONTRAST-SALPINGOGRAPHY

Grayscale Hy-Co-Sy always begins with instillation of isotonic saline, which clearly outlines the hyperechogenic surface of the endometrium.[10,25] The uterine cavity, which in most cases will still be dilated by the anechoic solution instilled previously, is then slowly filled with the echogenic ultrasound contrast medium. If the tube is patent, constant flow in a pattern resembling a point, spot or streak is seen. Further intermittent injections of volumes of 1-2 ml, given slowly and continuously, using lateral sweeps of the ultrasound probe, allow visualization of the intraluminal or intratubal flow. This is visualized under normal anatomical conditions via the pars intramuralis into the medial and distal segments of the tubes. For the diagnosis of tubal patency, two or three observation phases per tube are needed, with an observation period of a continuous flow for about 10 seconds (while contrast medium is slowly injected). Although visualization of a longer segment of the tube beyond the pars intramuralis is convincing for tubal patency, one should carefully examine the adnexal regions for filling of the distal segments of the tube to exclude sactosalpinx. Examination of the pouch of Douglas for any increase in retrouterine fluid, comparing it with the initial image obtained at the start of the evaluation, completes the examination procedure.

PULSED DOPPLER ANALYSIS OF TUBAL PATENCY

Findings obtained by B-mode ultrasound may be confirmed by pulsed Doppler wave from analysis. If the examination during B-mode reveals evidence suggesting tubal occlusion or if a segment of the tube measuring less than 2 cm in length is not visualized, a pulsed Doppler examination should be performed.[10,25] After the Doppler gate has been positioned over the area of interest, the gate width is reduced to measure only the flow noise from pertubation and not vascular or other noise. In case of tubal patency, brief injections (lasting approximately 5 seconds) of contrast medium produce a long, drawn-out and initially hissing, broad "noise band" on the monitor. The width of the band that slowly decreases after the injection indicates that the tube is patent. Thus, unobstructed flow is characterized by a short filling phase with a rapid, steep increase in Doppler shift and a slow, uniform fall in Doppler shift along the time axis, indicating unobstructed free distal outflow. The absence of these acoustic signals indicates obstruction of tubal flow or tubal occlusion. In this case, there is only a short, steep Doppler shift with no subsequent noise signals. This indicates an absence of outflow of the contrast medium distal to the Doppler gate. Deichert et al, tried to determine whether the additional use of pulsed wave Doppler can improve the accuracy of Hy-Co-Sy.[10] They studied 17 patients with infertility problems. Following Hy-Co-Sy by gray-scale and pulsed wave Doppler patients underwent chromolaparoscopy (n = 16) and HSG (n – 1). The diagnostic efficacies of gray-scale and pulsed wave Doppler were compared with each other and with a conventional procedure (chromolaparoscopy or HSG). The gray-scale findings were confirmed by pulsed wave Doppler in five cases on one side; confirmed by pulsed wave Doppler in seven cases on both sides; corrected by pulsed wave Doppler in one case on one side and confirmed on the other side by pulsed wave Doppler. In all 17 cases, the tubal findings after pulsed wave Doppler were confirmed by chromolaparoscopy or HSG. Therefore, the additional use of pulsed wave Doppler in hysterosalpingo-contrast-sonography (Hy-Co-Sy) is recommended as a supplement to gray-scale imaging in cases of suspected tubal occlusion, and in patients in whom intratubal flow was demonstrated only over a short distance.

When Hy-Co-Sy was compared to conventional HSG or laparoscopy with dye, 87.5% concordance with other techniques, predicted 100% of tubal occlusions and detected 86% of patent tubes. According to Ayida et al,[26] saline contrast hysterosonography as a screening test for uterine cavity abnormalities, has 87.5% sensitivity, 100% specificity, 100% positive predictive value and a 91.6% negative predictive value.

COLOR DOPPLER HYSTERO-CONTRAST-SALPINGOGRAPHY

Transvaginal color Doppler HSG is a safe and efficacious method for evaluation of Fallopian tube patency without exposure to radiation or contrast dyes. The cost of the procedure is significantly lower than for x-ray HSG and it gives immediate results. It is advisable that all the scans are recorded electronically on DVD, vide-recorder or Polaroid films. Further advantages of transvaginal sonosalpingography include the possibility of performing the procedure on an outpatient basis. This has significantly altered the need for inpatient facilities at some infertility departments. Similar to X-ray HSG, bleeding, pregnancy and presence of adnexal masses on pelvic or ultrasound examination are contraindications to color Doppler HSG.

Equipment needed to perform color Doppler HSG includes an ultrasound unit with color Doppler capability and an intrauterine catheter. The intrauterine cannula is placed into the uterus with one balloon placed at the level of the internal cervical os, while another one is fixed at the level of external cervical os. Two to five ml of sterile saline is instilled into the uterine cavity. After the observation of the morphology of the uterus end endometrial lining, color Doppler is directed at the cornual region where the tubal catheter is located (Figure 10.3). The exact placement of the catheter is sonographically controlled. Color signals passing through the Fallopian tube indicate its patency (Figure 10.4), while the absence of such signals is interpreted as tubal occlusion.[6,27] Accumulation of the fluid in the cul-de-sac on the side of injection controlled by transvaginal color and pulsed Doppler is an accurate indicator of ipsilateral tubal patency. In most cases spill of the contrast medium is visualized in color signals. Selective tubal injection increases the accuracy of the procedure and appropriateness of the interpretation. The procedure is repeated on the contralateral side. Difficulty in making the diagnosis of tubal occlusion arises in patients with dilated fluid filled tubes (hydrosalpinx) because flow through the proximal portion of the tube may stimulate spillage on the Doppler ultrasonography screen.[9,28] To avoid this error, the sonographer should carefully observe both adnexa before the procedure. Using our modified technique, we compared

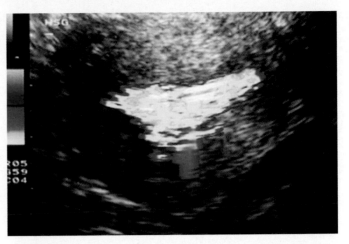

FIGURE 10.3: Transvaginal color Doppler scan of the uterus after injection of the isotonic saline solution. The triangular uterine cavity is clearly outlined by color flow imaging.

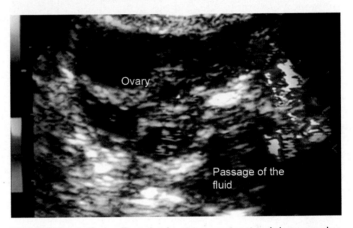

FIGURE 10.4: Color Doppler hystero-contrast-salpingography. The color flow is from saline passing through the right tube, indicating normal tubal patency. Accumulation of the anechoic fluid is visualized in the cul-de-sac.

the findings of color Doppler HSG with chromopertubation at the time of laparoscopy.[9] Forty-three out of 47 (91.48%) color Doppler HSG findings agreed with observations at chromopertubation. In only one patient, color Doppler ultrasound did not demonstrate color flow signals. Indirect diagnosis of tubal patency was performed by observing free fluid accumulation in the cul-de-sac. The increased incidence of conception during the three months period after the procedure (in our study, two patients) may be an effect of a mechanical lavage of the uterus by dislodging the mucous plugs, breakdown of the peritoneal adhesions or a stimulatory effect on the tubal cilia. No serious side effects were observed during and after the transvaginal color Doppler HSG procedure. Eighteen patients complained of mild pain that continued for 2-10 minutes after the procedure. No medication were required for these cases. The shortest time taken for the transvaginal color Doppler HSG was 5 minutes, while the longest time was 14 minutes. After removing the instruments, the cervix should be inspected for hemostasis and pressure applied to the tenaculum site whenever necessary.

REVIEW OF LITERATURE

To assess the accuracy of the diagnosis of tubal occlusion with the use of color Doppler flow ultrasonography and HSG, Peters and Coulam[6] studied 129 infertile women. When results of Hy-Co-Sy were compared with X-ray HSG, 69 of 85 (81%) studies showed a complete agreement. In addition, fifty out of 58 (86%) ultrasound HSG findings agreed with observations at chromopertubation. The frequency of comparable findings between X-ray HSG and chromopertubation was 75%.

Richman et al[13] evaluated tubal patency in 36 infertile women. They compared ultrasound findings with conventional hysterosalpingograms, which were performed simultaneously. Ultrasound demonstrated bilateral occlusion, with a sensitivity of 100% and tubal patency with a specificity of 96%.

Tüfekci et al[20] studied 38 women with infertility complaints. The results obtained from transvaginal sonosalpingography and laparoscopies were completely consistent for 29 cases (76.32%) and partially consistent for eight cases (21.05%). Only one case showed inconsistent result. Complete consistence means that the passage through both Fallopian tubes is identical by both methods. Partial consistence indicated identical results for only either the left or the right tube. Transvaginal sonosalpingography correctly indicated tubal patency or non-patency in 37 of 38 cases.

Heikkinen et al[29] evaluated the advantages and accuracy of transvaginal sonosalpingography in the assessment of tubal patency with regards to laparoscopic chromopertubation. Sixty-one Fallopian tubes were examined by both techniques, with a concordance of 85%. By transvaginal sonosalpingography, 45 tubes were found to be patent and 16 occluded. On chromopertubation, 50 tubes were patent and 11 were occluded. Bilateral tubal patency was detected by transvaginal sonosalpingography in 17 cases and by laparoscopy in 22 cases. Bilateral occlusion was found in three cases using either technique. Transvaginal sonosalpingography with the combination of air and saline is a low-cost, reliable, safe and comfortable examination method that can be used for primary investigation of infertility on an outpatient basis.

Jeanty et al[30] assessed the use of air as a sonographic contrast agent in the investigation of tubal patency by sonohysterography. They examined 115 women assessed for infertility. After a saline sonohysterography, small amounts of air were insufflated and the tubal passage of bubbles was monitored. Air-sonohysterography and laparoscopy with chromopertubation showed an agreement in 79.4%. In 17.2% of patients, the tubes were not visualized by air-sonohysterography when they were patent. Air sonohysterography is a comfortable, simple and inexpensive first line tubal patency investigation yielding high accuracy (85.7% sensitivity and 77.2% specificity).

Battaglia et al[31] found that correlation between color Doppler Hy-Co-Sy and X-ray HSG with chromolaparoscopy was 86% and 93%, respectively.

Boudghene et al[32] compared the efficiency of air-filled albumin microspheres (Infoson) with saline solution in determining Fallopian tube patency during Hy-Co-Sy. Hy-Co-Sy was performed with a 7-MHz transvaginal probe using both B-mode and color Doppler. Tubal patency was demonstrated by the appearance of the contrast agent in the peritoneal cavity adjacent to the ovaries. Infoson Hy-Co-Sy provided a significantly larger number of correct diagnoses (20/22 Fallopian tubes) than did saline Hy-Co-Sy (12/24 Fallopian tubes). A positive ultrasound contrast agent appears to be more efficient than saline solution at determining Fallopian tube patency in infertile women by means of Hy-Co-Sy and was as efficient as an iodinated contrast agent in the same population explored by X-ray HSG.

Stern et al[8] administered saline transcervically during transvaginal color Doppler sonography in 238 women. Traditional X-ray HSG was performed in 89 women. Laparoscopy with chromopertubation was performed in 121 women. Forty-nine women had all three procedures performed. Correlation between color Doppler HSG and X-ray findings with chromopertubation occurred in 81% versus 60% ($p = 0.0008$) of all women studied. In forty-nine women who had all three procedures performed, color Doppler HSG results correlated with chromopertubation more often than X-ray HSG (82% versus 57%, $p = 0.0152$). Their previous report,[6] noted discrepancies between color ultrasound HSG and chromopertubation findings in a patient with unilateral tubal patency. Therefore, these authors have recommended that color ultrasound HSG should be repeated before making a diagnosis of unilateral occlusion.

Allahbadia reported a 92.6% agreement between color Doppler hystero-contrast-salpingography (Hy-Co-Sy) compared with HSG and laparoscopy.[33] The same author also described the so-called Sion procedure or hydrogynecography. This procedure takes approximately 15 minutes as compared to the 5-6 minutes for sonosalpingography. After accomplishing sonosalpingography, sterile normal saline is injected until approximately 350 ml have flooded the pelvis. With the adnexa and uterus submerged in a fluid medium, the pelvis is rescanned. The saline fills up the pelvis and delineates various types of adhesions. All the patients undergoing this procedure were given prophylactic antibiotics.

Contrary to optimistic results of different ultrasound techniques for evaluation of tubal patency, Balen and colleagues[34] found the use of ultrasound contrast HSG using both sterile saline and Echovist contrast media insufficiently accurate and inferior to conventional X-ray HSG. False-positive rates in the range of 9% and false-negative rates in the range of 20% have been reported in the diagnosis of tubal obstruction by color Doppler HSG.[8] Based on the data presented in the review of literature, all abnormal Hy-Co-Sy studies should undergo laparoscopic or hysteroscopic follow-up.

However, normal X-ray or color Doppler HSG does not rule out the need for diagnostic laparoscopy. While X-ray HSG is the most accurate method for the diagnosis of the intramural or intraluminal abnormalities of the Fallopian tube, at this moment color and pulsed Doppler HSG is the only available noninvasive method for the evaluation of the tubal motility and function. To obtain optimal information, the procedure should be performed by a well-trained physician who is familiar with the color Doppler investigation and who is capable of manipulating the instruments, the patient's reproductive tract and the rate of injection of the contrast medium.

THREE-DIMENSIONAL HYSTERO-CONTRAST-SALPINGOGRAPHY

Basic structural information provided by conventional scans in longitudinal and transverse planes can now be augmented by the new 3D ultrasound. This provides an additional view of the coronal or C-plane, which is parallel to the transducer face.[35,36] The computer generated scan is displayed in three perpendicular planes. Presentation of the three perpendicular planes on one screen allows free scrolling of an endless amount of frames through the volume of interest. The coronal or C-plane view allows a more detailed

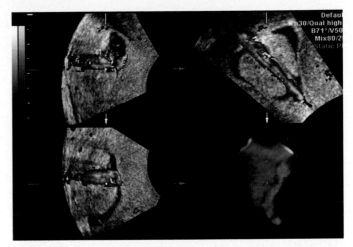

FIGURE 10.5: Three dimensional power Doppler scan of the uterus after injection of the isotonic saline solution. The triangular uterine cavity is clearly outlined by power flow 3D imaging.

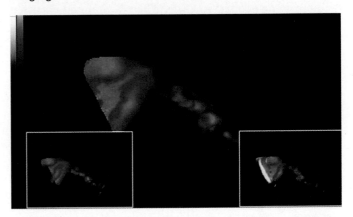

FIGURE 10.6: Three-dimensional power Doppler hystero-contrast-salpingography. Triangular uterine cavity and passage of the contrast through the left Fallopian tube are shown in color.

analysis of the uterus and for the first time, the endometrial cavity between the uterine angles can be visualized (Figures 10.5 and 10.6). Translation or rotation can be carried out in one plane while maintaining the perpendicular orientation of all three planes. The images produced by the transvaginal ultrasound are superior to those produced by the transabdominal ultrasound because vaginal transducers are in closer proximity to the tissues.[36] Because vaginal transducers are in closer proximity to the tissues, higher frequencies are used and artifactual echoes caused by multiple reflections from intervening tissues are minimized.

Demonstration of the coronal plane is mandatory for the diagnosis of uterine congenital anomalies, such as septate, arcuate, bicornuate, duplex or unicornuate uterus and provides the most exact measurements of the endometrial width when transected in a midperpendicular manner. During 3D hysterosonography, the typical triangulated uterine cavity appears in its full shape.[37] Surface rendering, maximal/minimal and X-ray renderings provide even more information on the uterine findings, such as uterine anatomy, uterine cavity volume and its content. There are two techniques to accomplish this goal: "native" approach and the use of contrast medium. The use of contrast medium is especially useful for the demarcation of the uterine cavity abnormalities. Due to the combined consistency of the endometrium and myometrium, the uterus acts an excellent ultrasonic medium. The endometrium and myometrium have different acoustic impedance, which permits the visualization of the size and shape of the uterus and its cavity. In addition, a contrast medium is mandatory in cases where a thin endometrium or pathologic content of the uterine cavity precludes its visualization.

The negative contrast medium, normal saline, is used for the demonstration of the entire uterine cavity, which includes its shape, pathology and the frame of the myometrial mantel, whereas for demonstration of the permeability of the Fallopian tubes, a positive contrast medium (Echovist) is used (Figures 10.7 and 10.8).

Weinraub and Herman[37] were the first to evaluate the findings of various uterine pathologies using 3D hysterosonography. With the use of the three perpendicular planes on one screen, wherein the left upper plane is coronal and is termed "a", the right upper plane is sagittal and is termed "b", and the left lower plane is transverse and is termed "c" the sonographer can detect numerous causes of infertility. For example, by visualizing the fundal region in "a", a very important small indentation, which is pathognomonic for an arcuate uterus, is not overlooked. The maximal endometrial width is easily measured in the sagittal plane. When the transverse section demonstrates separated uterine cornua, this finding can be typical of a septate uterus. Clear concavity in the middle of the uterine fundus exceeding 1 cm or more with a division of the uterine cavity is suggestive of a bicornuate uterus.

Hydrosonography is very useful for the detection of uterine abnormalities, such as adhesions, submucosal fibroids, endometrial polyps or endometrial carcinoma. The same method may be used for the visualization of displaced intrauterine devices (IUDs). Multiplanar imaging following the instillation of the saline is as effective as hysteroscopy

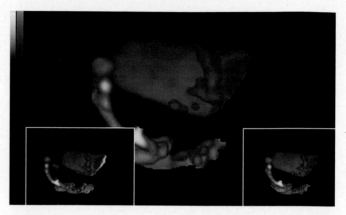

FIGURE 10.7: Three-dimensional power Doppler hystero-contrast-salpingography. Note the regular shape of the uterine cavity, right tubal patency and spillage of the contrast medium into the cul-de-sac.

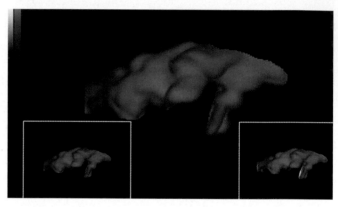

FIGURE 10.8: Three-dimensional power Doppler Hy-Co-Sy demonstrating regular tubal patency.

in preoperative grading of submucosal fibroids.[37] This modality improves spatial anatomic orientation and is superior to conventional ultrasound in mapping the uterine fibroids in patients undergoing surgical enucleation.

Due to its tortuosity, the tube can rarely be seen completely in a single scanning plane and the echo-contrast medium is, therefore, observed in small sections. The position of the tube is very variable and distended bowel may prevent the visualization of the distal parts of the tubes. Therefore, usually only the tubal ostia and proximal parts of the tubes are visualized by gray-scale two-dimensional (2D) ultrasound imaging. Free spread of the dye is difficult to visualize because of the surrounding bowel that produces strongly echogenic signals. Instead of visualizing the echo contrast with gray-scale ultrasound, Sladkevicius et al.[38] used 3D power Doppler technology sensitive to slow flow. If the tube is patent, Doppler signals are obtained along the tube and free spill from the fimbrial end is identified.

The aim of their study was to evaluate the feasibility of three-dimensional power Doppler imaging (3D-PDI) in the assessment of the patency of the Fallopian tubes during hysterosalpingo-contrast-sonography (Hy-Co-Sy). Hysterosalpingo-contrast-sonography using the contrast medium Echovist was performed in 67 women. Findings on 2D gray-scale scanning and 3D power Doppler imaging were compared. The first technique visualizes positive contrast in the Fallopian tube; while the second demonstrates flow of the medium through the tube. Free spill from the fimbrial end of the Fallopian tubes was demonstrated in 114 (91%) tubes using the 3D-PDI technique and in 58 (46%) of tubes using conventional Hy-Co-Sy. The mean duration of the imaging procedure was significantly shorter with 3D-PDI, but the operator time, which included post-procedure analysis of the stored information, was similar. A significantly lower volume of contrast medium (5.9 ± 0.6 mL) was used for 3D-PDI in comparison to the volume (11.2 ± 1.9 mL) used for conventional 2D Hy-Co-Sy. The authors concluded that color coded 3D-PDI with surface rendering allows visualization of the flow of the contrast medium throughout the entire tubal length. Free spill of the contrast is clearly identified in the majority of cases. Three-dimensional PDI methods have significant advantages over the conventional Hy-Co-Sy technique, especially in terms of visualization of the free spill from the distal end of the tube, which was achieved twice as often with the 3D technique. Although the design of the investigation does not allow for the comparison of the side effects of the two techniques, the shorter duration of the imaging and lower volume of the contrast medium used suggest that the 3D-PDI technique might have a better side-effect profile. In addition, 3D-PDI technique allows for better storage of the information for re-analysis and archiving than conventional Hy-Co-Sy.

Ayida and colleagues[39] compared conventional 2D and 3D ultrasound scanning of the uterine cavity with and without saline contrast medium. The 2D scanning suggested uterine cavity abnormalities in 4 of 10 women (3 fibroids and one hyperechoic thick endometrium). The 3D ultrasound scanning confirmed all four uterine cavity abnormalities and revealed one additional abnormality suggestive of a uterine septum. The 2D scanning with saline injection diagnosed a 5 of 10 abnormalities (one uterine septum, 3 fibroids and one endometrial polyp). The 3D contrast scanning with saline did not add any further information to 2D contrast scanning with saline. In this pilot study, a 3D ultrasound contrast scanning appeared to offer no advantages over conventional 2D contrast sonography.

Weinraub et al.[40] have demonstrated the feasibility of a combined 3D ultrasound and saline contrast hysterosonography. Since volume sampling has a short pick-up time of a few seconds, the examination is completed immediately after the uterus is reasonably distended. As this is a very uncomfortable examination, such an advantage should not be underestimated. Evaluation of the uterine cavity at a later time allows the operator to manipulate the data at leisure and scrutinize findings in desired planes, which were not available during the initial examination. Simultaneous display of the three perpendicular planes offers a more comprehensive overview of the examined area and gives access to the planes that are unobtainable by conventional 2D ultrasound examination. Surface rendering may confirm the presence of pathological findings in equivocal cases and characterize their appearance, size, volume and relationship to the surrounding structures. Surface rendering of the polypoid structures shows echogenic masses on a pedicle protruding into the uterine cavity.

Submucosal fibroids appear as mixed echogenic lesions bulging into the cavity. Intrauterine synechiae appear as bands of varying thickness traversing the uterine cavity. This method is useful when deciding on treatment options, such as conservative management vs. surgery and can be a valuable tool in surgical procedures carried out under the ultrasonographic guidance.

Kiyokava et al.[41] evaluated 25 infertile patients using 3D Hy-Co-Sy with saline. X-ray HSG was used as a reference for the efficacy assessment in this study. The positive predictive value, negative predictive value, sensitivity and specificity of predicting tubal patency by 3D Hy-Co-Sy were 100, 33.3, 84.4 and 100%, respectively. The full contour of the uterine cavity was depicted in 96% of cases by 3D Hy-Co-Sy and 64% by X-HSG (P < 0.005). The uterine cavity area measured on 3D Hy-Co-Sy correlated well with the volume of the contrast medium required on X-HSG. Three-dimensional Hy-Co-Sy enabled better assessment of the uterine cavity over X-HSG. Three-dimensional Hy-Co-Sy was well tolerated, required no sedation or anesthesia and was well completed during the reduced examination time. Thus, 3D Hy-Co-Sy with saline as a contrast medium could be incorporated as a part of the routine outpatient procedure in the initial evaluation of infertile women.

Three-dimensional ultrasound technique offers simultaneous visualization of the uterine cavity and the fallopian tubes, shortens the procedure time and decreases the discomfort of the patient (Figures 10.6 and 10.7). Transvaginal 3D examination time is similar to 2D sonography, but has the advantage of reviewing certain specific parts of the examination, such as measurements, reconstruction of the planes of interest or tomography and surface rendering at a later time and offline. The acquired volumes of the most appropriate planes of interest are stored on a removable hard disk for additional re-evaluations and documentation. Ultrasonic tomography can be performed using one panel control, producing parallel sections in increments of less than 1 mm. 3D ultrasound systems have the ability to produce serial scans that can be stored for subsequent analysis, perform 3D reconstruction, accurate volume assessment, and the demonstration of a coronal plane for detailed analysis of the uterus and endometrial cavity.

More recently Kupesic and Plavsic[42] evaluated the diagnostic efficacy of 2D B-mode, color and pulsed Doppler Hy-Co-Sy and 3D B-mode and power Doppler Hy-Co-Sy. One hundred and fifty-two women were evaluated by 2D B-mode, color and pulsed Doppler Hy-Co-Sy and 116 other women were recruited into the 3D B-mode and power Doppler Hy-Co-Sy study. The sensitivity, specificity, PPV and NPV of 2D hysterosonography compared to hysteroscopy were 93.6, 97.3, 98.2 and 97.3%, respectively. The sensitivity, specificity, PPV and NPV of 3D hysterosonography compared to hysteroscopy were 97.9, 100, 97.9 and 100%, respectively. The addition of color and pulsed Doppler to 2D Hy-Co-Sy and power Doppler to 3D Hy-Co-Sy contributed to diagnostic precision in detection of tubal patency. The sensitivity, specificity, PPV and NPV of 3D power Doppler Hy-Co-Sy in detection of tubal patency compared to laparoscopy and dye intubation were 100, 99.1, 99.2 and 100%, respectively. Hy-Co-Sy performed by 3D US is a superior screening method for the evaluation of infertile patients.[43,44] Screening positives should be directed to operative hysteroscopy and/or laparoscopy.

CONCLUSION

Color Doppler and 3D Hy-Co-Sy are safe and efficacious methods for the evaluation of the uterine cavity and fallopian tube patency without exposure to radiation. These procedures allow the physician to interpret the results immediately on an outpatient clinic basis and review them offline, without the presence of the patient.

REFERENCES

1. Hill ML. Infertility and reproductive assistance. In Neiberg, DA, Hill LM, Bohm-Velez M and Mendelson EB (Eds). Transvaginal Ultrasound. St Louis: Mosby Year Book, 1992; 43-6.
2. Arronet GH, Eduljee SY and O'Brien JR . A 9 year survey of Fallopian tube dysfunction in human infertility. Diagnosis and therapy. Fertil Steril 1969;20(6):903-18.
3. Page H.. Estimation of the prevalence and incidence of infertility in a population: a pilot study. Fertil Steril.1989; 51(4), 571-7.
4. Kerin JF, Williams DB, San Roman GA, et al. Falloposcopic classification and treatment of fallopian tube lumen disease. Fertil Steril 1992;57(4):731-41.
5. Thurmond AS, Rosch J. Nonsurgical fallopian tube recanalization for treatment of infertility. Radiology 1990; 174(2):371-4.
6. Peters AJ, Coulam CB. Hysterosalpingography with color Doppler ultrasonography. Am J Obstet Gynecol 1991;164 (6 Pt 1):1530-2.
7. Volpi E, Zuccaro G, Patriarca S, et al. Transvaginal sonographic tubal patency testing using air and saline solution as contrast media in a routine infertility clinic setting. Ultrasound Obstet Gynecol 1996;7(1):43-8.
8. Stern J, Peters AJ, Coulam CB. Color Doppler ultrasonography assessment of tubal patency: a comparison study with traditional techniques. Fertil Steril 1992;58(5):897-900.
9. Kupesic S, Kurjak A. Gynecological vaginal sonographic interventional procedures – what does color add? Gynecol Perinatol 1994;3:57-60.
10. Deichert U, Schlief R, van de Sandt M, et al. Transvaginal hysterosalpingo-contrast sonography for the assessment of tubal patency with gray scale imaging and the additional use of pulsed wave Doppler. Fertil Steril1992;57(1):62-7.
11. Rubin I. Differences between the uterus and tubes as a cause of oscillations recorded during uterotubal insufflation. Fertil Steril 1954;5:147-53.
12. Nannini R, Chelo E, Branconi F, et al. Dynamic echohysteroscopy: a new diagnostic technique in the study of female infertility. Acta Eur Fertil 1981;12(2):165-71.
13. Richman TS, Viscomi GN, deCherney A, et al. Fallopian tubal patency assessed by ultrasound fluid injection. Work in progress. Radiology 1984;152(2):507-10.
14. Randolph JR, Ying YK, Maier DB, et al. Comparison of real-time ultrasonography, hysterosalpingography and laparoscopy/hysteroscopy in the evaluation of uterine abnormalities and tubal patency. Fertil Steril 1986; 46(5):828-32.
15. Davison GB, Leeton J. A case of female infertility investigated by contrast-enhanced echo-gynecography. J Clin Ultrasound 1988;16(1):44-7.
16. Allahbadia GN. Fallopian tubes and ultrasonography. The Sion experience. Fertil Steril 1992:58;901-7.
17. Broer KH, Turanli R. Überprüfung des Tubenfaktors mitels Vaginalsonographie. Ultraschall Klin Prax 1992;7:50-3.

18. Bonilla-Musoles F, Simón C, Sampaio, et al. An assessment of Hysterosalpingosonography (HSSG) as a diagnostic tool for uterine cavity defects and tubal patency. J Clin Ultrasound 1992; 20(3):175-81.

19. Deichert U, Schlief R, van de Sandt M, et al. Transvaginal hysterosalpingo-contrast sonography (Hy-Co-Sy) compared with conventional tubal diagnostics. Hum Reprod 1989; 4(4):418-24.

20. Tüfekci EC, Girit S, Bayirli MD, et al. Evaluation of tubal patency by transvaginal sonosalpingography. Fertil Steril 1992; 57:336-40.

21. Gramiak R, Shah PM. Echocardiography of the aortic root. Invest Radiol 1968:3(5);356-66.

22. Meltzer RS, Tickner EG, Sahines, et al. The source of ultrasound contrast effect. J Clin Ultrasound 1980;8(2):121-7.

23. Suren A, Puchta J, Osmers R. Fluid instillation into the uterine cavity. In. Osmers, R, Kurjak A. (Eds). Ultrasound and the Uterus. Carnforth, UK. Parthenon Publishing, 1995;45-51.

24. Schlief R. Ultrasound contrast agents. Radiology 1991; 3:198-207.

25. Deichert U, van de Sandt M. Transvaginal hysterosalpingo-contrast sonography (Hy-Co-Sy). The assessment of tubal patency and uterine abnormalities by contrast-enhanced sonography. Advances in Echo-Contrast 1993;2:55-8.

26. Ayida G, Chamberlain P, Barlow D, et al. Uterine cavity assessment prior to in vitro fertilization: comparison of transvaginal scanning, saline contrast hysterosonography and hysteroscopy. Ultrasound Obstet Gynecol 1997;10(1): 59-62.

27. Peters JA, Stern JJ, Coulam, et al. Color Doppler hysterosalpingography. In: Jaffe R and Warsof SL (Eds). Color Doppler in Obstetrics and Gynecology. New York: McGraw Hill, 1992;283.

28. Groff TR, Edelstein JA, Schenken RS. Hysterosalpingography in the preoperative evaluation of tubal anastomosis candidates. Fertil Steril 1990;53(3):417-20.

29. Heikkinen H, Tekay A, Volpi E, et al. Transvaginal salpingosonography for the assessment of tubal patency in infertile women: methodological and clinical experiences. Fertil Steril 1995;64(2):293-8.

30. Jeanty P, Besnard S, Arnold A, et al. Air-contrast sonohysterography as a first step assessment of tubal patency. J Ultrasound Med 2000;19(8):519-27.

31. Battaglia C, Artini PG, D'Ambrogio G, et al. Color Doppler hysterosalpingography in the diagnosis of tubal patency. Fertil Steril 1996;65(2):317-22.

32. Boudghène FP, Bazot M, Robert Y, et al. Assessment of Fallopian tube patency by Hy-Co-Sy: comparison of a positive contrast agent with saline solution. Ultrasound Obstet Gynecol 2001;18(5):525-30.

33. Allahbadia GN. Fallopian tube patency using color Doppler. 1993: 40(3): Int J Gynecol Obstet 1993;40(3):241-4.

34. Balen FG, Allen CM, Siddle NC, et al. Ultrasound contrast hysterosalpingography–evaluation as an outpatient procedure. Br J Radiol 1993;66:592-99.

35. Raga F, Bonilla-Musoles F, Blanes J, et al. Congenital Müllerian anomalies: diagnostic accuracy of three-dimensional ultrasound. Fertil Steril 1996;65(3):523-8.

36. Kyei-Mensah A, Zaidi J, Pittrof R, et al. Transvaginal three-dimensional ultrasound: accuracy of follicular volume measurements. Fertil Steril 1996;65(2):371-6.

37. Weinraub Z, Herman A. Three-Dimensional Hysterosal-pingography. In: Merz E (Ed). 3D Ultrasonography in Obstetrics and Gynecology. Philadelphia:Lippincott Williams & Wilkins, 1998;57-64.

38. Sladkevicius P, Ojha K, Campbell S, et al. Three-dimensional power Doppler imaging in the assessment of Fallopian tube patency. Ultrasound Obstet Gynecol 2000;16(7):644-7.

39. Ayida G, Kennedy S, Barlow D, et al. Conventional sonography for uterine cavity assessment: a comparison of conventional two-dimensional with three-dimensional transvaginal ultrasound; a pilot study. Fertil Steril 1996;66(5):848-50.

40. Weinraub Z, Maymon R, Shulman A, et al. Three-dimensional saline contrast hysterosonography and surface rendering of uterine cavity pathology. Ultrasound Obstet Gynecol 1996; 8(4):277-82.

41. Kiyokawa K, Masuda H, Fuyuki T, et al. Three-dimensional hysterosalpingo-contrast sonography (3D Hy-Co-Sy) as an outpatient procedure to assess infertile women: a pilot study. Ultrasound Obstet Gynecol 2000;16(7):648-54.

42. Kupesic S, Plavsic BM. 2D and 3D hysterosalpingo-contrast-sonography in the assessment of uterine cavity and tubal patency. Eur J Obstet Gynecol Reprod Biol 2007; 133(1):64-9.

43. Watermann D, Denschlag D, Hanjalic Beck A, et al. Hystero-salpingo-contrast-sonography with 3D ultrasound — a pilot study. Ultraschall Med 2004;25(5):367-72.

44. Chan CC, Ng EH, Tang O, et al. Comparison of three-dimensional hysterosalpingo-contrast-sonography and diagnostic laparoscopy with chromopertubation in the assessment of tubal patency for the investigation of subfertility. Acta Obstet Gynecol Scand 2005;84(9):909-13.

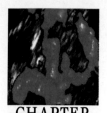

S Kupesic Plavsic
A Kurjak, N Zafar

CHAPTER 11

Color Doppler and 3D US Imaging in Normal and Abnormal Early Pregnancy

The introduction of two-dimensional (2D) and three-dimensional (3D) transvaginal and color Doppler ultrasound has, for the first time enabled in vivo studies of early embryonic, fetal and uteroplacental circulations. This technological improvement has helped us to better understand vascular changes associated with early implantation and formation of the definitive placenta.

A positive pregnancy test offers more questions than answers. It suggests that there is most likely an intrauterine pregnancy, but there may be an abnormal intrauterine or an ectopic pregnancy. Production of human chorionic gonadotropin (hCG) may also be caused by tumors (dysgerminoma, choriocarcinoma) or a maldevelopment of pregnancy (ectopic or molar pregnancy).[1]

If the clinical data supplied by the history, physical examination and beta hCG are incomplete for the diagnosis of early intrauterine pregnancy, it is the sonographer's role to assist the clinician in the evaluation of the pregnancy. Improvement of ultrasound technology and computerization has enabled introduction of an early pregnancy screening.[2] One of the major advantages of 3D ultrasound is the ability to examine the embryos and fetuses in any arbitrary plane after acquisition by the transabdominal or transvaginal transducer. The examination time is short and does not increase the patient's discomfort. Doppler waveform recordings may be obtained following the visualization of uteroplacental and fetal vessels. Color-coded Doppler is helpful in locating the arterial, intracardiac and venous blood flow during early pregnancy. Therefore, it is not surprising that in a relatively short period, this new technique has gained a great popularity. Pulsed Doppler studies have provided us with data about the hemodynamic changes, which occur in all three trimesters of pregnancy.

In this chapter, we will review the role of 2D, color Doppler and 3D ultrasound in the assessment of normal and abnormal early pregnancy.

ULTRASOUND STUDIES OF THE UTERUS FROM OVULATION TO IMPLANTATION

It is well known that normal early human development depends on uterine perfusion, implantation mechanisms and the chromosomal structure of the embryo. Inadequate implantation and poor uterine blood flow can be noninvasively detected by color Doppler technique. After ovulation, there is a small window of time during, which endometrial receptivity is at its maximum. During these few days, a blastocyst traveling to the uterine cavity can establish a physical contact with the endothelial lining and eventually implant. At the time of its initial attachment, the blastocyst is oriented with the inner cell mass toward the endometrium. Proteolytic enzymes produced by the trophoblast results in the penetration and erosion of the uterine mucosa. During implantation, the trophoblast erodes adjacent to maternal capillaries and maternal blood comes into direct contact with the embryo. The intercommunicating lacunar network becomes the intervillous space of the placenta.

During the 4th week, the migrating trophoblast penetrates the spiral arteries and invades the superficial arterioles and venous sinusoids of increasing size. Trophoblastic cells may be detected within the spiral arteries at about the 6th week after fertilization. Increasing blood flow causes progressive distension of these arteries into the uteroplacental arteries capable of accommodating the increasing blood supply.

Ultrasound Findings

With 3D ultrasound, we are able to quantify the endometrial volume and predict the likelihood of implantation in patients undergoing medically assisted reproduction. Studies presented in the chapter on infertility elaborate why quantitative volume measurements may be more precise than estimation of the endometrial thickness. Results presented by Kupesic et al.[3] suggest that quantification of endometrial volume and vascularity by 3D power Doppler ultrasound is the best way to predict pregnancy rates following IVF/ET procedures.

Ovaries

Following implantation luteal flow is characterized with high velocity and low vascular impedance blood flow signals. At 8 weeks gestation, luteal flow becomes less detectable and the visualization rate is 60% to 80%[3]. There is no correlation between the 2D ultrasonographic and Doppler characteristics of the corpus luteum and first trimester pregnancy outcome.[4] The role of 3D ultrasound in the evaluation of the corpus luteum morphology and vascularity is still to be investigated.

UTERINE FINDINGS FOLLOWING IMPLANTATION

The earliest visible sign of pregnancy is a gestational sac that can be visualized during the 5th week of amenorrhea. Ultrasonographically, it presents as a hypoechoic oval structure, surrounded by a hyperechoic ring. At this time the yolk sac and embryonic pole could not be identified. The gestational sac, located asymmetrically in the uterine cavity, measures approximately 5 mm and grows 1-2 mm per day (Figure 11.1).

As the fetal and placental structures develop, their vascular network becomes more pronounced. Hence, during pregnancy it is possible to observe three separate and yet unified units: The maternal, placental and fetal portions of circulation.

Maternal Portion

The maternal portion of placental circulation consists of the main uterine arteries and their branches. These branches spread throughout the uterus until they reach the decidual plate of the placenta. The main uterine arteries originate from the internal iliac arteries, and give off branches, which extend inward for about a third of the myometrial thickness without significant branching. They subdivide into an arcuate wreath, encircling the uterus. From this network,

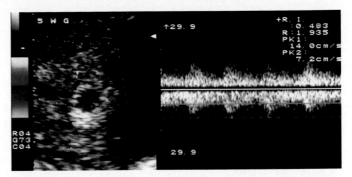

FIGURE 11.1: Transvaginal color Doppler image of a gestational sac at 5 weeks gestation. Color Doppler displays blood flow signals derived from the spiral arteries and intervillous space. Note low vascular impedance blood flow signals obtained from spiral arteries (RI = 0.48).

smaller branches called the radial arteries arise and are directed towards the uterine lumen. The radial arteries branch into basal arteries and spiral arteries as they pass through the myometrial-endometrial junction. Basal arteries are relatively short and terminate in a capillary bed that serves the basal layer of the endometrium. The spiral arteries project further into the endometrium and terminate in a vast network of capillaries that serves as the functional layer of the endometrium.

All these vessels can clearly be identified in the pregnant uterus by their anatomic position and characteristic waveform profile. Intrauterine placental development requires adaptive changes of the uterine vascular environment. The fact that the uterine vascular network elongates and dilates throughout the pregnancy is a well known from anatomical studies.[5]

Doppler Findings

Flow velocity waveforms from small arteries show significantly lower pulsatility and blood velocity as compared to the main uterine artery. Branching of the uterine circulation and increased total vascular cross-sectional area, which results in lower impedance to blood flow, is the background of this phenomenon. Most authors have demonstrated a progressive decrement in the impedance to blood flow in all the segments of the uterine circulation during early pregnancy.[6-9] Transvaginal color and pulsed Doppler allows identification of the uterine vascular transformation. Invasion of larger maternal blood vessels with higher pressure results in higher velocity and more prominent diastolic component of Doppler waveform. Kurjak et al.[10] demonstrated uterine vascular changes even before visualization of the gestational sac. There is evidence that impedance to blood flow decreases from the main uterine to spiral arteries. At the same time, an increase in blood flow by means of peak systolic velocity has a decreasing trend starting from the uterine, through to the arcuate and radial and finally to the spiral arteries.

Uterine Artery Blood Flow in Nonpregnant and Pregnant Patients

The main uterine artery is visualized at the level of the internal cervical os, as it approaches the uterus laterally and curves upward alongside the uterine body. Pulsed Doppler waveform profile of the main uterine artery is characteristic, being comprised of a high peak-systolic component that has a characteristic notch in the protodiastolic part and a very low-end diastolic flow. Numerous Doppler studies have demonstrated a gradual decrement in the uterine artery resistance index during the first trimester of pregnancy.[6-9] The characteristic notch in the protodiastolic part of the sonogram gradually disappears; diastolic flow is characterized by high velocity, and the difference between systolic and diastolic flow velocities decreases with gestational age. These hemodynamic changes reflect trophoblast invasion. This decrement continues during the second trimester of pregnancy and is observed in all the segments of the uteroplacental circulation.

Arcuate and Radial Arteries

Arcuate arteries are visualized within the outer third of the myometrium, while the radial arteries are identified within the two inner third of the myometrium. Doppler sonograms of the arcuate and radial arteries are very similar, with moderate peak systolic and diastolic components of blood flow. However, differences exist in the values of the resistance (RI) or pulsatility (PI) indices. These are lower in the radial than in the arcuate arteries, corresponding to the lower peripheral impedance to blood flow.

Spiral Arteries

During early pregnancy, the spiral arteries are progressively converted to nonmuscular dilated tortuous channels. Their thin normal musculoelastic wall is replaced with a mixture of fibrinoid material and fibrous tissue. Spiral arteries are visualized above the chorion (near the placental implantation site). Their Doppler waveform is characterized with a low resistance index and high peak systolic velocity (Figure 11.1).

This kind of flow is typical for wide tortuous blood vessels and has the hemodynamic characteristics of an arteriovenous shunt. The active trophoblast induces vascular adaptation, which ensures adequate blood supply to the growing embryo.

The spiral artery sonogram characterized by low impedance to blood flow and a characteristic spiky outline presents the blood flow from more than one spiral artery. The spiral arteries change their wall structure with gestation and become vessels with completely different hemodynamics in relation to other arteries of the uteroplacental circulation.

PLACENTA

Primary chorionic villi develop between 13th and 15th day after the ovulation (during 4th week of gestation), and mark the beginning of the placental development. At the same time, the formation of blood vessels starts in the extraembryonic mesoderm of the yolk sac, the connecting stalk and the chorion.[11] By 18-21 days (during 5th week) of gestation, the villi have become branched and the mesenchymal cells within the villi have differentiated into blood capillaries and formed an arteriocapillary venous network. By the end of the 8th week, chorionic villi cover the entire surface of the gestational sac. At that time, the villi on the side of the chorion proliferate towards the decidua basalis to form the chorion frondosum, which develops into the definitive placenta. The villi in contact with the decidua capsularis begins to degenerate and form an avascular shell, known as the chorion laeve or smooth chorion. The placenta is mostly derived from fetal tissues. The maternal component contributes little to the architecture of the definitive placenta.

Normal placentation requires a progressive transformation of the spiral arteries and an infiltration of trophoblastic cells into the placental bed. These physiological changes normally extend into the inner third of the myometrium, and in normal pregnancies, all the spiral arteries are transformed into uteroplacental arteries before 20 weeks of gestation.[12] In some cases of early pregnancy failure and pregnancy-induced hypertension, there is an inadequate placentation with a defective transformation of spiral arteries.[13]

2D Ultrasound Features of the Placenta

During and after the implantation, the inner cytotrophoblast and the outer syncytiotrophoblast layers proliferate rapidly. Sonographically, they are the source of the somewhat enhanced echogenicity of the chorionic sac wall. The endometrium, which is also echogenic (in the late secretory phase), is invaded by the trophoblast, giving rise to the decidua basalis and chorion frondosum on one side, and the decidua capsularis and parietalis on the other side. The echodense structure around the chorionic sac is thus formed. It is possible that the ring-like echogenicity of the chorionic sac is generated by the fuzzy villi surrounding the sac itself. The entire chorionic sac appears to have the same thickness and echogenicity, without any indication as to the differentiating process of a specific chorionic area.

Doppler Studies of Intervillous Circulation

Development of the placenta begins after the first contact between trophoblast and decidua has been established. There are two waves of trophoblast invasion. The first occurs at eight weeks of pregnancy. It is characterized by the invasion of the interstitial trophoblasts invasion into the myometrium and cytotrophoblasts (endothelial trophoblast) invasion into the complete decidua, but not myometrium. The second wave is characterized just by the invasion of the endothelial trophoblasts into the myometrium, which occurs between 16 and 18 weeks of gestation.[14] The intervillous space, combined with the villi, is the functional unit of the human placenta, where maternal fetal metabolic exchange occurs.[15] During the second month, the intervillous space increases as the result of the extensive branching of the villi. During this period, many terminal portions of the spiral arteries adjacent to the intervillous space contain plugs of cytotrophoblastic cells. At the same time, centrally placed communications between the decidual veins are numerous and large. After 40 days, spiral arteries show direct openings into the intervillous space and the cytotrophoblastic cells appear within their lumen. The maternal blood reaches the intervillous space through the gaps between the cells of the endovascular trophoblasts. These events may be nicely studied by 2D and 3D color and power Doppler ultrasound (Figure 11.2). Pulsed Doppler analysis demonstrates two types of waveforms obtained from the intervillous space: Pulsatile arterial-like and continuous venous flow-like. The lumen of the spiral arteries is never completely obstructed by the trophoblastic plugs. This data indicates that establishment of the intervillous circulation is a continuous process rather than an abrupt event at the end of the first trimester. Hafner et al.[16] performed a cross-sectional study in a group of 25 patients in gestational age ranging from 5 to 11 weeks. After acquisition of the 3D power Doppler volume data of the pregnant uterus, they evaluated signals obtained from the chorion. Vascular 3D measurements were expressed by

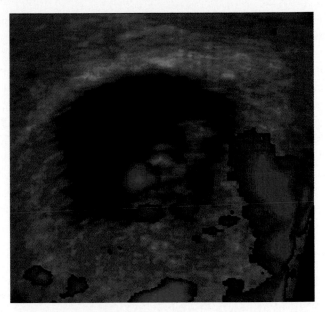

FIGURE 11.2: Three-dimensional power Doppler scan of a gestational sac at 6 weeks gestation. Note embryonic heart activity and blood flow signals obtained from intervillous space and maternal circulation.

Vascularization Index (VI) and Vascularization Flow Index (VFI). The volume of the chorion increased exponentially throughout observation period. The VI and VFI positively correlated with the crown-rump length (CRL) and chorionic volume and showed gradual increment throughout the investigation period.

Spiral arteries are identified by their anatomical position and their typical pulsed Doppler waveform. Impedance in spiral arteries decreases during early pregnancy from 5 to 6 weeks gestation. The continuous decrease of spiral artery vascular impedance suggests continuous cytotrophoblast invasion, indicating that the physiological changes are not yet completed. Decrement is detected until the 18th week of gestation, and after that period there is no significant change in terms of vascular impedance of the spiral arteries. These hemodynamic changes obtained by Doppler analysis are in correlation with the second wave of the trophoblast invasion.[14] It has been reported that circulatory changes in spiral arteries and within the intervillous space may assist in detection of the pregnancy-induced hypertension and intrauterine growth restriction.

Kurjak and Kupesic[15] analyzed intervillous blood flow and blood flow in spiral arteries in normal and abnormal early pregnancies. Pulsed Doppler signals obtained from the intervillous arteries showed low impedance values and a characteristic spiky outline.

This type of a waveform profile is indicative of high turbulence and a tortuous vessel with an irregular wall and is similar to profiles obtained from the spiral arteries. However, both the RI and PI obtained from the intervillous space in normal pregnancy (RI 0.36 ± 0.02, PI 0.72 ± 0.04) were significantly lower than vascular indices obtained from the spiral arteries (RI 0.45 ± 0.02, PI 0.80 ± 0.06). Continuous intervillous blood flow pattern was another type of pulsed Doppler signals obtained from the intervillous space. These Doppler signals are marked by low velocity for up to 10 weeks of gestation. As the gestation advances, venous type signals become more prominent and randomly dispersed throughout the placenta. Blood-flow velocity values obtained from these vessels in the normal pregnancy group increased significantly from 11 weeks gestation (8.0 ± 0.9 versus 12.2 ± 1.4 cm/sec).

UMBILICAL AND FETAL PORTION

The assessment of the fetal portion of circulation includes evaluation of the umbilical and fetal circulation. Hemodynamic changes in the umbilical artery represent the placental side of the uteroplacental circulation. Signals from the umbilical artery may be clearly visualized at the embryo's distal edge, which is connected to the placenta. The fetal circulation is usually analyzed by the assessment of the fetal heart, fetal aorta, carotid arteries and intracranial circulation (middle cerebral artery in particular) (Figure 11.3). The appearance of blood flow in these arteries is described separately for every gestational week and compared to the main histological and conventional gray-scale ultrasound findings.

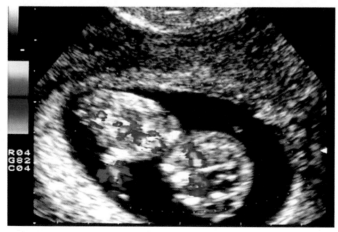

FIGURE 11.3: Transvaginal color Doppler scan of the fetal circulation at 9 weeks gestation. Note color Doppler signals obtained from the umbilical and fetal circulation.

Kurjak and Kupesic[17] used B-mode, color and power Doppler imaging to evaluate fetal growth and development of fetal circulation. The study included 270 normally developing pregnancies analyzed by digitized three-dimensional ultrasound power Doppler ultrasound. Different rendering modalities were used in color-coded data processing and presentation. Minimum-intensity modality was used to create a translucent image, while maximum-intensity modality was applied for the demonstration of surface rendered vascular images. The former was superior in the assessment of the spatial inter-relationship of the vascular structures, and the latter was useful in the assessment of the morphology and outer surface of a confined vascular structures.

Now, we will demonstrate typical 2D and 3D ultrasound and color/power Doppler findings corresponding to every gestational week during the first trimester of pregnancy.[17-30]

The 5th Week

Embryologic Findings

At this gestational age, the deep neural groove and the first somites are present. The embryo is almost straight and the somites produce conspicuous surface elevation. The heart prominence is distinct and the optic pits are present. The attenuated tail with its somites is also a characteristic feature.

2D Ultrasound Findings

At five weeks of gestation, the gestational sac can be detected by transvaginal ultrasonography as a tiny ring-shaped structure. The gestational sac is usually located within the "shining" endometrium on one of the sides of the uterine cavity line. A clear and accurate display of the gestational ring is suggestive of a normal intrauterine pregnancy. It is important to point out that at this gestational age, the distinction between the real gestational sac and other ring-like structures, such as the "pseudogestational sac" of an ectopic pregnancy may be difficult.

3D Ultrasound Findings

Multiplanar mode is helpful in distinguishing an early intraendometrial gestational sac from the collection of fluid between the endometrial leafs (pseudogestational sac). Also, it enables a precise measurement of the exponentially expanding gestational sac volume during the first trimester. At the beginning of the 5th week, the gestational sac exceeds 8 mm.[18] The small secondary yolk sac is visible as the earliest sign of a developing embryo. There is an incremental increase of the yolk sac volume until 10 weeks of gestation. After reaching the maximum size, it remains stable for a week and then decreases.

Kupesic and coworkers[19] found that 3D ultrasound measurement of the yolk sac volume and vascularity may be predictive of a pregnancy outcome. Using this non-invasive modality and in only few seconds, the sonographer can obtain multiplanar and surface images. Surface images are beneficial in the evaluation of the yolk sac echogenicity and detection of the hyperechoic yolk sac, which is associated with chromosomal abnormalities. Automatic and manual volume calculation allows for analysis of the precise relationship between the yolk sac and gestational sac volumes, as well as the assessment of the correlation between yolk sac volume and CRL measurements.

Multiplanar imaging is useful for evaluation of the embryo. The embryo is detected 24 to 48 hours after visualization of the yolk sac, approximately 33 days after the onset of menstruation. The embryo is seen adjacent to the yolk sac as a small straight line measuring 2 to 3 mm.[20]

Transvaginal Color Doppler Findings

Color signals from the spiral arteries are visualized in close proximity to the gestational sac. The blood flow velocities in systole and diastole are very low. Using this sensitive modality it is possible to obtain color Doppler signals from the hyperechoic endometrium, where the future gestational sac will be developed.[21]

3D Power Doppler Findings

Three-dimensional power Doppler ultrasound reveals intensive vascular activity surrounding the chorionic shell starting from the first sonographic evidence of the developing pregnancy during the 5th week of gestation. Color-coded sprouts penetrating its borders interrupt the hyperechoic chorionic ring and represent the areas of the developing intervillous circulation.

The 6th Week

Embryologic Findings

The embryo has a C-shaped curve. The growth of the head (caused by the rapid development of the fetal brain) exceeds that of the other regions.

2D Ultrasound Findings

At this gestational age, the gestational sac is always visible on the transvaginal ultrasound and is surrounded by a broad, echodense asymmetrical ring. This double line is an important characteristic of the early gestational sac, differentiating it from intracavitary blood collection or the "pseudogestational sac". At this gestational age, the origin of the double contour or double ring may be attributed to the rapidly proliferating inner cytotrophoblasts and outer syncytiotrophoblasts. The gestational sac is therefore easily measurable, but a prognosis cannot yet be made as to the outcome of the pregnancy. The yolk sac becomes clearly visible and measures 3 to 4 mm. Using the vaginal probe, the embryo crown-rump length (CRL) can be measured and varies from 3 to 5 mm. Embryonic heartbeats can be detected as early as 5 weeks and 4 days of the gestational age. The structures, such as fetal head or trunk, usually cannot be visualized by ultrasound at this stage.

3D Ultrasound Findings

A rounded bulky head and thinner body characterize three-dimensional ultrasound image of an embryo during the 6th week of pregnancy. The head is prominent due to the developing forebrain. Limb buds are rarely visible on ultrasound at this stage of pregnancy. However, the umbilical cord and the vitelline duct are always clearly seen. At six weeks of gestation, the ductus omphalomesentericus can be as much as three to four times the length of the embryo itself. The amniotic membrane may be clearly demonstrated, initially, at the dorsal part of the embryo. A few days later, it surrounds the embryo but not the yolk sac, which remains in the extracelomic cavity.

Transvaginal Color Doppler Findings

Transvaginal color Doppler sonography accurately indicates the position of the embryonic heart pulsations. Pulsed Doppler signals from the aorta and umbilical artery demonstrate absent end-diastolic flow, while umbilical vein blood flow is pulsatile. Spiral artery blood flow, intervillous circulation and intraovarian luteal flow are also clearly visualized.

3D Power Doppler Findings

Aortic and umbilical blood flow is well depicted. The initial branches of the umbilical vessels are visible at the placental umbilical insertion.

The 7th Week

Embryologic Findings

The head of an embryo is now much larger in relation to the trunk and is bent over the cardiac prominence. The trunk and neck have begun to straighten. The hand and foot plates are formed and the digital or finger rays have started to appear.

2D Ultrasound Findings

The gestational sac occupies approximately one-third of the uterine volume. The main landmark is now an echogenic fetal pole consisting of a 5 to 9 mm embryo adjacent to the yolk sac. Between 6 and 7 weeks of gestation, the embryo passes the 5 mm limit and the crown-rump length (CRL) can be measured with certainty. During the 7th week, the embryonic length is from 7 to 12 mm and the yolk sac has an average diameter of 5 mm. At this gestational age, the yolk sac is clearly separated from the embryo, which is most likely related to the growth of the vitelline duct. The cephalic pole becomes distinguishable and a single hypoechoic cavity can be seen, corresponding to a part of the primitive cerebral ventricle in the rhombencephalic area, which represents the future fourth ventricle. Fetal heartbeats are seen from the 6th gestational week onward.

3D Ultrasound Findings

During the 7th gestational week, the spine gradually becomes visible, as well as the limb buds, on the lateral sides of fetal body. The amnion is visualized as a spherical hyperechoic membrane, which is close to the embryo. The chorion frondosum can be distinguished from the chorion laeve. During this gestational age, there is a fast development of the rhombencephalon (hindbrain). This process gives even more prominence to the embryonic head, which then becomes the dominant structure. Using the multiplanar mode, developing vesicles of the brain are depicted as anechoic structures within the head. The most prominent is rhombencephalon, which is placed on the top of the head (vertex). The head is strongly flexed, the anterior portion being in contact with the chest. At this juncture of time, the hypoechogenic brain cavities can be identified, including the separated cerebral hemispheres. The lateral ventricles are shaped like small round vesicles. The cavity of the diencephalon (future third ventricle) runs posterior. The medial telencephalon forms a continuous cavity between the lateral ventricles. The future foramina of Monro are wide. In the sagittal plane, the height of the cavity of the diencephalon (future third ventricle) is slightly bigger than that of the mesencephalon. Thus, the wide border between the cavities of the diencephalon and the mesencephalon is indicated. The curved tube-like mesencephalic cavity (the future Sylvian aqueduct) lies

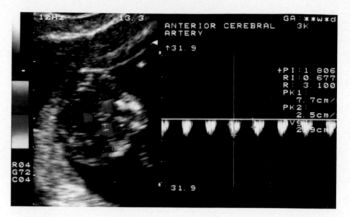

FIGURE 11.4: Transvaginal color Doppler scan of intracranial circulation at 7/8 weeks gestation. Note the absence of end-diastolic flow, which is a typical finding for this gestational age.

anterior, with its rostral part pointing caudal. It straightens considerably during the following weeks.

Transvaginal Color Doppler Findings

By the completion of the 6th gestational week, the villous vascularity is connected to the primitive heart. In addition, the embryonic circulation through the umbilical cord is established. The blood flow signals in the umbilical artery and fetal aorta are clearly demonstrated. Intracranial circulation becomes visible as early as the 7th week of gestation (Figure 11.4). At this time, discrete pulsations of the internal carotid arteries are detectable at the base of the skull. Power Doppler demonstrates vascularity at the periphery of the rhombencephalic cavity at 7-8 weeks of gestation, while spectral Doppler detects low velocity and the absence of the diastolic flow.

3D Power Doppler Findings

Besides the aorta and umbilical blood flow, at the end of the 7th week, 3D power Doppler depicts the features of early vascular anatomy on the base of the fetal skull. Vessels are evolving laterally to the mesencephalon and cephalic flexure. Apart from the embryonic circulation, 3D power Doppler may demonstrate blood flow signals within the intervillous space.

The 8th Week

Embryological Findings

By the beginning of the 8th week, the embryo has developed a skeleton, which is mostly cartilaginous and gives form to its body. The communication between the primitive gut and the yolk sac has been reduced to a relatively small duct (the yolk stalk).

2D Ultrasound Findings

By the 8th week, an embryo's length is between 10 and 16 mm, and the crown-rump length (CRL) is easily measured. The lower limb buds, which are short but discernible, are seen more clearly; the upper limb buds are harder to visualize because the echoes from the chest sometimes conceals them. The folding of the hypoechoic cerebral vesicle limits the lateral recesses of the rhombencephalic cavity. The placental site can also be identified by following the umbilical cord from the abdominal wall of the embryo (to the placenta). By the end of the 8th week, discrete undulating body movements can be sporadically seen on real time imaging. The heart motion is clearly detectable within the central area of the curved embryo. At this time, the heart beat ranges between 110 and 140 beats per minute.

3D Ultrasound Findings

The most characteristic finding at this gestational age is a complete visualization of the fetal limbs. Thick areas at the end of each extremity correspond to the future hands and feet. The shape of the face begins to appear but is not clearly visualized. The great majority of embryos demonstrate a cranial pole flexion that conceals visualization of the fetal face. The insertion of the umbilical cord is visible on the anterior abdominal wall. During the 8th week of pregnancy, there is expansion of the ventricular system of the brain (lateral, third and midbrain ventricles). Due to this process, the head erects extends from the anterior flexion. The vertex is now located over the position of the midbrain. Structures of the viscerocranium are not visible due to their small size. Blaas et al.[22] evaluated an embryo at 7 weeks and 5 days of gestation whose brain structures were analyzed in detail by 3D ultrasound. They described the process depicting distinct hemispheres of the rhombencephalic cavity (the future fourth ventricle), deepening gradually with the growth of the embryos, while simultaneously decreasing its length.[22] At this time, rhombencephalon has a pyramid-like shape with a central deepening of the pontine flexure at the peak of the pyramid.[13]

During the 8th and 9th weeks, the developing intestines are being herniated into the proximal umbilical cord. This can be assessed using ultrasound.

Transvaginal Color Doppler Findings

The visualization rates of the fetal aorta and umbilical artery are now higher. Blood flow in the fetal heart and aorta, as well as in the umbilical artery and spiral arteries are clearly

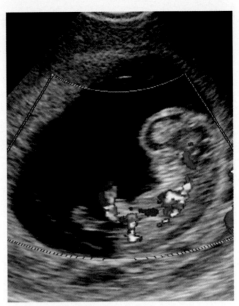

FIGURE 11.5: Transvaginal color Doppler scan of the entire fetal circulation at 9 weeks gestation.

visualized. There are no significant hemodynamic changes in blood vessels in comparison to that of the earlier period of pregnancy, in either the uteroplacental or fetal circulation. From the 8th week it is possible to obtain blood flow signals from the internal carotid and vertebral arteries (Figure 11.5). The internal carotid arteries, upon reaching the brain, branch into the anterior, middle and posterior cerebral arteries supplying cortical areas of the fetal brain. Vertebral arteries supply cerebellum and the brain stem.[24]

3D Power Doppler Findings

Three-dimensional power Doppler imaging allows visualization of the entire fetal circulation (Figure 11.6).

The 9th and 10th Weeks

Embryologic Findings

At this gestational age, the head is more rounded and constitutes almost half of the embryo. The hands and feet approach each other. The upper limbs develop faster than the lower limbs and toward the end of the 9th week, the fingers are almost entirely formed. The abdominal cavity becomes too small to contain all the intestinal loops and they enter extraembryonic coelom in the umbilical cord (physiologic midgut herniation).

2D Ultrasound Findings

The fetal structures are now clearly discernible. The size of the fetal head surpasses the diameter of the yolk sac.

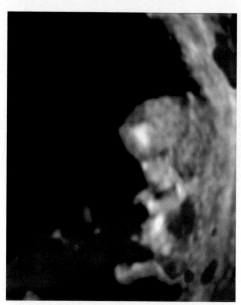

FIGURE 11.6: Three-dimensional power Doppler image of the fetal and umbilical vessels at 9 weeks gestation.

The fetal head often measures two-thirds of the entire body. The physiologic (ventral) midgut herniation is seen and the size of the cord insertion containing the midgut is at least 1.5 times the size of the cord thickness. Fetal kidneys and adrenal glands can be imaged by transvaginal ultrasound since their size is within the resolution of today's equipment. Anatomic structures within the head, such as the hyperechoic falx and choroid plexuses and a hypoechoic heart-shaped structure corresponding to the cerebral peduncles are also visible. The placenta becomes more demarcated and its relationship to the uterine cavity may be evaluated with greater accuracy.

3D Ultrasound Findings

Merz et al.[25] provided striking images of the fetal face at this gestational age. Using transvaginal 3D ultrasound they were able to demonstrate remarkably well-defined facial images at 9 weeks gestation. Using 3D surface imaging even the external ear can be depicted. Herniation of the midgut is still present as it is a consequence of the rapid growth of the bowel and liver before the closure of the abdominal wall. Although this is a physiologic phenomenon, it does not appear in every fetus. At 10 weeks, the bowel undergoes two 180 degrees turns, returning to its original position. At the same time, development of the abdominal wall ends. The dorsal column, the early spine, can be examined in its entire length. The arms with elbows and legs with knees are clearly visible, while the feet can be seen approaching

the midline. At this gestational age the size of the lateral ventricles increases rapidly. While the third ventricle is still relatively wide at the beginning of this week, its antero-medial part narrows due to the growth of the thalami. In fetuses whose CRL measured 25 mm or more, there is a clear gap between the rhombencephalic and mesencephalic cavity due to the growing cerebellum. The cavity of the diencephalon decreases in the larger fetuses (CRL = 25 mm) and becomes narrow, especially at its upper anterior part. The spine is still characterized by two echogenic parallel lines.

Transvaginal Color Doppler Findings

From the 9th gestational week, arterial pulsations can be detected on a transverse section, lateral to the mesencephalon and cephalic flexure. It is not always possible to distinguish between the internal carotid and middle cerebral arteries. At this time, blood flow through the full length of the fetal aorta and umbilical artery can be visualized. A characteristic waveform profile, the systolic component, with an absent end-diastolic frequency, is visible from the 7th to the 10th gestational week, suggesting a high vascular resistance. Within the symmetrical cerebellar hemispheres, intracerebellar arteries can be visualized. Blood flow signals from the intracerebellar arteries can be obtained from the 9th week of gestation. The posterior lateral choroidal artery is derived from the posterior cerebral artery, whereas the lateral choroidal arteries are derived from the middle cerebral artery and internal carotid artery. The choroid plexus vessels can be visualized starting from the 9th week of gestation. Subtle color and pulsed Doppler signals are obtained at the inner edge of the choroid plexus. Choroid plexus vascularity during the 9th and 10th weeks of gestation has two typical patterns: a prominent venous blood flow and an absence of diastolic flow in the arterial signal.[24] Thereafter, low vascular impedance signals are easily obtainable. Continuous pan-diastolic blood flow emerges in the cerebral vessels on the base of the skull.[26] At that time, the aorta and the umbilical arteries are still characterized by the absent end-diastolic blood flow (Figures 11.7 and 11.8). Until the end of the 8th week of gestation all embryonic/fetal arteries demonstrate absence of diastolic flow. After that time a progressive increase is observed first in all the cerebral arteries. Between the 9th and 10th weeks of gestation, diastolic velocities begin to emerge, but they are incomplete and inconsistently present. After the 9th week of gestation blood flow signals may also be obtained from the cranial veins.[24]

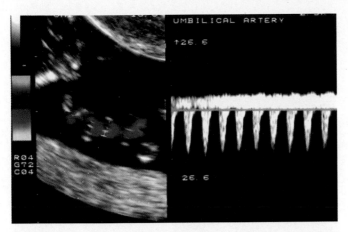

FIGURE 11.7: Transvaginal color Doppler image of the umbilical circulation: umbilical artery demonstrating absence of diastolic flow and venous component of the circulation.

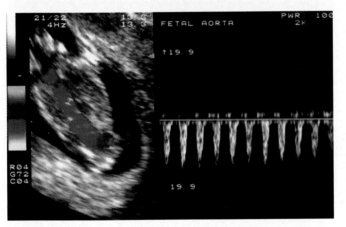

FIGURE 11.8: Transvaginal color Doppler image of the fetal aorta demonstrating absence of diastolic flow.

3D Power Doppler Findings

The umbilical cord vessels, fetal aorta, circle of Willis and its major branches are easily depicted by 3D power Doppler ultrasound.

The 11th Week

Embryologic Findings

The midgut herniation disappears and fetal kidneys produce urine that is excreted into the amniotic fluid.

2D Ultrasound Findings

At this stage, with the increasing differentiation of the fetus and rapid progression of ossification, fetal biometry becomes easier. Although measurable during the 8th week of pregnancy, the biparietal diameter becomes an accurate

and reliable parameter at 11 weeks of gestation. For practical applications, it is best to use both: Crown-rump length (CRL) and biparietal diameter (BPD) measurements. From now on, a more detailed fetal anatomy survey is obtained, including evaluation of cerebral anatomy, cardiovascular system, digestive and urinary tracts. The midgut is no longer herniated and can be seen as a hyperechoic round image within the abdominal cavity, which is located in the median region of the lower abdomen.

3D Ultrasound Findings

During the 11th week of pregnancy development of the head and neck continues. Facial details, such as the nose, orbits, maxilla and mandibles are often visible. The herniated midgut returns into the abdominal cavity. Its persistence after the 11th week of gestation is presumptive of an omphalocele. Multiplanar mode enables a detailed analysis of the fetal body with visualization of the stomach and urinary bladder. Kidneys are often visible. The arms and legs continue with development. Hata et al.[27] conducted a study on visualization of the fetal limbs by 2D and 3D sonography. The ability to visualize fetal hands/fingers and feet/toes was better with 3D that with 2D ultrasonography during the late first trimester (detection rates were 65% and 41% by 3D ultrasonography for hands and feet, respectively and 41% and 12%, by 2D ultrasonography). A detailed 3D ultrasound analysis of the fetal spine, chest and limbs is obtainable by using the transparent, X-ray like mode. Starting at the 13th gestational week, with the use of the transparency mode, medullary canal, each vertebra and rib can be visualized, and even the intervertebral disks can be precisely measured. This opens unexpected possibilities for early diagnosis of skeletal malformations.

Transvaginal Color Doppler Findings

At this stage, the pulsations of the middle cerebral artery are easily detected. Until the end of the first trimester, the absence of end-diastolic blood flow in fetal and placental components of the circulation is a normal physiologic finding. Establishment of the end-diastolic component of the blood flow is in direct correlation with an increment of blood flow velocities in the maternal arteries. A significant decrease of pulsatility index (PI) is observed in intracranial vessels with the advancing gestational age (Figure 11.9). Continuous end-diastolic flow is present two weeks earlier than in other parts of the fetal circulation and umbilical artery. This data suggests that the low vascular impedance in the fetal brain does not depend on changes in the vascular

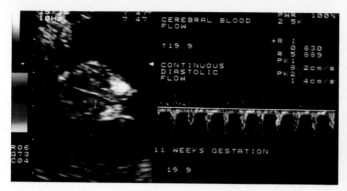

FIGURE 11.9: The cerebral artery at 9 to 10 weeks' gestation. Pulsed Doppler waveform analysis indicates permanent diastolic flow and significantly lower impedance to blood flow (RI = 0.83) than in other fetal vessels.

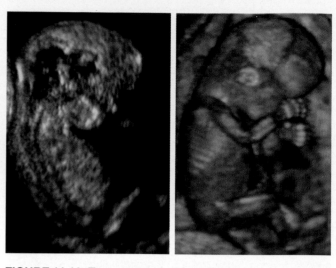

FIGURE 11.10: Two and three-dimensional images of a normal embryo during the end of first trimester. Note the anterior flexion of the head and clear image of the limb buds.

resistance of the fetal trunk or uteroplacental circulation. This apparently independent, autoregulatory mechanism provides an adequate blood supply to the growing fetal brain. This physiologic response is similar to the "brain-sparing effect" which has been described in hypoxic fetuses in the late second and third trimesters of pregnancy. It has been suggested that the full establishment of the intervillous circulation may lead to increased oxygen transport and decreased resistance in the peripheral embryonic circulation.[21]

The 12th Week

Embryological Findings

At 12 weeks of gestation, the neck is well defined, the face is broad and the eyes are widely separated. By the end of the 12th week, erythropoeisis decreases in the liver and commences in the spleen. The decidua capsularis adheres to the decidua parietalis. Fetal sex is clearly distinguishable by 12 weeks.

2D Ultrasound Findings

By transvaginal ultrasound fetal head, heart, diaphragm, stomach, kidney, urinary bladder, spine and extremities can be evaluated.

3D Ultrasound Findings

Visualization by 3D ultrasound enables a more detailed analysis of fetal anatomy, and especially of the limbs (Figure 11.10). It is possible to count fetal fingers and toes. The growing cerebellum is also clearly visible. The lateral ventricles dominate the brain.[28]

Transvaginal Color Doppler Findings

From this period, the umbilical vein blood flow is visible as a continuous flow. Between the 10th and 14th weeks, the diastolic velocities in the fetal blood vessels begin to emerge, but are incomplete and inconsistently present. The umbilical artery and fetal aorta are still the most prominent vessels for color Doppler assessment. After the 11th gestational week, the lowest RI values are obtained from the intracerebellar and choroid plexus arteries. A significantly lower RI (p < 0.05) for the intracerebellar artery than for the carotid arteries and cerebral arteries were demonstrated. However, the difference in RI between the choroid plexus artery and intracerebellar artery was not statistically significant (p > 0.05).[29] Wladimiroff et al.[30] analyzed the blood flow velocity waveform recordings in the umbilical artery, fetal descending aorta and intracerebral arteries between 11 and 13 weeks of gestation. Although flow velocity waveforms in the descending aorta and umbilical artery displayed absent end-diastolic flow, the flow velocity waveforms in the intracerebral arteries were characterized by forward flow throughout the cardiac cycle. Van Zalen-Sprock et al.[31] analyzed blood flow in the fetal aorta, umbilical artery and cerebral arteries between 6 and 16 weeks of gestation. The cerebral arteries showed a positive end-diastolic velocity in all fetuses after 10 weeks gestation. In the cerebral artery, the pulsatility index (PI) showed a mild gradual decrease towards the 16th week of pregnancy. This data suggests lower vascular impedance in the fetal brain, independent of the vascular resistance of

Color Doppler and 3D US Imaging in Normal and Abnormal Early Pregnancy

the fetal trunk and uteroplacental circulation. This apparently independent and autoregulatory mechanism thus provides an adequate blood supply to the growing fetal brain. Our data is in agreement with the results of the groups of Wladimiroff and Van Zalen-Sprock and prove that the cerebral vessels are a separate hemodynamic system, which is independent from other parts of the fetal circulation and exists from the start of the pregnancy.[21,28-31] Owing to this mechanism, the fetal brain is probably well protected from hypoxia even in early pregnancy. Hyett et al.[26] conducted a morphometric analysis of the great fetal vessels in early gestation. They performed examinations of the heart and great vessels of 61 specimens obtained after surgical termination of pregnancy for psychosocial reasons. The terminations occurred between 9 and 18 weeks of gestation. Doppler studies have demonstrated that at 11 to 13 weeks impedance in the cerebral vessels is only marginally higher than in the late second trimester. In contrast, in the descending aorta and umbilical arteries, there is a major decrease in impedance during the second trimester. This is thought to be due to the vascular changes in the placenta.[32-34] It could be hypothesized that preferential blood flow to the fetal head during the first and early second trimester of pregnancy is accomplished by the early development of low-resistance vessels in the cerebral circulation, at a stage when the resistance in other fetal parts and the placenta is high. Some authors suggested that there is an additional mechanism supporting preferential growth of the fetal head by a relative narrowing of the aortic isthmus so that left ventricular output is preferentially directed to the head.[23,30,31,33]

3D Power Doppler Findings

With the use of the 3D power Doppler, it is possible to depict major branches of the aorta: Such as the common iliac and renal arteries. In addition the Circle of Willis and its branches are also easily visualized (Figure 11.11).

First Trimester Screening for Chromosomal Anomalies

Yolk Sac

With the formation of the extraembryonic celomic cavity at the end of the 4th week, the primary yolk sac is replaced with a newly formed secondary yolk sac. During the organogenesis and before the placental circulation is established, the yolk sac is the primary source of exchange between the mother and the embryo. It has nutritive,

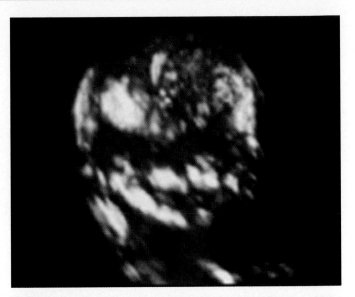

FIGURE 11.11: Three-dimensional power Doppler image of the fetus at 12 weeks gestation. Note two major vessels supplying the fetal brain: Carotid and vertebral arteries.

metabolic, endocrine, immunologic, excretory and hematopoietic functions.

At the beginning of the 5th week, it becomes visible as the first structure within the chorionic cavity. At this time, the yolk sac, a circular, well-defined, sonolucent structure measures 3-4 mm in diameter,[35] while the gestational sac measures about 8-10 mm. The yolk sac grows slowly until it reaches a maximum diameter of approximately 5-6 mm at 10 weeks. Its stalk can be followed from its origin all the way to the embryonic abdomen. As the gestational age advances and the amniotic cavity expands, being an extraembryonic structure, the yolk sac is gradually separating itself from the embryo. Different theories exist about the destiny of the yolk sac. Until recently, it was assumed that yolk sac gets caught and compressed between the amnion and chorion and disappears during the second trimester of pregnancy. Recent studies emphasized that the yolk sac degenerates first and then consequently disappears.

The ultrasound appearance of the yolk sac has already been proposed as a prognostic parameter for pregnancy outcome. Kurjak et al.[36] evaluated the yolk sac appearance in a normal and an abnormal early pregnancy. They found that the yolk sac is always visualized before the viable embryo; it measures 4.0 to 5.0 mm in diameter until 7 to 8 weeks of gestation and reaches 6.0 to 6.5 mm by the end of the 9th week. Their results suggest that sonographic detection of abnormal yolk sac morphology may predict an abnormal fetal outcome. Absence of the yolk sac, its abnormal size, echogenicity, shape and number are predictive indicators of early pregnancy failure. All these parameters should be defined and assessed during an early pregnancy ultrasound scan.

Abnormal yolk sac size may be the first sonographic indicator of chromosomal anomaly and pregnancy failure. Primarily, the presence of an embryo without the visible yolk sac before the 10th gestational week is considered abnormal. In normal pregnancies before the 10th gestational week the inner diameter of the yolk sac should always measure less than 5.6 mm. Lyons[37] has established the ratio between the gestational sac and yolk in normal pregnancy. In patients with mean gestational sac diameter of less than 10 mm, the yolk sac diameter should measure less than 4 mm.[37] In 15 patients who had abnormally large yolk sacs, six had no embryos, five aborted spontaneously and only one pregnancy was continued. Out of nine others with embryo and large yolk sac, eight patients aborted and in one patient trisomy 21 was detected at 24 weeks of gestation.[37]

The yolk sac can be too small and this feature is also accepted as a marker of poor pregnancy outcome. Green and Hobbins[38] analyzed a group of patients between 8 and 12 weeks of gestation with a yolk sac diameter of less than 2 mm. This measurement was associated with an adverse outcome. It is unknown whether the abnormalities of the yolk sac are related primarily to the yolk sac or are secondary to the embryonic maldevelopment. Clearly, the yolk sac plays an important role in maternofetal transportation in early pregnancy. Changes in size and shape could indicate or reflect the significant dysfunction of this system and therefore could influence early embryonic development. Currently, major benefits of the sonographic evaluation of the yolk sac are the following:

1. Differentiation between potentially viable and nonviable gestations.
2. Confirmation of an intrauterine pregnancy vs. a decidual cast.
3. Indication of a possible fetal abnormality.

Kupesic et al.[39] performed a transvaginal color Doppler study of the yolk sac vascularization and volume estimation by 3D ultrasound. This study evaluated 150 patients with uncomplicated pregnancy whose gestational age ranged from 6 to 10 weeks. Transvaginal 3D and power Doppler examination was performed before the termination of pregnancy. The termination of pregnancy was performed for psychosocial reasons. The highest visualization rates for yolk sac vessels were during the 7th and 8th gestational weeks, reaching a value of 90.71%. Doppler waveform

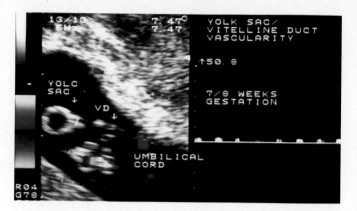

FIGURE 11.12: Transvaginal color Doppler image of the yolk sac at 7 weeks' gestation. Pulsed Doppler signals isolated from the connection of the yolk sac and vitelline duct demonstrate absence of diastolic flow.

analysis extracted from the wall of the yolk sac was characterized with low velocity (5.8 ± 1.7 cm/s) and absence of the diastolic flow (Figure 11.12). The pulsatility index (PI) showed a mean value of 3.24 ± 0.94 without significant changes between the gestational age subgroups. There was a positive correlation between the gestational age and volume of the yolk sac until 10 weeks of gestation.

At the end of the first trimester, the yolk sac volume remained constant, while the gestational sac volume continued to grow. Surface renderings by three-dimensional ultrasound may significantly contribute to "in vivo" observation of the yolk sac's "honeycomb" surface pattern (Figure 11.13). Increased echogenicity of the yolk sac walls was reported as a sign of dystrophic changes that occur in nonviable cellular material indicating early pregnancy loss.[40] Volume calculation by 3D ultrasound enables assessment of the relationship between the gestational sac and yolk sac volumes. The same method is used to obtain the correlation between the yolk sac volume and CRL measurements. Kupesic et al.[19] measured the gestational sac volume and yolk sac volume and vascularity in 80 women with uncomplicated pregnancy between 5 and 12 weeks of gestation. Regression analysis revealed an exponential growth of the gestational sac volume throughout the first trimester of pregnancy. It is well known that the gestational sac volume measurements are used for estimation of the gestational age in early pregnancy. Therefore, abnormal gestational sac volume measurement could potentially be used as a prognostic marker for pregnancy outcome. The yolk sac volume was found to increase from the 5th to the 10th gestational weeks. However, when the yolk sac reaches

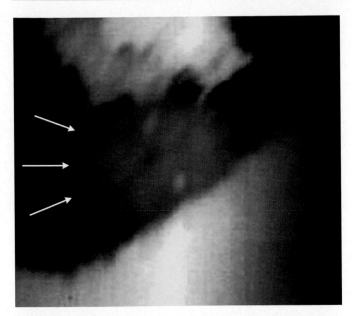

FIGURE 11.13: Transvaginal three-dimensional ultrasound scan of the yolk sac. Note the regular outer contours and "honeycomb" surface pattern of the yolk sac.

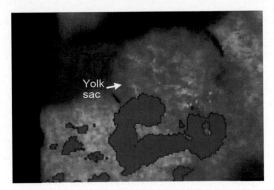

FIGURE 11.14: Three-dimensional power Doppler image of the yolk sac and its turgescent blood vessels.

its maximum volume at around 10 weeks of gestation it has already started to degenerate, which could be indirectly assessed by a significant reduction in visualization rates of the yolk sac vascularity.[19,39] As suggested earlier, the disappearance of the yolk sac in normal pregnancies is probably the result of yolk sac degeneration rather than a mechanical compression of the expanding amniotic cavity. These events suggest that an evaluation of the biologic function of the yolk sac by measuring the diameter and/or the volume is limited. Therefore, a combination of color and power Doppler ultrasound and volumetric studies is necessary to noninvasively study functional and morphologic events during early pregnancy. Although, the reports on yolk sac and vitelline circulation are very exciting, it should be noted that such studies are not ethically feasible in ongoing human pregnancies since the secondary yolk sac is a source of primary germ cells and blood stem cells.[41]

3D ultrasound and power Doppler will allow us to study turgescent blood vessels, which were on the surface of the yolk sac (Figure 11.14). The same technique may be used to study the evolution of the embryo-vitelline towards the embryo-placental circulation. Since, yolk sac and vitelline blood vessels are prerequisites for the oxygen transfer, absorptive and transfer processes during the first trimester, alterations in this early circulatory system may have some prognostic value for predicting pregnancy outcome.

3D ULTRASOUND MEASUREMENT OF NUCHAL TRANSLUCENCY

The unsuccessful nuchal translucency (NT) measurements were reported in many studies. [42,43] Clear guidelines and establishment of a training regimen for NT measurement as reported by Monni et al.[44] and Braithwaite et al.[45] may overcome some of the methodological problems. Kurjak et al.[46] demonstrated that 3D transvaginal ultrasound enables depiction of the most appropriate midsagittal section of the fetus in all the patients examined between 11 and 13 weeks of gestation. Precise NT measurement was possible due to the ability of 3D ultrasound to reorient the fetal position using multiplanar imaging. Better intraobserver reproducibility was obtained for 3D than for 2D ultrasound. The three-dimensional transvaginal ultrasound improves the accuracy of nuchal translucency measurement allowing appropriate midsagittal section of the fetus and clear distinction of the nuchal region from the amniotic membrane.

DOPPLER ASSESSMENT OF DUCTUS VENOSUS

The ductus venosus (ductus Arantii), foramen ovale and ductus arteriosus represent specific shunts during the intrauterine life. The ductus venosus (DV) connect the umbilical circulation with inferior vena cava. It originates from the umbilical vein and enters the inferior vena cava at the level of the hepatic veins, just below the diaphragm, forming the subdiaphragmatic venous vestibulum.[47] The main function of DV is the distribution of the oxygenated blood through foramen ovale into the left atrium. In normal conditions, approximately 53% of the umbilical blood flows through the ductus venosus.[48] It has been demonstrated that in hypoxic fetuses about 70% of the umbilical blood flows through ductus venosus.[49] The introduction of color Doppler has enabled the assessment of DV blood flow. Ductus venosus blood flow signals are depicted in the right sagittal section of the fetal abdomen, as a continuation of the umbilical vein towards the inferior vena cava.[50] In normal fetuses, the DV waveform shows a peak velocity during the ventricular systole, another peak during the ventricular diastole and a nadir during the atrial contraction. The DV pulsatility index is independent of the insonation angle and has proved to be the most reproducible parameter for flow assessment in these minute vessels.[51] Changes have been reported in the DV waveform in different hemodynamic situations. In fetuses with cardiac failure without structural defects, reversed flow during atrial contraction was observed in ductus venosus.[52] Similar findings were reported in growth-restricted fetuses.[53,54] More recently, abnormally increased DV pulsatility index was found to be associated with a significant prediction of chromosomal defects during early pregnancy.[55] The results from Antolín et al.[56] demonstrate the usefulness of a combined assessment of nuchal translucency and DV pulsatility index in an unselected population. Combining ductus venosus pulsatility index and NT in screening for chromosomal anomalies, the overall sensitivity decreased to 55%, but specificity reached 99.3% with a negative predictive value of 99.3%. When only autosomal trisomies were considered, the detection rate was similar to NT with a decrease in the false-positive rate. These results suggest that NT may be used as a first line-screening test in order to maintain the sensitivity, while examination of the DV blood flow may be used as a second line test in order to reduce the false-positive rate. Using this approach the need for invasive testing was reduced to less than 1%.[57] Increased DV pulsatility index (using the 95th percentile) may be explained by early cardiac failure.[58] Transient changes in DV waveform have been noted in chromosomally abnormal fetuses early in pregnancy, with a reversed flow during atrial contraction. Huisman and Bilardo[58] reported a case of twin pregnancy, where the fetus with trisomy 18 had increased nuchal translucency thickness and reversed end-diastolic DV flow. It was hypothesized that transient cardiac failure may be involved in the physiology of the NT thickness. Early cardiac dysfunction can produce a transient fluid accumulation in the back of the neck and a temporary increase in DV pulsatility index.[59] However, normal DV hemodynamics were reported for cardiac anomalies, involving the left atrium or ventricle, even though blood flow from this vessel is preferentially directed across the foramen ovale into the left heart. Abnormal DV parameters were demonstrated in association with right ventricular pathology.[60] Malformations involving the right ventricular inlet or outlet are more commonly associated with changes in the DV waveform during atrial contraction than in isolated septal defects.[51] Zoppi et al.[60] found reduced, absent or reversed flow in DV during late diastole, coinciding with atrial contraction. This was considered a sign of early fetal cardiac function impairment and was observed in first trimester fetuses with chromosomal abnormalities and cardiac defects. Because of the high prevalence of cardiac defects in fetuses with chromosomal abnormalities, it is clear that some signs of heart failure may be evident during the first trimester and DV seems to be an essential structure for evaluation of this manifestation.

The conclusion of this study was that DV pulsatility index should not be used as a first line screening test because it does not increase the number of cases detected by NT.[60] However, it can be useful as a second line test in screen-positive cases with increased NT in order to increase the specificity and reduce the need for invasive testing. In chromosomally normal fetuses with an abnormal DV waveform pattern, a careful follow-up ultrasound scan, including echocardiography done by a specialist is recommended.

FIRST TRIMESTER SCREENING FOR CHROMOSOMOPATHIES: NASAL BONE AND FETAL HEART

Nasal Bone

It has been reported that in combination with NT and biochemical markers, ultrasound detection of absent nasal bone may indicate a chromosomal anomaly.[61] The most common chromosomal anomaly associated with this finding is trisomy 21, Down syndrome. The nasal bone should be assessed between 11 and 14 weeks gestation. In normal fetuses, the nasal bone is visualized in the sagittal section using medial orbital angle. Cicero et al.[61] reported that the nasal bones were visualized in 99.5% of chromosomally normal fetuses. In 73% of cases of trisomy 21, the nasal bones were not demonstrated. The sensitivity of nasal bone detection, when used in combination with NT thickness and maternal serum biochemical screening achieved 90%.[61]

Fetal Heart Assessment

Simpson and Sharland[62] analyzed the association between congenital heart defects and increased NT. Their data indicate that normal nuchal translucency scans cannot exclude karyotyping abnormalities or serious cardiac malformations. Bronshtein and Zimmer[63] suggest that the transvaginal ultrasound examination of the fetal heart should be performed in at least in two main planes of four chambers and three specific images of the vessels (X,P,Y) during the period between 14 and 16 weeks of gestation. Earlier diagnosis enables the entire spectrum of diagnostic and therapeutic options, including genetic studies when indicated or therapeutic abortion. In cases of severe cardiac malformations, early detection may prevent unnecessary invasive procedures.[63]

PATHOLOGY OF EARLY PREGNANCY

Threatened Abortion

Early pregnancy failure defines a pregnancy that ends spontaneously before the fetus has reached a viable gestational age. The most common symptom in early pregnancy is vaginal bleeding. Threatened abortion is the clinical term used to describe this symptom during the first 20 weeks of pregnancy in women whom, on the basis of clinical evaluation, are considered to have a potentially living embryo. The main problem in management of these patients is to assess fetal viability. When vaginal bleeding occurs every clinician should ask several questions that can radically alter patient's management:

1. Is the patient pregnant?
2. Is the fetus viable?
3. What is the gestational age?
4. Is there any evidence to suggest that the pregnancy is an ectopic pregnancy?
5. In case of an abortion, is it complete or incomplete?
6. Is there any associated pelvic mass?

After such a detailed evaluation, it is possible to proceed with proper therapeutic measures, in cases where a normal pregnancy outcome can be expected. After an accurate diagnosis is performed, the selection of possible therapeutic measures is easier. At present, ultrasonography is considered the best diagnostic method for evaluation of early pregnancy complications. The skill of the sonographer is put to the test, since a verdict of pregnancy failure will often result in surgical intervention.

In patients with a normal intrauterine pregnancy, bleeding from the chorion frondosum is undoubtedly the most common source of vaginal bleeding during the first trimester. Sonographic evidence of such a bleeding can be identified as a perigestational hemorrhage in 5 to 22% of women with symptoms of threatened abortion. However, some precautions must be taken because the perigestational hemorrhage is occasionally difficult to distinguish from a blighted twin. The prognostic significance of identifying perigestational hemorrhage during the first trimester remains uncertain. Most of the small hemorrhages resolve without clinical consequences, while in some cases spontaneous abortion may occur. Pellizari et al.[64] analyzed blood flow in patients with vaginal bleeding during the first trimester. RI and PI did not show any difference between the patients with vaginal bleeding during the first trimester and patients with normal pregnancy (control group). However, the peak systolic velocity (PSV) has significantly increased with gestational age in a control group, but not in the group presented with vaginal bleeding.

Intrauterine Hematoma

A sonolucent crescent or wedge-shaped structure between the uterine wall and chorion is defined as a subchorionic hematoma. The hematoma represents a separation of the chorionic plate from the underlying decidua. In these patients, the decidua surrounding the gestational sac may demonstrate irregular echogenicity, subdecidual bleeding and fragmentation. The gestational sac may be detached from the decidual wall and the chorion may appear crumpled and flat. It is likely that if bleeding occurs at the level of the definitive placenta (located under the cord insertion), it may result in placental separation and subsequent hematoma. In addition, only by detaching from the membrane opposite to the insertion of the umbilical cord can a subchorionic hematoma reach a significant volume before it affects normal pregnancy development. In the ultrasound studies, much emphasis has been placed on the volume of the hematoma, but not on the location of the hemorrhage. Kupesic et al.[65] used color Doppler to visualize the spiral arteries in patients presenting with vaginal bleeding during the first trimester of pregnancy. Blood flow velocity waveforms were analyzed by the means of pulsed Doppler. Parameters used in the study were the resistance index and peak systolic velocity. The significant factor was the presence of the hematoma in the corpus or fundus of the uterus. Since, this is the region of the placental site in most cases, it suggests a possible disruption of placental function. This study demonstrated that patients with intrauterine hematomas have significantly higher vascular resistance in the ipsilateral spiral arteries, indicating decreased subchorionic flow. In cases with large subchorionic hematomas Doppler measurements showed

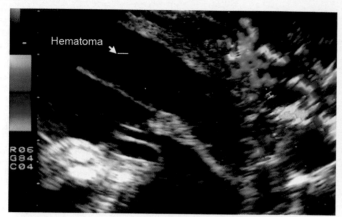

FIGURE 11.15A: Transvaginal color Doppler scan of hematoma, visualized as an echo free area in a close proximity to the gestational sac. Color signals are obtained from adjacent spiral arteries.

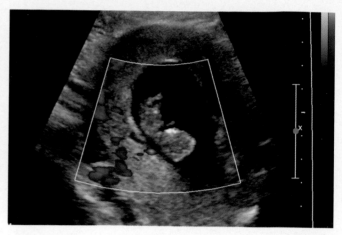

FIGURE 11.16: Transvaginal power Doppler scan of a missed abortion at 10 weeks gestation. Absence of a fetal cardiac activity is clearly demonstrated by power Doppler ultrasound.

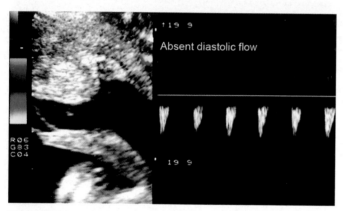

FIGURE 11.15B: The same patient as in figure 15A. Absence of diastolic flow (RI = 1.0) is detected in the spiral arteries close to the perigestational hemorrhage.

lack of diastolic flow and RI of 1.0 (Figures 11.15A and 11.15B). In patients with normal pregnancy outcome, these indices returned to normal values. Similarly, patients with a subchorionic hematoma had significantly lower peak systolic velocities detected in ipsilateral spiral arteries. It is likely that the subchorionic hematoma compresses the spiral arteries and reduces the velocity in underlying vessels. With continuation of pregnancy and reabsorption of hematoma, impedance to blood flow returns to normal values. In this study improvement of blood flow was predictive for normal pregnancy outcome, while decreased spiral artery perfusion indicated increased risk of first- and early second-trimester loss.[65] Since, patients with a subchorionic hematoma did not show increased risk for preterm delivery, it is expected that the elevated impedance to blood flow is a transitory consequence of a compression of the spiral arterial walls by the nearby hematoma. Clearly, transvaginal color and pulsed Doppler studies have the potential to detect the patients with altered spiral artery blood flow who are at increased risk for spontaneous abortion and may require hospitalization, bed rest and medical treatment.

Missed Abortion

The diagnosis of missed abortion is based on the visualization of the fetus with no evidence of heart activity or motion. It is relatively easy to make this diagnosis by means of a transvaginal color Doppler ultrasound (Figure 11.16). The main parameter is the absence of fetal heartbeats, which should be detected in all embryos after 6 weeks of gestation. Histological studies performed on some patients with missed abortion detected insufficient trophoblastic invasion into the spiral arteries. These findings may suggest defective transformation of spiral arteries as a possible cause of a spontaneous abortion. However, Doppler studies did not confirm increased spiral artery impedance in patients with spontaneous abortion. Being aware that chromosomal anomalies are one of the most important causes of a spontaneous abortion, occurring in more than 50% of patients, it is not surprising that Doppler studies did not demonstrate any significant difference in terms of vascular resistance between normal pregnancies and missed abortions. Pellizzari et al.[64] concluded that a blood flow analysis of the uterine artery blood flow does not contribute to the clinical management of patients with vaginal bleeding in early pregnancy. During normal and abnormal early pregnancy, sensitive color Doppler equipment may demonstrate two types of blood flow velocity waveforms from the intervillous space (pulsatile arterial-like and continuous venous-like patterns).[65-68] Doppler studies did not show any difference in terms of RI and PI for the intervillous arterial flow between women with missed abortion and patients with normal pregnancy.[68,69] However, in a long-standing demise, the cessation of the embryonic portion of placental circulation leaves the fluid pumping action of the trophoblast unaffected as it remains nourished by the maternal intervillous blood.[68] Consequently, the embryonic circulation no longer drains a trophoblast conveyed fluid in the villous stroma. Progressive accumulation of the fluid may result in a significant reduction of the intervillous blood flow impedance. Lower impedance to blood flow, observed in spiral arteries, indicates that a massive and continuous infiltration of the maternal blood without effective drainage causes further disruption of the maternal embryonic interface resulting in an abortion.[15] Therefore, changes in the vascular pattern, as well as changes in yolk sac appearance (size, shape and echogenicity) seem to be a consequence of poor embryonic development or even embryonic death rather than a primary cause of an early pregnancy failure.[69] Changes in vascularization of the yolk sac noticed in missed abortions are probably caused by a resorption of the embryo through the vitelline duct.[15] Abnormal patterns of the yolk sac vascularity can be related to the decreased vitelline blood flow, which may cause a progressive accumulation of nutritive secretions not utilized by an embryo. This process ends with the enlargement of the yolk sac indicative of an early pregnancy failure. This data indicate that there is an interaction between the yolk sac vascularity and intervillous circulation in patients with a missed abortion.[66,68]

Blighted Ovum

Blighted ovum (anembryonic pregnancy) refers to a gestational sac in which the embryo either failed to develop or died at a stage too early to visualize. The diagnosis of anembryonic pregnancy is based on the absence of embryonic echoes within the gestational sac large enough to be visible independent of the clinical data or date of the last menstrual bleeding. Advances in transvaginal sonography have allowed us to detect this kind of abnormality at a mean sac diameter of 1.5 cm.[67] If the volume of the gestational sac is less than 2.5 ml in a pregnancy which fails to increase in size by at least 75% over a period of 1 week, a pregnancy could be diagnosed

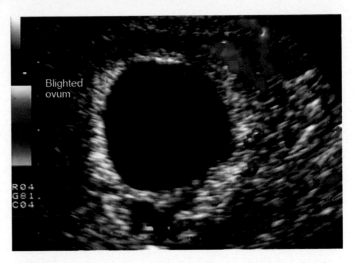

FIGURE 11.17: Transvaginal color Doppler ultrasound of an anembryonic pregnancy (blighted ovum). Note dilated spiral arteries in a close proximity to the empty gestational sac.

as a blighted ovum.[70] When a large empty sac measuring from 12 to 18 mm in mean diameter is detected, absence of a living embryo is suspicious for nonviability, but this finding should be correlated with other clinical and sonographic data, including the presence of a yolk sac (Figure 11.17). However, transvaginal sonography can clearly detect a nonliving embryo (embryonic demise) in some cases that would have been, undoubtedly, diagnosed as blighted ovum if the transabdominal sonography was the only examination performed. What the sonographer would detect on the screen during the ultrasound examination depends on the stage of development of the pregnancy or resorption of the embryo. Sometimes even the embryos that measure 1cm by transvaginal sonography may be completely absorbed after prolonged retention. In an anembryonic pregnancy, a fertilized ovum develops into a blastocyst, but the inner cell mass and resultant fetal pole never develops. The gestational sac invades the endometrium and acts partly like a normally developing pregnancy. The syncytiotrophoblast invades the endometrium and produces human chorionic gonadotropin, which results in a positive pregnancy test, enlarged tender breasts and other clinical stigmata of pregnancy. The normal appearances, however, are short-lived. The gestational sac fails to grow and develop normally, and the uterus fails to develop as expected. The incidence of chromosomal abnormality in patients with anembryonic pregnancy is high. It is estimated that about 15-20% of all human pregnancies diagnosed before the end of the first trimester terminate as spontaneous abortion.[70] Falling levels of human chorionic gonadotropin, progesterone and estrogen, lead to disappearance of the feeling of being pregnant. Since, clinical impression and beta hCG values are variable, the diagnosis of an anembryonic pregnancy is performed by ultrasound. Two-dimensional real time ultrasound performed accurate diagnosis of an anembryonic pregnancy in 100% of cases when the examination was performed one week apart.[70] Doppler studies on intervillous circulation demonstrated lower vascular resistance of the arterial like signals in patients with blighted ovum when compared to normal pregnancies.[15,66,68] This finding may be explained by a massive and continuous infiltration of the maternal blood without an effective drainage, resulting in lower vascular impedance of the arterial type blood signals within the intervillous space.

CONCLUSION

The introduction of 2D and 3D transvaginal sonography and color Doppler has, for the first time, enabled in vivo studies of early embryonic and uteroplacental circulations. One of the major advantages of 3D ultrasonography is the noninvasive evaluation of the developing embryo/fetus using a multiplanar view, surface reconstruction, volume calculation, storage of the data for retrospective analysis and telemedicine.

Color Doppler ultrasound enables noninvasive evaluation of the embryonic, uterine and ovarian vessels. There is evidence of a gradual decrease of the uterine artery resistance index during the first trimester of pregnancy. Decrease of the vascular impedance continues during the second trimester of pregnancy and is observed in all the segments of the uteroplacental circulation. During early pregnancy spiral arteries are progressively converted to non-muscular dilated tortuous channels. This alteration may be demonstrated even before the gestational sac is visualized on ultrasound. Estimation of the circulatory changes in the spiral arteries and intervillous space may be potentially useful to detect patients who will later develop pregnancy induced hypertension and intrauterine growth restriction. The earliest visible sign of pregnancy by transvaginal ultrasonography is a ring-shaped gestational sac that can be seen during the 5th week of amenorrhea. It is important to distinguish between the gestational sac and other ring-like sonolucent intracavitary structures, such as the "pseudogestational sac" of an ectopic pregnancy. When the gestational sac reaches about 8 to 10 mm, the yolk sac becomes visible. At 6 of weeks of gestation, the embryo is C-shaped and its crown rump length is about 3 to 4 mm.

Color Doppler signals accurately indicate the position of the fetal heart. During the 7th week of gestation, the gestational sac occupies about one-third of the uterine volume. At this gestational age, the main landmark is an echogenic embryonic pole measuring between 5 and 9 mm. During the 8th gestational week an embryo's length is between 10 and 16 mm. Discrete undulating body movements can sporadically be seen on real time ultrasound. At this gestational age, expansion of the ventricular system of the brain is evident. During the 9th and 10th weeks of gestation the fetal structures are clearly discernible and are represented by distinct parts of the fetal body, such as the head, trunk and limbs. The physiologic (ventral) midgut herniation can be seen. From the 11th week of gestation, a more detailed fetal anatomy survey can be obtained, including the cerebral, cardiovascular, digestive and urinary systems, including the urinary tracts. At this point the midgut is no longer herniated. At 12 weeks of gestation, using transvaginal ultrasound, it is possible to visualize the fetal head, heart, diaphragm, stomach, kidney, urinary bladder, spine and extremities. At this period of time, the umbilical vein flow is visible as a continuous flow. As the gestational sac grows and the amniotic cavity expands, the yolk sac is gradually separated from the embryo. The ultrasound appearance of the yolk sac is one of the prognostic parameters for the outcome of the pregnancy. Currently, the major benefits of the sonographic evaluation of the yolk sac are differentiation of the potentially viable and nonviable gestations, confirmation of the presence of an intrauterine pregnancy and indication of a possible chromosomal abnormality.

Some studies indicate that the three-dimensional transvaginal ultrasound improves accuracy of the nuchal translucency measurement, allowing the appropriate mid-sagittal sections of the fetus with clear distinction of the nuchal region from the amniotic membrane. The ductus venosus pulsatility index assessment is a useful second line test in screen-positive cases with NT to increase the specificity, reduce the need for invasive testing of chromosomal anomalies. The prognostic significance of identifying perigestational hemorrhage during the first trimester remains uncertain. Most of the small hemorrhages resolve without clinical sequelae, while in some cases spontaneous abortion may occur. A subchorionic hematoma is visualized as an echo free area between the amniotic membrane and the uterine wall. Fundal corporeal location is considered a high risk location of subchorionic bleeding. Color Doppler may aid follow-up of the blood flow changes that occur in spiral arteries as a consequence of the mechanical compression of the nearby hematoma. The diagnosis of a missed abortion is determined by identification of a fetus, which does not demonstrate any heart activity or motion. Blighted ovum (anembryonic pregnancy) refers to a gestational sac in which the embryo either failed to develop or died at a stage too early to visualize. The diagnosis of anembryonic pregnancy is based on the absence of the embryonic pole within the gestational sac large enough to be visualized by ultrasound (≥ 1.5 cm), independent of the clinical data or last day of menstrual bleeding.

Early human development could be evaluated in vivo using 3D sonography[71]. There is a significant correlation between the embryo volume and the gestational age and CRL measurements.[72] Therefore, the embryo volume may become an important parameter for the early diagnosis of growth disorders. Placental volume has also demonstrated a strong correlation with the gestational age.[73] Using 3D power Doppler ultrasound, the placental volume and vascularity could be simultaneously assessed and evaluated. It was demonstrated that intervillous and uteroplacental blood flow increases throughout the first trimester of pregnancy.[74] It has been demonstrated that intervillous circulation is abnormally increased in patients with a miscarriage. However, more studies are needed to address the practical value of these observations.

REFERENCES

1. Jukic J. Pathology of women's reproductive system. AGM, Zagreb. 1999.
2. Zoppi MA, Ibba RM, Floris M, et al. Fetal nuchal translucency screening in 12495 pregnancies in Sardinia. Ultrasound Obstet Gynecol 2001;18(6):649-51.
3. Kupesic S, Kurjak A, Hafner T, et al. Events of ovulation to implantation studied by three-dimensional ultrasound. J Perinat Med 2002;30(1):84-98.
4. Frates MC, PM Doubilet, SM Durfe, et al. Sonographic and Doppler characteristics of the corpus luteum: Can they predict pregnancy outcome? 2001;20(8):821-7.
5. Itskovitz J, Lindenbaum ES, Brandes JM. Arterial anastomosis in the pregnant human uterus. Obstet Gynecol 1980;55(1):67-71.
6. Kurjak A, Zudenigo D, Funduk-Kurjak B, et al. Transvaginal color Doppler in the assessment of the uteroplacental circulation in normal early pregnancy. J Perinat Med 1993;21(1):25-34.
7. Kurjak A, Kupesic-Urek S, Predanic M, et al. Transvaginal color Doppler assessment of the uteroplacental circulation in normal and abnormal early pregnancy. Early Hm Dev 1992;29(1-3):385-9.
8. Jauniaux E, Jurkovic D, Campbell S. In vivo investigations of anatomy and physiology of early human placental circulation. Ultrasound Obstet Gynecol 1991;1:435-45.
9. Jaffe R, Warsof SL. Transvaginal color Doppler imaging in the assessment of uteroplacental blood flow in the normal first trimester pregnancy. Am J Obstet Gynecol 1991;164(3):781-5.
10. Kurjak A, Kupesic-Urek S, Predanic M, et al. Transvaginal color Doppler in the study of early pregnancies associated with fibroids. J. Matern. Fetal Invest 1992;2:81-87.
11. Pijnenborg R, Bland JM, Robertson WB, et al. Uteroplacental arterial changes related to interstitial trophoblast migration in early human pregnancy. Placenta 1983;4:397-414.
12. Pijnenborg R, Dixon G, Robertson WB, et al. Trophoblastic invasion of human decidua from 8 to 18 weeks of pregnancy. Placenta 1980;1(1):3-19.
13. Kanayama N. Trophoblast injury: A new etiological and pathological concept of preeclampsia. Croat Med J 2003;44(2):148-56.
14. Matijevic R, Kurjak A, Hafner T. Terminal parts of uteroplacental circulation in pregnancy: Assessment by color/pulsed Doppler ultrasound; Ultrasound Rev Obstet Gynecol 2001;262-74.
15. Kurjak A, Kupesic S. Doppler assessment of the intervillous blood flow in normal and abnormal early pregnancy. Obstet Gynecol 1997;89(2):252-6
16. Hafner T, Kurjak A, Funduk-Kurjak B, et al. Assessment of early chorionic circulation by three dimensional power Doppler. J Perinat Med 2002;30(1):33-9.
17. Kurjak A, Kupesic S, Banovic I, et al. The study of morphology and circulation of early embryo by three-dimensional ultrasound and power Doppler. J Perinat Med 1999;27(3):145-57.
18. Bree RL, CS Marn. Transvaginal sonography in the first trimester: Embryology, anatomy, and hCG correlation. Semin Ultrasound CT MR 1990;11(1):12-21.
19. Kupesic S, Kurjak A, Ivancic-Kosuta M. Volume and vascularity of the yolk sac studied by three-dimensional ultrasound and color Doppler. J Perinat Med 1999;27(2):91-6.
20. Bonilla-Musoles, et al. Demonstration of Early Pregnancy with Three-Dimensional Ultrasound. In: Merz E (Ed). 3D Ultrasound in Obstetrics and Gynecology. Philadelphia, New York, Baltimore. Lippincott Williams & Wilkins 1998;31-7.
21. Kurjak A. An atlas of transvaginal color Doppler. London, New York. The Parthenon Publishing group, 1994.
22. Blaas HG, Eik-Nes SH, Kiserud T, et al. Three-dimensional imaging of the brain cavities in human embryos. Ultrasound Obstet. Gynecol 1995;5(4):228-32.
23. O.Rahilly R, Mueller F. Ventricular system and choroid plexuses of the human brain during the embryonic period proper. Am J Anat 1990;189(4):285-302.
24. Kupesic S, Kurjak A. Early cerebral circulation assessed by color Doppler. In: Kurjak A, Kupesic S (Eds). An Atlas of Transvaginal Color Doppler; 2nd edition. New York, London: Parthenon publishing New York, London 2000;59-63.
25. Merz E, Weber G, Bahlmann F, et al. Application of transvaginal and abdominal three-dimensional ultrasound for the detection

or exclusion of fetal malformations of the fetal face. Ultrasound Obstet Gynecol 1997;9(4):237-43.

26. Hyett J, Moscoso G, Nicolaides K. Morphometric analysis of the great vessels in early fetal life. Hum Reprod 1995; 10(11):3045-8.

27. Hata T, Aoki S, Akiyama M, et al. Three-dimensional ultrasonographic assessment of fetal hands and feet. Ultrasound Obstet Gynecol 1998;12(4):235-9.

28. Kurjak A, Zodan T, Kupesic S. Three-dimensional sonoembryology of the first trimester. In: Clinical application of 3D sonography. Kurjak A, Kupesic S. (Eds) NY, London: The Parthenon publishing, 2000;109-21.

29. Kupesic S, Kurjak A, Babic MM. New data on early cerebral circulation. Prenatal Neonatal Med 1997;2:48-55.

30. Wladimiroff JW, Huisman TW, Stewart PA. Intracerebral, aortic, and umbilical artery flow velocity waveforms in the late-first trimester fetus. Am J Obstet Gynecol 1992;166(1 Pt 1):46-9.

31. VanZalen-Sprock MM, Van Vugt JM, Colenbrander GJ, et al. First trimester uteroplacental and fetal blood flow velocity waveforms in normally developing fetuses: A longitudinal study. Ultrasound Obstet Gynecol 1994;4(4):284-8.

32. Kurjak A and Kupesic S. Ultrasound of the first trimester CNS development (structure and circulation). In: Levine M (Ed). Fetal and Neonatal Brain. London: Harcourt Health Sciences; 1999.

33. Wladimiroff JW, Huisman TWA, Stewart PA. Fetal cardiac flow velocities in the late first trimester of pregnancy: A transvaginal Doppler study. J Am Coll Cardiology 1991;17:1357-9.

34. Wladimiroff JW, Huisman TW, Stewart PA. Fetal and umbilical flow velocity waveforms between 10-16 weeks' gestation: A preliminary study. Obstet Gynecol 1991;78:812-4.

35. Lindsay DJ, Lovett IS, Lyons EA, et al. Endovaginal appearance of the yolk sac in pregnancy: Normal growth and usefulness as a predictor of abnormal pregnancy outcome. Radiology 1992; 183:115-18.

36. Kurjak A, Kupesic S, Kostovic L. Vascularization of yolk sac and vitelline duct in normal pregnancies studied by transvaginal color and pulsed Doppler. J Perinat Med 1994;22(5):433-40.

37. Lyons EA. Endovaginal sonography of the first trimester of pregnancy. Proceedings of the 3rd International Perinatal and Gynecological Ultrasound Symposium Ottawa, Ontario, 1994; 1-25.

38. Green JJ, Hobbins JC. Abdominal ultrasound examination of the first trimester fetus. Am J Obstet Gynecol 1988;159(1):165-75.

39. Kupesic S, Kurjak A. Volume and vascularity of yolk sac assessed by three-dimensional and power doppler ultrasound. Early Pregnancy 2001;5(1):40-1.

40. Harris RD, Fvincent LM, Askin FB. Yolk sac calcification: A sonographic finding associated with intrauterine embryonic demise in the first trimester. Radiology 1988;166(1 Pt 1):109-10.

41. Witschi E. Migration of the germ cells of human embryos from the yolk sac to the primitive gonadal folds. Contrib Embryol Carnegie Inst 1948;32:67.

42. Bewley S, Roberts LJ, Mackinson AM, et al. First trimester nuchal translucency: Problems with screening the general population. Br J Obstet Gynaecol 1995;102(5):386-8.

43. Haddow JE and Palomokie GE. Down's syndrome screening. Lancet 1996;347:1625.

44. Monni G, Zoppi MA, Ibba RM, et al. Fetal nuchal translucency test for Down's syndrome. Lancet 1997;350:1631.

45. Braithwaite JM and Economides DL. The measurement of nuchal translucency with transabdominal and transvaginal sonography- success rates, repeatability and level of agreement. Br J Obstet Gynaecol 1995;68:720-3.

46. Kurjak A, Kupesic S, Ivancic-Kosuta M. Three-dimensional transvaginal ultrasound improves measurement of nuchal translucency. J Perinat Med 1999;27(2):97-102.

47. Huisman TWA, Gittenberger-de Groot AC, Wladimiroff JW. Recognition of fetal subdiaphragmatic venous vestibulum essential for fetal venous Doppler assessment. Pediatric Res 1992; 32(3):338-41.

48. Edelstone DI. Regulation of blood flow through the ductus venosus. J Dev Physiol 1980;2(4):219-38.

49. Meyers RL, Paulick RP, Rudolph CD, et al. Cardiovascular responses to acute, severe hemorrhage in fetal sheep. J Dev Physiol 1991;15(4):189-97.

50. Antolin E, Comas C, Carrera JM. Doppler velocimetry of the ductus venosus in the first trimester of pregnancy. In: The Embryo as a Patient; Kurjak A, Chervenak FA, Carrera JM, (Eds). New York London: Parthenon Publishing Group, 181-5.

51. Hecher K, Campbell S, Snijders R, et al. Reference ranges for fetal venous and atrioventricular blood flow parameters. Ultrasound Obstet Gynecol 1994;4(5):381-90.

52. Kiserud T, Eik-Nes SH, Hellevik LR, et al. Ductus venosus blood velocity changes in fetal cardiac diseases. J Matern Fetal Invest 1993;3:15-20.

53. Kiserud T, Eik-Nes SH, Blaas HG, et al. Ductus venosus blood velocity and the umbilical circulation in seriously growth-retarded fetus. Ultrasound Obstet Gynecol 1994;4(2):109-14.

54. Hecher K, Campbell S, Doyle P, et al. Assessment of fetal compromise by Doppler ultrasound investigation on the fetal circulation. Arterial, intracardiac and venous blood flow velocity studies. Circulation 1995 91:129-38.

55. Matias A, Montenegro N, Areas JC, et al. Anomalous fetal venous return associated with major chromosomopathies in late first trimester of pregnancy. Ultrasound Obstet Gynecol 1998; 11(3):209-13.

56. Antolion E, Comas C, Torrents M, et al. The role of ductus venosus blood flow assessment in screening for chromosomal abnormalities at 10-16 weeks of gestation. Ultrasound Obstet Gynecol. 2001;17(4):295-300.

57. Montenegro N, Matias A, Areias JC, et al. Increased nuchal translucency: Possible involvement of early cardiac failure. Ultrasound Obstet Gynecol. 1997;10(4):265-8.

58. Huisman TW, Bilardo CM. Transient increase in nuchal translucency thickness and reversed end-diastolic ductus venosus flow in a fetus with trisomy 18. Ultrasound Obstet Gynecol.1997;10(6):397-9.

59. DeVore GR and Horenstein J. Ductus venosus index: A new method for evaluating right ventricular preload in the second trimester fetus. Ultrasound Obstet Gynecol.1993;3:338-42.

60. Zoppi MA, Putzolu M, Ibba RM, et al. First trimester ductus venosus velocimetry in relation to nuchal translucency thickness and fetal karyotype. Fetal Diagn Ther 2002;17(1):52-7.

61. Cicero S Curcio, Papageorghiou A, Sonek J, et al. Absence of nasal bone in fetuses with trisomy 21 at 11-14weeks of gestation: An observational study. Lancet 2001; 358(9294):1665-7.

62. Simpson JM, Sharland GK. Nuchal translucency and congenital heart defects: Heart failure or not? Ultrasound Obstet Gynecol 2000;16(1):30-6.

63. Bronshtein M, Zimmer EZ. The sonographic approach to the detection of fetal cardiac anomalies in the early pregnancy. Ultrasound Obstet Gynecol 2002;19(4):360-5.

64. Pellizari P, Pozzan C, Marchiori S, et al. Assessment of uterine artery blood flow in normal first trimester pregnancies and in those complicated by uterine bleeding. Ultrasound Obstet Gynecol 2002;19(4):366-70.

65. Kupesic S, Kurjak A. Physiology of uteroplacental and embryonic circulation. In: Kurjak A (Ed). Textbook of Perinatal Medicine. New York, London: Parthenon Publishing; 1998.

66. Kurjak A, Kupesic S. Blood flow studies in normal and abnormal early pregnancy. In: Kurjak A, Kupesic S (Eds). An Atlas of transvaginal color Doppler. London New York: Parthenon Publishing 2000;41.

67. Kurjak A, Dudenhausen J, Hafner T, et al. Intervillous circulation in all three trimesters of normal pregnancy assessed by color Doppler. J Perinat Med 1997;25(4): 373-80.

68. Kurjak A, Kupesic S. Parallel Doppler assessment of yolk sac and intervillous circulation in normal pregnancy and missed abortion. Placenta 1998;19:619-23.

69. Hustin J, Jauniaux: Implantation and the yolk sac. In: Kurjak A (Ed). Textbook of Perinatal Medicine. New York, London: The Parthenon Publishing Group, 1998;960.

70. de Crepigni LC. Early diagnosis of pregnancy failure with transvaginal ultrasoud. Am J Obstet Gynecol 1988;159(2):408-9.

71. Kim MS, Jeanty P, Turner C, et al. Three-dimensional sonographic evaluations of embryonic brain development. J Ultrasound Medicine 2008;27:119-24.

72. Rolo LC, Nardozza LM, Araujo Junior E, et al. Measurement of embryo volume at 7-10 weeks' gestation by 3D-sonography. J Obstet Gynecol 2009;29(3):188-91.

73. Nowak PM, Nardozza LM, Araujo Junior E, et al. Comparison of placental volume in early pregnancy using multiplanar and VOCAL methods. Placenta 2008;29(3):241-5.

74. Merce LT, Barco MJ, Alcazar JL, et al. Intervillous and uteroplacental circulation in normal early pregnancy and early pregnancy loss assessed by 3D power Doppler angiography. Am J Obstet Gynecol 2009;200(3):315.

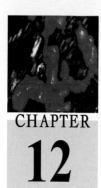

S Kupesic Plavsic
A Kurjak, N Zafar

CHAPTER
12

Ectopic Pregnancy

An ectopic pregnancy occurs when a fertilized ovum implants itself at a place other than the uterine cavity. Although an ectopic pregnancy is most often localized in the fallopian tubes (95%), the remaining ectopic gestations implant elsewhere, such as abdominal, ovarian, intraligamentous, cornual, intramural or cervical sites.[1-4] The incidences of ectopic pregnancies are usually calculated from the overall number of deliveries, being different for each country/state. The rate of ectopic pregnancies in developed countries is one ectopic pregnancy for every 100 to 200 normal pregnancies.[1] The exact cause of blastocyst implantation and development outside the endometrial cavity is unknown. There has been an increased incidence of ectopic pregnancies during the last decades,[5,6] but fortunately, there has been a reduction of fatal outcomes by up to 75%. The increased incidences in ectopic pregnancies have been mainly attributed to a greater degree of socially acceptable sexual behavior. This, in turn, has led to an increased incidence of sexually transmitted and pelvic inflammatory diseases. Among the mechanical factors that have been implicated as the cause of ectopic pregnancy are low-grade pelvic infections, salpingitis and peritubal adhesions. Of note, ectopic pregnancies do occur in totally normal tubes. This would suggest that abnormalities of the conceptus or maternal hormonal changes are possible etiological factors.[7] Logistic regression analysis has identified tubal factors of infertility and previous myomectomy to have a predictive power for an ectopic pregnancy.[8] Risk factors for ectopic pregnancy are given in Table 12.1.

It is essential to identify risk factors in order for health care professionals to identify, provide timely treatment, develop preventive strategies[13-15] and provide patients with adequate information regarding an ectopic pregnancy.

TABLE 12.1: Risk factors for ectopic pregnancy

Risk factors	
STD–PID[9,10]	Surgical procedures in pelvis[11]
Assisted reproductive techniques	IUD[12]
Abnormalities of the conceptus	Previous ectopic
Uterine malformations	Fibroids
Maternal hormonal changes	Cigarette smoking

The main problem of an ectopic pregnancy is the clinical presentation. This condition is well known as the great masquerader.[16] Symptoms can vary from vaginal spotting to hypovolemic shock, such as hemoperitoneum.[17,18] The classic triad of delayed menses, irregular vaginal bleeding and abdominal pain are commonly not encountered. The exact frequency of clinical symptoms and signs is hard to assess.[1] Atypical clinical presentation can mimic all kinds of diseases, which have no connection with pathology of the reproductive system. In many cases, ectopic pregnancy is confused with an early abortion because of similar symptoms. Delayed menses, enlarged and softened uterus and vaginal bleeding can be found in a uterine abortion and an ectopic pregnancy, respectively (Table 12.2).

Early and reliable diagnosis of an ectopic pregnancy remains a challenge for every clinician. An undiagnosed

TABLE 12.2: Differential diagnosis of ectopic pregnancy

Differential diagnosis	
Intrauterine pregnancy	Salpingitis
Spontaneous abortion	Adnexal torsion
Ruptured ovarian cyst	Perforated appendicitis
Hemorrhagic cyst	Gastroenteritis
Endometriosis	Diverticulitis

ectopic pregnancy can lead to a fatal outcome for a woman. Significance of an early diagnosis leads to the possibility of applying conservative methods of treatment. These methods are crucial for preserving further reproductive capabilities.[19] Diagnostic procedures are divided into the two groups:

Noninvasive: History, general physical, including pelvic examination and investigations (serum quantitative beta HCG and pelvic ultrasound).

Invasive: Culdocentesis,[20] curettage[21] and laparoscopy.

THE ROLE OF BIOCHEMICAL MARKERS IN ECTOPIC PREGNANCY

Starting on the 8th day postconception, human chorionic gonadotropin (hCG), a glycoprotein hormone, is released into the circulation by human placental trophoblastic cells. Its concentration in the blood rises 1.7 times per 24 hours.[22] As soon as implantation occurs, the trophoblast starts to produce beta hCG. In general, urine hCG tests turn positive when the serum concentration of hCG is equal to or higher than 1000 IU/ml. This, in turn, corresponds to a positive urine hCG result occurring approximately 10-14 days postconception.[1] Causes of false positive results are usually due to proteinuria, erythrocyturia, gynecological tumors, tubo-ovarian abscess[23] or drug intake (e.g. tranquilizers). In the case of an ectopic pregnancy, the embryo usually disappears, gets resorbed and an empty gestational sac, producing smaller amounts of beta hCG is visualized at an ectopic location. For an ectopic pregnancy, only in cases of a living embryo, it can normal levels of beta hCG be found. This occurs in 5 to 8% of ectopic pregnancies.[22]

Because of the low concentrations of human chorionic gonadotropin, only 40 to 60% of ectopic pregnancies have a positive urine test result. Therefore, the more sensitive serum hCG test should be performed. This becomes positive 10 days postconception.[22] For an ectopic pregnancy, the absolute value of serum hCG levels in the circulation are much lower than in normal intrauterine pregnancies of the same gestational age.[24,25] Dynamics of the serum titer show a slower rise of the circulating concentrations and a prolonged doubling time. The most important use of the quantitative hCG determination is its use in conjunction with ultrasonography and in understanding the value of the hCG "discriminatory zone." The discriminatory zone represents that level of hCG above which all normal intrauterine gestational sacs should be detected by ultrasound. At present, the consensus is that the discriminatory zone is approximately 1000 mIU/ml with the use of transvaginal probe of 5 MHz.[26-29]

THE ROLE OF ULTRASOUND IN THE DIAGNOSIS OF TUBAL ECTOPIC PREGNANCY

Ultrasound has made a dramatic impact on the evaluation of patients suspected of an ectopic pregnancy. Ultrasonography (more precisely, transvaginal sonography), has become the "gold standard" modality for the effective and fast diagnosis of an ectopic pregnancy. An important advantage of the most currently used transvaginal transducers is the ability to perform simultaneous and spectral Doppler studies, allowing easy identification of the ectopic peritrophoblastic flow. In comparison to transvaginal sonography, transabdominal ultrasound is reserved for a very small number of oddly located ectopic pregnancies, mainly high-up in the pelvis, outside the effective reach of a 5 MHz vaginal probe.[30]

Transabdominal Ultrasound

With the use of transabdominal ultrasonography, the gestational sac of a normal intrauterine pregnancy becomes visible at 6 weeks. In patients with positive beta hCG in whom an intrauterine gestational sac is not visualized, a clinician should always suspect and rule out an ectopic pregnancy. At present, abdominal ultrasonography cannot reliably diagnose ectopic pregnancy. One of the exceptions, being a live fetus demonstrated outside the uterine cavity with real time equipment. It is estimated that an ectopic gestational sac with embryonic echoes and clear heart activity can be demonstrated in only 3 to 5% of the cases.[31] A probe with a frequency of 3.5 MHz, with a large contact area is used for transabdominal ultrasonographic imaging. In addition, a full bladder aids in the role of an acoustic window. The resolution of a transabdominal probe is somewhat lower than a transvaginal probe, but the penetration is much deeper.

With the use of the following criteria, the best results confirming an intrauterine pregnancy can be obtained:
* A normal size, shape and location of the gestational sac in the uterine cavity
* A double ring surrounding the gestational sac
* Embryonic parts with clearly marked heart activity.

Ultrasound criteria for an ectopic pregnancy can be divided into the uterine and extrauterine signs (some signs are suggestive and others are diagnostic).

The diagnostic signs are:
* Absence of an intrauterine gestational sac, including the double ring surrounding it

- Absence of the fetal structures within the gestational sac
- Presence of an extraovarian adnexal structure.

The suggestive signs include:
- Uterine enlargement with a thickened endometrium
- Blood or coagulum in the cul-de-sac, appearing as anechoic or hyperechoic retrouterine echoes.[31]

Transabdominal ultrasound has a low sensitivity, specificity, positive and negative predictive values for the detection of an ectopic pregnancy. This method identifies an ectopic gestational sac with a live embryo in 11.8% of patients and without an embryo in 30.4%.[32,33] A mixed solid or cystic nonspecific adnexal mass is detected in 57.8% of ectopic pregnancies. This modality still has some value in successful detection of a small proportion of ectopic pregnancies with a bizarre location, such as being high in the pelvis.

Transvaginal Ultrasound

The enhanced resolution obtained through the use of a high frequency vaginal transducer has become the method of choice for the evaluation of suspected ectopic pregnancies. In comparison with transabdominal approaches, transvaginal ultrasound enables a much better imaging of the morphological features in the pelvis due to the higher frequencies probes and probe location in the immediate vicinity of the examined area. Hopp and colleagues[34] studied the diagnostic reliability of transvaginal ultrasound in an ectopic pregnancy and found that sensitivity of transvaginal sonography was 96%, the specificity 88%, the positive predictive value 89% and the negative predictive value 95%. Hertzberg and Kliewer[35] have described data on the ultrasonographic diagnosis of an ectopic pregnancy, emphasizing the potential pitfalls in image interpretation. Intrauterine gestational sac surrounded by a double ring with a clear embryonic echo is considered to be strong evidence against an ectopic pregnancy because heterotopic, intrauterine and ectopic pregnancies rarely coincide. However, this possibility should not be ignored, especially in patients undergoing assisted reproduction.

Intrauterine sonographic findings in women with ectopic pregnancy are variable.

Uterine findings include:
- An empty uterus, with or without increased endometrial thickness, which is the most common finding
- A central hypoechoic area or a sac like structure inside the cavity, the so called pseudogestational sac

- A concurrent intrauterine pregnancy–which is an extremely rare occurrence.

An empty uterus with a variable thickness of the endometrial layer is considered suggestive for the diagnosis of an ectopic pregnancy. However, similar findings are common in early intrauterine pregnancy and a recent spontaneous abortion.[3] A pseudogestational sac has a mixed echo pattern of the endometrium that results from a decidual reaction, fluid or both. It can be demonstrated in 10 to 20% of patients with an ectopic pregnancy.[3] Careful scrutiny of uterine findings usually permits a reliable distinction between the pseudogestational sac and normal gestational sac. The pseudogestational sac is detected in the middle of the uterine cavity, has only one echogenic ring, which is characterized by shape changes, owing to myometrial contractions. In differentiating a real gestational sac from a pseudogestational sac, transvaginal color and pulsed Doppler ultrasound have been shown to be very useful.

Adnexal sonographic findings in women with an ectopic pregnancy are variable.

Adnexal findings include:
- Gestational sac in the adnexal region with clear embryonic echo and heart activity, which directly demonstrates an ectopic pregnancy (15 to 28% of the cases)
- Visualization of the adnexal gestation sac with or without embryonic echo (without heart activity)
- A tubal ring 1 to 3 cm in diameter, consisting of a concentric ring of 2 to 4 mm of echogenic tissue surrounding a hypoechoic center [36] visualized adjacent to the ovary. This finding is detected in 46 to 71% of unruptured tubal pregnancy cases[37]
- An unspecific complex adnexal tumor
- Free fluid in the cul-de-sac (40 to 83% of cases).

It should be pointed out that the examiner's experience has a strong effect on the diagnostic accuracy of the ultrasound examination. Adnexal abnormalities may be difficult to identify because of the confusion with the loops of bowel or other pelvic structures.[38]

Sonographic features of intrauterine and ectopic pregnancies are given in Table 12.3.

Timor-Tritsch and colleagues[39] described four adnexal structures that may mimic an ectopic pregnancy that should be correctly identified and include:

1. *The corpus luteum*: Which is eccentrically located within the ovary, surrounded by an ovarian tissue and possibly creating the impression of a sac like structure. A corpus luteum cyst tends to be more eccentrically located

TABLE 12.3: Sonographic features of intrauterine and ectopic pregnancies

Intrauterine pregnancy		Ectopic pregnancy	
• Intrauterine gestational sac • Eccentric location • Double ring • Yolk sac • Embryonic/fetal pole • Positive fetal heart activity	**Uterine findings**	**Diagnostic signs**	• Absence of the gestational sac • Absence of embryo and yolk sac
		Suggestive signs	• Enlarged uterus • Thick endometrium • Free fluid in the cul-de-sac
	Adnexal findings	• Ectopic gestational sac with or without a living embryo • Mixed solid and/or cystic mass	

within the rim of ovarian tissue as opposed to the concentric ring created by ectopic pregnancy surrounding the chorionic sac. In addition, the hemorrhagic corpus luteum usually shows a hypoechoic rather than a cystic central region. This differentiates the two structures in most instances.[40]

2. A thin-walled ovarian follicle.
3. The small intestine.
4. *Tubal pathology conditions*, such as hydrosalpinx containing fluid.

Bernhart and colleagues[41] described a diagnostic algorithm, consisting of a clinical examination, serum beta hCG assay and transvaginal ultrasound examination. Using this protocol, diagnosis of an ectopic pregnancy can be made with a sensitivity of 100% and specificity of 99%.

About 85% of ectopic pregnancies are formed on the same side as the corpus luteum.[42] This raises an important differential diagnostic issue, how to differentiate between a tubal pregnancy from an ipsilateral corpus luteum. The corpus luteum is found in the ovary and its echogenicity is slightly (or at times even substantially) lower than that of the trophoblastic tissue of the tubal ring.

Patients undergoing medically assisted reproduction procedures or simple hormonal superovulation pose a challenge for early and accurate detection of ectopic pregnancy. Besides having an increased risk for an ectopic pregnancy, these patients have multiple artificial corpora luteal and hemorrhagic cysts, which may cause pelvic pain and imitate tubal rings of ectopic pregnancy. Sometimes, cystic adnexal masses (ovarian cystadenoma, cystadenofibroma, endometrioma, teratoma and pedunculated fibroids) may cause significant diagnostic dilemmas.

Cul-de-sac Findings

Free intraperitoneal fluid is one of the most common sonographic findings in women with an ectopic pregnancy. This cannot only be demonstrated in 40 to 83% of ectopic

pregnancy cases, but also in up to 20% of normal intrauterine pregnancies.[37] In the cases of tubal abortion, echogenic echoes suggest the presence of blood clots. Tubal rupture is associated with a homogeneous, a hypoechoic retrouterine echo that represents a blood collection. The possibility of an ectopic pregnancy increases, if the amount of fluid is moderate to large, but the absence of blood does not exclude its diagnosis.

With the aid of serum beta hCG monitoring, an ectopic pregnancy can be suspected at a very early gestational age, at such a time when the transvaginal ultrasound scan may not be able to demonstrate the site of pregnancy. Under these circumstances, laparoscopic examination is needed to exclude the possibility of an ectopic pregnancy. However, even laparoscopic examination may not be able to achieve a precise diagnosis, especially when the ectopic pregnancy is very small or when there are coexisting pathologies, such as hydrosalpinx, adhesions or fibroids. Some reports have demonstrated that laparoscopic ultrasound can facilitate the diagnosis of the site of an ectopic pregnancy intraoperatively, even if it is as small as 3.9 mm.[43] Laparoscopic ultrasound should be used when the site of an ectopic pregnancy cannot be determined or is obscured by other pathologies during the laparoscopic examination.

COLOR DOPPLER IN EARLY DIAGNOSIS OF TUBAL ECTOPIC PREGNANCY

Transvaginal color Doppler ultrasound is an excellent and rapid modality when searching for blood flow signals in the entire pelvis. Once the anatomical region of interest is identified and blood flow confirmed by color Doppler, a pulsed Doppler waveform analysis is used to quantify the observed hemodynamic events (Figure 12.1). The results are interpreted by means of waveform analysis and calculation of different indices, such as the resistance index (RI), the pulsatility index (PI) and systolic/diastolic ratio. The color flow pattern associated with an ectopic pregnancy is variable. It usually presents as randomly dispersed

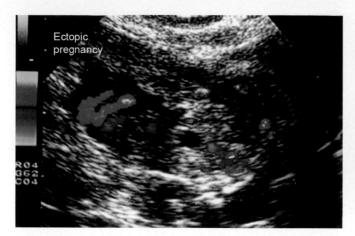

FIGURE 12.1: Transvaginal color Doppler scan of a small gestational sac in the adnexal region measuring 8-10 mm. Note the dilated tubal vessels, indicating the pathophysiological site of ectopic pregnancy, within the tube.

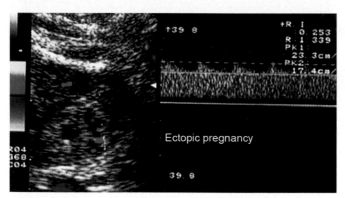

FIGURE 12.2: The same patient as in Figure 12.1. Blood flow velocity waveforms depicted from the area of peritrophoblastic flow show high velocity (23.3 cm/s) and low-vascular resistance (RI = 0.25).

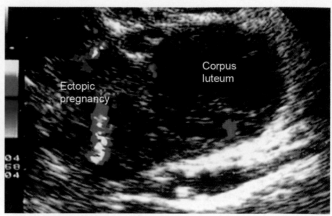

FIGURE 12.3: The same patient as in Figures 12.1 and 12.2. An ipsilateral corpus luteum is demonstrated laterally to the ectopic gestational sac.

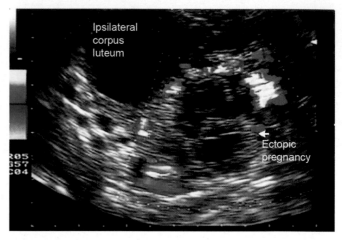

FIGURE 12.4: Color Doppler facilitates visualization of randomly dispersed tubal arteries indicating prominent peritrophoblastic flow and trophoblastic invasiveness. Note the ipsilateral corpus luteum.

multiple small vessels within the adnexa, showing high-velocity and low impedance signals, which are clearly separated from the ovarian tissue and corpus luteum (Figures 12.2 and 12.3). The sensitivity of transvaginal color and pulsed Doppler in the diagnosis of an ectopic pregnancy ranges from 73 to 96% and the specificity is from 87 to 100%.[3,4,37,44]

Visualization of the ipsilateral corpus luteum blood flow may aid in diagnosis of an ectopic pregnancy. Zalud and Kurjak[45] studied luteal blood flow in pregnant and nonpregnant women. Typical luteal low impedance blood flow was detected in 82.8% of normal cases of early pregnancy, 80.8% of ectopic pregnancies and 69.3% of nonpregnant women during the luteal phase of the menstrual cycle. The lowest RI (0.42 ± 0.12) of the luteal

flow was found in cases of nonpregnant women and the highest RI (0.53 ± 0.09) in cases of early intrauterine pregnancy. The RI in the cases of an ectopic pregnancy was 0.48 ± 0.07. In 96.4% of the patients with proven ectopic pregnancy, luteal flow was detected on the same side as the ectopic pregnancy (Figure 12.4). This observation can be used as a guide in searching for an ectopic pregnancy.

The importance of the "between-side" difference in tubal artery blood flow was also documented. There was a significant increase in the tubal artery blood flow on the side of tubal gestation. The mean reduction of the RI on the side with the ectopic pregnancy compared to the opposite side was 15.5%.[4] These changes appear to be due to trophoblastic invasion and showed no dependence on the gestational age. A bright color on the screen while using

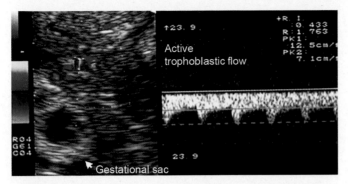

FIGURE 12.5: Transvaginal color Doppler image of ectopic pregnancy. Note color signals indicative of invasive trophoblast (left). Pulsed Doppler waveform analysis (right) demonstrates low resistance index (RI = 0.43).

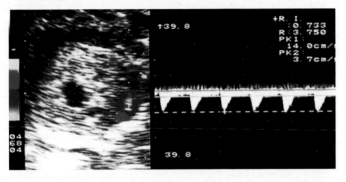

FIGURE 12.6: Gestational sac measuring 12 mm visualized in the left adnexal region. Color Doppler depicts a small area of angiogenesis characterized by a moderate to high resistance index (RI = 0.73). This finding is indicative of tubal abortion.

the pulsed Doppler facility is due to a very high speed of the peritrophoblastic blood flow and low impedance (RI = 0.36-0.45) (Figure 12.5). It should be stressed that patients with a tubal abortion demonstrate significantly higher vascular impedance of the peritrophoblastic flow (RI > 0.60) and less prominent color signals (Figure 12.6).

The main diagnostic importance of the transvaginal color and pulsed Doppler ultrasound is in differentiating the nature of a nonspecific adnexal mass as the diagnostic certainty in the cases of ectopic gestational sac with living embryo is high. Doppler analysis of the uterine circulation in intrauterine pregnancies demonstrates a decreased vascular resistance of the uterine and spiral arteries.[46] In patients with an ectopic pregnancy uterine and spiral artery resistance remained constant.[46] The peak systolic blood flow velocity in the uterine artery increased with increasing gestational age in intrauterine pregnancies, and the values were significantly higher than in ectopic pregnancies.[47] The difference in peak systolic velocity reflects a decreased

blood supply to the ectopic pregnancy. Intrauterine gestational sacs show prominent peritrophoblastic vascular signals (RI = 0.44-0.45), while pseudogestational sacs do not demonstrate increased blood flow (RI > 0.55). It has been suggested that velocities below 21 cm/s are diagnostic for a pseudogestational sac and can successfully rule out the trophoblastic flow of a normal intrauterine pregnancy.[48] Corpus luteum vessels are demonstrated in 88% of women with intrauterine pregnancy compared to 100% in those with an ectopic pregnancy.[46] Corpus luteum RI values are similar in ectopic and normal pregnancies.

The intravascular ultrasound contrast agent has a recognizable effect on Doppler ultrasonographic examination of the adnexal circulation. It appears to be most helpful when examining ectopic pregnancies where the findings in color flow imaging is ambiguous. The use of a contrast agent may also facilitate visualization of the trophoblastic tissue in hemorrhagic adnexal lesions.[49]

As with other diagnostic methods, transvaginal color and pulsed Doppler studies include both, false-positive and false-negative findings. A false-positive diagnosis arises predominantly from the corpus luteum, but in exceptional cases some adnexal lesions may also mimic an ectopic pregnancy. A false-negative result may arise from technical inadequacy, lack of experience or the patients' non-compliance. The other possibility is a nonvascularized ectopic gestation, as these are associated with low beta hCG values.

Some authors compared technical errors with improper setting of color flow parameters.[50] The color velocity scale, color priority, color gain, color sensitivity and color wall filter should be adjusted to optimize color flow information. Technical errors may result in false diagnosis of an ovarian torsion, a malignancy and an ectopic pregnancy.

The diagnosis of an ectopic pregnancy still remains a challenge to the clinician despite advances in ultrasound and biochemical technology. Frequently the diagnosis remains uncertain until laparoscopy or D&C are performed. With the increasing tendency towards conservative therapy, the distinction between ectopic pregnancies that will resolve spontaneously and those that will rupture is essential.[51] Patients without acute symptoms, characterized by declining human chorionic gonadotropin (hCG) values may be treated conservatively.[52] However, secondary ruptures have been reported in patients with low initial hCG concentrations.[53] The differentiation between viable ectopic pregnancies with trophoblastic activity and dissolving tubal abortions could facilitate the decision to proceed with conservative or operative treatment.

After implantation in the mucosa of the endosalpinx, which consists of the lamina propria and the muscularis, the blastocyst continues to grow mainly between the lumen of the tube and its peritoneal covering.[54] Growth occurs both parallel to the long axis of the tube and circumferentially around it. As the trophoblast invades the surrounding vessels, intensive blood flow and or intraperitoneal bleeding occur. The intensive ring of vascular signals could be a criterion for the viability of an ectopic pregnancy that can be determined rapidly and easily and seems to be independent of hCG values.[55] In patients with a viable ectopic pregnancy who require immediate treatment, this method could provide another diagnostic modality/investigation in addition to the hCG values. Color Doppler ultrasound may also be used for follow-up treatment, especially in cases where hCG levels slowly normalize. In this way, duration of hospitalization may be shortened and the cost of treatment reduced. In cases of persisting high hCG levels after operative removal of the ectopic pregnancy, Doppler sonography can provide evidence for the presence of viable trophoblast remnants. On the contrary, in asymptomatic patients with hypoperfused and/or avascular ectopic gestational sac and decreased values of hCG, expective treatment can be established.

3D ULTRASOUND IN THE ASSESSMENT OF TUBAL ECTOPIC PREGNANCY

The first generation of three-dimensional (3D) ultrasound technology, during the early 1980s, provided a pseudo-3D image by a simultaneous display of three orthogonal planes. This offered some advantages over conventional two-dimensional (2D) sonographic imaging.[56,57] Modern systems are capable of generating surface and transparent views depicting the sculpture-like reconstruction of surfaces or transparent images of the structure's content.

Three-dimensional ultrasound helps in a spatial delineation of the pelvic structures. Any scanned volume can be rotated in all three planes and thus it is possible to observe the borders of the tissues and the organs. Three-dimensional ultrasound renders a feasible simultaneous visualization of all three perpendicular planes. Planar mode tomograms are helpful in distinguishing the early intraendometrial gestational sac from a collection of free fluid between the endometrial leaves (pseudogestational sac).

Rempen[58] conducted a prospective follow-up study in order to evaluate the potential utility of 3D ultrasound to differentiate the intrauterine from extrauterine gestations. Fifty-four pregnancies with a gestational age <10 weeks and with an intrauterine gestational sac < 5 mm in diameter were evaluated. The configuration of the endometrium in the frontal plane of the uterus was correlated with eventual pregnancy outcome. After exclusion of three patients with a poor 3D ultrasound image quality, the endometrial shape was found to be asymmetrical with regard to the median longitudinal axis of the uterus in 84% of intrauterine pregnancies, whereas the endometrium showed symmetry in the frontal plane in 90% of extrauterine pregnancies. Intrauterine fluid accumulation may distort the uterine cavity, thus being responsible for false-positive, as well as false-negative results. The evaluation of the endometrial shape in the frontal plane appeared to be a useful additional means of distinguishing intrauterine from ectopic pregnancies, especially when a gestational sac was not clearly demonstrated with a conventional ultrasound.

Harika and coworkers[59] conducted a 3D imaging study for the early diagnosis of ectopic pregnancy. Twelve asymptomatic patients before six weeks of amenorrhea and with no typical features of intrauterine or ectopic pregnancy were examined with conventional 2D ultrasound. Three-dimensional transvaginal ultrasonography preceding a laparoscopy showed a small ectopic gestational sac in four cases. The fallopian tube on the side of the ectopic pregnancy was imaged in all nine cases of ectopic pregnancies. This was possible because the fallopian tube on the side of the ectopic pregnancy was surrounded by a fine hypoechogenic border, an apparently specific feature that had not been reported previously. These preliminary data suggest that 3D sonography is an effective procedure for the early diagnosis of ectopic pregnancy in asymptomatic patients before six weeks of amenorrhea.

The possible use of 3D power Doppler is the monitoring of the vascularity of ectopic pregnancy. The hypoperfusion, quantified by indices of vascularity (VI) and flow (FI) could indicate that the ectopic pregnancy is undergoing spontaneous resorption and that laparoscopy may be postponed. Using this technique, the conservative approach to ectopic pregnancy may rely on more precise and easily obtainable data. In the case of hyperperfusion, the patients may be subjected to immediate laparoscopy or medical treatment.

Shih and colleagues[60] described the use of 3D color/power angiography in two cases in which an arteriovenous malformation of mesosalpinx was diagnosed following the involution of an anembryonic ectopic gestation. The diagnosis of arteriovenous malformations has traditionally been made by arteriography. Recently, it has also been diagnosed by a noninvasive method, such as contrast enhanced CT, MRI and color Doppler ultrasound. The advantage of 3D color/power angiography imaging is better spatial and anatomic orientation and fast reconstruction of the vessels (within 1 minute), especially in the areas where complex structures are present. Therefore, unlike MRI, digital subtraction angiography or contrast enhanced CT, 3D color/power angiography allows the physician to examine the vascular anatomy immediately and without radiation exposure.

Most tubal gestations are not ongoing viable gestations. They are usually in the involutional phase of tubal abortion within a confined area, which results in the extrusion of the products of conception through a ruptured site or fimbriae.[60]

The major difference between the uterine implantation and tubal gestation is that endosalpingeal stroma usually fails to undergo decidualization. The chorionic villi of the tubal pregnancy cause a direct invasion of the tubal wall and mesentery (mesosalpinx). The vascularization within the ectopic pregnancy is an analog of the placenta increta.[61] In such situations cytotrophoblasts may invade the contiguous artery and vein of the mesosalpinx with destruction of the vessels' walls and thus may induce an arteriovenous malformation in situ or nearby. Possibly, the secretion of angiogenic factors (by trophoblasts) and the increasing afterload of an arteriovenous shunt may induce the rapid growth of a small pre-existing congenital arteriovenous malformation.[60] B-mode and color Doppler ultrasound provides information on the uterine vasculature and assists in noninvasive and rapid diagnosis of the arteriovenous malformation. Three-dimensional color/power angiography further improves understanding of the complex vascular anatomy and refines the diagnosis.

Even though the exact role of 3D ultrasound in the pathology of early pregnancy is yet to be established, promising results of already published papers are encouraging. Unlimited numbers of sections are easily obtained without the need of excessive manipulation with the probe. Additional advantage of 3D ultrasound is off-line analysis of the previously stored 3D volumes and Cartesian elimination of surrounding structures and artifacts. Three-dimensional reconstruction of the stored volumes and telemedicine are the most impressive benefits of 3D ultrasound scanning.

OTHER SITES OF IMPLANTATION

About 5% of ectopic pregnancies implant in sites other than the tubes.[1] These locations are more difficult to detect, may rupture and cause significant bleeding, leading to higher morbidity and mortality than the tubal ectopic pregnancy.

Cornual/Interstitial Pregnancy

Interstitial pregnancy occurs in 1.1-6.3% of all ectopic pregnancies.[1,53] Clinically, the diagnosis is based on the findings of abdominal pain and a tender, asymmetrically enlarged uterus. Often the diagnosis is not reached until the rupture of the uterine horn has occurred, which may result in a massive hemorrhage.

Implantation of the fertilized ovum is more likely to occur in the interstitial part of the fallopian tube following in vitro fertilization (IVF) and previous salpingectomy.[53] However, in most cases there are no apparent risk factors. Previously, interstitial pregnancies were diagnosed only at laparotomy following the tubal rupture. Many women suffered major hemorrhage and hysterectomy rate was as high as 40%.[50] In recent years, the routine use of ultrasound for the assessment of patients with early pregnancy complications has enabled a noninvasive diagnosis of interstitial pregnancy. Early diagnosis allows the use of more conservative management, such as medical treatment or laparoscopic surgery.

A viable interstitial pregnancy may, occasionally, be misinterpreted as a normal intrauterine pregnancy. Therefore, it is important that strict diagnostic criteria are used in every case. An interstitial pregnancy should be diagnosed in women with an empty uterine cavity and chorionic sac that is seen separately and more than 1 cm from the most lateral edge of the uterine cavity and surrounded by a thin myometrial layer.[54]

Approximately 15% of patients with an interstitial pregnancy have a heterotopic pregnancy.[54] In these cases, intrauterine findings may be misleading and should be interpreted with caution, rather than being used as a primary diagnostic criterion. Visualization of the interstitial part of the tube adjoining the endometrium and trophoblast improves the diagnosis of an interstitial pregnancy.[55] It also confirms that the pregnancy is located outside the uterine cavity, facilitating the differential diagnosis between an interstitial pregnancy and unusual forms of intrauterine pregnancy such as angular pregnancy or pregnancy in the cornu of an anomalous uterus. Rarely, small intramural

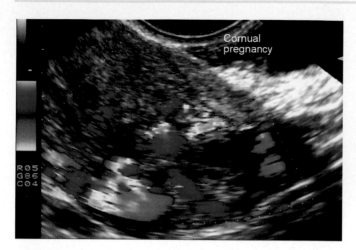

FIGURE 12.7: Color Doppler ultrasound facilitates early diagnosis of cornual pregnancy by exposing peritrophoblastic blood vessels.

fibroids are located in the vicinity of the interstitial part of the tube, which may be misinterpreted as a solid interstitial pregnancy.[56] In women with fibroids, the intramural part of the tube is displaced and can be visualized, bypassing the mass, thus preventing the false-positive diagnosis of the interstitial pregnancy. Color Doppler facilitates the diagnosis of a cornual pregnancy by exposing low resistance peritrophoblastic flow (Figure 12.7).

Three-dimensional ultrasound has the advantage of providing multiplanar view of the uterus.[57] In the coronal section, the position of the interstitial pregnancy in relation to the uterine cavity can be studied in detail. The visualization of the proximal section of the interstitial tube is facilitated, which increases diagnostic confidence.[55] A 3D ultrasound is a helpful diagnostic tool for women with suspected interstitial pregnancy and should be considered in patients with uncertain diagnosis on conventional transvaginal scan.[58]

Most cornual/interstitial ectopic pregnancies are treated by laparotomy and laparoscopy. Lately, transvaginal sonographic puncture and even conservative medical treatment of a cornual ectopic pregnancy have been advocated. Local injection of methotrexate has been used to treat both viable and nonviable interstitial pregnancies, with no failure reported in 14 cases described in literature.[54,55] Data reported in the literature suggest the superiority of local therapy, in regards to both the safety aspect and the success rate. A likely explanation for the increased effectiveness of the local injection of methotrexate is higher concentration of the therapeutic agent achieved at the target tissue.[59] Although absorption

of methotrexate into the circulation does occurs after both local and systemic administration, a lower dose of methotrexate is used locally, leading to lower systemic levels and therefore fewer side-effects.[60] Color Doppler plays an extremely important role in approaching the cornual pregnancy from the medial aspect and traversing the thicker myometrial layer through which rupture or bleeding are less likely to occur.[61] In these cases, color Doppler guidance during the instillation of methotrexate enables better visualization of blood vessels and avoidance of intraprocedural complications.

Viable heterotopic/interstitial pregnancies are often treated by a local injection of potassium chloride, which is not teratogenic. All six reported cases of heterotopic pregnancies in the literature were successfully treated with local injection of methotrexate, resulting in three (50%) intrauterine pregnancies progressing normally to full term.[4]

Expectant management of interstitial pregnancy has also been reported.[54,56] All three of the nonviable interstitial pregnancies managed in this way were resolved spontaneously and without any need for intervention. Expectant management can be a useful option in selected cases. Although it may take longer for the pregnancy to resolve spontaneously, an important advantage is the elimination of the risk associated with medical treatment.

Cervical Pregnancy

Cervical pregnancy is defined as the implantation of the conceptus below the level of the internal os. It is a rare condition that occurs in one in 50,000 pregnancies.[4] The incidence has been increasing in recent years, but is likely to be even higher, as a significant number of cervical pregnancies remain an important cause of maternal morbidity and mortality. Intrauterine adhesions, Cesarean sections, fibroids, previous therapeutic abortions and IVF treatment have all been associated with increased cervical implantation.

Traditionally, the diagnosis of cervical pregnancy was based solely on clinical findings and case history reports after a hysterectomy. Therefore, it is likely that only the most severe cases were diagnosed and a significant number of cervical pregnancies were undiagnosed or treated as incomplete miscarriages. In the past two decades, ultrasound has become the method of choice for diagnosis of early pregnancy disorders and has certainly contributed to the recent increase in number of reported cervical pregnancies.

The diagnosis of cervical pregnancy is based on the following criteria:

- No evidence of an intrauterine pregnancy
- Ballooned cervical canal
- Presence of a gestational sac or placental tissue within the cervical canal
- Closed cervical internal os.

Early diagnosis may explain the milder clinical symptoms and better prognosis of cervical pregnancy today as compared to the preultrasound era.

The level of the insertion of the uterine arteries should be used to identify the internal os and thus may facilitate the diagnosis of a cervical pregnancy.[62] The extensive vascular blood supply to the trophoblastic tissue originating from the adjacent maternal arteries at the implantation site (within the cervix) is easily visualized by transvaginal color Doppler (Figures 12.8 and 12.9). Abortion in progress is easily differentiated from the cervical pregnancy due to visualization of the opened internal cervical os and lack of peritrophoblastic flow (the gestational sac is detached from its implantation site and does not demonstrate color Doppler signals).[62] Conversely, even a small amount of placental tissue in a true cervical pregnancy remains highly vascular on color Doppler examination.[63] This facilitates the differential diagnosis between the cervical pregnancy and ongoing abortion. Color Doppler analysis may improve follow-up of the patients undergoing conservative medical treatment. In addition, color Doppler ultrasound may assist during the course of an interventional procedure (i.e. instillation of potassium chloride and monitoring the fetal heart activity). Because of better anatomic orientation and multiplanar sections of the uterus and cervix, 3D ultrasound may further improve the diagnosis of an ectopic pregnancy.

A local injection of methotrexate or potassium chloride appears to be the most effective way of treating an early viable cervical pregnancy regardless of the gestational age. There are virtually no data on the use of local injection in nonviable pregnancies and it is uncertain whether the treatment would be as effective as in viable pregnancies.[62,63] Systemic treatment in patients with cervical pregnancy and no evidence of fetal heart activity is simple and highly effective. Local injection does not seem to offer any advantage.

The regiments and dosages of methotrexate used for systemic therapy vary considerably. There is no clear correlation between the dose and therapeutic success and it is therefore logical to use as little methotrexate as possible to minimize side-effects.[62] The usual regiment should be two intramuscular injections of 1 mg/kg methotrexate followed by the folic acid rescue. For local injection, 25 mg

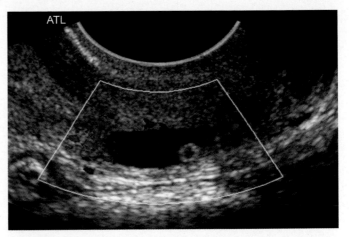

FIGURE 12.8: Color Doppler ultrasound of a cervical pregnancy. Prominent blood flow signals are suggestive of invasive trophoblast.

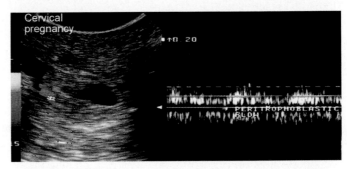

FIGURE 12.9: Pulsed Doppler waveform analysis obtained from peritrophoblastic flow in a patient with cervical pregnancy demonstrates low vascular impedance blood flow signals.

methotrexate into the gestational sac appears to be sufficient. Dosages of Potassium chloride from 3 to 5 mEq are equally successful and less likely to cause side effects.[4]

Surgical intervention should only be limited to cases where medical treatment has failed. Dilatation and curettage in combination with cervical cerclage with the insertion of a Foley catheter into the cervical canal is probably the best choice for a general gynecologist. This is as effective as more complicated and expensive interventions for the prevention of uncontrollable hemorrhage.[61]

Ovarian Pregnancy

The sonographic diagnosis of ovarian pregnancy is extremely difficult to establish. It has been calculated that an ovarian pregnancy accounts for less than 3% of ectopic pregnancies.[1,3,4] The sonographic diagnosis is made upon the finding of a hyperechoic trophoblastic ring detected within the ovarian tissue and the fact that it is impossible to separate the ectopic gestational sac from the ovary by a gentle transabdominal pressure from either the examiner's hand or transvaginal ultrasound probe.[64] Color Doppler facilitates detection of peritrophoblastic flow, which can speed up the entire diagnostic procedure.

Abdominal Pregnancy

An intra-abdominal pregnancy is a rare occurrence, constituting only 1% of all ectopic gestations.[65] Its complications, however, can be devastating. These include massive hemorrhage due to disseminated intravascular coagulation (DIC) and placental separation resulting in fetal demise. Although maternal morbidity and mortality are high, the outlook for the fetus is even worse, since perinatal mortality may reach 75 to 90%.[66] The diagnosis of an abdominal pregnancy is not easy, especially in the early stages. Characteristically, patients present with abdominal pain, vaginal bleeding and gastrointestinal complaints.[67] Ultrasound is the most valuable diagnostic tool for this rare type of ectopic pregnancy.[4,64] If the fertilized oocyte implants directly into the peritoneal surface of the abdominal cavity, this is called a primary abdominal pregnancy. If, however, an early tubal pregnancy dislodges and aborts into the pelvis, adhering to the peritoneal surface, it is termed a secondary abdominal pregnancy through the secondary nidation (implantation). The sonographic image of abdominal pregnancy is no different from any other ectopic pregnancy (i.e. empty uterus and hyperechoic ectopic gestational sac containing embryonic/fetal structures and extraembryonic structures with or without active heart beats). In advanced cases, sonography reveals oligohydramnios and no uterine myometrial mantle around the fetus and the placenta.

A time-honored treatment for an abdominal pregnancy following its diagnosis is surgery. The placenta should never be extracted, but rather left *in situ*. This is mainly because, in many instances, the placenta is attached to the vital organs or vascular sites, which could be seriously damaged during the placental separation. No serious complications have occurred when placenta was left *in situ*.[68] An additional important factor is that most abdominal pregnancies where diagnosed relatively late in pregnancy, when the placenta and its area of the attachment were larger. More recently, however, there have been cases of abdominal pregnancies that were diagnosed earlier. In one case, the diagnosis was made at six weeks of amenorrhea.[3,4,68] Early diagnosis allows the possibility of these pregnancies to be removed laparoscopically. Possible advantages of such a

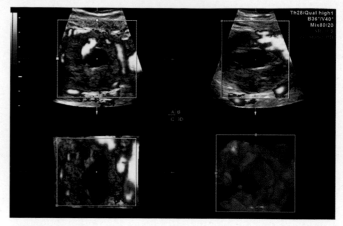

FIGURE 12.10: Three-dimensional power Doppler image of ectopic pregnancy. Power Doppler depicts peritrophoblastic blood flow signals, indicative of invasive trophoblast.

therapeutic approach include lower maternal morbidity and mortality, as well as better future fertility potential. Because only a limited number of cases of abdominal pregnancies have been diagnosed in the early stages of pregnancy, the safety of operative laparoscopy can only be guaranteed in appropriately selected cases.[67,68] Similar cases further demonstrate the importance of the first trimester ultrasound examination in diagnosing early pregnancy complications. The importance of sonographic imaging in cases of an acute abdomen during pregnancy cannot be over-stressed.

Although there are no available data on the use of color Doppler and 3D ultrasound in this field, we believe that these novel modalities may add additional information about the implantation site and attachment of the placenta to the surrounding structures (Figure 12.10).

THERAPY

Historically, the treatment of an ectopic pregnancy has been emergency laparotomy, which included salpingectomy. In order to preserve the fertility, alternatives to laparotomy and salpingectomy include observation, laparoscopic removal of ectopic pregnancy and systemic or local use of methotrexate or other feticidal agents. As medical therapy for an ectopic pregnancy becomes a common practice, familiarity with its side effects may lead to greater success rates. The decision to abandon medical treatment and proceed with surgery should be based on defined guidelines, such as the dimensions of the gestational sac, presence of fetal heart activity, development of peritoneal signs, decreasing hemoglobin levels or hemodynamic instability.[62,68]

Methotrexate may be administered systemically[63,65], locally[64,66] or in combination.[67] Local application is performed either laparoscopically or transvaginally under ultrasound needle puncture.[39] In the latter approach, methotrexate is injected directly into the gestational sac. The success rate of systemic, single-dose methotrexate (83 to 96%) is similar to that of local administration under laparoscopic guidance (89 to 100%), but the success rate of methotrexate under ultrasound guidance seems to be lower (70 to 83%).[66] Local injection of methotrexate under control of color Doppler imaging may increase the success rate.[4] The use of color and pulsed Doppler enables visualization of the trophoblastic adnexal flow with high-velocity and low impedance pulsed Doppler (RI < 0.40). The needle can be inserted into the area of maximum color signal, which marks the trophoblastic invasiveness and vitality.

Pharmacological management of an unruptured, size-appropriate ectopic pregnancy is now an established standard of care. The present protocol recommends a single-dose of methotrexate.[67] This form of methotrexate has proven to be a successful and cost-effective alternative to the traditional surgical management of an ectopic pregnancy.[68] In view of the risk of standard therapy and patient's desire for fertility, methotrexate treatment may be a therapeutic alternative in cervical pregnancy as well. Recent reports have affirmed that ectopic pregnancies have become a medical, rather than a surgical disease.[4,62,66,67,69,70]

Puncture injections are valid and reasonable alternative to a traditional surgical approach, especially in patients with an interstitial, cervical or heterotopic pregnancy. In these particular cases, puncture procedures guided by transvaginal ultrasound can efficiently replace surgical treatment and save the patients from unnecessary hysterectomy.

Early diagnosis using diagnostic algorithms combining serial beta hCG measurements and transvaginal ultrasound is the key to effective nonsurgical treatment. With color Doppler ultrasound, it is possible to identify the activity, invasiveness and vitality of the trophoblast. The information mentioned above is extremely important for selective management of patients with an ectopic pregnancy. This allows differentiation between the patients who require immediate treatment, versus those who may benefit from an expectative option. A single dose methotrexate injection is a cost saving, nonsurgical fallopian tube sparing treatment alternative for patients with an ectopic pregnancy.[71]

Methotrexate treatment is recommended in the asymptomatic patient with serum beta hCG levels of less than 2000 IU/ml, a tubal diameter of < 2 cm, and absence of fetal heart activity. The patient's understanding of her condition and compliance are mandatory. However, in many cases, ectopic pregnancy does not meet suitable medical criteria and still requires surgery. In cases suspicious of tubal abortion with a high impedance signal (RI > 0.55) and beta hCG below 1000 IU/ml, local administration of methotrexate is not advised.

Laparoscopic salpingostomy, the surgical gold standard, is an effective therapy in patients who are hemodynamically stable and wish to preserve their fertility. The reproductive performance after salpingostomy appears to be equal to, or better than salpingectomy, but the recurrent ectopic pregnancy rate is slightly higher.[3] A variable systemic dose of methotrexate produces outcomes close to those of laparoscopic salpingostomy in similar patients.[72]

CONCLUSION

The introduction of beta hCG testing and transvaginal ultrasound has changed our approach to the patient suspected of an ectopic pregnancy. An important advantage of the most currently used transvaginal transducers is the ability to perform simultaneous color and spectral Doppler studies, allowing an easy identification of the ectopic peritrophoblastic flow. Therefore, color should be applied whenever a finding is suggestive of ectopic pregnancy.

Further progresses in diagnostic procedures were made when 3D ultrasound was introduced. Transvaginal 3D ultrasound enables the clinician to perceive the true spatial relations and thus easily distinguish the origin of an adnexal mass, while 3D power Doppler allows detailed analysis of the vascularization.

Transvaginal color and pulsed Doppler imaging may be potentially used for detection of the patients with less prominent tubal perfusion, suitable for the expectant management of an ectopic pregnancy. It is expected that with the increased sensitivity of the serum beta hCG immunoassay, the high resolution transvaginal B-mode, color Doppler ultrasound and more recently 3D ultrasound with power and power Doppler facilities will allow even earlier detection and conservative management of ectopic pregnancies. It is therefore expected that fertility outcomes and number of women attempting to conceive after ectopic pregnancy will further increase.

REFERENCES

1. Ectopic pregnancy. In Speroff L, Glass RH, Kase NG (Eds). Clinical gynecologic endocrinology and infertility. London: Williams and Wilkins, 1999;1149-67.

2. Timor-Tristch IE, Monteagudo A. Ectopic pregnancy. In Kupesic S, de Ziegler D (Eds). Ultrasound and Infertility. London: Partenon Publishing group 2000;215-39.

3. Kurjak A, Kupesic S. Ectopic pregnancy. In Kurjak A (Ed) Ultrasound in obstetrics and gynecology. Boston: CRC Press, 1990;225-35.

4. Kupesic S, Kurjak A. Color Doppler assessment of ectopic pregnancy. In Kurjak A, Kupesic S (Eds). An atlas of Transvaginal Color Doppler. London: Parthenon Publishing 2000;137-47.

5. Boufous S, Quartararo M, Mohsin M, et al. Trends in the incidence of ectopic pregnancy in New South Wales between1990-1998. Aust NZJ Obstet Gynecol 2001; 41(4):436-8.

6. Rajkhowa M, Glass MR, Rutherford AJ, et al. Trends in the incidence of ectopic pregnancy in England and Wales from 1966 to1996. BJOG 2000;107(3):369-74.

7. Nederlof KP, Lawson H W, Saftlas AF, et al. Ectopic pregnancy surveillance. Morbid Mortal Weekly Rep 1990;39:9.

8. Strandell A, Thorburn J, Hamberger L. Risk factors for ectopic pregnancy in assisted reproduction Fertil Steril 1999;2:282-6.

9. Kamwendo F, Forslin L, Bodin L, et al. Epidemiology of ectopic pregnancy during a 28 years period and the role of pelvic inflammatory disease. Sex Transm Infect 2000;76(1):28-32.

10. Barlow RE, Cooke ID, Odukoya O, Heatley MK, Jenkins J, Narayansingh G, Ramsewak SS, Eley A. The prevalence of chlamydia trachomatis in fresh tissue specimens from patients with ectopic pregnancy or tubal factor infertility as determined by PCR and in situ hybridisation. J Med Microbiol 2001; 50:902-8.

11. Brown WD, Burrows L, Todd CS. Ectopic pregnancy after cesarean hysterectomy. Obstet Gynecol 2002;99(5 pt 2):933-4.

12. Bouyer J, Rachou E, Germain E, et al. Risk factors for extrauterine pregnancy in women using an intrauterine device. Fertil Steril 2000;74(5):899-908.

13. Mol BW, van der Veen F, Bossuyt PM. Symptom-free women at increased risk of ectopic pregnancy: Should we screen? Acta Obstet Gynecol Scand 2002;81(7):661-72.

14. Kalinski MA, Guss DA. Hemorrhagic shock from a ruptured ectopic pregnancy in a patient with a negative urine pregnancy test result. Ann Emerg Med 2002;40(1):102-5.

15. Mertz HL, Yalcinkaya TM. Early diagnosis of ectopic pregnancy. Does use of a strict algorithm decrease the incidence of tubal rupture? J Reprod Med 2001;46(1):29-33.

16. Sagaster P, Zojer N, Dekan G, et al. A paraneoplastic syndrome mimicking extrauterine pregnancy. Ann Oncol 2002;13(1):170-2.

17. Hick JL, Rodgerson JD, Heegaard WG et al. Vital signs fail to correlate with hemoperitoneum from ruptured ectopic pregnancy. Am J Emerg Med 2001;19(6):488-91.

18. Birkhahn RH, Gaeta TJ, Bei R, et al. Shock index in the first trimester of pregnancy and its relationship to ruptured ectopic pregnancy. Acad Emerg Med 2002;9(2):115-9.

19. Wong E, Suat SO. Ectopic pregnancy—A diagnostic challenge in the emergency department. Eur J Emerg Med 2000; 7(3):189-94.

20. Dart R, McLean SA, Dart L. Isolated fluid in the cul-de-sac: How well does it predict ectopic pregnancy? Am J Emerg Med 2002;20(1):1-4.

21. Barnhart KT, Katz I, Hummel A, et al. Presumed diagnosis of ectopic pregnancy. Obstet Gynecol 2002;100(3):505-10.

22. Sheppard RW, Patton PE, Novy MJ. Serial beta hCG measurements in the early detection of ectopic pregnancy. Obstet. Gynecol 1990;7:417-20.

23. Levsky ME, Handler JA, Suarez RD, et al. False-positive urine beta-hCG in a woman with a tubo-ovarian abscess. J Emerg Med 2001;21(4):407-9.

24. Dumps P, Meisser A, Pons D, et al. Accuracy of single measurements of pregnancy-associated plasma protein-A, human chorionic gonadotropin and progesterone in the diagnosis of early pregnancy failure. Eur J Obstet Gynecol Reprod Biol 2002;100(2):174-80.

25. Poppe WA, Vandenbussche N. Postoperative day 3 serum human chorionic gonadotropin decline as a predictor of persistent ectopic pregnancy after linear salpingotomy. Eur J Obstet Gynecol Reprod Biol 2001;99(2):249-52 .

26. Timor-Tristch IE, Rottem S, Thale I. Review of transvaginal ultrasonography: Description with clinical application. Ultrasound 1988;6:1-32.

27. Peisner DB, Timor-Tritsch IE. The discriminatory zone of beta hCG for vaginal probes. J Clin Ultrasound 1990;18(4):280-5.

28. Fossum GT, Dvajan V, Kletzky DA. Early detection of pregnancy with transvaginal ultrasound. Fertil Steril 1988; 49(5):788-91.

29. Bernascheck G. Euaelstorfer R, Csaicsich P. Vaginal sonography versus serum human chorionic gonadotropin in early detection of pregnancy. Am J Obstet 1988;158(3 Pt 1):608-12.

30. Albayram F, Hamper UM. First trimester obstetric emergencies: Spectrum of sonographic findings. J Clin Ultrasound 2002; 30(3):161-77.

31. Kurjak A, Zalud I, Volpe G. Conventional B-mode and transvaginal color Doppler in ultrasound assessment of ectopic pregnancy. Acta Med 1990;44(2):91-103.

32. Rubin GL, Petersin HB, Dorfman SF. Ectopic pregnancy in the United States 1970-1978. J Am Med Assoc 1983; 249:1725-9.

33. Bolton G. Cohen F. Detecting and treating ectopic pregnancy. Contemp Obstet Gynecol 1981;18:101-4.

34. Hopp H, Schaar P, Entezami M. Diagnostic reliability of vaginal ultrasound in ectopic pregnancy. Geburtshilfe Frauenheilkd 1995;55(12):666-70.

35. Hertzberg BS, Kliewer MA. Ectopic pregnancy: ultrasound diagnosis and interpretive pitfalls. South Med J 1995;88:1191-8.

36. Thoma ME. Early detection of ectopic pregnancy visualizing the presence of a tubal ring with ultrasonography performed by emergency physicians. Am J Emerg Med 2000;18(4):444-8.

37. Nyberg D. Ectopic pregnancy. In Nyberg DA, Hill LM, Bohm-Velez M (Eds.) Transvaginal Sonography. St. Luis: Mosby Year Book 1992;105-35.

38. Wojak JC, Clayton MJ, Nolan TE. Outcomes of ultrasound diagnosis of ectopic pregnancy. Dependence on observer experience. Invest Radiol 1995;30(2):115-7.

39. Timor-Tritsch IE, Yeh MN, et al. The use of transvaginal ultrasonography in the diagnosis of ectopic pregnancy. Am J Obstet Gynecol 1989;161:167-70.

40. Fleischer AC, Pennell RG, McKee MS. Ectopic pregnancy: Features at transvaginal sonography. Radiology 1990;174:375-8.

41. Bernhart K, Mennuti MT, Benjamin D, et al. Prompt diagnosis of ectopic pregnancy in an emergency department setting. Obstet Gynecol 1994;84(6):1010-5.

42. Pellerito JS, Taylor KJW, Quedens-Case C. Ectopic pregnancy: Evaluation with endovaginal color flow imaging. Radiology 1992;183(2):407-11.

43. Leung TY, Ng PS, Fung TY. Ectopic pregnancy diagnosed by laparoscopic ultrasound scan. Ultrasound Obstet Gynecol 1999; 13:281-6.

44. Kurjak A, Zalud I, Shulman H. Ectopic pregnancy: Transvaginal color Doppler of trophoblastic flow in questionable adnexa. J Ultrasound Med 1991;10:685-9.

45. Zalud I, Kurjak A. The assessment of luteal blood flow in pregnant and non-pregnant women by transvaginal color Doppler. J Perinat Med 1990;18(3):215-21.

46. Jurkovic D, Bourne TH, Jauniaux E, et al.. Transvaginal color Doppler study of blood flow in ectopic pregnancies. Fertil Steril 1992;57:68-73.

47. Wherry KL, Dubinsky TJ, Waitches GM, et al. Low-resistance endometrial arterial flow in the exclusion of ectopic pregnancy revisited. J Ultrasound Med 2001;20:335-42.

48. Dillon EH, Feyock AL, Taylor KJ. Pseudogestational sacs: Doppler US differentiation from normal or abnormal intrauterine pregnancies. Radiology 1990;176:359-64.

49. Orden MR, Gudmundsson S, Helin HL, Kirkinen P. Intravascular contrast agent in the ultrasonography of ectopic pregnancy. Ultrasound Obstet Gynecol 1999;14:348-52

50. Pellerito JS, Troiano RN, Quedens-Case C, et al. Common pitfalls of endovaginal color Doppler flow imaging. Radiographics 1995;15(1):37-47.

51. Lurie S, Katz Z. Where a pendulum of expectant management of ectopic pregnancy should rest? Gynecol Obstet Invest 1996; 42(3):145.

52. Stovall TG. Ling FW. Expectant management of ectopic pregnancy. Obstet Gynecol Clin North Am 1991;18(1):135-44.

53. Laurie S, Insler V. Can the serum beta hCG level reliably predict likelihood of a ruptured tubal pregnancy? Isr J Obstet Gynecol 1992;3:152-544.

54. Budowich M, Johnson TRB, Genadry R. The histopathology of developing tubal ectopic pregnancy. Fertil Steril 1980;34:169-73.

55. Kemp B, Funk A, Hauptmann S, Rath W. Doppler sonographic criteria for viability in symptomless ectopic pregnancies. Lancet 1997;349(9060):1220-1.

56. Baba K, Stach K, Sakamoto S, et al. Development of an ultrasonic system for three- dimensional reconstruction of the fetus. J Perinat Med. 1989;17(1):19-24.

57. Fredfelt KE, Holm HH, Pedersen JF. Three-dimensional ultrasonic scanning. Acta Radiol Diagn 1995;25:237-40.

58. Rempen A. The shape of the endometrium evaluated with three-dimensional ultrasound: An additional predictor of extrauterine pregnancy. Hum Reprod 1998;13(2):450-4.

59. Harika G, Gabriel R, Carre-Pigeon F, et al. Primary application of three-dimensional ultrasonography to early diagnosis of ectopic pregnancy. Eur J Obstet Gynecol Reprod Biol 1995;60(2):117-20.

60. Shih JC, Shyu MK, Cheng WF, et al. Arteriovenous malformation of mesosalpinx associated with a 'vanishing' ectopic pregnancy: Diagnosis with three-dimensional color power angiography. Ultrasound Obstet Gynecol 1999;13(1):63-6.

61. Mazur MT, Kurman RJ. Disease of the fallopian tube. In: Kerman RJ (Ed). Blaustein's pathology of the female genital Tract, 4th edn. New York: Springer-Verlag 1994;541-3.

62. Thoen LD, Crenin MD. Medical treatment of ectopic pregnancy with methotrexate. Fertil Steril 1997;68:727-30.

63. Lipscomb GH, Meyer NL, Flynn DE, et al. Oral methotrexate for treatment of ectopic pregnancy. Am J Obstet Gynecol 2002;186(6):1192-5.

64. Haimov-Kochman R, Sciaky-Tamir Y, Yanai N, et al. Conservative management of two ectopic pregnancies implanted in previous uterine scars. Ultrasound Obstet Gynecol 2002;19(6):616-9.

65. el-Lamie IK, Shehata NA, Kamel HA. Intramuscular methotrexate for tubal pregnancy. J Reprod Med 2002;47(2):144-50.

66. Yao M, Tulandi T. Current status of surgical and non-surgical management of ectopic pregnancy. Fertil Steril 1997;67(3): 421-33.

67. Powell MP, Spellman JR. 1996 Medical management of the patient with an ectopic pregnancy. J Perinat Neonat Nurs 1997;9:31-43.

68. Luciano AA, Roy G, Solima E, et al. Ectopic pregnancy from surgical emergency to medical management. Acad Sci 2001; 943:235-54.

69. Ben-Sholmo I, Eliyahu S, Yanai N, et al. Methotrexate as a possible cause of ovarian cyst formation: Experience with women treated for ectopic pregnancies. Fertil Steril 1997; 67(4):786-8.

70. Jurkovic D, Hacket E, Campbell S. Diagnosis and treatment of early cervical pregnancy: A review and a report of two cases treated conservatively. Ultrasound Obstet Gynecol 1996; 8(6):373-80.

71. Morlock RJ, Lafata JE, Eisenstein D. Cost-effectiveness of single-dose methotrexate compared with laparoscopic treatment of ectopic pregnancy. Obstet Gynecol 2000;95:407-12.

72. Tulandi T, Sammour A. Evidence-based management of ectopic pregnancy. Curr Opin Obstet Gynecol 2000;12:289-92.

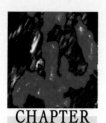

U Honemeyer, A Kurjak
B Ahmed, S Kupesic Plavsic

CHAPTER
13

The Assessment of Normal Fetal Anatomy

INTRODUCTION

More recent technological breakthroughs in diagnostic ultrasound have surpassed all expectations. With these advances, clinicians now have the tools needed to contend with many significant diagnostic challenges. However, these new technologies are so numerous and have been introduced in such rapid succession that considerable confusion surrounds their operation and application.

Indeed, with the advent and evolution of three-dimensional (3D) ultrasound technology over the last 15 years, we now stand at a new threshold in noninvasive diagnosis. The progression from two to three dimensions has brought with it a variety of new options for imaging, storing and postprocessing of the ultrasound data. This technology gives ultrasound, the multiplanar capabilities that were previously reserved for computed tomography (CT) and magnetic resonance imaging (MRI). In addition, it can generate surface-rendered and transparent views that provide entirely new diagnostic capabilities.

The main advantages of this new technology in obstetrics include improved assessment of the complex anatomic structures, surface-scan analysis of fetal fingers and toes, three-dimensional examination of the fetal skeleton, spatial presentation of blood flow information and volumetric measurements of the fetal organs. When operating in multiplanar mode, the three-dimensional orientation of tomograms is unlimited, even with limited probe manipulation or inadequate position of the fetal structures. These imaging capabilities are extremely important during the first trimester of pregnancy when manipulations with the vaginal probe are restricted and obtainable ultrasound sections are limited.

During the transabdominal scanning, frontal planes parallel to the fetal abdominal wall that are unobtainable with conventional ultrasound became visible. Additional progress has been achieved through the possibility of eliminating surrounding structures. It has to be emphasized that, rather than representing an alternative, the three-dimensional technique is complementary to the conventional ultrasound technique in the field of prenatal diagnosis. However, 3D imaging is superior in solving specific diagnostic problems. A comparison of two-dimensional (2D) and 3D techniques shows that in a large percentage of cases 3D offers a diagnostic gain owing to the possibility of surface- and transparent mode imaging.

As with any new technique, 3D ultrasound scanning has some limitations. For example, fetal and maternal movements during the scanning process lead to motion artifacts that can degrade the image quality. Fetal surface rendering primarily depends on sufficient amniotic fluid volume in front of the region of interest (ROI). In some cases, oligohydramnios and superimposed structures like umbilical cord or limbs make surface rendering impossible.

TECHNOLOGICAL IMPROVEMENTS IN PRENATAL DIAGNOSIS

Three-dimensional sonography (3D US) provides completely new modalities of sonographic scanning, including coronal section imaging, 3D reconstruction and volumetric calculation. Improved visualization rate, depiction of spatial relationship, "sculpture like" plastic imaging and volume measurement are the main benefits of new technology.

Three-dimensional Multiplanar Imaging

Multiplanar imaging offers an option of synchronous scanning in three orthogonal sections, including even coronal section (Figure 13.1). Computer data processing

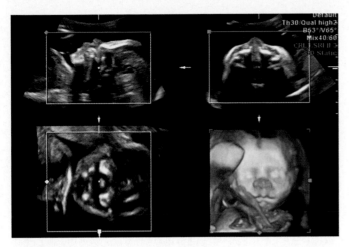

FIGURE 13.1: Multiplanar view of the normal fetal face. Three orthogonal planes (frontal, sagittal and transverse) and the final 3D reconstruction are visible.

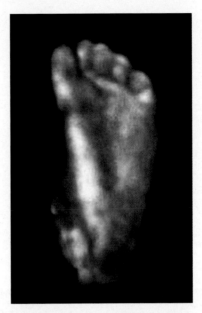

FIGURE 13.2A: Surface rendered fetal foot in plantar projection.

provides numerous sections unobtainable by 2D sonography (2D US). Multiplanar view results in a simultaneous display of three sections, one orthogonal to the others. Two of them (transverse and longitudinal) are dependent on the angle of insonation, whereas the third one (coronal) is not. This section is orthogonal to the insonation beam.

Three-dimensional Spatial Reconstruction

Integration of data obtained by volume scanning can be used to depict 3D plastic (sculpture-like) reconstruction of region of interest (ROI). Three-dimensional reconstruction can be presented in surface or transparent mode. In the surface mode, only the signals from the surface of the ROI are extracted and displayed in plastic appearance (Figure 13.2A). In transparent mode, the signals of highest and lowest echogenicity are extracted from the entire volume, resulting in possibility of spatial reconstruction of internal structure of ROI (Figure 13.2B).[1] This mode is particularly useful for spatial reconstruction and imaging of fetal skeletal parts and their topographic relationship.

Spatiotemporal Image Correlation Mode (STIC)

The breathtaking speed of progress in the development of computer technology with fast processors has led to the further advancement of the ultrasound systems. Since 3D fetal echocardiography contributes significantly to the detection of cardiac malformations by visualization of the cardiac structures, which cannot be demonstrated by 2D echocardiography alone (C plane in multiplanar imaging)

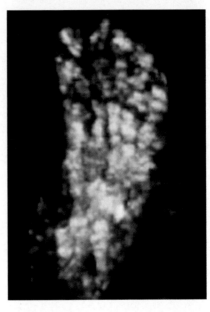

FIGURE 13.2B: Changing to transparent mode: normal skeletal structure and soft tissue are visualized.

and because 3D ultrasound is less dependent on the angle of acquisition, the introduction of the STIC technique to overcome nongated acquisition artifacts in the reconstructed volume data due to the beating heart, was long awaited. The most promising aspect of this modality is the possibility of storing and compressing a volume of 3D information for later offline evaluation by an expert, with the option of telemedicine.

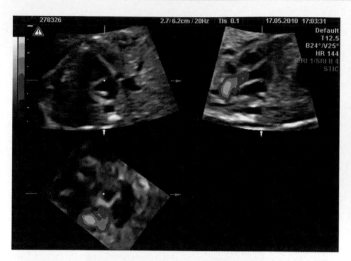

FIGURE 13.3A: Left ventricular outflow tract (LVOT).

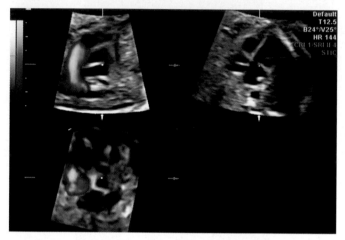

FIGURE 13.3B: Right ventricular outflow tract (RVOT). LVOT and RVOT images are generated offline from the STIC volume data set after the patient has left.

Spatiotemporal Image Correlation Mode enables automatic volume acquisition by time-gated production of multiple slices of the beating fetal heart, which are then ordered according to their temporal and spatial reference within the heart cycle. The result is the volume of a complete fetal cardiac cycle displayed in motion in an endless 3D cine loop sequence. To achieve this, a single sweep recording 3D data set over an area of 15 to 40° is performed. This data set of multiple time-gated slices contains information of the entire fetal heart in motion, including the surrounding structures. If the acquisition begins at the level of the four-chamber view, which is usually recommended as a standard approach, a real-time motion sequence of a sweep from 15 to 40° cranially and caudally from the four-chamber view is stored. This volume

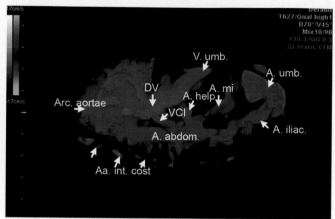

FIGURE 13.4: Fetal vascular system visualized by 3D color Doppler technique. Spatial reconstruction of the three orthogonal planes. Color coding (blue = flow direction away from probe, red = flow direction towards probe) facilitates identification of vessels.

provides a multiplanar view of the heart in motion. Hemodynamic insights are gained by combining STIC with color and/or power Doppler mode. In addition, all existing rendering modes can be utilized to improve the diagnostic precision[2,3] (Figures 13.3A and B).

Three-dimensional Angio Mode

Three-dimensional angio mode operates on technological basis of high-energy powered Doppler. Its greater sensitivity is related to direction independent scanning and better detection of smaller vessels. This mode provides optimal visualization and selective 3D reconstruction even of tortuous parts of vessels and of the blood flow arborization (Figure 13.4).

DV=Ductus venosus, VCI = Vena cava inferior, A. umb. = Arteria umbilicalis, V. umb. = Vena umbilicalis, A. mi = Arteria mesenterica inferior, A. hep = arteria hepatica.

More recently, 3D reconstruction of the vascular signals has been accomplished utilizing the Doppler amplitude mode.[4,5] The implementation of the 3D color and power Doppler imaging permits the physician to investigate the anatomy and topography of hemodynamics within particular organ or ROI.

Volumetric Calculations

Three-dimensional measurement of organ volume (volumetry) is obtainable using sequential slice-stepping measurements of areas through the volugram of a targeted organ (Figure 13.5).

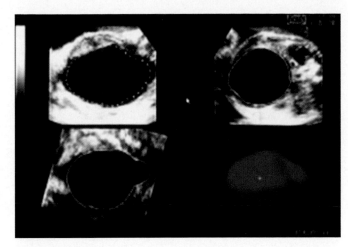

FIGURE 13.5: Technique of volume measurement. The margins of a full fetal bladder are traced with cursor in three orthogonal planes. Volume of the bladder is automatically calculated.

TABLE 13.1: Visualization rates of fetal structures with 2D and 3D ultrasound

Structure	2D US (%)	3D US (%)
Tooth germs[9]	8.8	31.0
Upper lip[2]	93.0	100.0
Palate[2]	41.0	86.0
Distal extremities[3]	52.0	85.0
Fetal digits[4]	74.3	52.9

The volume assessment by 2D US includes the approximation of volume based on the assumption that fetal organs have an ideal geometric shape. This however could be erroneous.

VISUALIZATION OF NORMAL FETAL ANATOMY

Two-dimensional sonography (2D US) is routinely used in obstetrics and has proved to be a powerful tool in clinical diagnosis and management. However, the ability to obtain certain views of the fetus may be limited because of its position or limited probe manipulations. Three- and four-dimensional ultrasound is advantageous in the workup of fetal anomalies involving the face, limbs, thorax, spine and central nervous system.[6] More realistic images contribute to the bonding effect between the parents and their future offspring. In addition, consulting specialists understand fetal pathology better and, if necessary, could better plan postnatal interventions. It is hoped that in the coming years, this technique will be accepted by a large number of obstetricians, maternal fetal specialists and imaging specialists.[6]

Using 3D US, any desired plane through the fetus is obtainable regardless of the fetal or probe position. Only the quality of imaging can be different, depending on various sections. Therefore, in case of unsuccessful 2D US visualization, additional information confirming normal fetal anatomy can be obtained by 3D US. The most common difficulties in 2D US scanning are related to the visualization rates of the fetal face, mandible, lip, palate,

tooth germs, distal part of the extremities, fingers and toes.[7-10] Depiction rate of these structures is significantly higher with 3D US (Table 13.1).[2,3,4,9]

The data presented in Table 13.1 indicate that 3D US examination should be performed whenever 2D US is incapable to visualize these structures. Improved visualization rates of the detailed anatomy of the fetal face and extremities are closely related to the use of multiplanar imaging. Moreover, 3D US has greater potential to facilitate depiction of the distal segments of the upper and lower extremities and digits than 2D US. Depiction rate of the distal parts of the extremities is significantly higher with 3D US (85% vs. 52%).[7] Ploeckinger-Ulm et al., reported that the depiction rate of all digits was 74.3% by 3D US, compared to 52.9% by 2D US.[8]

An interesting point in the ongoing comparison of 2D and 3D/4D ultrasound was reached with the study of Goncalves et al.[11] They reviewed 706 articles on the use of 3D/4D ultrasound from the field of obstetrics. Their research concluded that 3D US compared with 2D, provided additional diagnostic information for facial anomalies, evaluation of the neural tube defects and skeletal malformations. They concluded that more studies were required to find out, if the image information contained in a volume data set would alone be sufficient to evaluate fetal biometric measurements and diagnose congenital anomalies.[11]

One year later, the same research group evaluated a paradigm shift—"What does 2D imaging add to 3D/4D obstetrical ultrasound?" After an initial 3D/4D volume sonography, 99 fetuses were then examined with 2D ultrasound. The frequency of agreement and diagnostic accuracy of the two modalities were calculated and compared to postnatal outcome. There was no significant difference in sensitivity and specificity between 3D/4D and 2D ultrasound. The authors concluded that diagnostic information provided by 3D/4D volume data sets alone did not exceed the information obtained by 2D ultrasonography.[12]

After Goncalves review in 2005, Kurjak et al., analyzed the data from the literature published on the use of 3D US and 4D US in perinatal medicine. Out of 575 articles identified, 438 were relevant to their research definition. Their analysis revealed that 3D and 4D US is advantageous in evaluation of the facial anomalies, neural tube defects, skeletal malformations, congenital heart disease, central nervous system (CNS) anomalies and fetal neurodevelopmental impairment perceptible by abnormal behavior in high-risk fetuses.[13]

Visualization of the fetal face became one of the major interests in the domain of 3D ultrasonography. Due to their affection in malformation syndromes and chromosomal abnormalities, regions of special interest are fetal maxilla, mandible arch, ear and nose. Ulm et al, reported better visualization rate of tooth germs with 3D US than 2D US (31% vs 8.8%).[9] Merz et al, studied 125 fetuses to examine the effect of 3D US imaging on evaluation of the axis of facial profile.[10] They found that in 30.4% of the results, the profile section of 2D US facial profiles had a bias of 3° to 20° compared with an optimal midsagittal section obtained by 3D US. As a result, 2D US was able to obtain profile in only 69.6% of the fetuses. The importance of this finding should not be underestimated. When midsagittal plane could not be visualized, anomalies may be easily missed. Clearly, main improvement of 3D US is primarily related to facilitated visualization of the morphological details and complex anatomical structures.[14-16]

Fetal Head and Face

Assessment of the fetal head is an essential part of routine sonographic examination.[17] Even under optimal conditions, the position of the fetal head makes it difficult to obtain adequate images with 2D ultrasonography and many cross sectional images are required to imagine the complete structure of the fetal head. Normal anatomy and major anomalies of the fetal head, such as exencephaly, anencephaly, encephalocele and holoprosencephaly can be recognized by detailed observation of the skull shape.[18] There are numerous reports about first trimester diagnosis of these anomalies using high-frequency 2D transvaginal sonography.[19-21] Surface rendering enables assessment of the shape of the fetal head and detailed evaluation of the cranial flat bones, orbits, ears, nose and lips.[22] However, 3D sonography does not provide significant improvement regarding early diagnosis of major malformations. Surface rendered "sculpture-like" 3D images represent the most impressive way of fetal visualization, easily acceptable and

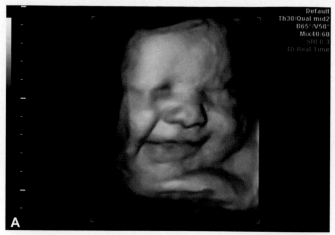

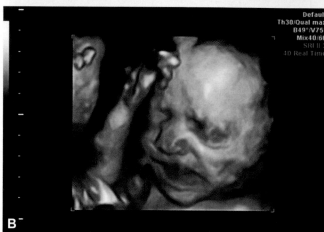

FIGURES 13.6A AND B: Different fetal facial expressions: (A) demonstrates fetal smile; (B) visualizes scowling.

recognizable even by parents. Ji et al, conducted a study comparing the maternal-fetal bonding after 2D and 3D US imaging.[23] They found that 3D had a more positive influence on maternal-fetal bonding than 2D US.

Kurjak et al,[24] evaluated the potential of 3D/4D US for the assessment of the structural and functional development of the fetal face. They considered fetal face as a "diagnostic window" for fetal diseases and syndromes, especially in relation to the central nervous system (CNS). They found that 3D US has improved the evaluation of the fetal facial anomalies. Four-dimensional ultrasonography allowed visualization of facial expressions that might be useful in evaluation of the fetal behavior and contributed significantly to maternal-fetal bonding (Figures 13.6A and B).

Surface mode is particularly useful for the investigation of the neurocranium, sutures and fontanels, which are flat and curved structures.[25] Cranial bone and suture assessment by 3D US is an important step in confirming normal morphology of the fetal skull.

Cranial sutures and fontanels are spaces between the fetal skull plates that allow progressive growth of the brain and skull bones during fetal development. At 12 weeks, premature cranial bones and sutures in between are detectable. The sagittal suture, lambda sutures and posterior fontanel can be recognized from 13 weeks. Therefore, fetal skull anomalies, such as craniosynostoses can be excluded in late first and early second trimesters of pregnancy.[26]

Sutures and fontanels can be identified with 2D sonography when experienced sonographers target them. Unfortunately, sometimes it is difficult to assess the structural continuity of the sutures and fontanels with 2D US in a single plane because of physiological cranial curvature.[26,15] In general, real time 2D imaging permits the recognition only of their parts, whereas final impression about their integrity is a matter of sonographer's abstract thinking. 3D surface rendering of the fetal neurocranium allows visualization of the sutures, fontanels and flat bones on a single reconstructed image.

Fetal face can be identified using 2D and 3D transvaginal sonography even at 10 weeks gestational age.[27] However, detailed observation and evaluation of the face can be accomplished between 22 and 24 gestational weeks.[28,29]

Facial examination can be performed only to a limited extent by 2D sonography because of the facial curvatures and limitations of probe manipulation. Moreover, an unfavorable fetal position can make it impossible to visualize minute facial structures, such as nose, eyes, periorbital region and orbits. Surface rendered images depict the entire face and relationship between the facial structures, such as the nostrils, opened or closed eyelids and mouth on a single image. Moreover, depiction and observation of the orbital region and status of the fetal eyelids can be easily performed using this modality (Figure 13.7).

Assessment of the facial structures is useful to detect unusual abnormalities.[30] Depiction of fetal eyelids is particularly good on a surface rendered view, as demonstrated in Figure 13.8.

Surface rendering of the fetal face allows images that are easy to understand. Perceiving the integrity of a face and interpreting facial expressions is an intuitive process that happens instantly. Therefore, it is much easier to use surface rendered images of the face in helping parents to

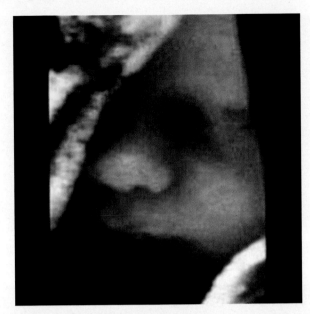

FIGURE 13.7: Surface rendered mode reconstruction of the fetal face. Facial structures and their spatial relationships are clearly visualized.

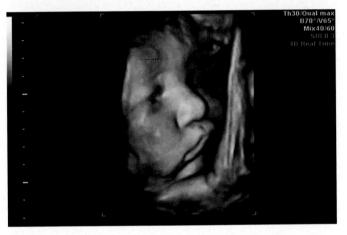

FIGURE 13.8: Surface rendered face of a fetus with opened eyes.

understand the extent of craniofacial malformations of the fetus. Both 2D and 3D US are used to diagnose a cleft lip, however 3D US is superior to 2D in the detection and exact description of a cleft palate.[29]

Campbell et al,[31] reported on the use of "3D reverse face view" (3D RF) as an improved approach for the assessment of hard palate, not visible in the surface view of the face. The surface rendered frontal view of the face is rotated 180 degrees around the vertical axis until the face is seen "from behind". This technique assists in the

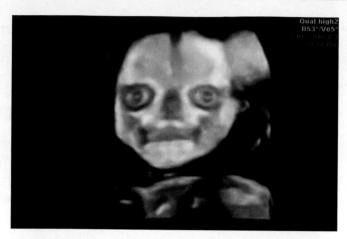

FIGURE 13.9A: Normal 3D reverse face view (3D RF) of the fetus seen in Figure 13.1.

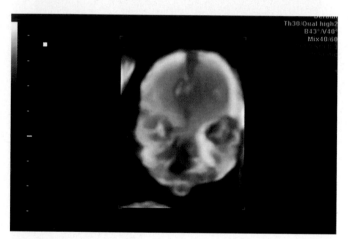

FIGURE 13.9B: Abnormal 3D RF view of the fetus with cleft palate.

antenatal categorization of the hard palate clefts (Figures 13.9A and B).

Besides normal morphology the following anomalies can be detected by surface rendered examination of the fetal face: anophthalmia, microophthalmia, hypotelorism, hypertelorism, anterior or frontal encephalocoele, exophthalmia, periorbital tumors, epignatus, teratoma and hemangioma. Sagittal view of the fetal face, facial profile, allows observation of the spatial relationship between the surface structures of the forehead and viscerocranium. Moreover, evaluation of the relationships between the structures of the viscerocranium, including nose, lips and chin is easily performed (Figures 13.10A to D).

Even, the slight retraction of the inferior lip and chin in relationship to the upper lip can be recognized. A view of the profile allows prenatal diagnosis of the following anomalies: absence of the nose or nasal bridge, micrognatia and macroglossia. Clearly, the surface rendered image of the face is much more informative than a 2D image. This is of special interest in patients with family history of facial anomalies or in cases of maternal consumption of teratogens. Unfortunately, optimal visualization by this mode can be achieved only in 72% fetuses scanned between 20 and 35 weeks.[14]

Surface rendering image in combination with multiplanar views can reassure the ultrasonographer that lost signals in facial defects are not due to transducer angulation and that the view of the face is symmetric. Rotational images are particularly comprehensive to parents, because they allow better understanding of the fetal anatomy and anomalies, if present.[28] It is well documented that anomalous shape, size and position of the fetal ears are associated with a number of morphological and chromosomal syndromes. Prenatal assessment of the ear includes the evaluation of ear morphology, size and position.

Unfortunately, due to the complex shape, ear examination can be performed only to a limited extent by 2D US. In most of the cases, 2D images are inadequate for precise evaluation of the ear morphology. Since only auricular geometry is visualized, the differentiation between variants of normal morphology and a dismorphic ear is difficult. Surface rendering provides spatial reconstruction of the auricle and improves evaluation of the ear morphology (Figure 13.11).

Furthermore, evaluation of the spatial relationship between the neurocranium and fetal ear can be obtained, including orientation regarding axis, location, length, width and area of the fetal ear.[16,32] By determination of the line between the orbits and peak of the auricle of the fetal ear, we can assess normal and low-set ears. Low-set ears are associated with aneuploidies.[33]

Assessment of the fetal brain is an essential part of routine sonographic examination.[11] However, fetal brain can be examined only to a limited extent by 2D US. Observation of the fetal brain offers sagittal and coronal sections of the brain from fetal parietal direction through the fontanels and/or sagittal suture as ultrasound windows.[34,35]

Three-dimensional sonography provides multiplanar analysis of the fetal intracranial anatomy. Moreover, rotating the brain volume image produces multiplanar image analysis of the intracranial structures in any cutting section. It is possible to demonstrate not only the sagittal and coronal sections but also the axial section of the brain, which cannot

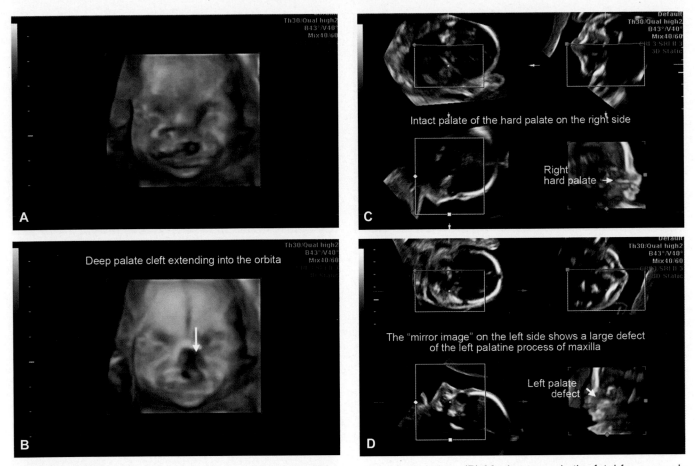

FIGURES 13.10A TO D: (A) Unilateral left facial cleft, surface rendered frontal view; (B) Moving towards the fetal face reveals deep cleft palate; (C) 3D multiplanar rendering demonstrates an intact hard palate on the right side; (D) Rendering the "mirror image" on the left depicts the partial lack of the hard palate.

be demonstrated from the parietal direction by conventional 2D transvaginal sonography[36] (Figure 13.12).

The most impressive advancement achieved by 3D ultrasonography concerning prenatal neurosonography is the possibility to visualize the entire lateral ventricle, including the anterior, posterior and inferior horns on single image. This section is called "the three horn view" and it is particularly useful for the longitudinal evaluation of dimensions of the fetal ventricles.[37]

Transvaginal 2D sonography with color and power Doppler demonstrates sagittal and coronal images of the brain circulation.[38,39] Power Doppler images in midsagittal section obtained via the anterior fontanel demonstrate the internal carotid artery, the anterior cerebral artery, the pericallosal artery, the calloso-marginal artery and their branches. In coronal section, power Doppler images show the bilateral internal carotid arteries, the branches of the middle cerebral arteries and the anterior cerebral artery.

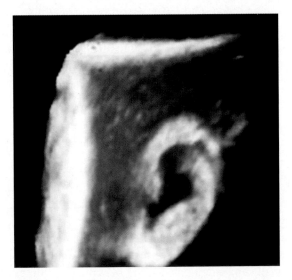

FIGURE 13.11: Surface rendered mode reconstruction of the fetal ear. Ear morphology, position and size are easily evaluated.

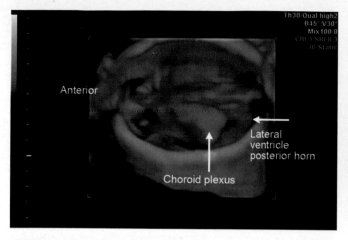

FIGURE 13.12: Intracranial structures visualized by 3D ultrasound.

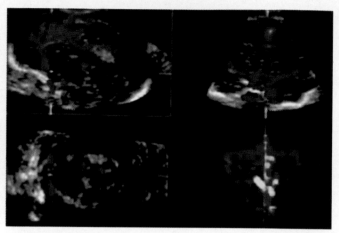

FIGURE13.13A: Three-dimensional power Doppler image of the fetal brain (multiplanar analysis). In sagittal section pericallosal artery with branches is clearly visualized.

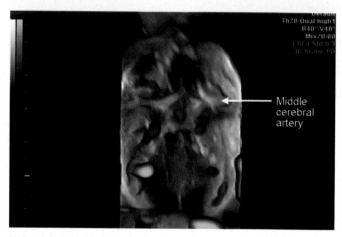

FIGURE 13.13B: 3D power Doppler glass body rendering of the circulus arteriosus Willisi.

Through the sagittal suture of the fetal cranial bone, power Doppler imaging demonstrates the intracranial venous circulation, including the superior sagittal sinus, the internal cerebral vein, the vein of Galen and the straight sinus. The main steam and the branches of the middle cerebral artery run in different directions and both main line and branches cannot be detected in the same coronal section. This shortcoming of 2D US imaging has been overcome by reconstruction of the 3D power Doppler volume data showing the configuration of the brain vessels in three dimensions (Figures 13.13A and B).

The internal carotid artery, anterior cerebral artery, bilateral middle cerebral arteries and their branches, can be demonstrated simultaneously on one image. Ultrasound angiography of the fetal brain allows noninvasive assessment of the brain circulation. Since 3D vascular images can be rotated in any direction, the vessels can be observed from the frontal, occipital, lateral, oblique, parietal or basilar part of the brain.

Fetal Thorax and Abdomen

Due to the curvature of the thoracic bones detailed evaluation of the thoracic skeleton is often difficult with 2D US.[40] Three-dimensional US transparency mode reduces the echogenicity of the soft tissues, leaving only echogenic structures, namely the bones, which enables visualization of the fetal ribs. The curvature and relationship of the ribs ending in the vertebral bodies and the anterior chest wall can be demonstrated in the entire length. Achiron et al, evaluated specific advantages of certain 3D imaging and rendering modes for the optimal diagnostic display of

certain malformations.[41-44] Volume datasets of 23 fetuses with thoracic anomalies were acquired with static 3D and cine peripheral pulmonary segments. Especially the right lung can be assessed even with little experience. Mitchell et al, used color, pulsed and power Doppler to image the fetal pulmonary vasculature in normal pregnancies, but also in patients with pulmonary hypoplasia.[45] Compared to the normal fetuses, fetuses with pulmonary hypoplasia had a significantly higher resistance pattern of the Doppler signals obtained from the peripheral pulmonary arteries.

Power Doppler ultrasound produces impressive anatomic imaging with excellent demonstration of the fetal heart anatomy and delineation of heart borders. The anatomy of the great vessels is better understood by visualizing the crossing over of the vessels with easy assessment of their size, course and shape. Visualization of the crossing of the aorta and pulmonary artery is facilitated with power Doppler technique due to the sharp edge definition. Another striking capability is display of both the left and right pulmonary veins draining into the left atrium. Such a clarity of images is difficult to achieve with conventional color Doppler imaging (Figure 13.14).

Using 3D power Doppler, Chaoui and Kalache demonstrated the fetal heart at 28 weeks' gestation in longitudinal view of the great vessels showing the right and left ventricular outflow tracts in their spatial relationship.[45] The aortic arch and the crossing of the pulmonary trunk was clearly seen, as well as the connection of the ductus arteriosus to the descending aorta. The left pulmonary artery arises before the origin of the ductus arteriosus. Three-dimensional power Doppler approach enables imaging of the blood flow mainly in the center of the vessel, which assists in the spatial separation of the aorta and pulmonary artery despite high persistence. The expectation that 3D fetal echocardiography would include 3D power Doppler in addition to 3D or 4D gray scale, has come true with the introduction and perfection of STIC. It is expected that this modality will improve our understanding of the malformations such as hypoplastic left heart syndrome (HLHS), right heart syndrome or other malformations with a singular ventricle and hypoplasia of the great arteries. The majority of the complex congenital heart anomalies show a steadily progression of the pathological changes during the course of pregnancy, including subsequent secondary phenomena such as arrhythmias or myocardial insufficiency. 3D/4D ultrasound is a tool of choice for follow-up of such a progression and may have a significant input in prenatal treatment of an abnormal fetus. Better understanding of the pathophysiological causa may encourage some researchers to explore new minimally invasive therapeutic options in terms of early pre- and postnatal cardiac palliation.[46]

Three-dimensional surface mode enables sculpture-like reconstruction of the abdominal wall and normal umbilical cord insertion. The complete abdominal surface is invisible by conventional 2D technology, unless the abdominal surface is scanned in a survey-like manner, involving serial tomographic sections in sagittal and transverse planes. Using 3D surface mode we are able to visualize the complete abdominal surface, including a umbilical cord insertion, in a single image. Using surface rendering mode continuity of the fetal skin can be easily confirmed.

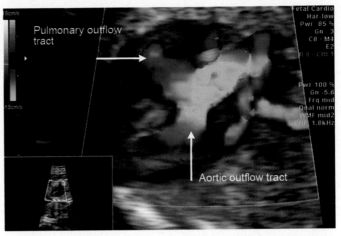

FIGURE 13.14: "Crossing over of the fetal aorta and pulmonary artery" in color Doppler mode. "Color coding" of flow direction enables differentiation of the two outflow tracts.

Moreover, fetal fat deposits can be easily differentiated from abnormal protrusion caused by malformations and cutaneous or subcutaneous tumors.[47,48] Postprocessing offers opportunity for surface imaging of the fetal intra-abdominal structures. Multiplanar imaging enables construction of the planes nearly parallel to the mother's abdominal wall, thus, making it possible to observe the esophageal-gastric junction and pylorus. The electronic scalpel or electronic rubber is used to "cut out" the overlying body segments, producing either a longitudinal or transverse section. Once this has been done, the pathologic organ can be evaluated separately. Three-dimensional ultrasound confirms suspected multicystic dysplastic kidney, as well as renal agenesis and abnormal pelvi-ureteral junction.[49]

Fetal intra-abdominal vessels are numerous and most of them can be visualized by color and power Doppler ultrasound.[50] The main veins of interest are the intrahepatic umbilical vein, the hepatic veins, the ductus venosus and the inferior vena cava. Other arteries that are commonly evaluated are the descending aorta and the superior mesenteric, renal, splenic, iliac and umbilica. Owing to different velocities in these vessels and their different course, the examiner can focus on the region of interest by choosing the appropriate setting of the velocity scale as well as the insonation angle. Intrahepatic vessels are best obtained when the fetus is lying in the dorsoposterior position[38] (Figure 13.15).

A. mi = inferior mesenteric artery; A. ren = renal arteries; A. hep. d = right hepatic artery; A. umb. = umbilical arteries

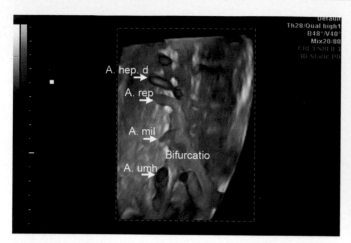

FIGURE 13.15: Abdominal aorta and its branches in power Doppler glass body rendering.

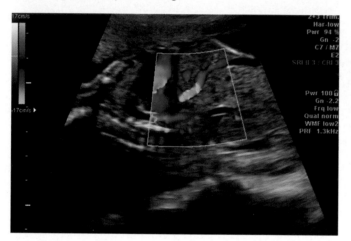

FIGURE 13.16: Ductus venosus in color Doppler mode. Note the aliasing phenomenon in the continuation of the umbilical vein near the diaphragm, indicated by changing the colors from blue to orange. This color Doppler finding indicates turbulent jet in ductus venosus.

Longitudinal approach renders the best images of the insertion of the umbilical cord, the intra-abdominal course of the umbilical vein into the ductus venosus towards the heart, and the assessment of the relationship between the aorta and the inferior vena cava (Figure 13.16).

In the lower abdomen, a sagittal view allows the visualization of the umbilical arteries circling the urinary bladder (Figures 13.17A and B).

The renal vascular tree is well visualized in a coronal plane, with the descending aorta showing a horizontal course.[38] Depending on the pulse repetition frequency setting, the vessels can be seen from the main artery with some ramifications to the peripheral cortical vessels, including arteries and veins (Figures 13.18A and B).

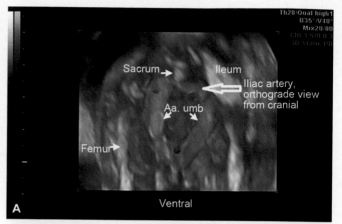

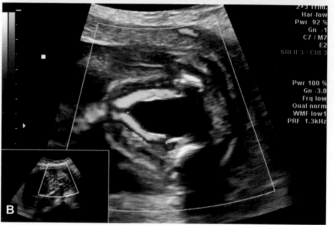

FIGURES 13.17A AND B: Umbilical arteries circling the urinary bladder in power Doppler 3D glass body rendering (A) and gray scale power Doppler mode (B).

The examiner should be aware of the possible false information given by the visualization of more ventrally situated abdominal arteries (inferior mesenteric artery and celiac trunk vessels).[26] These might be misinterpreted as renal arteries in some planes.

This can be avoided by choosing a narrow sweep volume to avoid the imaging of nonrenal vessels. To date, power Doppler imaging has been applied in fetal medicine as a qualitative imaging tool, while attempts at quantifying fetal blood flow have centered on comparing velocity measurements or ratios using spectral Doppler ultrasound. Modern digital imaging techniques nowadays allow extraction of the numerical information from the ultrasound images. Welsh and Fisk[51] assessed fetal renal perfusion by power Doppler digital analysis, choosing a region of renal cortex for examination as the region of interest and extracting energy flow information. Integrated energy is plotted for the given region of interest where periodicity reflects fluctuations in a vascular volume within the arteries

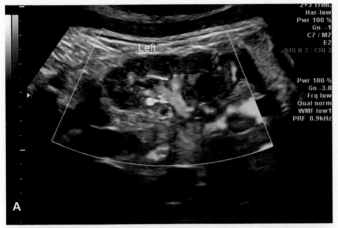

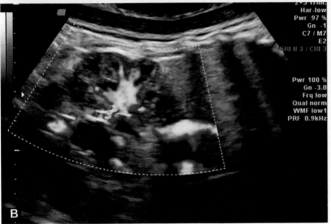

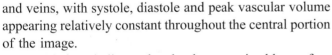

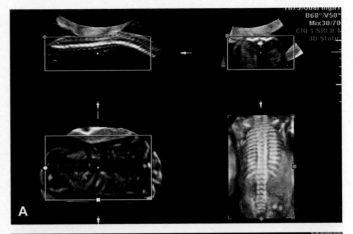

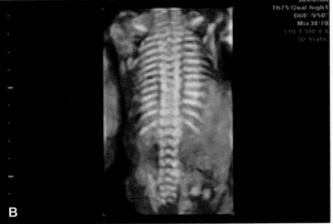

FIGURES 13.18A AND B: Power Doppler image of the renal artery and its arborization within the left and right kidney.

FIGURES 13.19A AND B: Fetal spine in maximum mode. (A) Multiplanar display; (B) Maximum mode reconstruction from the three orthogonal planes.

and veins, with systole, diastole and peak vascular volume appearing relatively constant throughout the central portion of the image.

External genitalia can be clearly recognized by surface rendering and complex malformations or developmental anomalies are diagnosed easily and much earlier than it was possible by the use of conventional ultrasound.[52]

Spine and Extremities

Particular importance should be given to visualization of the anatomy, spatial relationship and angulations of the fetal skeleton by volume rendering using transparent mode, maximum mode and "X-ray-like" imaging.[53] This technique includes the volume rendered imaging possibilities between minimum and maximum intensity method (Figures 13.19A and B).

3D ultrasonography using transparent mode allows imaging of the fetal skeleton and enables detection of the

fetal skeletal malformations in spatial orientation. The vertebral column is originally curved anteroposteriorly. In fetuses with pathological lateral curvature, 2D ultrasound cannot display the entire vertebral column in one 2D tomogram. The advantage of 3D ultrasound is the ability to visualize both curvatures at the same time. Anomalies, such as scoliosis, kyphosis, lordosis and spina bifida may be overlooked by 2D ultrasound, but are easily recognized using 3D maximum mode. Congenital malformations of the fetal spine and ribs can be identified earlier using 3D surface imaging and transparent mode reconstruction, simultaneously. Specific vertebral body level can be accurately identified by instantaneous demonstration of the axial planes within a volume rendered image or within the coronal plane image. It may be difficult to acquire the entire spine in a single volume and thus, multiple volumes are often necessary to completely evaluate the spine. An impressive example for transparent mode reconstruction is the complete skeletal "baby-gram."[22,15]

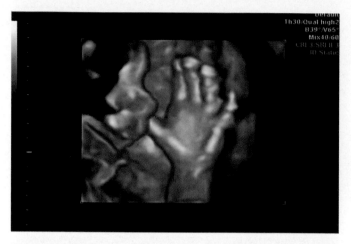

FIGURE 13.20A: Normal fetal hand reconstructed in surface rendered mode.

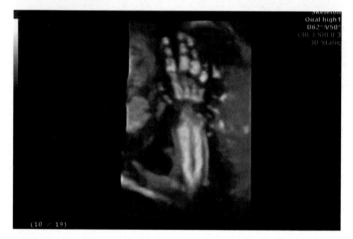

FIGURE 13.20B: Transparent mode reconstruction of the same hand and underarm, with clearly visible skeletal structures and soft tissue.

Extremities consist of the three parts: the proximal, medial and distal part. Using this modality, all three segments and spatial relationships between them could been analyzed in three dimensions. Therefore, deviation of the normal anatomical axis seen as pathological angulations of the fetal hands and feet can be excluded by 3D US examination.[54]

Three-dimensional images can be presented in two modes. If one is interested in spatial relationship between the segments of the fetal extremities, surface rendered mode should be used (Figures 13.20A and B).

However, if the focus of interest is the relationship between the bone elements of the fetal extremity then transparent mode should be used (Figure 13.20B).

By combining these two modalities, more detailed analysis of the fetal anatomy is achieved. Distal parts of

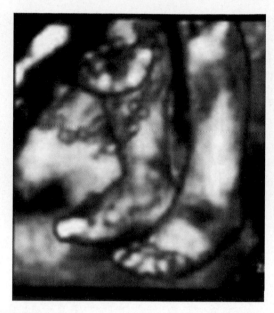

FIGURE 13.21: Surface rendered mode of the fetal legs. Normal anatomy and topographic relationships of the lower extremities are clearly depicted.

fetal extremities are clearly visualized by surface rendered reconstruction (Figure 13.21).

Spatial relations between medial and distal segment of the fetal leg can also be assessed in surface rendering mode. Normal anatomical axis and axis deviations can be confirmed. Using 3D ultrasound sonographer can evaluate fetal extremities from the external appearance to complex inner and intratopographic bone relations. Surface of the skin and external spatial relations are shown on surface rendering image, while complex anatomy of bone elements is better evaluated by transparent mode.

VOLUMETRY—ORGAN VOLUME MEASUREMENTS

Before the introduction of 3D US, organ volume measurements have not been widely used for the assessment of fetal growth and organ abnormalities, because of limitations of 2D US in estimating volumes of irregular structures. Comparing with 2D US, 3D US enables organ volume measurement by stepping through the fetal organs slice-by-slice. The area of interest can be traced by means of a cursor in each plane of the object. The total volume calculation is equal to the sum of the individual slice's volumes. Riccabona et al, demonstrated both in vitro and in vivo that 3D US provides more accurate volume estimation of the structures with irregular shapes compared with 2D US.[55,56]

The feasibility of calculating the volumes of the following structures and/or organs has been reported: fetal lungs and fetal heart from second trimester to full term, placental volume, fetal arms, thighs, and renal and cerebellar volume for estimation of the fetal weight.[57-59] Of special interests are measurements of the fetal lung volumes in order to confirm or exclude fetal lung hypoplasia or immaturity.[60]

Three-dimensional US enables more sophisticated volume measurements of the irregularly shaped organs.[46,47] Lung and hepatic volume normograms have been published, showing that the volume of these organs increases with gestational age and weight.[58-60] After upper abdominal circumference, the best prediction of fetal growth restriction is the hepatic volume.[61] Therefore, hepatic volume may become a new useful parameter in the assessment of fetal growth. For many years, fetal weight calculation has been mainly based upon abdominal circumference measurement. Among all possible sections and parameters of the fetal trunk, abdominal circumference has been chosen because it reflects changes of the liver size. This method does not consider the amount of the fetal fat tissue and there is still no better discriminator for fetal growth aberrations.[62-64]

Although neonatal fat mass represents only 14% of birth weight, it explains 46% of its variance.[65] Birth weight prediction based on limb volumetry, including upper arm and thigh seems to be more accurate.[66,67]

CONCLUSION

The main advantages of 3D sonography in prenatal diagnosis are:

- Improved visualization and diagnosis (evaluation of the image planes that cannot be obtained with conventional 2D imaging due to anatomic constraints and/or fetal position).
- Easy demonstration of the coronal plane (the third plane, which cannot be displayed by conventional 2D ultrasonography).
- Transparent mode (particularly useful for imaging of the fetal skeleton).
- Improved orientation and improved anatomic relationship by interactive rotation of volume rendered images.
- Volume assessment.
- Three-dimensional power Doppler reconstruction of fetal, placental and uterine vasculature.
- Analysis of fetal movement patterns by real-time 3D (4D) ultrasound.[68]

REFERENCES

1. Jurkovic D, Jauniaux E, Campbell S. Three dimensional ultrasound in obstetrics and gynecology. In. Kurjak A, Chervenak F, (Eds.) The Fetus as a Patient. Carnforth, UK: Parthenon Publishing, 1994;135-140.
2. Volpe P, De Robertis V, Campobasso G, et al. Evaluation of the fetal heart by four dimensional echocardiography. Donald School Journal of Ultrasound in Obstetrics and Gynecology 2007;1(3):49-53.
3. Szymkiewicz-Dangel J. 3D/4D echocardiography-STIC. Donald School Journal of Ultrasound in Obstetrics and Gynecology 2008;2(4):22-8.
4. Downey DB, Fenster A, Williams JC. Clinical utility of three-dimensional US. Radiographics 2000;20:559-71.
5. Downey DB, Fenster A. Vascular imaging with a three-dimensional power Doppler system. Am J Roentgenoll. 995;165:656-58.
6. Timor-Tritsch IE, Platt LD. Three-dimensional ultrasound experience in obstetrics. Curr Opin Obstet Gynecol 2002 Dec;14(6):569-575.
7. Budorick NE, Pretorius DH, Johnson DD, et al. Three-dimensional ultrasonography of the fetal distal lower extremity: Normal and abnormal. J Ultrasound Med. 1998;17(10):649-60.
8. Ploeckinger-Ulm B, Ulm MR, Lee A, et al. Antenatal depiction of fetal digits with three-dimensional ultrasonography. Am J Obstet Gynecol 1996;175(3 Pt 1):571-74.
9. Ulm MR, Kratochwil A, Ulm B, et al. Three-dimensional ultrasonographic imaging of fetal tooth buds for characterization of facial clefts. Early Hum Dev 1999;55(1):67-75.
10. Merz E, Weber G, Bahlmann F, et al. Application of transvaginal and abdominal three-dimensional ultrasound for the detection or exclusion of malformations of the fetal face. Ultrasound Obstet Gynecol 1997;9(4):237-43.
11. Gonçalves LF, Lee W, Espinoza J, et al. Three- and 4-dimensional ultrasound in obstetric practice:does it help? J Ultrasound Med. 2005;24(12):1599-624.
12. Gonçalves LF, Nien JK, Espinoza J, et al. What does 2-dimensional imaging add to 3- and 4-dimensional obstetric ultrasonography? J Ultrasound Med 2006;25(6):691-9.
13. Kurjak A, Miskovic B, Andonotopo W, et al. How useful is 3D and 4D ultrasound in perinatal medicine? J Perinat Med 2007;35(1):10-27.
14. Pretorius DH, Nelson TR. Fetal face visualization using three-dimensional ultrasonography. J Ultrasound Med 1995;14(5):349-56.
15. Pretorius DH, Nelson TR. Prenatal visualization of cranial sutures and fontanelles with three-dimensional ultrasonography. J Ultasound Med. 1994;13(11):871-6.
16. Shih JC, Shyu MK, Lee CN, et al. Antenatal depiction of the fetal ear with three-dimensional ultrasonography. Obstet Gynecol 1998;91(4):500-5.
17. Baba K, Okai T. Clinical applications of three dimensional ultrasound in obstetrics. In: Baba K, Jurkovic D, (Eds.) Three dimensional ultrasound in obstetrics and gynecology. Carnforth, UK: Parthenon Publishing 1997;29-44.

18. Benoit B, Hafner T, Kurjak A, et al. Three-dimensional sonoembryology. J Perinatal Med 2000;30(1):63-73.

19. Achiron R, Achiron A. Transvaginal fetal neurosonography: The first trimester of pregnancy. In: Chervenak FA, Kurjak A, Comstock CH (Eds.) Ultrasound of the fetal brain. London-New York: Parthenon Publishing, 1995; 95-102.

20. Pooh RK. B-mode and Doppler studies of the abnormal fetus in the first trimester. In: Chervenak FA, Kurjak A, (Eds.) Fetal Medicine: The clinical care of the fetus as a patient. London-New York: Parthenon Publishing, 1999; 46-51.

21. Weissman A, Achiron R. Ultrasound diagnosis of congenital anomalies in early pregnancy. In: Jurkovic D, Jauninaux E, (Eds.) Ultrasound and early pregnancy. Canforth, UK: Parthenon Publishing, 1996;95-119.

22. Benoit B. Three dimensional surface mode for demonstration of normal fetal anatomy in the second and third trimester. In: Merz E (Ed.) 3D Ultrasound in obstetrics and gynecology. Philadelphia: Lippincott Williams and Wilkins, 1998, 95-100.

23. Ji EK, Pretorius DH, Newton R, et al. Effects of ultrasound on maternal-fetal bonding: A comparison of two- and three-dimensional imaging. Ultrasound Obstet Gynecol. 2005;25(5): 473-7.

24. Kurjak A, Azumendi G, Andonotopo W, et al. Three- and four-dimensional ultrasonography for the structural and functional evaluation of the fetal face. Am J Obstet Gynecol 2007;196(1): 16-28.

25. Pooh RK. Fetal cranial bone formation: Sonographic assessment. In: Margulies M, Voto LS, Eik-Nes S, (Eds.) Proceedings of 9th World congress of Ultrasound in Obstetrics and Gynecology. Bologna, Italy:Monduzzi Editore,1999; 407-410.

26. Patel MD, Swinford AE, Filly RA. Anatomic and sonographic features of fetal skull. J Ultrasound Med 1994;13:251-7.

27. Bonilla-Musoles F, Raga F, Blanes J, et al. Three-dimensional ultrasound in reproductive medicine: Preliminary report. Human Reprod update. Vol. 1, 4 item 21 CD Rom 1995.

28. Johnson DD, Pretorius DH, Budorick NE, Jones MC, Lou KV, James GM, Nelson TR. Fetal lip and primary palate: three-dimensional versus two-dimensional US. Radiology 2000;217: 236-9.

29. Chmait RH, Hull AD, James TR, Nelson TR, Pretorius DH. Three-dimensional ultrasound evaluation of fetal face. Ultrasound Rev Obstet Gynecol 2001;1:138-143.

30. Osborne N, Bailao L, Abad L Jr, Bonilla-Musoles F. Macadores ecográficos de infección fetal: In. Bonilla- Musoles F y Machado L. (Ed.) Ecografía y Reproducción. Panamericana. Madrid, 1999;5:205-231.

31. Campbell S, Lees CC. The three-dimensional reverse face (3D RF) view for the diagnosis of cleft palate. Ultrasound Obstet Gynecol 2003;22:552-4.

32. Chang CH, Chang FM, Yu CH, et al. Fetal ear assessment and prenatal detection of aneuploidy by the quantitative three-dimensional ultrasonography. Ultrasound Med Biol 2000;26(5): 743-9.

33. Shih JC, Chen CP, Hsieh FJ. Three-dimensional ultrasonography in genetic screening and counselling. Ultrasound Rev Obstet Gynecol 2001;1:120-7.

34. Monteagudo A, Timor-Tritsch IE, et al. In utero detection of ventriculomegaly during the second and third trimesters by transvaginal sonography. Ultrasound Obstet Gynecol 1994;4(3): 193-9.

35. Pooh RK, Maeda K, Pooh KH, Kurjak A. Sonographic assessment of the fetal brain morphology. Prenatal Neonat Med 1999;4:18-25.

36. Pooh RK, Pooh K, Nakagawa Y, et al. Clinical application of three-dimensional ultrasound in fetal brain assessment. Croat Med J 2000;41(3):245-51.

37. Timor-Tritsch IE, Monteagudo A, Mayberry P. Three-dimensional ultrasound evaluation of the fetal brain: The three horn view. Ultrasound Obstet Gynecol 2000;16(4):302-6.

38. Pooh RK, Aono T. Transvaginal power Doppler angiography of the fetal brain. Ultrasound Obstet Gynecol 1996;8(6):417-21.

39. Pooh RK, Pooh KN, Nakagawa Y. Transvaginal Doppler assessment of fetal intracranial venous flow. Obstet Gynecol 1999;93(5 Pt 1):697-701.

40. Nelson TR, Pretorius DH. Visualization of the fetal thoracic skeleton with three-dimensional sonography: A preliminary report. AJR Am J Roentenol 1995;164(6):1485-8.

41. Achiron R, Gindes L, Zalel Y, et al. Three- and four-dimensional ultrasound: new methods for evaluating fetal thoracic anomalies. Ultrasound Obstet Gynecol 2008;32(1):36-43.

42. Zosmer N, Gruboeck K, Jurkovic D. Three dimensional fetal cardiac imaging. In: Baba K, Jurkovic D (Eds.) Three-dimensional ultrasound in obstetrics and gynaecology. New York: Parthenon Publishing, 1997;45-53.

43. Nelson T, Sklansky M, Pretorius DH. Fetal heart assessment using three dimensional ultrasound. In: Merz E (Ed.) 3D Ultrasound in Obstetrics and Gynecology. Philadelphia: Lippincott, Williams and Wilkins, 1998;125-133.

44. Chaoui R, Kalache KD. Three-dimensional power Doppler ultrasound of the fetal great vessels. Ultrasound Obstet Gynecol 2001;17(5):455-6.

45. Mitchell JM, Roberts AB, Lee A. Doppler waveforms from the pulmonary arterial system in normal fetuses and those with pulmonary hypoplasia. Ultrasound Obstet Gynecol 1998;11(3): 167-72.

46. Nelle M, Raio L, Pavlovic M, et al. Prenatal diagnosis and treatment planning of congenital heart defects–possibilities and limits.World J Pediatr 2009;5(1):18-22.

47. Hosli I, Holzgreve W, Danzer E, et al. Two case reports of rare fetal tumors: An indication for surface rendering? Ultrasound Obstet Gynecol 2001;17(6):522-6.

48. Senoh D, Hanaoka U, Tanaka Y, et al. Antenatal ultrasonographic features of fetal giant hemangiolymphangioma. Ultrasound Obstet Gynecol 2001;17(3):252-4.

49. Hata T, Aoki S, Hata K, et al. Three-dimensional ultrasonographic assessement of umbilical cord during the 2nd and 3rd trimesters of pregnancy. Gynecol Obstet Invest 1998; 45(3):159-164.

50. Chaoui R, Kalache K, Bollmann R. Three-dimensional color power Doppler in the assessment of fetal vascular anatomy under normal and abnormal conditions. In: Kurjak A (Ed.) Three-dimensional power Doppler in obstetrics and gynecology. New York-London: Parthenon Publishing Group; 2000;113-119.

51. Welsh AW, Fisk NM. Assessment of fetal renal perfusion by power Doppler digital analysis. Ultrasound Obstet Gynecol. 2001;17(1):89-91.

52. Kurjak A, Kupesic S. Slide Atlas of Three-dimensional sonography in Gynecology and Obstetrics. Carnforth, UK:Parthenon Publishing, 1998.

53. Linney AD, Deng J. Three-dimensional morphometry in ultrasound. Proc Inst Mech Eng H 1999;21(3):235-45.

54. Kurjak A, Hafner T, Kos M, et al. Three-dimensional sonography in prenatal diagnosis: A luxury or a necessity? J Pernatal Med 2000;28(3):194-209.

55. Riccabona M, Nelson TR, Pretorius DH, et al. Distance and volume measurement using three-dimensional ultrasonography. J Ultrasound Med 1995;14(12):881-6.

56. Riccabona M, Nelson TR, Pretorius DH. Three-dimensional ultrasound: Accuracy of distance and volume measurements. Ultrasound Obstet Gynecol 1996;7(6):429-34.

57. Pöhls UG, Rempen A. Fetal lung volumetry by three-dimensional ultrasound. Ultrasound Obstet Gynecol 1998;11(1):6-12.

58. Laudy JA, Janssen MM, Struyk PC, et al. Fetal liver volume measurement by three-dimensional ultrasonography: A preliminary study. Ultrasound Obstet Gynecol 1998;12(2):93-6.

59. Lee W, Deter RL, Ebersole JD, et al. Birth weight prediction by three-dimensional ultrasonography: Fractional limb volume. J Ultrasound Med 2001;20:1283-92.

60. Osada H, Iitsuka Y, Masuda K, et al. Application of lung volume measurement by three-dimensional ultrasonography for clinical assessment of fetal lung development. J Ultrasound Med 2002; 21(8):841-7.

61. Boito SM, Laudy JA, Struijk PC, et al. Three-dimensional US assessment of hepatic volume, head circumference, and abdominal circumference in healthy and growth-restricted fetuses. Radiology 2002;223:661-5.

62. Deter RL, Nazar R, Milner LL. Modified neonatal growth assessment score: a multivariate approach to the detection of intrauterine growth retardation in the neonate. Ultrasound Obstet Gynecol 1995;6(6):400-10.

63. Vintzileos AM, Campbell WA, Rodis JF, et al. Fetal weight estimation formulas with head, abdominal, femur, and thigh circumference measurements. Am J Obstet Gynecol 1987; 157(2):410-14.

64. McLean F, Usher R. Measurements of live born fetal malnutrition infants compared with similar gestation and with similar birth weight normal controls. Biol Neonate 1970;16(4):215-21.

65. Catalano PM, Tyzbir ED, Allen SR, et al. Evaluation of fetal growth by estimation of neonatal body composition. Obstet Gynecol 1992;79(1):46-50.

66. Liang RI, Chang FM, Yao BL, et al. Predicting birth weight by fetal upper-arm volume with use of three-dimensional ultrasonography. Am J Obstet Gynecol 1997;177(3):632-8.

67. Chang FM, Liang RI, Ko HC, et al. Three-dimensional ultrasound-assessed fetal thigh volumetry in predicting birth weight. Obstet Gynecol 1997;90(3):331-9.

68. Kurjak A, Pooh RK, Tikvica A, et al. Assessment of fetal neurobehavior by 3D/4D ultrasound. In: Pooh RK, Kurjak A, (Eds.) Fetal Neurology. New Delhi: Jaypee Brothers Medical Publishers (P) Ltd, 2009;222-85.

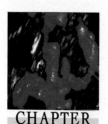

A Kurjak, B Ahmed
U Honemeyer, S Kupesic Plavsic

CHAPTER

14

The Assessment of Abnormal Fetal Anatomy

INTRODUCTION

Various studies have already shown that three-dimensional ultrasound (3D US) can detect or exclude not only major anomalies, but also subtle fetal abnormalities. Besides an impressive demonstration of normal fetal structures, 3D US is adding a "new window" to the diagnosis of fetal malformations. During the second and third trimester, 3D US makes possible a completely new way of visual perception of unborn baby. Reconstructions and sculpture-like images, generated from surface-rendering mode, are the most impressive presentations. Three-dimensional imaging of the fetal surface greatly refines and expands our capabilities in the evaluation of normal anatomy (Figure 14.1) and in the detection of fetal anomalies.[1-11]

Fetal surface abnormalities can be selectively visualized and the extension of the defect can be determined in all spatial dimensions. The additional information is obtained by means of improved visualization rate, possibility of volume measurement and visualization of spatial relations between the surface and inner structures. Therefore, 3D US examination is a complementary technique for the evaluation of fetal malformations, after the initial assessment with two-dimensional ultrasound (2D US). As shown by Dyson et al, 3D US images provide additional information in 51%, in 45%, they are equivalent to 2D US and in 4% inapt for the depiction of certain anomalies.[1] 3D US is most helpful in evaluating the fetuses with facial anomalies,[2-5] hand and foot abnormalities,[6,7] spinal and neural tube defects.[1]

HEAD AND NECK

Fetal head evaluation is the important part of sonographic examination due to various physiological variations and association with malformations and chromosomal abnormalities.[9-11] Even under optimal conditions, the position of fetal head may not permit to produce adequate images with 2D US. In addition, many cross sectional images are required to obtain a complete impression about the structure of the fetal cranium. Volume rendered 3D images of the fetal head can be rotated into various spatial positions. This allows the evaluation of different projections of the head in a rapid and repeatable manner from the earliest stage of pregnancy. 3D US can demonstrate two basic anatomic parts of the head: the neurocranium, containing the brain and viscerocranium, composed of facial structures and skeleton. Even during the early second trimester, scanning with 3D probe enables the visualization of major head anomalies, such as acranius and anencephaly (Figures 14.2A and B).[9,10]

Dysmorphic appearance of the fetal cranium and anencephaly is better understood when fetal head and neck

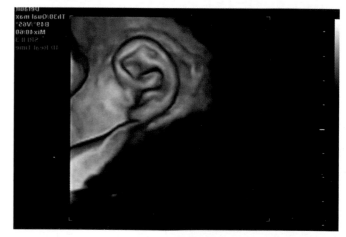

FIGURE 14.1: 3D surface rendering of the fetal ear at 38 weeks.

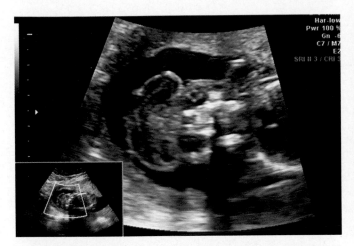

FIGURE 14.2A: Acranius-anencephalus sequence visualized by B-mode ultrasound at 17 weeks gestation.

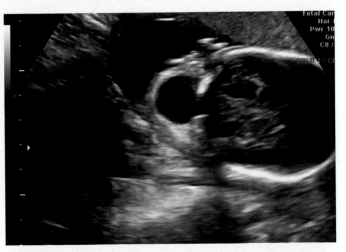

FIGURE 14.3A: B-mode ultrasound of an encephalocele.

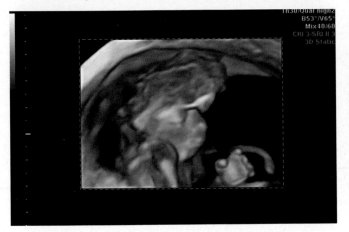

FIGURE 14.2B: Acranius-anencephalus sequence demonstrated by surface-rendering mode.

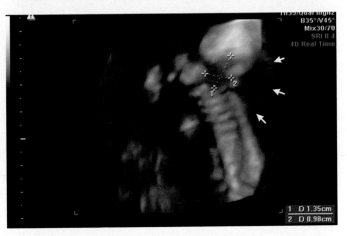

FIGURE 14.3B: 3D maximum mode for the evaluation of occipital bone defect in a fetus with encephalocele.

are demonstrated by 3D volume scanning.[9] In acrania, we can clearly differentiate the fetal brain as area cerebrovasculosa covering the skull and orbits in form of protuberances on the top of the head.

Simultaneous display of three orthogonal planes provides the better visualization of encephalocele.[1] Despite its relatively high sensitivity, 2D US is inferior to 3D US in evaluation of the exact location of the extracranial mass and amount of extracranial tissue (Figures 14.3A and B).

Fetal hydrocephaly is one of the most common malformations detected by ultrasonography, also assessed by 3D US.[9,11] 3D reconstruction of intracranial contents offers insight view of dilated bilateral ventricles and thin brain mantle (Figures 14.4A and B).

It has been demonstrated that cases of unilateral ventriculomegaly are better assessed with 3D US. This technique permits better delineation of the anatomic level

of brain malformation.[9,10] Intracranial echo-free spaces, such as dilated ventricles, enlarged cisterna magna and Dandy-Walker cyst are necessary for obtaining adequate 3D acoustic window.[11,12] If holoprosencephaly is present, 3D surface images of CNS structures can be obtained by electronically eliminating the calvaria from the image.

3D sonography is particularly useful for the evaluation of the midline anomalies, due to the reconstruction of the midsagittal plane by using multiplanar or volume-contrast-imaging (VCI) mode. The midsagittal view of the fetal brain enables simultaneous visualization of the structures, such as corpus callosum and cerebellar vermis. A combination of sonographic appearance of these two structures is helpful in differentiating the cause of ventriculomegaly: failure to demonstrate corpus callosum means partial or complete corpus callosum-agenesis. Posterior fossa, small and funneling, could be a sign for Chiari II—malformation.

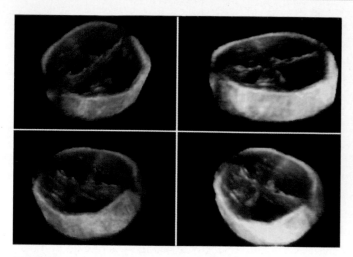

FIGURE 14.4A: Surface rendering of hydrocephaly. The midline echo and choroid plexus are normal, while brain tissue is significantly reduced.

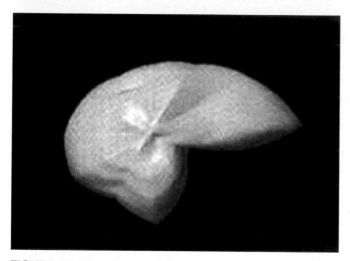

FIGURE 14.4B: 3D volume extraction and volumetric analysis of a dilated lateral ventricle (*Courtesy:* V D'Addario).[12]

Cerebellar vermis, hypoplastic and upward rotated, with enlarged 4th ventricle, could signalize a Dandy-Walker malformation. 3D US has become a fundamental tool for a complete neurosonographic examination, especially when 4D-evaluation of fetal behavioral patterns is included by applying recently introduced KANET score: structural analysis completed by functional analysis.[12,13]

Absent interhemispheric fissure, common ventricle and thalamic fusion are characteristics of holoprosencephaly (HPE). Three-dimensional ultrasound assists in detection and classification of this defect.[14] With incidence of one in ten to twenty-thousand live born children,[15] HPE is the most common fetal forebrain malformation. Categorization of HPE is based on the degree of separation of the forebrain (telencephalon). *Alobar* HPE is diagnosed, if a single ventricle is seen, whereas *semilobar* HPE shows at least some separation of the forebrain. *Lobar* HPE shows the highest degree of forebrain separation and is likely to be missed on standard ultrasound examination.[15] The most severe facial malformations are usually associated with alobar holoprosencephaly. Most fetuses with holoprosencephaly have associated craniofacial fusion defects, such as cleft lip/palate, hypotelorism, cyclopia, cebocephaly, and ethmocephaly.[16] Since 3D US is the method of choice for the evaluation of the fetal face, the 3D exam could be useful in the determination of severity and extent of this malformation.[14]

A relatively new display technique of 3D inversion rendering inverts anechoic structures (brain ventricles) that are displayed in black by conventional gray-scale, into colorized cast-like appearance, as described in 2008 by Timor-Tritsch et al.[15] The resulting display enables a 3D perception of the normal or deviant ventricular system of the brain. 3D inversion rendering constitutes a new tool to define brain anomalies and is especially useful in the classification of HPE.[15]

Examination of the fetal face is the basic part of ultrasonic examination for low-risk and high-risk pregnancies. Unfortunately, it can be analyzed only to a limited extent by conventional 2D sonography. Fetal position, gestational age, movements, hands covering the face, maternal obesity and technical limitations are the reasons for difficulties in diagnosis of facial abnormalities. During the second trimester, the examination of fetal face includes a complete impression of the head, face and profile followed by identification of normal frontal bones and forehead, orbits, eyelids, nose, philtrum, upper and lower lip, chin and cheeks. Some defects with prominent superficial changes, such as cleft lip, facial dysmorphia, anophthalmia and proboscis are easier to depict with 3D surface mode.[2,3,16] These facial deformities are important markers for chromosomal abnormalities and 3D US technology may be useful in increasing the selectivity of ultrasound screening.[2,17,18] Three-dimensional surface-mode provides clear image of all structures and deformities previously mentioned, particularly if associated with the appropriate amount of amniotic fluid in front of the fetal face.[19] To obtain the best surface-mode rendering, the face has to be directly oriented toward the transducer and the pocket of amniotic fluid should be located between the transducer and surface of the face. Because of this practical

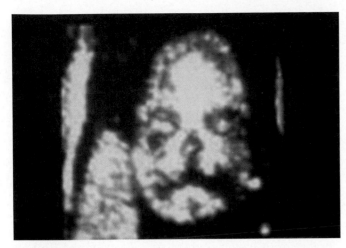

FIGURE 14.5A: Cleft lip and palate demonstrated by transparent mode.

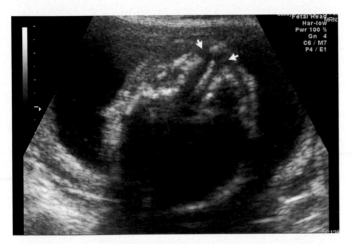

FIGURE 14.5B: Bilateral cleft demonstrated by B-mode ultrasound.

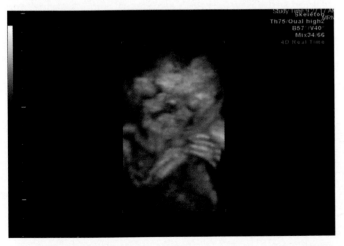

FIGURE 14.5C: Surface rendering/maximum mode of the bilateral cleft defect.

problem, multiplanar view has become the most important modality for the evaluation of the normal and abnormal anatomy of the fetal face during the past few years.[20]

One of the first investigators who reported about 3D ultrasound imaging of the fetal face were Pretorius and coworkers.[3] They were able to obtain satisfactory images of fetal face in 24 of 27 studied fetuses. Higher quality images were produced only in scans after 19 weeks of gestation, possibly due to the better anatomic definition of fetal structural details.

Malformations of palate and lips (fetal cleft lip/palate) are among the most frequent craniofacial malformations with an estimated incidence of about 0.1% births.[21] Before the introduction of 3D US detection rates of cleft lip/palate were very low (21 to 30%).[22] Three-dimensional ultrasound is helpful in the visualization of these abnormalities. Using this modality, the investigator can rotate the image to gain the impression about the depth of the defect (Figures 14.5A to C). A simple cleft lip, for example, can be reliably differentiated from a more severe cleft involving the lip, maxilla and palate.

With time, multiplanar view became fundamental for the detection of the facial malformations. Volume rendered data offer a real benefit for the analysis of some "subsurface" structures within the fetal head. It is possible to obtain three orthogonal slices of palate, pharynx and soft tissues regardless of intrauterine head position. In evaluation of these anomalies, lips may be better assessed by 3D US. Johnson and coworkers correctly detected cleft lip in all affected fetuses with 3D and in 93% with 2D US.[20] The opportunity to see the fetal face in the standard anatomic orientation on surface rendered image allows a more confident interpretation. Sequential transverse views may be obtained easily with 3D US and in the area of the upper lip they could confirm the presence of a cleft lip and help in the precise detection of the location. Appearance of the tooth germs can provide important diagnostic clues for cleft palate and are evaluated as parameters of normal development. In affected fetuses underdeveloped, supernumerary, or missing lateral maxillary incisors may be detected. Ulm and coworkers reported that 3D US allowed the visualization of tooth germs in 31% of the fetuses.[23] On the other hand, tooth germs were obtained in only 8.8% fetuses using 2D ultrasonography. There are also several advantages of 3D US in evaluation of the fetal palate. By using the interactive display, planar views may be manipulated without concern for fetal movement. Also surface-rendering image in combination with planar views could ensure that the loss of signal in fetuses with palate defect is not due to the insonation angle, and that the view of the face is symmetrical. With combination of these modalities, it is easy to differentiate the maxilla from the mandible. Another advantage is better understanding of the defect by the parents. Recent studies demonstrated that primary cleft palate could be diagnosed by 3D US in 86% of the cases.[20] Therefore, 3D US is not only a good tool for identification, but also for better localization of the defects.

Lee and coworkers proposed a standardized approach for evaluation of the cleft lip and palate by 3D US.[24] They used multiplanar view for examination of the upper lip, and axial views for evaluation of the maxillary tooth bearing alveolar ridge and anterior tooth socket alignment. Combination of multiplanar view and surface-rendering view was the best combination for the successful detection of premaxillary protrusion. Incomplete integrity of the alveolar ridge was used as a sign of cleft palate and a presence of premaxillary protrusion as a sign of bilateral cleft lip and palate. Surface rendering has increased diagnostic confidence by confirming findings that were initially suspected by multiplanar views.[24] Using this method, the authors analyzed seven fetuses with facial clefting anomalies. For example, in fetuses with unilateral cleft lip/palate positive predictive value was up to 100%. On the other hand, in the group with bilateral cleft lip/palate, positive predictive value was only 75%. A combined use of different 3D US modalities gives opportunity to easily assess rare morphological anomalies, such as single nostril, flat nose, proboscis, cyclopia, hypertelorism and hypotelorism.[2,17,23,25] The anomalies of the fetal mandible can be also recognized and confirmed by 3D US. They are a common feature of many chromosomal and genetic syndromes.[26] For example, micrognatia is associated with Robins, Treacher-Collins, Pena-Shokier, Seckel and many other syndromes.

Advantages of 3D US in visualization of fetal mandible are:

- Reduced time for evaluation of the fetal mandible.
- Increased precision of the measurements.
- Better assessment of the posterior displacement and restriction in size of the fetal mandible.
- Multiplanar imaging and ability to store the representative volumes provide opportunity to make objective diagnosis and teleconsultation.[27]

Surface rendering and multiplanar imaging by 3D US were used by Rotten and coworkers to assess the most common anomalies of fetal mandible, such as retrognathia and micrognathia. Retrognathia (posterior displacement of the fetal mandible) was assessed by the measurement of the inferior facial angle. All fetuses with anomalies of the mandible had an inferior facial angle below the cut-off value of 50 degrees. The sensitivity for predicting retrognathia was 100%, specificity 98%, positive predictive value 75% and negative predictive value 100%.[27]

Lateral head abnormalities, such as auricular deformities and low-set ears could also be detected using the same imaging strategy.[28] Development of the ears includes migration into the final temporal location and axis rotation from an anterior-transverse to a lateral-vertical orientation. Because of the complex embryonic development, fetal ear abnormalities are frequent and there are numerous physiological variations and minor ear malformations. Usually, they are without clinical significance. On the other hand, most severe ear abnormalities are associated with complex syndromes, chromosomopathies and acquired embryopathies due to infections, ischemia and toxic exposure.[29] Therefore, whenever malformation of the fetal ear is suspected or recognized, a systematic fetal anatomy scan is recommended. It is difficult to recognize a congenital anomaly of the fetal ear in utero, due to its complex embryonic development and the inability of 2D US to demonstrate auricular geometry. However, with 3D US, it appears that ear abnormalities may be detected by the end of second trimester. Shih and coworkers showed new possibilities of 3D US in the systematic analysis of the fetal ear and achieved better detection rates than with 2D US (84% versus 52.8%).[2] One of the most important advantages of 3D US is evaluation of the auricula. Due to surface rendering auricula structures, such as helix and tragus are better visualized.

Spatial information, such as location and axis orientation can also be evaluated by 3D US. The major axis of normal auricula is vertical and parallel to the head. The normal orientation is anterolateral, with the superior border pointing towards the cranium. Spatial information allows the detection of low-set ears and ear asymmetry. Dysplastic ears are present in 60% fetuses with Down syndrome[30] and trisomy 18.

Chang and coworkers developed charts of normal fetal ear-growth indices (ear length, ear width and ear area) and evaluated their efficacy in the diagnosis of fetal aneuploidy.[30] Combination of these three measurements increased the sensitivity and specificity in the detection of fetal trisomies to 57.1% and 83.2%, respectively.

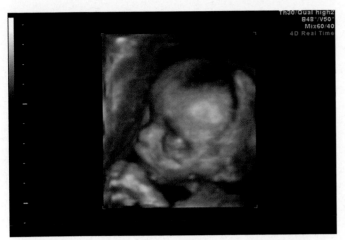

FIGURE 14.6A: Surface rendering of frontal bossing in a fetus with achondroplasia.

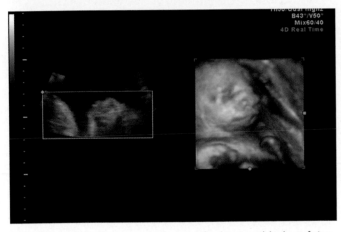

FIGURE 14.6B: Surface rendering of micrognathia in a fetus with Edwards' syndrome.

Clearly 3D ultrasound is superior to conventional sonography in the following cases:
- Fetal cleft lip and palate.
- Abnormal curvature of fetal face in a profile reconstruction.
- Minor defects of fetal face related to chromosomal abnormalities.
- Fetal face/profile dysmorphism related to chromosomal, systemic or metabolic disorders (pterygium syndrome, skeletal dysplasias) (Figures 14.6A and B).
- Facial profile investigation: micrognathia, absent nose and frontal bossing.
- Fetal tooth germs investigations (oligodontia or anodontia).

In the neck region, ultrasound can detect increased nuchal thickness, cystic hygromas, occipital cephalocele, thyroid tumors, etc.[18, 31]

FETAL SPINE

3D surface rendering enables accurate surface analysis of the fetuses with dorsal cleft anomalies. Using multiplanar and surface rendering the level and the extent of protrusive lesion are precisely assessed.[17] Complete rachischysis, isolated spina bifida, myelomeningocele, and some other defects of the spinal column are easily depicted (Figures 14.7 to 14.9).

The optimal period for the evaluation of the fetal spine is between 12 and 16 weeks gestation. Sometimes the

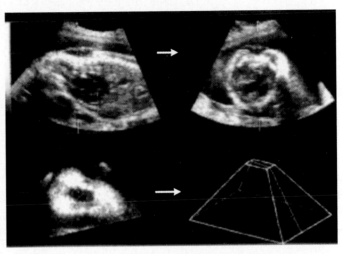

FIGURE 14.7: Lumbar myelomeningocele by multiplanar view. The surface of the fetal skin and open neural tube defect are clearly demonstrated.

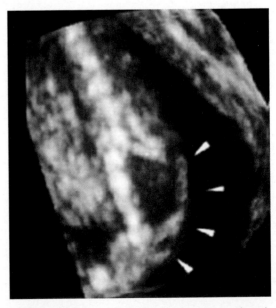

FIGURE 14.8: Myelomeningocele by surface rendered mode. Neural tube defect at the lumbar level is clearly visualized.

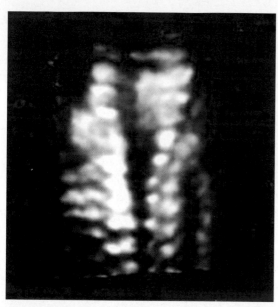

FIGURE 14.9. Severe rachischysis by transparent mode. In the upper thoracic spine widening of ossification centers of the vertebral bodies are visualized.

examination of the area of interest is not possible due to unfavorable fetal position. Therefore, indirect intracranial signs of spinal malformations like the so called "botanical signs" are used, such as "lemon and banana sign." Screening for these signs of spinal malformations is a part of the routine prenatal sonographic exam. "Banana sign" is present in up to 70% of cases with open spina bifida during the second trimester, with a sensitivity of up to 99%.[32] False negative findings were documented in fetuses with smaller and skin-covered lesions. Other areas of superiority of 3D US imaging are visualization of scoliosis and subtle neural tube defects with minimal or no changes in bone structures. For all practical purposes, 3D US can help the less experienced sonographer to successfully detect these anomalies in a low-risk group of patients. Accurate identification of the level of spina bifida, and of the extent of the defect is very important in counseling the families, and has significant impact on decision about the termination of pregnancy and obstetric management.

The practical steps of 3D image evaluation include the use of the surface rendering, and sagittal and/or coronal planar views for the assessment of the transverse view through the vertebral bodies. Simultaneous multiplanar view through the same vertebral body offers a more accurate identification of the level of the neural tube defect.[33] In fetuses with myelomeningocele, the sac can be "electronically resected" to demonstrate the actual surface defect, even if the orifice is quite small.

HEART

Congenital heart anomalies are one of the most commonly occurring congenital malformations. The four-chamber view of the fetal heart is used for screening and is included in the standard views of ultrasound examination of the fetal heart. By visualization of a normal four-chamber view only 40% or less fetal congenital heart defects can be excluded.[34] The search for a more improved type of cardiac examination providing better assessment of cardiac anatomy, especially in low-risk population, led to the implementation of guidelines for basic and extended cardiac examination, by adding standard views like left ventricular outflow tract (LVOT), right ventricular outflow tract (RVOT) and three-vessel view.[35]

Using 3D US, Bonilla-Musoles and coworkers were able to visualize the fetal heart in 11% of cases. They were able to visualize outer contours but no internal structures.[36] With 2D US, fetal heart and four-chamber view was clearly depicted in 97% of cases.[36] Zosmer and coworkers observed intracardiac anatomy by transparency display, and were able to obtain high quality cardiac images as early as 20 weeks of gestation.[37] When 3D US examination of the adult heart with the regular rhythm is performed, 3D data are usually acquired over a period of many heart beats, monitored by an electrocardiogram (ECG). A 3D image at each part of the cardiac cycle is constructed using data only from that particular part. For a fetus, an ECG for synchronization is not obtainable. Nelson and coworkers[38,39] solved this problem by using the movement of the heart wall/valve instead of the ECG and constructed 3D images of the fetal heart without distortion due to beating.[40] The same authors measured the cardiac output based on volume change of the lumen of the fetal heart.[41] However, much time was required to obtain 3D data and fetal movements were a significant problem. Meyer-Wittkopf and coworkers then developed a novel 3D US system with Doppler-based phasing of the fetal cardiac cycle.[40] Volume acquisition time is reduced to <30 sec and provides spatial and temporal assessment of the beating fetal heart. Using this technique scanning time is much reduced and does not require specialized scanning skills to obtain standard views. Unfortunately, 3D US with this new technique enabled visualization of standard cardiac views in only 19 of 30 fetuses.[40] The same views were well visualized in all but one fetus using 2D US. However, there was some additional information provided with 3D US, including structural depth, dynamic 3D perspective of valvular morphology and ventricular wall motion.

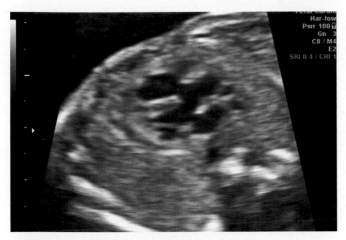

FIGURE 14.10A: B-mode ultrasound of the overriding aorta.

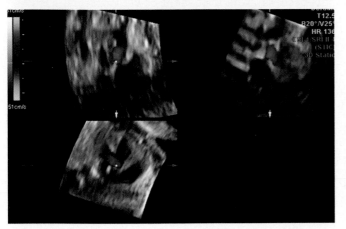

FIGURE 14.10B: STIC by color Doppler ultrasound of the overriding aorta. Navigation through three orthogonal planes increased diagnostic accuracy.

From 2003 onwards, four-dimensional (4D) visualization of the fetal heart became a practical reality with the incorporation of spatio-temporal image correlation (STIC) (Figures 14.10A and B) algorithms into commercially available equipment. This matured technique allows the acquisition of the fetal heart and visualization of the cardiac structures as a 4D cine sequence. Color and power Doppler can be incorporated into the examination and thus permit additional hemodynamic analysis of the volume dataset. Navigation through the *dataset* in the absence of the patient after obtaining the volume with a single sweep of the 4D probe opens completely new doors for expert review, telemedicine, interdisciplinary consultation with the pediatric cardiologist/surgeon, teaching students and counseling of the parents. Naturally, STIC cannot be used in fetuses with cardiac arrhythmias.

Also, *offline* analysis requires a second appointment to discuss results. In multiplanar mode, the simultaneously produced orthogonal planes A, B and C allow virtual views like coronal view of mitral and tricuspid valve, which are normally inaccessible.[41,42]

ABDOMEN

Omphalocele and gastroschisis are the most commonly identified malformations of the abdominal wall (Figures 14.11A to D). Other ventral abdominal wall defects (cloacal exstrophy, bladder exstrophy, bodystalk syndrome and pentalogy of Cantrell) occur in a much lower incidence than gastroschisis and omphalocele but they are much more severe. Distinction between these two anomalies has prognostic implications and can usually be accomplished with 2D US.[1] Omphalocele is a defect in the anterior abdominal wall with extrusion of abdominal contents into

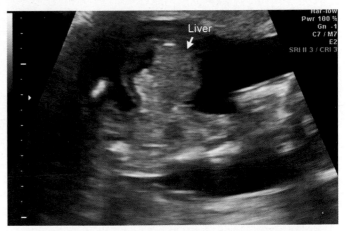

FIGURE 14.11A: B-mode sonogram, demonstrating an omphalocele at 16-weeks gestation.

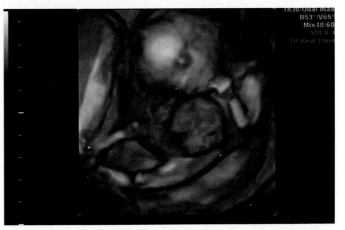

FIGURE 14.11B: 3D surface rendering of the same fetus with omphalocele.

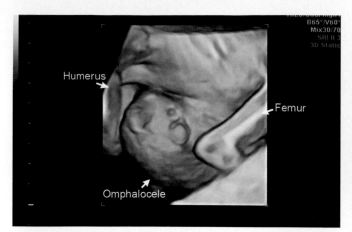

FIGURE 14.11C: Surface rendered view of omphalocele.

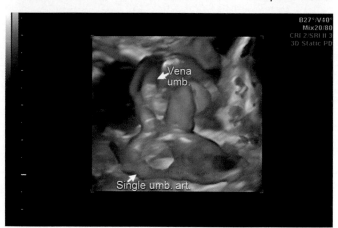

FIGURE 14.11D: The same fetus as in Figures 14.10A to C. Three-dimensional power Doppler glass body rendering of a single umbilical artery and vein and their separation/deviation due to omphalocele.

the base of the umbilical cord. The abdominal content is surrounded by a thin membrane, consisting of a parietal peritoneum and amnion.[43]

On contrast, in fetuses with gastroschisis intestinal loops float freely in the amniotic fluid without any covering membrane. The bowel prolapse occurs through a small paraumbilical defect that involves all layers of the abdominal wall and is mostly right sided. Gastroschisis (Figures 14.12A to C) is usually an isolated entity, rarely associated with other malformations and chromosomopathies. However, omphalocele is usually associated with chromosomal abnormalities, such as trisomy 18 and 13, triploidy and Klinefelter's syndrome. It can appear in a variety of syndromes, most notably, Beckwith-Wiedemann syndrome (omphalocele, macroglossia, organomegaly and neonatal hypoglycemia), pentalogy of Cantrell (midline

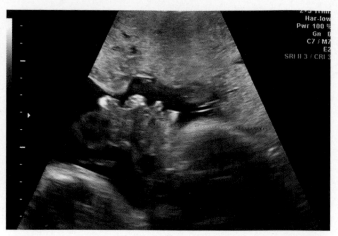

FIGURE 14.12A: Transverse axial plane of fetal abdomen with gastroschisis. Note uncovered bowel loops and uncertain umbilical cord position.

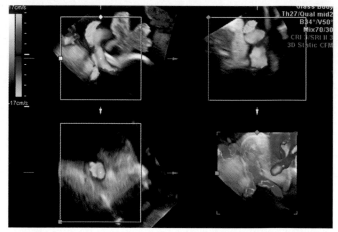

FIGURE 14.12B: The same fetus evaluated by 3D CD ultrasound. Note three orthogonal planes depicting abdominal wall defect on the right side of umbilical vessel entry/exit.

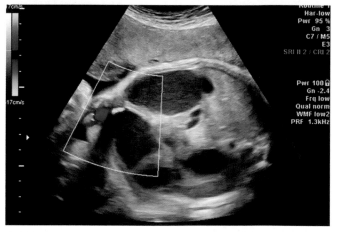

FIGURE 14.12C: 2D color Doppler image of the same fetus. Note distended intra-abdominal bowel segments suggestive of obstructive changes due to abdominal wall defect.

supraumbilical abdominal defect, sternal defect, intracardiac anomaly, deficiency of diaphragmatic pericardium and anterior diaphragm) and cloacal exstrophy (OEIS-complex: omphalocele, exstrophy of the bladder, imperforate anus and spina bifida). In fetuses with ventral body clefts, 3D US allows better visualization of the defect and prolapsed organs.[17] Although most of these defects are large and well depicted by 2D US, the rotational 3D display enables better view of the defect from multiple angles and gives much better impression about the extent and severity of the anomaly. Even in omphalocele and gastroschisis where depiction rate with 2D US is nearly 100%, 3D US has some advantages, such as surface-rendering view enabling sculpture-like reconstruction of the abdominal wall defects. Using this modality, the type, size and extension of the defect are precisely determined, as well as the umbilical cord position and the peritoneal coverage. The prognosis of the anterior wall defect depends on its association with other anomalies or chromosomal abnormalities. The prognosis is less dependent on the size of the defect or time of the diagnosis. However, the outcome is less favorable when there is evidence of bowel thickening, distension of bowel loops or other affected abdominal organs. In these cases, multiplanar view and volumetric evaluation of exteriorized abdominal contents may contribute to better prediction of neonatal outcome.

With the use of 3D US imaging, structural changes of the fetal skin surface also can be evaluated, enabling prenatal diagnosis of congenital ichthyosis.[44]

Image postprocessing enables surface imaging of the intra-abdominal structures. It is possible to construct any slice nearly parallel to the mother's abdominal wall in arbitrary section or orthogonal triple-section display. Using this approach, it is possible to observe the esophageal-gastric junction and pylorus. The electronic scalpel or electronic rubber may be used to "cut off" the overlying body segments. Longitudinal or transverse sections can also be evaluated.

Recent studies demonstrate that 3D US may aid in diagnosis of multicystic dysplastic kidney, renal agenesis and abnormalities of the uretero-vesical junction.[45] Surface rendering also provides anatomic details of normal and abnormal genitalia. Normal genitalia are best visualized in midsagittal plane.[45]

Abnormalities of the fetal genital system, such as ambiguous genitalia, hypospadia and bipartite scrotum could be precisely assessed by multiplanar view and surface rendering.[46]

SKELETON AND EXTREMITIES

3D US gives clear display of curved structures, such as fetal spine, ribs, skull and extremities in a single rendered image.[6,7,17,47] Using these techniques, it is possible to assess skeletal development and related abnormalities. Transparent mode, maximum mode and "X-ray like" imaging are particularly useful for the visualization of the fetal skeleton. This technique includes the volume rendering combining minimum and maximum intensity mode. Transparent mode allows imaging of the fetal skeleton and depiction of the skeletal malformations in spatial orientation.

The vertebral column is originally curved anteroposteriorly. If it is pathologically curved laterally, it is impossible that the entire vertebral column may be displayed in one two-dimensional (2D) tomogram. Anomalies, such as scoliosis, particularly related to neural tube defects and hemivertebra, kyphosis and lordosis may be difficult to demonstrate with conventional 2D US (Figures 14.13A and B). The advantage of 3D US is the ability to visualize both curvatures at the same time.[33]

The overall incidence of congenital skeletal anomalies is about 20 cases per 100,000 births.[48] A number of these disorders are lethal, such as thanatophoric dysplasia, achondrogenesis, osteogenesis imperfect type II, etc. Therefore, confident antenatal diagnosis would give an option to the patient to terminate the pregnancy. Other skeletal dysplasias are associated with mental retardation. This information is very important in prenatal counseling. Furthermore, in most cases 2D ultrasonography does not allow correct and precise prenatal diagnosis. Among all other skeletal disorders, shortened ribs and narrow chest have been seen in fetuses with skeletal dysplasias. Such a finding is significant because chest restriction leads to pulmonary hypoplasia, a frequent cause of death in these conditions.

These malformations can be better depicted using 3D surface imaging and transparent mode reconstruction together.[49] The curvature and relationship of the rib ends to the vertebral bodies and sternum can be visualized, as well as the entire spinal length. The transparent mode is useful for detecting abnormalities of the fetal thorax, but in some conditions, such as a very narrow thorax, surface mode could be of additional clinical importance. Rotation of rendered volume data is helpful in detecting significant thoracic disproportion relative to the abdomen.

Surface mode is useful for the investigation of the fetal cranial bone structures.[50] Starting from 12 weeks cranial bones and sutures in between, are easily detectable. The

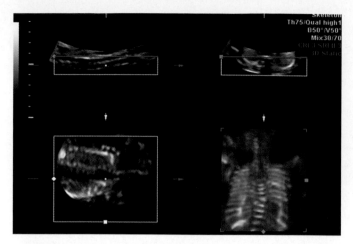

FIGURE 14.13A: 3D maximum mode demonstrating thoracic hemivertebra.

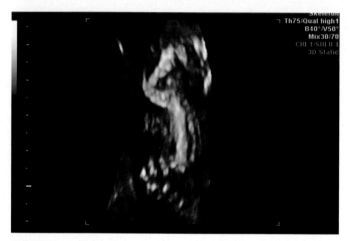

FIGURE 14.13B: 3D maximum mode demonstrating extreme kyphosis and lordosis of the vertebra in acranius-anencephalus sequence at 16-weeks gestation.

sagittal suture, lambdoid suture and posterior fontanelle are recognizable from 13 weeks onward.[3] Abnormalities of the sutures and fontanelles may be related to delayed closure or widening, craniosynostosis or abnormal cranial contours, such as cloverleaf skull. In fetuses with achondroplasia, widening of the frontal suture, caused by delayed ossification of the cranium, can be evaluated with 3D US.[51]

Abnormalities of fetal hands or feet may be associated with skeletal dysplasia and chromosomopathies, such as trisomy 13, 18 and 21.[6,7,51] 3D US clearly displays both normal and abnormal extremities[6,7,17] and allows improved visualization of the fetal hands and feet.

Surface-rendering mode can demonstrate changes of the normal anatomical axis of the extremities. With 3D US, two orthogonal sections can be displayed simultaneously.

The section at the exact midpoint of the limb can be obtained. Using this orientation, reversible or irreversible pathological angulations of the normal anatomical axis can be visualized.[17] Precise topographic relationship between the segments of each limb, but also of the wrist, hand and finger could be assessed. Fetal position and neurological damage can cause congenital deformities and contractures of joints and limbs. Their spatial relationship may be evaluated synchronously in three orthogonal planes. Using 3D US fingers and toes are very well observed, allowing prenatal diagnosis of syndactyly, polydactyly and overlapping fingers.[6,7]

Ploeckinger-Ulm and coworkers studied 72 fetuses from low-risk pregnancies and showed that 3D US enabled a complete visualization of all fingers in significantly higher proportion of the fetuses than 2D US (74.3% versus 52.9%), $p < 0.05$).[52] The optimal time for 3D US evaluation was between 20 and 23 weeks of gestation. With 2D US, one hand was visualized in 93% of cases and in 100% of cases using 3D US. According to these authors, advantages of 3D US were the following:

- The ability to rotate stored images into any plane until all fingers are evaluated.
- Rotation of stored 3D volume rendered images allows a more comprehensive evaluation of the fetal toes and fingers.
- Storage of the volume data allows systematic offline retrospective review and analysis of any structure of interest.

It is important to note that there are some fetuses in which it is not possible to scan adequate volumes of the hands and feet and accurately count digits due to rapid movements of extremities. This is to be stressed particularly for pregnancies less than 19 weeks.

Budorick et al, studied hands of 44 fetuses from high-risk pregnancies.[6] Hands and fingers were correctly diagnosed in all cases of normal and abnormal anatomy by both 3D US and 2D US. The advantages of 3D US were the following:

- Flexed fingers could be precisely assessed.
- The thumb could be evaluated simultaneously with the other fingers.
- The phalanges and metacarpals could be accurately counted and measured in normal hands, included even when fingers were flexed.[31,34]

In pathological cases, 3D US enabled better understanding of the spatial relationships between wrist, hand and fingers. In the study of Hata and coworkers, the percentage of visualization of the fetal digits with 3D US was 74%, which is in fair agreement with the report of Ploeckinger-Ulm and coworkers.[47,52] Optimal visualization of the fetal digits was achieved between 28 and 35 weeks of gestation. One of the reasons for this difference could be that Hata and coworkers used only the surface-rendering mode. Before 15 weeks or after 36 weeks, the respective percentages decreased. The ability to evaluate fetal fingers was better with 3D US than 2D US during the late first trimester and early second trimester. Evaluation of the distal extremity is difficult with 2D US because visualization of the relationship between tibia/fibula and the hind foot and forefoot is required. Optimal 2D US evaluation of the distal extremities needs a sagittal plane through the lower part of the leg. This plane is of crucial importance for the evaluation of the relationship of the tibia and fibula to the ankle and enables evaluation of the pathological angulations in fetuses with clubfoot and arthrogryposis.

According to Budorick and coworkers, normal legs were better assessed with 3D US than 2D US (85% versus 52%).[7] Rotation of the rendered volumes of the distal extremities provided additional information in assessing and understanding foot position. Although 3D US did not significantly improve the ability to distinguish normal from abnormal distal extremities, the authors stressed a significant shortening of the learning curve for less experienced sonographers in evaluating lower limb anomalies. The list of abnormalities of distal extremities included: clubfoot, rocker bottom feet, polydactyly and single bone short leg.

Kos and coworkers studied 41 out of 347 high-risk patients with initial diagnosis of limb abnormalities by 2D US.[53] The abnormal distal extremities were observed in 28 out of 41 suspected cases. According to these authors, positive predictive value for 2D US in detection of clubfoot was lower in comparison to the positive predictive value of 3D US (67.8% versus 89.9%) (Table 14.1). Three-dimensional US accurately visualized angular limb deformities (clubfoot), contracture of the limbs, shortening and bowing of the limbs, polydactyly and overlapping fingers (Figures 14.14A to D).

Best spatial reconstruction by 3D US was achieved in the case of fetal arthrogryposis associated with extremely reduced movements.

According to Kos et al.[53], the advantages of 3D US in the assessment of fetal skeletal anomalies are the following:

• Transparent-mode reconstruction is useful in the detection of polydactyly since it emphasizes strong reflecting surfaces of additional fingers and related skeleton.

• Surface mode provides additional help in the assessment of the surface anatomy and integrity of the skin cover. It is the most efficient modality for the diagnosis of

TABLE 14.1: Initial diagnosis obtained by 2D ultrasound compared to 3D sonography and diagnosis at the time of delivery

Suspected anomaly	2D US	3D US	Diagnosis at birth
Clubfoot	28	17	19
Hand polydactyly	5	3	3
Overlapping finger	0	1	1
Upper limb contractures	3	2	2
Lower limb contractures	1	1	1
Micromelia	4	4	4
Total	41	28	30

(With permission from reference Kos et al.[53])

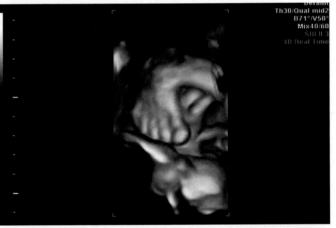

FIGURE 14.14A: 3D surface rendering of the right clubfoot. Note medial angulation of the foot.

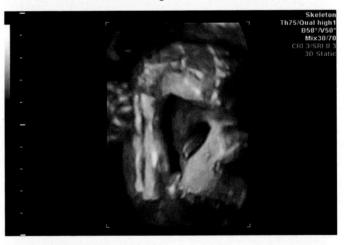

FIGURE 14.14B: Right leg in maximum mode. Note pathological angulation of tibia/fibula with the foot.

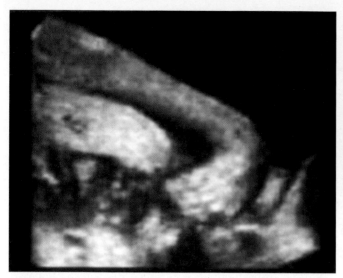

FIGURE 14.14C: Clubfoot by surface rendered mode. Note severe medial angulation of the foot and contracture of the knee joint with fixed hyperextension.

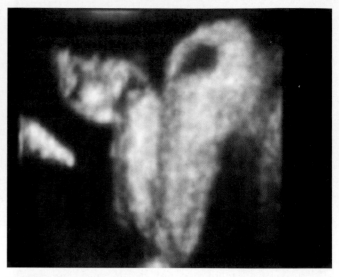

FIGURE 14.15A: Reconstruction of the fetal arm by surface rendered mode. Irreversible adductional contracture of the elbow-joint and flexion of the wrist are visualized.

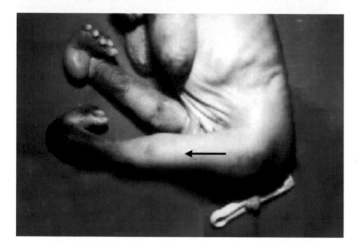

FIGURE 14.14D: Pathomorphological specimen of the aborted fetus with congenital arthrogryposis.

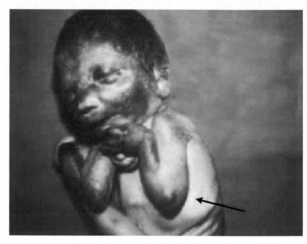

FIGURE 14.15B: Pathomorphological specimen of the same fetus with congenital arthrogryposis.

angular deformation and joint contractures especially in cases with optimal amount of amniotic fluid (Figures 14.15A to 14.17C).

Bone structures of the fetal skeleton can be depicted by 3D transparent mode, maximum mode and "X-ray like" mode, providing clear images of the structures with highest echogenicity. Using these modalities of 3D imaging, it was possible to perform a spatial reconstruction of the affected skeletal parts. These techniques enable detailed analysis of the normal skeletal anatomy, but also the reconstruction of the structural and topographic abnormalities in fetuses with skeletal dysplasias. Using maximum mode imaging and volume rendering of the data allows for visualization of the surface features, soft tissues and internal skeletal structures. The most advanced application of 3D sonography is real-time 3D or 4D ultrasonography. This modality enables better functional evaluation of the fetal joints and related segments of the musculoskeletal system. Surface rendering is very useful for the evaluation of the shortened and curved "bulky" extremities, in fetuses with severe

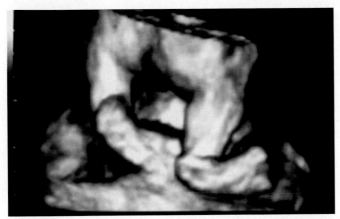

FIGURE 14.16: Severe micromelia by surface rendered mode. Note shortening, bowing and pathological angulation of the lower extremities.

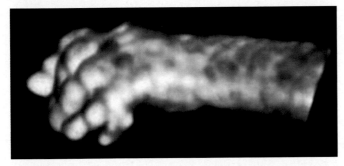

FIGURE 14.17A: Surface reconstruction of the fetal forearm, wrist and fingers with postaxial polydactyly.

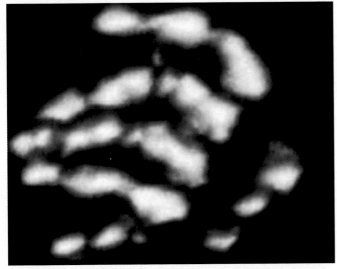

FIGURE 14.17B: Fetal metacarpals and phalanges by transparent mode. An extra digit is clearly visible.

micromelic dwarfism. Using "maximum-mode" or "X-ray-like" postprocessing features, the reconstruction of the fetal skeleton results in a complete "baby-gram".

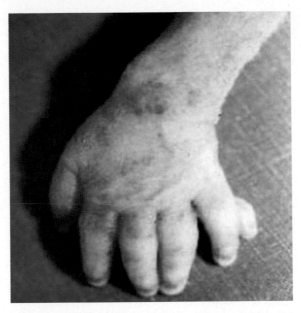

FIGURE 14.17C: Pathomorphological specimen of the aborted fetus: Fetal hand with postaxial polydactyly.

ROLE OF COLOR AND POWER DOPPLER ULTRASOUND

Despite the advances in 2D ultrasound imaging, assessment of the hemodynamic characteristics of blood flow in different organs and body systems was not possible without the use of the Doppler technology. Two-dimensional color Doppler (2D CD) and power Doppler ultrasound (2D PD) were shown to improve the prenatal diagnosis of malformations involving vascular system and topography of the fetal circulation. Also, it has been clearly confirmed that 3D US does offer wider possibilities of intrauterine orientation and topographic evaluation, particularly because of the volume rendering technology. Integration of 3D ultrasonography and power Doppler has resulted in three-dimensional power Doppler technology (3D PD), which was found to be useful in the evaluation of the vascular anatomy. The 3D power Doppler imaging technique is based on color powered ultrasound volume scanning, enabling noninvasive investigation of the normal and abnormal vascular anatomy and topography of circulation in 3D spatial orientation. Using this modality, we are able to depict 3D reconstructions of the intracranial aneurysms, umbilical knots and nuchal cords. Color and power Doppler ultrasound improves the prenatal diagnosis of malformations involving the cardiovascular system.[54,55] It provides additional information and facilitates the diagnosis by:

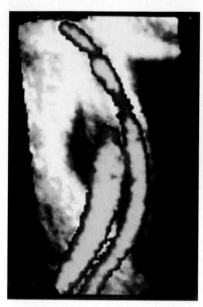

FIGURE 14.18: Umbilical cord with a single umbilical artery depicted by 3D power Doppler ultrasound. Note only one umbilical artery and umbilical vein.

- Establishing the topography and origin of a given anomaly.
- Depiction of the morphological defects of fetal circulation.
- Enabling precise differential diagnosis between malformations.
- Demonstration of the extracirculatory flow.[54]

Using 3D PD ultrasound, it is possible to differentiate the urinary bladder and other intra-abdominal cystic structures.[54] Two fetal hypogastric arteries surrounding the urinary bladder are identified with color Doppler ultrasound. Same modality provides information about the presence of only one umbilical artery[54,55] (Figure 14.18). Doppler also enables differential diagnosis to be made between obstructive intestinal pathology and bilateral megaureter by showing this circulation.[54]

The visualization of renal vessels is known to increase the accuracy of the diagnosis of kidney malformations. Renal arteries are easily recognizable using color and power Doppler ultrasound. Three-dimensional power Doppler ultrasound may aid in the diagnosis of renal agenesis, pelvic kidney and horseshoe kidney, detection of an accessory renal artery of a normal or a duplex kidney and depiction of abnormal vessel course in fetuses with cystic renal malformation.[55]

The absence of renal arteries confirms the diagnosis of renal agenesis in cases when such a diagnosis is unclear due to the poor image quality caused by oligohydramnios.[56] Sepulveda and coworkers assessed the role of power Doppler ultrasound in prenatal diagnosis of sirenomelia and sirenomelia sequence and fetuses with bilateral renal agenesis.[57] Both conditions were characterized by the absence of renal vessels. However, the two common iliac arteries were always visualized in the fetuses with renal agenesis, whereas absence of distal branching of the main abdominal vessel was a characteristic feature of sirenomelia. The conclusion of this study was that power Doppler ultrasound allows expeditious identification of the absent and/or nonfunctional renal arteries in fetuses with severe oligohydramnios.

An abnormal course and torsion of the intra-abdominal vessels shown by power Doppler ultrasound may be detected in fetuses with omphalocele, gastroschisis, congenital diaphragmatic hernia and hydrops.[55] In fetuses with right diaphragmatic hernia in whom the right liver lobe is herniated, the hepatic vessels with anomalous morphology of the portal system are clearly visualized by 3DPD.[54] Song and coworkers reported a case of bilateral congenital diaphragmatic hernia successfully diagnosed with color and power Doppler ultrasound at 33 weeks' gestation.[58]

Using 3DPD ultrasound, it is possible to detect dilatation of the umbilical vein and differentiate it from other pathology with the same appearance on B-mode ultrasound, such as hepatic, urachal, choledochal or mesenteric cysts.[54]

3D color Doppler may also be used for the evaluation of some heart anomalies, such as left isomerism and Scimitar syndrome.[55,59] Left isomerism is associated with an interruption of the inferior vena cava with the persistence of the azygous vein. Scimitar syndrome is a complex congenital cardiopulmonary anomaly. Michailidis and coworkers reported a case of Scimitar syndrome in which retrospective analysis of 3D color flow Doppler images of the fetal vasculature demonstrated the anomalous arterial supply of the right lung from the descending aorta.[59] The main feature was an anomalous vein draining blood from all or part of the right lung into the systemic venous circulation, usually the inferior vena cava. Associated features included hypoplasia of the right lung, secondary dextroposition of the fetal heart, anomalous systemic arterial supply to the right lung and other cardiac abnormalities. Scimitar syndrome was considered in the differential diagnosis of the cardiac malposition, but conventional 2D CD and 2D PD failed to identify any abnormal vessels arising from the descending aorta. Using 3D multiplanar mode the authors managed to acquire images of the abnormal artery supply of the right lower lobe and demonstrated its origin from the aorta at the level of the celiac axis, which was confirmed by angiography following the delivery.

In addition, 3D PD allows detection of the abnormalities of the intracerebral vessels, such as a vein of Galen aneurysm or intracranial arteriovenous fistulae.[55] Lee and coworkers were the first to describe the use of 3DPD ultrasound in the diagnosis of an aneurysm of the vein of Galen and visualization of its angioarchitecture *in utero*.[60] Aneurysm of the vein of Galen is a complex arteriovenous malformation consisting of multiple communications between the system of the vein of Galen and the cerebral arteries (carotid and vertebrobasilar systems). In order to understand the angioarchitecture of the vascular lesion, the fetus should be investigated with 3D PD. The vascular anatomy, including the supply and drainage, should be analyzed. A small contralateral aneurysm over the choroidal branches of the posterior cerebral artery also connected to the anterior and middle cerebral artery was found to feed the aneurysm. The venous drainage, including an aneurismatic falcine sinus, superior sagittal sinus, transverse sinus and occipital sinus were all clearly depicted by 3D-PD ultrasound. Three-dimensional PD is advantageous in interactive assessment of the lesions from different perspectives. The angioarchitecture depicted by 3D PD may help in identifying the neonates prone to poor prognosis. Abnormal venous drainage (falcine sinus) indicated fetal heart failure. Diagnosis of the Galen's aneurysm by identification of angioarchitecture, such as feeding and drainage vessels on 3D power Doppler may guide the postnatal treatment more precisely and may possibly help in identifying the fetus at high risk of neonatal congestive heart failure and poor prognosis. Three-dimensional PD ultrasound may also be helpful in evaluation of the intracerebral malformations, such as agenesis of the corpus callosum, holoprosencephaly and hydrocephaly.[54,55] In these cases, 3D reconstruction is helpful in obtaining an impression of the course of the intracranial vessels.

In the assessment of the umbilical cord, 3DPD ultrasound is found useful for detection of the nuchal cord, knots (false/true) and single umbilical artery (Figures 14.18 to 14.20).[54,55,61]

Presence of the nuchal cord is important for the management of the labor of the fetuses with breech presentation. In such cases, 3D PD can help to diagnose

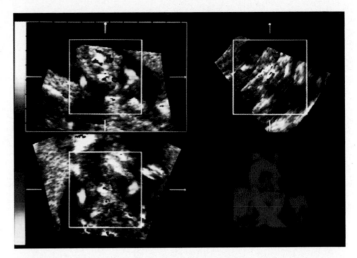

FIGURE 14.19: Multiplanar view of the nuchal cord by 3D power Doppler technique. Loops of the umbilical cord around fetal neck are visualized.

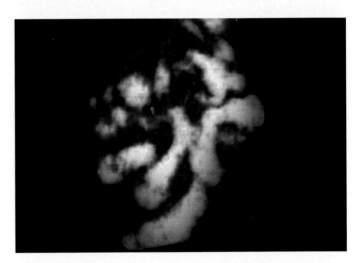

FIGURE 14.20: Umbilical cord knot by 3D power Doppler ultrasound.

the loops of the umbilical cord around the fetal neck. Sensitivity of color Doppler in detecting the nuchal cord is about 96%.[61]

Integration of 3D ultrasonography and power Doppler resulted in 3D PD, which was found to be useful in the evaluation of the vascular anatomy in fetuses with anomalies. The introduction of STIC with color and power Doppler provides new information in the field of fetal echocardiography with new possibilities of reconstructing the fetal heart, great vessels and analysis of their spatial relationship. The same technique may be efficiently utilized for the evaluation of normal and abnormal umbilical cord vessels.

CONCLUSION

Three-dimensional ultrasound is useful in the evaluation of the abnormal fetal anatomy. The major advantage of 3D US is the display of unlimited planes of the object of interest using multiplanar mode. This modality enables accurate measurements and detailed analysis of fetal malformations, especially of the fetal skeleton and face. Surface rendering improves the accuracy of prenatal ultrasound diagnosis and understanding of the spatial relationships. This modality is important in cases of complex surface anomalies. Transparent mode improves visualization of the fetal bones, their relationships and depiction of fetal skeletal anomalies. Three-dimensional power Doppler ultrasound is useful for detection of the cardiovascular anomalies, nuchal cord, umbilical cord knots and single umbilical artery.

REFERENCES

1. Dyson RL, Pretorius DH, Budorick NE, et al. Three-dimensional ultrasound in the evaluation of fetal anomalies. Ultrasound Obstet Gynecol 2000;16(4):321-8.
2. Shih JC, Shyu MK, Lee CN, et al. Antenatal depiction of fetal ear with three-dimensional ultrasonography. Obstet Gynecol 1998;91(4):500-5.
3. Pretorius DH, Nelson TR. Fetal face visualization using three-dimensional ultrasonography. J Ultrasound Med 1995;14(5):349-56.
4. Pretorius DH, House M, Nelson TR, et al. Evaluation of normal and abnormal lips in fetuses: comparison between three-and two-dimensional ultrasonography. Am J Roentgenol 1995;165(5):1233-7.
5. Lin HH, Liang RI, Chang FM, et al. Prenatal diagnosis of otocephaly using two-dimensional and three-dimensional ultrasonography. Ultrasound Obstet Gynecol 1998;11(5):361-3.
6. Budorick NE, Pretorius DH, Johnson DD, et al. Three-dimensional ultrasound examination of the fetal hands: normal and abnormal. Ultrasound Obstet Gynecol 1998;12(4):227-34.
7. Budorick NE, Pretorius DH, Johnson DD, et al. Three-dimensional ultrasonography of the fetal distal lower extremity: normal and abnormal. J Ultrasound Med 1998. 17(10):649-60.
8. Xu HX, Zhang QP, Lu MD, et al. Comparison of two-dimensional and three-dimensional ultrasonography in evaluating fetal malformations. J Clin Ultrasound 2002;30(9):515-25.
9. Kurjak A, Kos M. Three-dimensional ultrasonograhy in prenatal diagnosis. In: Chervenak FA, Kurjak A (Eds.): Fetal Medicine. New York: Parthenon Publishing Group 1999;102-8.
10. Merz E. Three-dimensional ultrasound in the evaluation of fetal malformations. In: Baba K, Jurkovic D, (Eds.) Three-dimensional ultrasound in obstetrics and gynecology. New York: Parthenon 1997;37-44.
11. Hata T, Yanagihara T, Matsumoto M, et l. Three-dimensional ultrasonographic features of fetal central nervous system anomaly. Acta Obstet Gynecol Scand 2000;79(8):635-9.
12. D'Addario V, Pinto V, Di Cagno L, et al. Three-dimensional ultrasound of the fetal brain. Donald School Journal of Ultrasound in Obstetrics and Gynecology 2007,1(3):17-25.
13. Kurjak A, Pooh RK, Tikvica A, Stanojevic M, Miskovic B, Ahmed B, Azumendi G. Assessment of fetal neurobehaviour by 3D/4D ultrasound. In: Pooh RK, Kurjak A (Eds.). Fetal Neurology. New delhi: Jaypee Brothers Medical Publishers (P) Ltd 2009;221-85.
14. Lai TH, Chang CH, Yu CH, et al. Prenatal diagnosis of alobar holoprosencephaly by two-dimensional and three-dimensional ultrasound. Prenatal Diagn 2000;20(5):400-3.
15. Timor-Tritsch, IE, Monteagudo A, Santos R. Three-dimensional inversion rendering in the first- and early second trimester fetal brain: its use in holoprosencephaly. Ultrasound Obstet Gynecol 2008;32(6):744-50.
16. Bonila-Musoles F, Machado LE, Osborne NG, et al. Three-dimensional visualization of the normal fetus- part I. In Bonila-Musoles F, Machado LE, Osborne NG (Eds.): Three-dimensional ultrasound for the new millennium. Text and atlas. Madrid: Marco Grafico S. L. 2000;89.
17. Merz E, Bahlaman F, Weber G, et al. Fetal malformations-assessment by three-dimensional ultrasound in surface mode. In Merz E (Ed.): 3D Ultrasound in obstetrics and gynecology. Philadelphia: Lippincot Williams and Wilkins 1998;109-20.
18. Kurjak A, Kupesic S, Di Renzo GC, et al. Recent advances in perinatal sonography. Prenat Neonat Med 1998;3:194-207.
19. Baba K, Okai T. Clinical applications of three-dimensional ultrasound in obstetrics. In: Baba K, Jurkovic D (Eds.): Three-dimensional ultrasound in Obstetrics and Gynecology. New York–London: The Parthenon Publishing Group 1997;29-44.
20. Johnson DD, Pretorius DH, Budorick NE, et al. Fetal lip and primary palate: three-dimensional versus two-dimensional US. Radiology 2000;217(1):236-9.
21. Clementi M, Tenconi R, Bianchi F, et al. Evaluation of prenatal diagnosis of cleft lip with or without cleft palate and cleft palate by ultrasound: experience from 20 European registers. Euroscan study group. Prenat Diagn 2000;20:870-5.
22. Crane JP, LeFevre ML, Winborn RC, et al. A randomized trial of prenatal ultrasonographic screening: impact on the detection, management, and outcome of anomalous fetuses. Am J Obstet Gynecol 1994;171(2):392-9.
23. Ulm MR, Kratochwil A, Ulm B, et al. Three-dimensional ultrasonographic imaging of fetal tooth buds for characterization of facial clefts. Early Hum Dev 1999;55(1):67-75.
24. Lee W, Kirk JS, Shaheen KW, et al. Fetal cleft lip and palate detection by three-dimensional ultrasonography. Ultrasound Obstet Gynecol 2000;16(4):314-20.
25. Pretorius D. The fetal face: 3D ultrasound. 2nd World Congress on 3D Ultrasound in Obstetrics and Gynecology (syllabus). Las Vegas, Nevada USA,1999.

26. Rotten D, Levaillant JM, Martinez H, et al. The fetal mandible: a 2D and 3D sonographic approach to the diagnosis of retrognathia and micrognathia. Ultrasound Obstet Gynecol 2002;19(2):122-30.

27. Rotten D, Levaillant JM, Martinez H, Ducou le Pointe H, Vicaut E. The fetal mandible: a 2D and 3D sonographic approach to the diagnosis of retrognathia and micrognathia. Ultrasound Obstet Gynecol 2002;19(2):122-30.

28. Bonila-Musoles F, Machado LE, Osborne NG, et al. Ear malformations. In Bonila-Musoles F, Machado LE, Osborne NG (Eds.): Three-dimensional ultrasound for the new millennium. Text and atlas. Madrid: Marco Grafico SL 2000;151-63.

29. Hall B. Mongolism in newborn infants. An examination of the criteria for recognition and some speculations on the pathogenic activity of the chromosomal abnormality. Clin Pediatr (Phila) 1966;5(1):4-12.

30. Chang CH, Chang FM, Yu CH, et al. Fetal ear assessment and prenatal detection of aneuploidy by the quantitative three-dimensional ultrasonography. Ultrasound Med Biol 2000;26(5):743-9.

31. Bonilla-Musoles F, Raga F, Villalobos, et al. First trimester neck abnormalities: three-dimensional evaluation. J Ultrasound Med 1998;17(7):419-25.

32. Watson WJ, Cheschier NC, Katz VL, et al. The role of ultrasound in the evaluation of patients with elevated maternal serum alpha-fetoprotein: a review. Obstet Gynecol 1991;78(1):123-8.

33. Riccabona M, Johnson D, Pretorius DH, et al. Three-dimensional ultrasound: display modalities in the fetal spine and thorax. Eur J Radiol 1996;22(2):141-5.

34. Hess DB, Hess LW, Carter GA, et al. Obtaining the four-chamber view to diagnose fetal cardiac anomalies. Obstet Gynecol Clin North Am 1998;25(3):499-515.

35. ISUOG. Cardiac screening examination of the fetus: guidelines for performing the "basic" and "extended" cardiac scan. Ultrasound Obstet Gynecol 2006;27:107-13.

36. Bonila-Musoles F, Machado LE, Osborne NG, et al. Three-dimensional visualization of the normal fetus-part II. In:Bonila-Musoles F, Machado LE, Osborne NG (Eds.). Three-dimensional ultrasound for the new millennium. Text and atlas. Madrid: Marco Grafico SL 2000;89.

37. Zosmer N, Gruboeck K, Jurkovic D. Three-dimensional fetal cardiac imaging. In Baba K, Jurkovic D (Eds.): Three-dimensional ultrasound in obstetrics and gynecology. New York: Parthenon 1997;45-53.

38. Nelson T, Sklansky M, Pretorius DH. Fetal heart assessment using three-dimensional ultrasound. In Merz E. (Ed.): 3D Ultrasound in obstetrics and gynecology. Philadelphia: Lippincot Williams and Wilkins 1998;125-33.

39. Nelson TR. Three-dimensional fetal echocardiography. Prog Biophys Mol Biol 1998;69(2-3):257-72.

40. Meyer-Wittkopf M, Rappe N, Sierra F, et al. Three-dimensional (3D) ultrasonography for obtaining the four and five chamber view: comparison with cross-sectional (2D) fetal sonographic screening. Ultrasound Obstet Gynecol 2000;15:397-402.

41. Volpe P, De Robertis V, Campobasso G, et al. Evaluation of the fetal heart by four-dimensional echocardiography. Donald School Journal of Ultrasound in Obstetrics and Gynecology 2007;1(3):49-53.

42. Szymkiewicz-Dangel J. 3D/4D echocardiography-STIC. Donald School Journal of Ultrasound in Obstetrics and Gynecology 2008;2(4):22-8.

43. Bonila-Musoles F, Machado LE, Osborne NG, et al. Three-dimensional (3D) ultrasound detection of abdominal wall defects. In Bonila-Musoles F, Machado LE, Osborne NG (Eds.): Three-dimensional ultrasound for the new millennium. Text and atlas. Madrid: Marco Grafico SL 2000;215-27.

44. Benoit B. Three-dimensional ultrasonography of congenital ichthyosis. Ultrasound Obstet Gynecol 1999;13(5):380-3.

45. Lev-Toaff AS, Ozhan S, Pretorius D, et al. Three-dimensional multiplanar ultrasound for fetal gender assignment: value of the mid-sagittal plane. Ultrasound Obstet Gynecol 2000;16(4):345-50.

46. Merz E, Miric-Tesanic D, Bahlmann F, et al. Prenatal diagnosis of fetal ambiguous gender using three-dimensional ultrasonography. Ultrasound Obstet Gynecol 1999;13(3):217-9.

47. Hata T, Aoki S, Akiyama, et al. Three-dimensional ultrasonographic assessment of fetal hands and feet. Ultrasound Obstet Gynecol 1998;12(4):235-9.

48. Pilu G, Rizzo N, Perolo A. Anomalies of the skeletal system. In: Chervenek FA, Isaacson GC, Cambell S (Eds.). Ultrasound in obstetrics and gynecology, Vol 2. Boston: Little Brown and Co 1993;981-97.

49. Nelson TR, Pretorius DH. Visualization of the fetal thoracic skeleton with three-dimensional ultrasonography: a preliminary report. AJR Am J Roentgenol 1995;164(6):1485-8.

50. Pooh RK. Fetal cranial bone formation: sonographic assessment. In Margulies M, Voto LS, Eick-Nes S (Eds.): Proceedins of 9th World congress of Ultrasound in Obstetrics and Gynecology. Bologna: Italy:Monduzzi Editore 1999;407-10.

51. Bonila-Musoles F, Machado LE, Osborne NG, et al. Thanatophoric dwarfism three-dimensional ultrasound diagnosis. In Bonila-Musoles F, Machado LE, Osborne NG (Eds.): Three-dimensional ultrasound for the new millennium. Text and atlas. Madrid: Marco Grafico SL 2000;229-45.

52. Ploeckinger-Ulm B, Ulm MR, Lee A, et al. Antenatal depiction of fetal digits with three-dimensional ultrasonography. Am J Obstet Gynecol 1996;175(3 Pt 1):571-4.

53. Kos M, Hafner T, Funduk-Kurjak B, et al. Limb deformities and three-dimensional ultrasound. J Perinat Med 2002;30(1):40-7.

54. Carrera JM, Torrents M, Muòoz A, et al. The role of Doppler in prenatal diagnosis. Ultrasound Rev Obstet Gynecol 2002;2:240-50.

55. Kupesic S, Kurjak A, Bjelos D. Power Doppler in prenatal diagnosis. Ultrasound Rev Obstet Gynecol 2002;2:261-73.

56. De Vore GR. The value of color Doppler sonography in the diagnosis of renal agenesis. J Ultrasound Med Biol 1995;14: 443-9.

57. Sepulveda W, Corral E, Sanchez J, et al. Sirenomelia sequence versus renal agenesis: prenatal differentiation with power Doppler ultrasound. Ultrasound Obstet Gynecol 1998;11(6): 445-9.

58. Song MS, Yoo SJ, Smallhorn JF, et al. Bilateral congenital diaphragmatic hernia: diagnostic clues at fetal sonography. Ultrasound Obstet Gynecol 2001;17:255-8.

59. Michailidis GD, Simpson JM, Tulloh RMR, et al. Retrospective prenatal diagnosis of scimitar syndrome aided by three-dimensional power Doppler imaging. Ultrasound Obstet Gynecol 2001;17(5):449-52.

60. Lee TH, Shih JC, Peng SSF, Lee CN, et al. Prenatal depiction of angioarchitecture of an aneurysm of the vein of Galen with three-dimensional color power angiography. Ultrasound Obstet Gynecol 2000;15:337-40.

61. Hanaoka U, Yanagihara T, Tanaka H, et al. Comparison of three-dimensional, two-dimensional and color Doppler ultrasound in predicting of a nuchal cord at birth. Ultrasound Obstet Gynecol 2002;19(5):471-4.

K Gersak

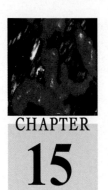

CHAPTER
15

First Trimester Ultrasonographic Screening and Prenatal Diagnostic Methods

FIRST TRIMESTER ULTRASONOGRAPHIC SCREENING

Chromosomal defects are considered as the important causes of perinatal mortality and the main reason for mental retardation in children. Every pregnant woman has a trisomy 21 risk in her fetus. Screening programs play a significant role in the assessment of fetal chromosomal defects and provide the appropriate prenatal counseling and diagnostic tests.[1]

At the beginning of the 1980s, the screening-based on a woman's age was introduced. With the cut-off age of 38 years, 5% of the pregnant women population was classified as "high-risk". However, only 30% of fetuses with Down's syndrome were detected in a "high-risk" group, meaning that 70% of trisomy 21 babies were born by mothers from a "low-risk" group. Later, biochemical screening tests in the second trimester became widely used. The test is based on the concentration of various fetoplacental products in the maternal circulation like alphafetoprotein (AFP), unconjugated estriol (uE3), human chorionic gonadotropin (hCG) and inhibin-A. This method of screening is more effective than maternal age alone and for the same rate of invasive testing (about 5%), it can identify about 50 to 70% of the fetuses with trisomy 21.[2,3]

In the 1990's, screening tests were moved to the first trimester. The woman's age was first combined with sonographic measurement of fetal nuchal translucency (NT). Currently, the most effective screening test combines maternal age and fetal NT with the assessment of fetal nasal bone and maternal serum biochemistry, including the maternal serum concentration of free β-hCG and pregnancy-associated plasma protein A (PAPP-A).[4] The detection rate for trisomy 21 is 95%, with a 5% rate of false positive results.

The first trimester screening includes the confirmation of fetal viability together with the accurate dating of the pregnancy, the detection of multiple pregnancies with identification of chorionicity and early diagnosis of major fetal abnormalities. It is essential that health professionals undertaking the first trimester scan are adequately trained and their results are subjected to an audit. The Fetal Medicine Foundation (FMF) has introduced a process of training and certification to help to establish high standards of scanning on an international basis.[3]

Nuchal Translucency

Nuchal translucency (NT) is the assessment of the amount of fluid behind the neck of the fetus, also known as the nuchal fold. An anechoic space is visible and measurable sonographically in all fetuses between the 11th and 14th week of pregnancy (Figure 15.1). Abnormal accumulation of nuchal fluid decreases after the 13th week. Enlarged NT has been shown to identify the fetuses at higher-risk for Down syndrome and other chromosomal abnormalities.[5,6]

Underlying pathophysiological mechanisms for nuchal fluid collection include cardiac dysfunction, venous congestion in the head and neck, altered composition of the extracellular matrix, failure of lymphatic drainage, fetal anemia or hypoproteinemia and congenital infection.[3]

The scan may be performed transabdominally but in some cases transvaginal approach may be beneficial. During the measurement, the fetus lies in a neutral position, with the head in line with the spine.[7] The assessment of the NT is obtained in a midsagittal view of the fetal profile. The fetal head and upper thorax occupy the whole screen. The

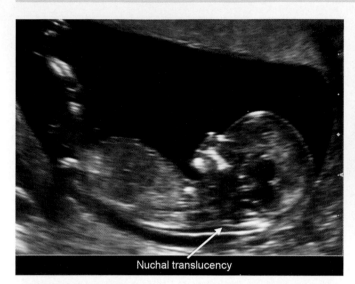

FIGURE 15.1: Fluid behind the neck of the fetus detected sonographically as nuchal translucency.

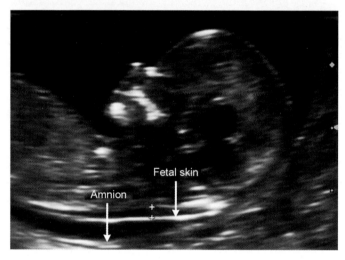

FIGURE 15.2: Measurement of the nuchal translucency.

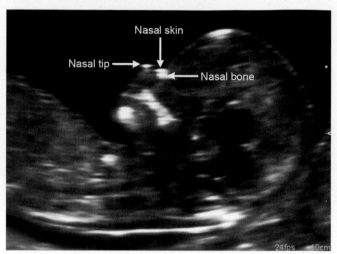

FIGURE 15.3: Assessment of the nasal bone in a mid-sagittal view of the fetal profile.

Nuchal translucency measurement has become a prenatal sonographic screening test suitable for all pregnant women. In the largest study, coordinated by the FMF, 100.311 singleton pregnancies were examined by 306 appropriately trained sonographers in 22 UK centers.[8] In all cases, the individual patient-specific risks, based on maternal age, gestational age and fetal NT were calculated. The estimated risk for trisomy 21 was 1 in 300 or more in 8% of the normal pregnancies and in 82% of those with trisomy 21. This method has enabled identification of about 75% of fetuses with trisomy 21 at a false positive rate of 5%.[3]

Nasal Bone

The nasal root depth is abnormally short in 50% of Down syndrome cases.[9] Sonographic studies at 15 to 22 weeks of gestation reported that about 65% of trisomy 21 fetuses had an absent or abnormally short nasal bone.[10] The fetal nasal bone can be visualized between 11 and 14 weeks of gestation, when CRL is between 45 mm and 84 mm.[11]

The assessment of the nasal bone should be obtained in a midsagittal view of the fetal profile (Figure 15.3).[11] The image of the nose includes three lines.[3] The top line represents the nasal skin, in continuity with the skin is the tip of the nose, and the bottom line, which is thicker and more echogenic, represents the nasal bone. The incidence of an absent nasal bone is related to NT, CRL and ethnic origin (Figure 15.4). It is absent in 60 to 70% of trisomy 21 fetuses. However, in chromosomally normal fetuses the incidence of absent nasal bone is less than 1% in Caucasian population and about 10% in Afro-Caribbeans.[12]

measurements are taken with the inner border of the horizontal line and calipers are placed on the line that defines the NT thickness. It is important to turn the gain down (Figure 15.2) in order to better distinguish between the fetal skin and amnion. Normally, NT increases with the crown-rump length (CRL). NT is evaluated in fetuses with CRL ranging from 45 to 84 mm.

In a fetus with a given CRL, every NT measurement represents a likelihood ratio, which is multiplied by the a priori maternal and gestational age-related risk to calculate a new risk. The larger the NT, the higher the likelihood ratio and, therefore the new risk becomes higher. In contrast, the smaller the NT measurement, the smaller the likelihood ratio, and therefore the new risk becomes lower.[3]

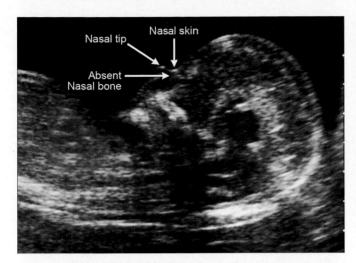

FIGURE 15.4: Assessment of the nasal bone.

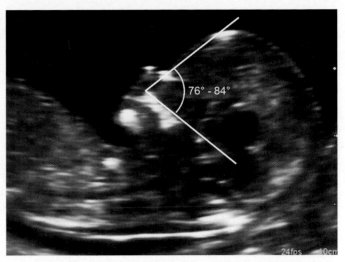

FIGURE 15.6: Measurement of the facial angle.

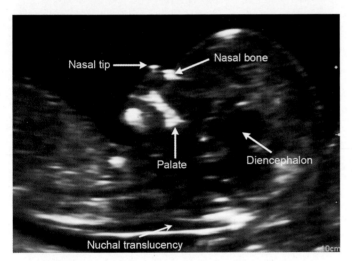

FIGURE 15.5: Assessment of the facial angle in a midsagittal view of the fetal profile.

In the screening combination with maternal age and measurement of NT, the detection of absent or abnormally short nasal bone increases the detection rate for trisomy 21 to 90%, at a false positive rate of 5%.[3]

Facial Angle

Down syndrome is associated with a flat face, which can be quantified by measurement of the frontomaxillary facial angle.[13] It is a new marker, which improves the performance of the first trimester screening tests for trisomy 21.

The assessment of the facial angle is obtained in a midsagittal view of the fetal profile. The midsagittal plane is defined by the echogenic tip of the nose, rectangular shape of the palate, translucent diencephalon in the center and nuchal fold, posteriorly (Figure 15.5). During the assessment of the angle, the fetal head and upper thorax should occupy the entire screen. The facial angle is measured between a line along the upper surface of the palate and a line which traverses the upper corner of the anterior aspect of the maxilla extending to the external surface of the forehead (Figure 15.6). In a recent study, the frontomaxillary facial angle was measured in 782 euploid and 108 trisomy 21 fetuses. In the euploid fetuses, the mean FMF angle decreased linearly with CRL from 83.5 degrees at a crown-rump length (CRL) of 45 mm to 76.4 degrees at a CRL of 84 mm.[13] Forty-five percent of fetuses with trisomy 21 have the facial angle above the 95th centile for existent CRL. Incorporating the angle in the first trimester combined screening with maternal age, measurement of NT, fetal heart rate and maternal serum free beta-hCG and PAPP-A, a detection rate has increased from 90 to 94% at a false positive rate of 5%.

Ductus Venosus Flow

Ductus venosus is a fetal vessel connecting the umbilical vein to the inferior vena cava. It plays a fundamental role in fetal hemodynamics. Highly oxygenated blood returns from the placenta in the umbilical vein. On approaching the fetal liver, between 20 to 50% of the blood under high pressure passes directly into the ductus venosus and bypasses the liver.[14] The pulsatility index of ductus venosus flow reflects its impedance.

Blood flow in the ductus has a characteristic waveform with high velocity during the ventricular systole (S-wave),

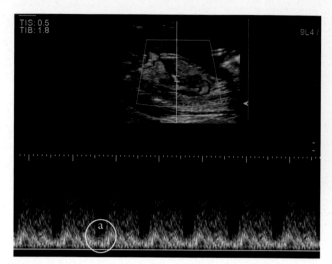

FIGURE 15.7: Assessment of ductus venosus flow; a-wave is forward flow during atrial contraction.

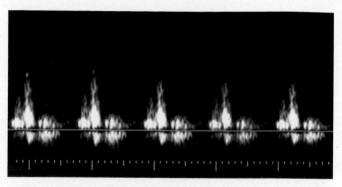

FIGURE 15.8: Assessment of tricuspid flow.

diastole (D-wave) and forward flow during the atrial contraction (a-wave). During the assessment, the ductus venosus flow (DVF), the fetal thorax and abdomen should occupy the entire screen. Ductus venosus is obtained in a right ventral midsagittal view of the fetal trunk using color and power Doppler imaging (Figure 15.7). Qualitative assessment of the blood flow is based on the appearance of the a-wave. Positive or absent a-wave is considered as normal, while a reversed one is defined as an abnormal finding.

Assessment of ductus venosus flow improves the performance of the first trimester screening for aneuploidies and major cardiac defects.[15,16] In a study including more than 19,000 pregnancies between 10 and 14 weeks gestation and 122 fetuses with trisomy 21, a reversed a-wave was observed in 66.4% of the fetuses with trisomy 21 and only 3.2% of the euploid fetuses. A detection of an abnormal a-wave increases the detection rate for trisomy 21 in a screening combination based on the maternal age, measurement of NT, fetal heart rate and maternal serum free beta-hCG and PAPP-A to 96% at a false positive rate of 3%.[15]

Abnormal a-wave may also be associated with a cardiac defect. In chromosomally normal fetuses with increased NT, the finding of an absent or reversed a-wave in the ductus venosus is associated with a three-fold increase in the likelihood of a major cardiac defect.[17]

Tricuspid Flow

The fetal tricuspid flow can be observed by pulsed wave Doppler analysis at 11 to 14 weeks of gestation (Figure 15.8). It has practical implications in the screening for both chromosomal abnormalities and major cardiac defects.[18]

During the assessment of tricuspid flow, the fetal thorax should occupy the whole screen. The tricuspid flow is obtained in an apical four-chamber view of the fetal heart. Tricuspid regurgitation is diagnosed if it is found during at least half of the systole.[7] The tricuspid valve could be insufficient in one or more of its three cusps. Tricuspid regurgitation was observed in 55% of the fetuses with trisomy 21 and only 1% of the euploid fetuses.[7,19] It is more common, if the fetal NT is high and the CRL is low.

The assessment of tricuspid flow increases the detection rate for trisomy 21 in a screening combination based on maternal age, measurement of NT, fetal heart rate and maternal serum free beta-hCG and PAPP-A to 96%, decreasing the false positive rate from 3 to 2.5%.[19]

Intracranial Translucency

Intracranial translucency is the assessment of the fourth ventricle between the 11th and 14th week of gestation (Figure 15.9). It is presented parallel to NT and delineated by two echogenic borders: the dorsal part of the brain stem anteriorly and the chorionic plexus of the fourth ventricle posteriorly.[20]

The assessment of the intracranial translucency is obtained in a midsagittal view of the fetal profile as used for the measurement of NT and assessment of the nasal bone. The fetal head and upper thorax should occupy the entire screen. After identification of the fourth ventricle, its anteroposterior diameter is measured (Figure 15.10).

The anteroposterior diameter increases linearly with gestation from a median of 1.5 mm at CRL of 45 mm to 2.5 mm at CRL of 84 mm. In the cases of spina bifida, the fourth cerebral ventricle was not visible.[20] Findings suggest

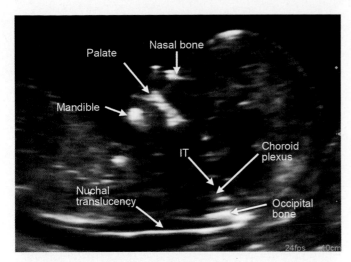

FIGURE 15.9: The forth ventricle detected sonographically as intracranial translucency.

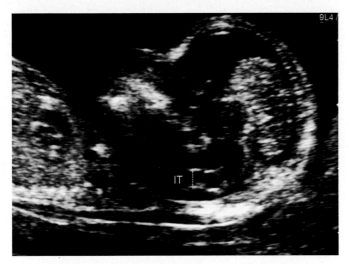

FIGURE 15.10: Measurement of the intracranial translucency.

that in open spina bifida, the caudal displacement of the brain is evident from the first trimester scan, resulting in a compression of the forth ventricle and loss of the normal intracranial translucency. Large prospective studies are needed to determine the association between intracranial translucency and open spina bifida.

PRENATAL DIAGNOSTIC METHODS

Introduction

Major advancement of medical genetics is due to the rapid development of different diagnostic methods and techniques for precise diagnosis, if genetic disorders *in utero*. It has altered the outlook for families at high-risk of having affected children, and has become one of the main options for patients undergoing genetic counseling.[21] The widespread use of screening tests in pregnancy means that a great majority of prenatal testing is undertaken in low-risk patients.

Several basic factors have to be examined when invasive prenatal diagnosis is being considered in genetic counseling. Firstly, the couple has to concern actively the wish for prenatal diagnosis. Sometimes, it may be suggested simply because it may be technically feasible and without providing adequate information.[21]

Before any prenatal procedures are contemplated, the acceptability of termination of pregnancy to a couple has to be determined. In some cases, it is unacceptable on religious grounds or because of the prevailing attitude of the community. In others, it is more a personal ethical view.[21] Unacceptability of termination has not to be considered as automatically ruling out prenatal diagnosis. In some instances, a couple may feel that they will gain by being able to prepare for an affected child. Serious ethical problems may arise, if prenatal diagnosis is undertaken for a late-onset disorders and/or if pregnancy continues.

The most commonly used invasive method for prenatal diagnosis is amniocentesis. However, in recent years additional invasive procedures have been introduced, such as chorionic villus sampling, early amniocentesis, fetal blood sampling and skin, muscle or other tissue biopsy for further assessment.[22]

Chorionic Villus Sampling

Chorionic villus sampling (CVS) is a procedure by which a sample of a chorionic tissue is obtained from the pregnant uterus during the course of the first trimester. It reduces the psychological stress of awaiting results until the second trimester of pregnancy.

It is performed transabdominally or transcervically under sonographic guidance and monitoring, at 11 to 13 weeks of gestation. During the procedure, 10 to 25 mg of tissue is usually aspirated. Maternal tissue is dissected away microscopically and the remaining villi consists only of the fetal tissue.

The fetal tissue can be used for karyotyping, molecular or biochemical analysis. Assays requiring only amniotic fluid cannot be performed.

Randomized studies have demonstrated that the rate of fetal loss following the first trimester transabdominal CVS is the same as with second-trimester amniocentesis, including bleeding, infection, rupture of the membranes and pregnancy loss.[23] Factors found to adversely influence fetal loss rates include fundal placenta, number of catheter's insertions, small sample size and previous bleeding during the current pregnancy.[24] Other obstetric complications do not exceed those in women not undergoing CVS. CVS should not be performed before 11 weeks because earlier CVS is associated with fetal transverse limb abnormalities, micrognathia and microglossia.[3] Maternal risks are usually minimal. Complications due to rhesus sensitization, perforation of intra-abdominal viscera with subsequent intra-abdominal infection and bleeding have been reported. Rh-negative mothers have to receive anti-D antibodies.

Amniocentesis

Amniocentesis is a procedure by which a sample of amniotic fluid and its cells is obtained from the amnion.

It is traditionally performed transabdominally under sonographic guidance and monitoring, at 15 to 17 weeks of gestation, when the volume of amniotic fluid is approximately 200 mL and the ratio of viable to nonviable cells in it is relatively high.[22] During amniocentesis, 20 to 30 mL of fluid is usually aspirated. First milliliters can contain maternal cells from the blood vessels, the abdominal wall or the myometrium. The blood, which is almost always maternal in origin, does not adversely affect amniotic cell growth. But brown or dark red colored amniotic fluid indicates previous intra-amniotic bleeding and is associated with a poor pregnancy outcome in about one third of cases.[22]

After the amniotic fluid is extracted, the fetal cells are separated from the sample. Amniotic cells can be used uncultured or cultured for karyotyping, molecular or biochemical analysis. The supernatant fluid is used for biochemical analysis.

The total fetal loss rate in a group of patients undergoing amniocentesis is about 1% higher than in ultrasonographically normal pregnancies without the procedure.[25,26] The most common intraoperative complications are membrane tenting and bleeding. Repeated procedures carry a much higher risk, estimated from 5 to 10%. Each center has to audit its own figures. Apart from a possibility of rhesus sensitization, maternal risks are minimal. Rh-negative mothers have to receive anti-D antibodies.

Early Amniocentesis

In some rare cases, early amniocentesis between 12th and 15th week of gestation is used as an alternative to chorionic villus sampling.

The amniotic cells can be used uncultured or cultured for karyotyping, molecular or biochemical analysis. The supernatant fluid is used for biochemical analysis.

The procedure-related complications are amniotic fluid leakage, postprocedure vaginal bleeding and fetal loss within 30 days of early amniocentesis. The fetal loss rate is about 2% higher and the incidence of talipes equinovarus is 1.6% higher than following the first trimester chorionic villus sampling or second-trimester amniocentesis.[3,25]

Fetal Blood and Tissue Sampling

Fetal Blood Sampling

Cordocentesis is a procedure by which a sample of fetal blood from the vein of the umbilical cord is obtained.

It is performed transabdominally under sonographic guidance and monitoring, during the second and third trimester, after 18th week of gestation. Usually, 5 mL of fetal blood is aspirated.

The fetal blood can be used for karyotyping, molecular and biochemical analysis, assessment of hematological indices, alloimmunization and prenatal diagnosis of viral, bacterial or parasitic infections of the fetus.[27] Despite maternal antibody titers, fetal serum analysis permits quantification of fetal antibody titers.[22]

The procedure-related complications are chorioamnionitis in 1%, bleeding from the puncture site, cord hematoma and bradycardia in 3 to 12% of cases.[27] Maternal risks are minimal, apart from a possibility of rhesus sensitization.

Fetal Tissue Sampling

Fetal biopsy is a procedure by which a sample of fetal skin, muscle, liver or other tissue and fluid is obtained.

It is performed transabdominally under sonographic guidance and monitoring, during the second and third trimester. Each skin biopsy specimen is approximately 1 × 1 mm in size. During the muscle or liver biopsy 10 to 20 mL of tissue is aspirated.[22]

A skin sample can be used for prenatal diagnosis of hereditary skin diseases by light and electron microscopy, while other tissues samples are used for molecular and biochemical analysis. For the detection of muscular dystrophies molecular analysis and histology of the fetal muscle is needed.

Fetal complications that may lead to fetal death or iatrogenic premature delivery include infection, premature rupture of membranes, hemorrhage, severe bradycardia, cord tamponade or thrombosis and placental abruption. The procedure related loss rate ranges between 1 and 1.5%.[22]

4D US AND PRENATAL DIAGNOSTIC METHODS

4D B-flow Sonography with Spatiotemporal Image Correlation (4D BF-STIC)

Spatiotemporal image correlation (STIC) is a recent technologic advance that allows dynamic multiplanar slicing and surface rendering of the fetal heart anatomy.[28] It provides clinicians with a new dynamic 3D sonoangiographic view of fetal intracardiac and extracardiac blood flow. Spatial and temporal information are combined to display dynamic 4D sequences of the fetal heart beating in a real time.[29] The examiner can navigate within the heart and produce all of the standard and unique planes necessary for comprehensive diagnosis.[30]

There have been a very few reports on 4D intracardiac blood flow observation of the fetal heart using 4D BF-STIC.[28,31,32] These observations describe normal fetal heart and congenital heart disease, extracardiac vessels, including the aorta, pulmonary artery, pulmonary veins and inferior vena cava. 4D BF-STIC might generate information about the anatomy and pathologic characteristics of the fetal heart that cannot be obtained with 2D fetal echocardiography and offline analysis of the acquired volume.[28,33] One significant limitation of fetal cardiac evaluation with 4D BF-STIC is the shadowing from the fetal bones. Further studies are required to confirm the diagnostic potential of this most recent ultrasound technology.

4D US in Fetal Invasive Procedures

During the course of invasive prenatal procedures ultrasound is a widely used method for visualization and guidance of the needle during the puncturing puncture. Conventional 2D sonography provides only one plane in an axial or sagittal display and a needle, apparently located in the correct position according to the sagittal image, may be found to be in a wrong position on axial imaging. Minimizing the time for correct positioning of the needle increases the safety and success of the invasive procedures. In patients with oligohydramnios undergoing amniocentesis, 2D ultrasound may not provide adequate information necessary for the correct positioning of the needle. Similar difficulties may occur in patients with thin placenta undergoing CVS and a narrow umbilical vein undergoing chordocentesis. As a consequence, it may not be possible to perform the intended procedure during the first attempt or the procedure may result in complications, such as premature rupture of membranes, pregnancy loss or preterm labor.[34,35] Four-dimensional (4D) ultrasound imaging during prenatal invasive procedures provides more information regarding needle position. The needle insertion can be performed in a safe and precise manner, with no increase of the procedure time.[35]

Multiplanar mode enabling simultaneous display of three orthogonal planes facilitates needle insertion but requires hand-eye coordination by an operator. Although 4D sonography provides an improved image of the amniotic cavity and reassures that no fetal parts are in the needle's path, the learning curve is longer than with 2D sonography.[36] Further refinements in 4D US technology, such as an enhanced multiplanar resolution, can further improve the needle placement and needle tip visualization, especially with free-hand guidance.

REFERENCES

1. Snijders RJM, Sebire NJ, Cuckle H, et al. Maternal age and gestational age-specific risks for chromosomal defects. Fetal Diag Ther 1995;10:356-67.
2. Wald NJ, Huttly WJ, Hackshaw AK. Antenatal screening for Down's syndrome with the quadruple test. Lancet 2003;361(3):835-6.
3. Nicolaides KH. The 11-13+6 weeks scan. London: Fetal Medicine Foundation, 2004.
4. Nicolaides KH. Nuchal translucency and other first trimester sonographic markers of chromosomal abnormalities. Am J Obstet Gynecol 2004;191(1):45-67.
5. Nicolaides KH, Azar G, Byrne D, et al. Fetal nuchal translucency: Ultrasound screening for chromosomal defects in the first trimester of pregnancy. BMJ 1992;304(6831):867-9.
6. Nicolaides KH, Brizot ML, Snijders RJM. Fetal nuchal translucency: Ultrasound screening for fetal trisomy in the first trimester of pregnancy. BJOG 1994;101:782-6.
7. Available from www://courses.fetalmedicine.com/fmf/ [Accessed May 2010].
8. Snijders RJM, Noble P, Sebire N, et al. UK multicentre project on assessment of risk of trisomy 21 by maternal age and fetal nuchal translucency thickness at 10-14 weeks of gestation. Lancet 1998;351:343-6.
9. Farkas LG, Katic MJ, Forrest CR, et al. Surface anatomy of the face in Down's syndrome: Linear and angular measurements in the craniofacial regions. J Craniofac Surg 2001;12:373-9.
10. Cicero S, Bindra R, Rembouskos G, et al, Integrated ultrasound and biochemical screening for trisomy 21 using fetal nuchal translucency, absent fetal nasal bone, free beta-hCG and PAPP-A at 11 to 14 weeks. Prenat Diagn 2003;23(4):306-10.
11. Cicero S, Sonek JD, McKenna DS, et al. Nasal bone hypoplasia in trisomy 21 at 15-22 weeks gestation. Ultrasound Obstet Gynecol 2003;21(1):15-8.

12. Cicero S, Rembouskos G, Vandecruys H, et al. Likelihood ratio for trisomy 21 in fetuses with absent nasal bone at the 11-14 weeks scan. Ultrasound Obstet Gynecol 2004;23(3):218-23.

13. Bronstein M, Persico N, Kagan KO, et al. Frontomaxillary facial angle in screening for trisomy 21 at 11+0 to 13+6 weeks. Ultrasound Obstet Gynecol 2008;32(1):5-11.

14. Moore KL, Persaud TVN. The cardiovascular system. In: Moore KL, Persaud TVN. The Developing Human. Clinically Oriented Embryology, 6th ed. Philadelphia: WB Saunders 1998:349-403.

15. Borrell A, Martinez JM, Seres A, et al. Ductus venosus assessment at the time of nuchal translucency measurement in the detection of fetal aneuploidy. Prenat Diagn 2003;23(11):921-6.

16. Maiz N, Valencia C, Kagan KO, et al. Ductus venosus Doppler in screening for trisomies 21, 18 and 13 and Turner syndrome at 11-13 weeks of gestation. Ultrasound Obstet Gynecol 2009; 33(5):512-7.

17. Maiz N, Plasencia W, Dagklis T, et al. Ductus venosus Doppler in fetuses with cardiac defects and increased nuchal translucency thickness. Ultrasound Obstet Gynecol 2008;31(3):256-60.

18. Huggon IC, DeFigueiredo DB, Allan LD. Tricuspid regurgitation in the diagnosis of chromosomal anomalies in the fetus at 11-14 weeks of gestation. Heart 2003;89(9):1071-3.

19. Kagan KO, Valencia C, Livanos P, et al. Tricuspid regurgitation in screening for trisomies 21, 18 and 13 and Turner syndrome at 11+0 to 13+6 weeks of gestation. Ultrasound Obstet Gynecol 2009;33(1):18-22.

20. Chaoui R, Benoit B, Mitkowska-Wozniak H, et al. Assessment of intracranial translucency (IT) in the detection of spina bifida at the 11-13-week scan. Ultrasound Obstet Gynecol 2009;34(3): 249-52.

21. Harper PS. Practical genetic counselling, 6th edn, London: Hodder Headline 2004.

22. Simpson JL, Elias S. Genetics in Obstetrics and Gynecology. Philedelphia: WB Saundres 2003.

23. Canadian Collaborative CVS-Aminocentesis Clinical Trial Group. Multicentre randomized clinical trial of chorion villus sampling. First report. Lancet 1989;1(8628):1-6.

24. Rhoads GG, Jackson LG, Schlesselman SE, et al. The safety and efficacy of chorionic villus sampling for early prenatal diagnosis of cytogenetic abnormalities. N Engl J Med 1989; 320(10):609-17.

25. Hanson FW, Tennant F, Hune S, et al. Early amniocentesis: Outcome, risks, and technical problems at less than or equal to 12.8 weeks. Am J Obstet Gynecol 1992;166 (6 Pt 1):1707-11.

26. Tabor A, Philip J, Madsen M, et al. Randomised controlled trial of genetic amniocentesis in 4606 low-risk women. Lancet 1986; 1(8493):1287-93.

27. Ghezzi f, Romero R, Maymon E, et al. Fetal Blood Sampling. In:Fleischer AC, Manning FA, Jeantry P, Romero R, (Eds.) Sonography in Obstetrics and Gynecology, 6th edn. New York: McGraw-Hill;2001:775-804.

28. Hata T, Dai SY, Inubashiri E, et al. Four-dimensional sonography with B-flow imaging and spatiotemporal image correlation for visualization of the fetal heart. J Clin Ultrasound 2008;36(4):204-7.

29. Goncalves LF, Lee W, Chaiworapongsa T, et al. Four-dimensional ultrasonography of the fetal heart with spatiotemporal image correlation. Am J Obstet Gynecol 2003;189:1792-802.

30. Vinals F, Poblete P, Giuliano A. Spatio-temporal image correlation (STIC): A new tool for the prenatal screening of congenital heart defects. Ultrasound Obstet Gynecol 2003;22(4):388-94.

31. Pooh RK, Korai A. B-flow and B-flow spatio-temporal image correlation in visualizing fetal cardiac blood flow. Croat Med J 2005;46(5):808-11.

32. Volpe P, Campobasso G, Stanziano A, et al. Novel application of 4D sonography with B-flow imaging and spatio-temporal image correlation (STIC) in the assessment of the anatomy of pulmonary arteries in fetuses with pulmonary atresia and ventricular septal defect. Ultrasound Obstet Gynecol 2006; 28(1):40-6.

33. Goncalves LF, Espinoza J, Lee W, et al. A new approach to fetal echocardiography: Digital casts of the fetal cardiac chambers and great vessels for detection of congenital heart disease. J Ultrasound Med 2005;24(4):415-24.

34. Timor-Tritsch IE, Platt LD. Three-dimensional ultrasound experience in obstetrics. Curr Opin Obstet Gynecol 2002;14(6): 569-75.

35. Kim SR, Won HS, Lee PR, et al. Four-dimensional ultrasound guidance of prenatal invasive procedures. Ultrasound Obstet Gynecol 2005;26(6):663-5.

36. Tonni G, Centini G, Rosignoli L, et al. 4D vs 2D ultrasound-guided amniocentesis. J Clin Ultrasound 2009;37(8):431-5.

K Gersak

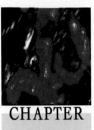

CHAPTER

16

Genetic Approach to Fetal Abnormalities

INTRODUCTION

History

For many centuries birth defects were seen as warnings or divine omens. They were a cause of wonderment considered as the "work of Gods" and such incorporated into mythology and legends. Children with congenital defects were often regarded as or confused with mythological beings.

Cyclop Polyphemus, the son of the Greek God Poseidon and the sea nymph Thoosa, was a giant with a single eye in the middle of his forehead. In the lethargic Lotus-Eaters country, he captured the Greek hero Odysseus who was on his long journey home to Ithaca. On the other hand, the Greek philosopher Anaximander speculated that mankind had sprung from an aquatic species of an animal called mermaid.

Later, the victims of sirenomelia and "monsters" became objects of interest to be collected, described and exhibited. Many museums of pathology still own collections of various fetal anomalies, although recently the display of such items has been regarded as inappropriate.

Today, the clinical recognition of structural abnormalities is an important element in patient care. When anomalies are identified sonographically, many questions arise. Parents want to know why they have appeared, which further tests are needed, what the prognosis for the fetus is and how high the risk of recurrence in future pregnancies may be. Collaboration of perinatologists, genetic counselors and nurses plays a significant role in the diagnosis and care for the patients affected by these anomalies.

Systematic Approach to Fetal Abnormalities

Dysmorphology is an area of clinical genetics that deals with clinical recognition of structural congenital anomalies.[1,2] Congenital abnormalities represent one of the most frequent and important reasons for seeking the genetic counseling. Until very recently, clinicians have had to rely almost entirely on their own skills and experience in making an accurate diagnosis. Laboratory studies were helpful in a minority of cases.[3] This is now changing rapidly and the underlying basis of congenital abnormalities is one of the most exciting and practically relevant fields of science and medicine.

There are several practical stages in the geneticist's approach to fetal structural abnormalities. An algorithmic or stepwise process of decision making includes at least four main steps:

- *Morphological* characterization of abnormalities,
- *Recognition* of patterns,
- *Establishment* of diagnosis, and
- *Assessment* of prognosis and recurrent risk.

MORPHOLOGICAL CHARACTERIZATION OF ABNORMALITIES

In the first step of the systematic approach to fetal abnormalities, an isolated abnormality has to be distinguished from multiple abnormal findings defined as either minor or major (Figure 16.1). Careful two-dimensional (2D) ultrasound imaging is the most important diagnostic method. With high resolution images, we can observe fine details, and can therefore better define the extent and severity of an anatomical defect.[4] However, improvement in resolution also creates many problems, since it permits the detection of minor abnormalities and normal variants that may eventually lead to the evocation of anxiety in parents and dilemmas of the geneticist.

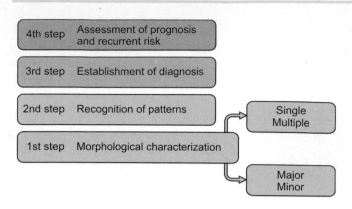

FIGURE 16.1: An algorithmic or stepwise approach to fetal abnormalities. In the first step an isolated abnormality has to be distinguished from multiple abnormal findings and defined as either minor or major.

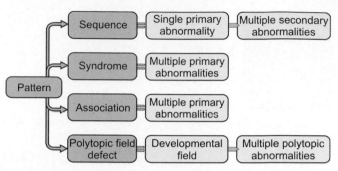

FIGURE 16.2: Multiple abnormalities represent either a random occurrence or a pattern, whereas a pattern can result from one or more primary abnormalities. On one hand some of these abnormalities repeatedly occur together due to a common known cause, while others emerge concurrently without any recognizable connection. In any pattern, the involved structures can derive either from one or all germ cell layers.

Single and Multiple Abnormalities

When an abnormality has been identified, the critical and careful scanning should search for other abnormalities, growth parameters and unusual fetal movements.[3] For each abnormality in an otherwise normal fetus, the type of anomaly has to be identified, such as malformation, deformation, disruption or dysplasia.[1,5] (see analysis of the type of congenital abnormalities).

When two or more abnormalities are detected, the embryonic origin of the tissue or organ involved has to be assessed.[5] Remnants of the primitive streak may persist and give rise to a large sacrococcygeal teratoma, while disturbance of neurulation may result in severe neural tube defects. Embryonic origin can be helpful in determining the possible cause and timing of their onset. The overall risk for genetic cause increases with the number of identified abnormalities.

Major and Minor Abnormalities

Both single and multiple abnormalities may be considered as minor or major defects.[1,4]

Major defects cause serious malfunctioning of an organ or organ system and require medical and/or surgical treatment. They could be lethal or are associated with severe handicaps. Major defects are often associated with multiple fetal abnormalities.

Minor defects or morphological variants are abnormalities that do not cause serious health problems and have no intrinsic functional or cosmetic significance. With high resolution images we can observe fine details and can therefore, better define the extent and severity of an anatomical defect.[4] Thus, the application of three-dimensional sonography in obstetrics has resulted in prenatal detection of a higher percentage of minor abnormalities and normal variants. Consequently it provides a more accurate genetic counseling.

RECOGNITION OF THE PATTERN OF MULTIPLE ABNORMALITIES

If multiple abnormalities are present, they may represent a random occurrence or a pattern (Figure 16.2).[1,5,6]

Sequence

A sequence is a pattern of multiple abnormalities that result from a single primary abnormality. For example, in Potter sequence, the primary defect is renal agenesis or oligohydramnios, which leads to fetal compression, characteristic face, abnormal position of the hands and feet and pulmonary hypoplasia. The cascade of abnormalities could be the result of any type of primary anomaly.

Syndrome

A syndrome is a recognizable pattern of multiple abnormalities when a common cause has resulted in a number of anatomically unrelated errors. Primary anomalies in two or more systems take a part of the syndrome. A well known example is Down syndrome, associated with brachycephaly, mild ventriculomegaly, nuchal edema, atrioventricular septal defect, duodenal atresia, echogenic bowel, mild hydronephrosis, sandal gap and shortening of the limbs.

Association

An association is a recognizable pattern of multiple abnormalities, which occur together more frequently than by chance alone. The initiating cause is not known, and neither are the abnormalities that are the results of a sequence.[6] An example is the combination of a mullerian duct aplasia, unilateral renal aplasia and cervicothoracic somite dysplasia known as MURCS association.

Polytopic Field Defect

A polytopic field defect is a pattern of abnormalities derived from a disturbance of a single developmental field or in one particular area of the body. In a pattern involving structures derived from all of the germ layers, it is likely that the defect is a consequence of abnormal blastogenesis. Because of shared molecular determinants, spatial contiguity and close timing of morphogenetic events during blastogenesis, most abnormalities are polytopic, involving two or more progenitor fields, e.g. acrorenal, cardiomelic, gastromelic or splenomelic anomalies.[7,8]

ESTABLISHMENT OF DIAGNOSIS

The diagnosis is the essential starting point for the appropriate genetic counseling of each individual case. Unfortunately, with recent knowledge it cannot be made in about half of the cases seen in a tertiary clinic not even with the additional information available after birth.[4] During the establishment of the diagnosis all available diagnostic methods, analysis techniques, literature and computerized databases should be used (Figure 16.3).

Although many aspects of the diagnostic approach to the fetal abnormalities are similar to genetic disorders, there are some significant differences.[9] Pregnancy history is of crucial importance, because it may reveal a specific nongenetic cause, such as teratogenic infection or drug-related issue, a mechanical uterine factor or factors, such as hydramnion or lack of fetal movement that may be a clue to the cause of abnormalities.[3] As in any other situation, where genetic counseling is needed, a full pedigree and information on relevant family members is essential. The extent and direction of prenatal diagnostic procedures is influenced by the history and pedigree.

Choice of a Diagnostic Method

Noninvasive Prenatal Diagnosis

Noninvasive methods for prenatal diagnosis include sonography, magnetic resonance and X-ray imaging (Figure 16.4).

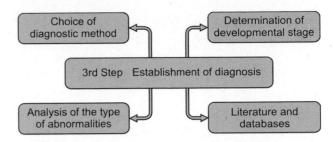

FIGURE 16.3: During the establishment of the diagnosis all available diagnostic methods, analysis techniques, literature and computerized databases are used.

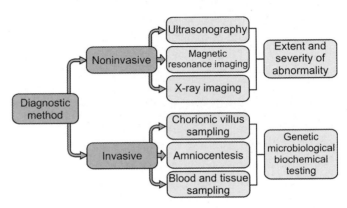

FIGURE 16.4: The two types of prenatal diagnostic methods are demonstrated. Noninvasive methods for prenatal diagnosis include sonography, magnetic resonance and X-ray imaging to expose fine details and define the extent and severity of the abnormality. Invasive fetal sampling is performed by amniocentesis, chorionic villus sampling and skin, muscle or other tissue biopsy for further assessment (karyotyping, molecular, biochemical or microbiological analysis).

Careful sonographic observation is the most important diagnostic method. When one abnormality is detected, the sonographer should search for additional markers. If only minor abnormalities are presented, unrecognized infection, teratogenic or genetic defect can be suspected.

High resolution color and pulsed Doppler imaging significantly contribute to better understanding of fetal physiology and circulation.[10] It is particularly useful in defining the structures and flow parameters of the fetal heart and great vessels. Using color flow modalities fetal heart defects and abnormalities associated with arteriovenous shunting are better diagnosed and explained. An important advance in prenatal diagnosis is the application of 3D and 4D sonography. It offers the possibility of surface analysis, acquired volume measurements and 3D reconstructions of the abnormalities and blood flow arborization (please refer to the chapter "Abnormal fetal anatomy").

During pregnancy magnetic resonance imaging (MRI) is a preferred method for the further evaluation of the fetal abnormalities that were first detected by ultrasonography. It is suitable for pelvimetry, examinations of maternal tumors and some fetal abnormalities.[11,12]

Radiography is often neglected. But it should not be underestimated in excluding particular disorders. Usually, it is performed on stillbirths with bone dysplasias.

Improvements in resolution and imaging provide more accurate genetic counseling. An important emphasis should be placed on the storage of the images and data. They supply accurate means of documentation and allow the retrospective analyses of abnormalities and evaluation of serial changes. Clinicians should make a habit of storing the most informative images, volumes and/or cine loops.

Invasive Prenatal Diagnosis

An accurate diagnosis should be made rapidly and prenatally, if possible (Figure 16.4). Prenatal diagnosis of abnormalities usually requires analysis of the fetal tissues.[3] Until today amniocentesis has been the most commonly used invasive technique for prenatal diagnosis. In recent years, additional invasive procedures have been introduced, such as chorionic villus sampling, early amniocentesis, fetal blood sampling and skin, muscle or other tissue biopsy for further assessment.[3,13] The prenatal methods are described in Chapter 15—First Trimester Ultrasonographic Screening and Prenatal Diagnostic Methods.

Fetus with major or multiple abnormalities should at least undergo prenatal cytogenetic testing. Even when the pattern seems to be of a nonchromosomal origin, karyotyping remains a valuable test for further analysis and genetic counseling. On the other hand, a normal cytogenetic result is not sufficient. The abnormalities caused by environmental agents or mutant genes are not immediately recognizable. Directed high-resolution techniques or molecular analysis, microbiological or biochemical testing may be required.

The most dynamic area is the study of metabolic and molecular pathways underlying normal development, along with the corresponding gene defects that produce congenital abnormalities.[3] Advance in this field, including the use of mouse and other models, have reached the point where a series of developmental pathways can be traced and congenital abnormalities grouped in families according to the specific type of molecular defect.

Analysis of the Type of Congenital Abnormalities

The process of establishing the diagnosis includes the analysis of the type of congenital abnormalities.[1,5,9] Acting factors have to be recognized and connected to the possible causes.

Every abnormality is a defect of morphogenesis. Morphogenesis is the process of formation and differentiation of tissues and organs and causes an organism to develop its shape. It arises because of the changes in the cellular structure or alterations in cell-cell interactions. Abnormalities in morphogenesis are classified into four main types, which lead to structural defects (Figure 16.5). However, not all variations of the development are abnormalities.

Malformation

Malformation is an irregular or abnormal structural development of an organ or region of the body, resulting from an intrinsically abnormal process of development. It is caused by genetic, environmental or a combination of factors. Underlying mechanisms include altered tissue formation (cell division, migration, apoptosis), growth or differentiation. Malformations are represented in different ways:

- Incomplete stage in the development, such as aplasia, hypoplasia, incomplete separation or closure, persistence of earlier location, incomplete migration or rotation (e.g. heart defects, duodenal atresia, omphalocele, hypospadia, cryptorchidism).
- Aberrant form that never exists in any stage of normal morphogenesis (e.g. aberrant skeletal pattern, pelvic spur).
- Accessory tissue (e.g. polydactyly, accessory spleen).[1]

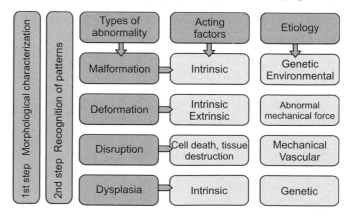

FIGURE 16.5: The process of establishing the diagnosis includes the analysis of the type of congenital abnormalities. Acting factors have to be recognized and connected to possible causes.

Deformation

Deformation is an abnormal form, shape or position of the body part caused by mechanical forces.[2] The force acting upon a normal developing or developed structure may be extrinsic or intrinsic. Extrinsic forces (e.g. uterine abnormalities) are related to typical secondary deformations. Intrinsic forces (e.g. fetal neuromyopathy) can also lead to primary deformations.

Disruption

Disruption is a morphologic defect of an organ or region of the body resulting from a destructive force, acting upon a normally developing or developed structure.[1,2] The result is a breakdown of a previously normal tissue. The mechanisms include cell death or tissue destruction due to vascular abnormalities, anoxia, teratogens, infections or mechanical forces (e.g. amelia, limb reduction, missing digit, disruption of bowel).

Dysplasia

Dysplasia is abnormal growth, development or function of cells, tissue or an organ.[1,5] There is a lack of normal organization of cells into tissue (dyshistogenesis), which leads to abnormal, often tumor-like tissues or abnormal function of cells because of mutations in specific genes (e.g. achondroplasia, Marfan's syndrome, neurofibromatosis).

Determination of Developmental Period When the Abnormality Occurred

If a firm diagnosis has not been established, it is important to determine the time when the abnormality occurred, so that the genetic counseling could be accurate and complete (Figure 16.3).

Fetal abnormality is related to the stage of embryogenesis at which the causal factor acted.[5] For each organ and organ system there is a critical period of susceptibility. If a specific harmful factor acts during the pre- and peri-implantation period, the loss of certain totipotent cells will neither induce any particular defect nor kill the embryo (an "all-or-nothing" effect).

Later, during the embryonic period and process of organogenesis, between 3rd and 8th week, most major abnormalities occur. Each gestational stage provides different patterns of abnormalities.

During the fetal period (beyond week 8 after conception), effects are most likely to be on growth or functional maturation and may continue after birth.

Literature and Databases

The transition from collecting the data and images to recognizing their implications for diagnosis, depends on the knowledge of diagnostic features of specific abnormalities and dysmorphic disorders.[3,4,9] As this information is too vast to commit to memory, books and other sources of information are available as reference materials for a successful diagnostic process.

The recognition and delineation of a new syndrome has benefited immensely from the development of databases of known and unknown disorders.[3] Several systems, regularly updated are now available, and are becoming clinical geneticists' essential tools.

By including information published or presented all over the world, the computerized and internet available databases are especially helpful in rare or atypical disorders. Also, molecular details and available tests are now being incorporated into these databases.

The OMIM database, London Dysmorphology database and POSSUM are the most applicable ones.[14-16] A list of possible diagnoses is generated by searching for combinations of clinical features. The main aim is to find a small number of possible diagnoses, review the features, photographs and abstracts from the database and original references to see whether the overall features of the condition fit into the pattern found in a tour case.[4]

ASSESSMENT OF PROGNOSIS AND RECURRENT RISK

The responsibility for establishing an accurate prognosis and providing a future care for a child is shared by the geneticists, obstetricians, perinatologists, neonatologists and surgeons. Nowadays, invasive prenatal and postnatal procedures can be planned and delivery can be timed more rigorously. The neonatal intensive care and surgery are highly sophisticated and available. Even without a specific diagnosis, the type of the defect may suggest the probable etiology and management of the offspring (Figure 16.6).

After appropriate testing of both the fetus and the parents, the genetic or nongenetic, either hereditary or sporadic basis of the abnormalities has to be determined.[1,3,13] The risk of passing a heritable disease to offspring varies widely. An understanding of the hereditary patterns (autosomal or X-linked, dominant or recessive, sporadic) is essential for counseling the parents regarding the risk of recurrence in future children. For instance, Mendelian risk estimates can only be given when a clear

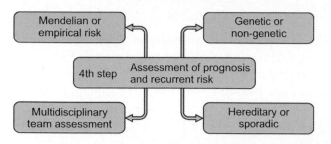

FIGURE 16.6: Every abnormality has its hereditary or sporadic (e.g. genetic or nongenetic) basis. Hereditary patterns are an essential basis for counseling parents about the risk of recurrence in future children. The responsibility of establishing an accurate prognosis and providing future care for the child is shared by geneticists, obstetricians, perinatologists, neonatologists and surgeons.

basis of a single gene inheritance is recognized. An autosomal recessive disorder has a 25% risk of recurrence with each pregnancy and a dominant or X-linked one has a 50% risk. Variability of expression can be a trap with an autosomal dominant inheritance.

Increasing range of abnormalities with specific developmental molecular defects prove to be new and genetically lethal dominant mutations. However, for a new mutation the recurrence risk might be negligible, almost 0%.

For most of the common nonmendelian or de novo chromosomal disorders, only the empirical risk is available. Frequently, such data are inadequate and the geneticist provides a genetic counseling without a secure basis on which he/she can estimate the risk of recurrence. The greatest potential for error lies when a disorder following mendelian inheritance, particularly autosomal recessive is mistaken for a similar, but nongenetic or polygenetic condition.[3] In general, the empirical risk of recurrence for a single primary abnormality is between 2% and 5%. A teratogen-induced abnormality does not recur, if the cause is removed.

REFERENCES

1. Graham JM (Ed). Smith's Recognizable Patterns of Human Deformation, 2nd edn. Philadelphia:WB Saunders 1988.
2. Jones KL Jr. (Ed). Smith's Recognizable Patterns of Human Malformation, 4th edn. Philadelphia:WB Saunders 1988.
3. Harper PS. Practical genetic counselling, 6th Edition. London: Hodder Headline 2004.
4. Twining P, McHugo JM, Pilling DW. Textbook of fetal abnormalities. London: Churchill Livingstone 2000.
5. Moore KL, Persaud TVN. The Developing Human. Clinically Oriented Embryology, 6th edn. Philadelphia:WB Saunders 1998.
6. Gilbert-Barness E, Debich-Spicer D. Embryo and Fetal Pathology. Color Atlas with ultrasound correlation. Cambridge: Cambridge University Press 2006.
7. Martinez-Frias ML, Frias JL, Opitz JM. Errors of morphogenesis and developmental field theory. Am J Med Genet 1998;76:291-6.
8. Delgado Luengo WN, Hernández Rodríguez ML, Valbuena Pirela I, et al. Human disorganization complex, as a polytopic blastogenesis defect: A new case. Am J Med Genet. 2004; 125A(2):181-5.
9. Nyhan WL. Structural abnormalities. A clinical approach to diagnosis. Clinical Symposia 1990;42:1-32.
10. Merz E, Welter C. 2D and 3D Ultrasound in the evaluation of normal and abnormal fetal anatomy in the second and third trimesters in a level III center. Ultraschall Med 2005;26(1):9-16.
11. Bardo D, Oto A. Magnetic resonance imaging for evaluation of the fetus and the placenta. Am J Perinatol 2008; 25(9):591-9.
12. Laifer-Narin S, Budorick NE, Simpson LL, et al. Fetal magnetic resonance imaging: A review. Curr Opin Obstet Gynecol 2007; 19(2):151-6.
13. Simpson JL, Elias S. Genetics in Obstetrics & Gynecology. Philadelphia: WB Saundres 2003.
14. Available from www3.ncbi.nlm.nih.gov/Omim/. Accessed on May 2010.
15. Winter R, Baraitser M. London Dysmorphology database, CD-ROM. Oxford: Oxford Medical Databases 2001.
16. Bankier A. POSSUM (Pictures of Standard Syndromes and Undiagnosed Malformations), CD-ROM. Melbourne: Murdoch Institute for Research into Birth Defect 2002.

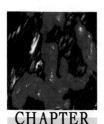

A Kurjak, M Stanojevic
B Ahmed, Tikvica Luetic

CHAPTER
17 Four-Dimensional Sonography in Perinatal Medicine

INTRODUCTION

Fetal behavior, defined as any observable action or reaction to an external stimulus by the fetus, reflects the activity of the fetal central nervous system (CNS). Insight in fetal behavior is crucial for the understanding of normal fetal well-being and in determining whether a fetus may be compromised. Since recently, maternal registration of fetal movements and obstetrician auscultation of fetal heartbeats were the only methods for judgement about fetal state in utero. This was changed with the development of real time two-dimensional (2D) ultrasound that enabled the direct visualization of fetal anatomy and achieved in observing fetal activity. This great accomplishment investigators used as a starting point for the analysis of fetal behavior in comparison with morphological studies, which led to the conclusion that fetal behavioral patterns directly reflect developmental and maturational processes of fetal central nervous system.[1,2] Therefore, it was suggested that the assessment of fetal behavior in different periods of gestation may provide the possibility to distinct between normal and abnormal brain development, as well as early diagnosis of various structural or functional abnormalities.[1] However, 2D ultrasound with poor image quality, especially at the beginning, was considered somewhat subjective method because information needs observer interpretation. The latest development of three-dimensional (3D) and four-dimensional (4D) sonography and their implementation into the clinical practice enable precise study of fetal and even embryonic activity. The use of this new technologies have shown that fetal activity appears as early as the late embryonic period, which is far earlier than a mother can sense it, what could be potentionally used in early embryonic neurobehavior assessment with great

implications in termination of pregnancy in a case of an abnormal finding. Since now the investigations of fetal neurobehavior seems inconceivable without the use of ultrasound, so fetal behavior can be defined as any fetal activity observed or recorded with ultrasonographic equipment.

FETAL MOTILITY AND 4D ULTRASOUND

Although 2D sonography enhanced our understanding of fetal neuromuscular development, the real breakthrough in studying fetal neurobehavior was achieved by 3D/4D ultrasound. This technique has important advantages, such as the ability to study fetal activity in the surface-rendered mode, it is particularly superior for the fast fetal movements and it is better in visualization of fetal face.[3] Fetal movements, such as yawning, swallowing and eyelid movements cannot be displayed simultaneously, while, with 4D sonography, the simultaneous facial movements can be clearly depicted.[4] Its additional advantage in comparison with 2D ultrasound is the ability to visualize the whole fetus continuously. The key benefit of 4D ultrasound lies in providing real-time 3D images of embryonic or fetal movements, previously limited by technological possibilities. The introduction of high-frequency transvaginal tranducers has resulted in remarkable progress in ultrasonographic visualization of early embryos and fetuses and the development of sonoembryology. For the first time, parallel analyses of structural and functional parameters in the first 12 weeks of gestation become possible.

3D ultrasound has been extensively used for more than ten years with the development of several different kinds of modes that have been created for different purposes. They include multiplanar imaging, volume rendering,

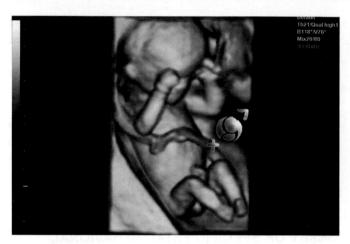

FIGURE 17.1: Three-dimensional ultrasound of fetus in the first trimester showing complex movements of body and limbs.

of the brain playing more subtle role in modulating quality and, perhaps, time patterning of the different movement patterns.[16] Isolated limb movements emerge almost simultaneously with the general movements and they could be seen from 8th to 9th weeks of gestation by 4D-US.[16] Organization of the appearance of the movement pattern occurs with the increasing frequency. It seems that fetal arms explore the surrounding environment and cross the midline, while the palmar surface is oriented towards the uterine wall. The fetal legs are extended to the uterine wall. From the 10th week onwards, the number and frequency of fetal movements increase and the repertoire of movements begins to expand. Breathing movements appearing between 10.5 and 12 weeks consist of the opening of the jaw, bending forward of the head and complex stretch movements, are added to the repertoire.[17]

To determine the accuracy of 4D sonography in the assessment of embryonic and early fetal motor activity in the first trimester of normal pregnancy, the Zagreb group conducted a study with fifty pregnant women and performed 2D and 4D recordings. Several movement patterns, such as sideway bending, hiccup, fetal breathing movements and facial movements could not be observed by 4D-US imaging technique, although they were clearly visible by 2D-US. The authors concluded that at the time, both 2D and 4D methods were required for the assessment of early fetal motor development and motor behavior. It was reasonable to expect that such technological improvement may provide some new information about the intrauterine motor activity and facilitate the prenatal detection of some neurological disorders.[17]

Detail observation of fetal hand and finger positioning by 3D/4D ultrasound revealed that at the beginning of the 10th week, fetal hands are located in front of the chest without movements of wrists or fingers. Active arm movements can be visualized from the middle of 10th week of gestation with changes in finger positioning from 11th week.[18]

In the first trimester, one could notice a tendency towards an increased frequency of fetal movement patterns with increasing gestational age. Only the startle movement pattern seemed to occur stagnantly during the early gestation.[19]

The Second Trimester

Only a few studies are available on fetal movement patterns during the second trimester.[15,35-37] In this period of gestation, the incidence of body movements increases considerably with longer periods of quiescence. The most active fetal behavioral pattern is arm movement, whereas the least active is mouth movement. Each fetal movement was shown to be synchronized and harmonized in this period of pregnancy.[20] Important movements that are most developed in the second trimester are eye movements with isolated eye blinking seen as consolidate movements from the 24th to 26th week of gestation, while facial grimaces are seen as sporadic movements with a limited frequency.[21] From a developmental point of view, one could say that in the second trimester, the development continues, but there are no new movements appearing for the first time.[22]

Using 4D sonography, the Zagreb group have found that from 13 gestational weeks onwards, a "goal orientation" of hand movements appears and a target point can be recognized for each hand movement.[23,24] All subtypes of hand to head movement could be seen from 13 weeks of gestation with fluctuating incidence (Figure 17.2).

Among facial expressions, two types could be easily differentiated: smiling and scowling. The authors concluded that 4D-US is superior over 2D real-time ultrasound for the qualitative, but inferior for quantitative analysis of hand movements. Thus, 4D-US makes it possible to determine exactly the direction of the fetal hand, but the exact number of each type of hand movements could not be determined. 2D sonography easily recognizes hand movements associated with body movements, but there are difficulties in the recognition and differentiation of isolated hand movements and hand movements associated with leg movements. In this situation, 4D-US is the method of choice for the reliable recognition of the isolated hand movements.

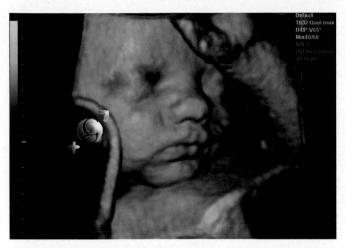

FIGURE 17.2: Example of 3D ultrasound of the fetal face and isolated hand movement in the second trimester.

Additionally, 4D sonography provides surface rendered images of the fetal head and visualization of hand movements in three dimensions that allows further differentiation of hand to head movements.[23,24]

Kurjak et al, reported the first study with the 4D-US techniques used for obtaining longitudinal standard parameters of fetal neurological development in all trimesters of a normal pregnancy.[25] Valid reference ranges appropriate for gestational ages are essential for comparisons with previous measurements of the same patients and among patients as well. The authors found a tendency towards an increase of fetal movement at the beginning of the 2nd trimester. All types of facial expressions display a peak frequency at the end of the 2nd trimester, except in isolated eye blinking, which increases at the beginning of 24th week. This longitudinal study established reference range of fetal movement patterns in different gestational ages in respected number of normal singleton pregnancies. Results from Yigiter and co are similar as they found a significant correlation between all head movements and hand to body contact patterns during the 2nd and the 3rd trimesters except for head anteflexion, which did not show a significant change during the second half of pregnancy.[19] It has also been suggested that there is a tendency towards decreased frequency of observed facial expressions and movement patterns with increasing gestational age.[25] All types of facial expressions display a peak frequency at the end of the 2nd trimester, except for isolated eye blinking, which increased at the beginning of 24th week.[25]

The Third Trimester

During this period of pregnancy, motor behavior becomes increasingly frequent and variable with an obvious developmental improvement in orienting responses. Prechtl showed that the development was intraindividually characteristic and consistent but at the same time variable.[26] In short, a rich variety of fetal and premature movements has been described and it has been shown that the repertoire of fetal movements consists exclusively of motor patterns, which can also be observed postnatally and that there is a high degree of continuity of behavior before and after birth. However, the behavioral repertoire of the newborn rapidly expands with patterns never observed in the fetus, such as the Moro reflex.

The concept of behavioral states has been used as a descriptive categorization of behavior in the third trimester as an explanatory concept in which the states are considered to reflect particular modes of nervous activity that modify the responsiveness of the infant.[27] These states consist of fetal heart rate pattern and eye and body movements.[27] The association of these movements increases steadily and, in the last weeks of pregnancy, authors stated that fetal behavior can almost completely be described in terms of behavioral states, which are stable overtime and recur repeatedly, not only in the same infant, but also in similar forms in all infants.[27,28]

By term, the number of general movements reduced as a result of cerebral maturation processes.[9] Simultaneously with this decrease, an increase in the facial movements, including opening/closing of the jaw, swallowing and chewing can be observed.[9] However, not only the changes in the quantity of movements but also in their quality are shown to be the result of maturational processes.

The incorporation of 3D-US technology into clinical practice has resulted in remarkable progress in visualization and anatomic examination of the fetal face. 4D-US, in turn, provided for the first time an opportunity to evaluate subtle fetal facial expressions, which can be used to understand fetal behavior[29] (Figure 17.3).

Because of its curvature and small anatomic details, the fetal face can be visualized and analyzed only to a limited extent with 2D-US, but 3D-US allows spatial reconstruction of the fetal face and simultaneous visualization of all facial structures, such as the fetal nose, eyebrows, mouth and eyelids. This technique does not replace conventional real-time 2D-US imaging but rather supplements it. Three-dimensional ultrasound requires an investment of additional

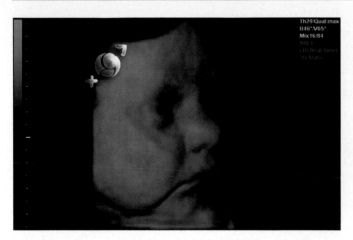

FIGURE 17.3: Example of 3D ultrasound of the fetal face in the third trimester, which provides the possibility to study a full range of facial expressions including smiling, crying, scowling and eyelid movements.

time in each case; therefore, it is predominately used, presently in conjunction with 2D-US, as a problem-solving tool.

It seems that facial movements, which are controlled by V and VII cranial nerves, appear around 10 and 11 weeks, however, the exact onset of facial expressions has not been determined and it is still unclear whether their appearance is gestational age related.[29] The possibility of studying such subtle movements might open a new area of investigation.

Zagreb group undertook the study to show the ability of 4D sonography to depict different facial expressions and grimacing, which might represent fetal awareness.[30] This was based on the consideration that "the face predicts the brain" because of the same embryologic origin for many facial and encephalic structures.[31] A tendency towards increased frequency of observed facial expressions with increasing gestational age was noted, but the difference between second- and third-trimester fetuses was not significant due to the low frequency of movements. As at that time the images were only near real-time, they were only able to study the quantity and not the quality of facial movement patterns with the possibility that some very subtle facial movements may have been missed.

Recently, Yan and his group found that mouthing was the most active facial expression from 28 to 34 weeks.[32] However, the frequency of eyelid blinking was lower compared to other studies may be due to the differences in the characteristics of the samples recruited and differences in interpreting the definition of each facial expression.[23,30]

NEW SCORING SYSTEM FOR FETAL NEUROBEHAVIOR ASSESSED BY 3D AND 4D SONOGRAPHY

In the recent study, the Zagreb group attempted to produce a new scoring system for fetal neurobehavior based on prenatal assessment by 3D/4D sonography.[33] That scoring system is a combination of prenatally visualized parameters by 4D-US from other previously used tests as fetal GM assessment and postnatal Amiel-Tison Neurological Assessment (ATNAT) at term.[34,35] The parameters were chosen based on developmental approach to the Neurological Assessment and on the theory of central pattern generators of GM emergence and were the product of multicentric studies conducted during several years (Table 17.1).[24,25]

The authors developed a three-point scale for isolated head anteflexion, isolated hand, leg, hand to face and finger movements, while for the assessment of cranial sutures, isolated eye blinking, facial alterations and mouth opening two-point scale was applied. The distinction between scores 0 and 2 is evident, whereas uncertainty may exist with regards to the assignation of a score of 1, indicating an abnormal result of moderate degree. The precise description of the moderate abnormal performance is included for each item in the record form.

In order to produce the new scoring test, Zagreb group identified severely brain damaged infants and those with optimal neurological findings by comparing fetal with neonatal findings. In the group of 100 low-risk pregnancies they retrospectively applied new scoring system. After delivery, postnatal neurological assessment (ATNAT) was performed[36] and all neonates assessed as normal reached a score between 14 and 20, which was assumed to be a score of optimal neurological development. New scoring system was applied in the group of 120 high-risk pregnancies in which, based on postnatal neurological findings, three subgroups of newborns were found: normal, mildly or moderately abnormal and definitely abnormal. Based on this, a neurological scoring system has been proposed. All normal fetuses reached a score in the range from 14 to 20. Ten fetuses who were postnatally described as mildly or moderately abnormal achieved prenatal score of 5 to 13, while another ten fetuses postnatally assigned as neurologically definitely abnormal had a prenatal score from 0 to 5. Among this group four had alobar holoprosencephally, one had severe hypertensive hydrocephaly, one had tanatophoric dysplasia and four fetuses had multiple malformations.

TABLE 17.1: Neurological scoring test for fetus

Sign	Score			Sign score
	1	2	3	
Isolated head anteflexion	Abrupt	Small range (0-3 movements)	Variable in full range, many alternation (> 3 movements)	
Cranial sutures and head circumference	Overlapping of cranial suttures	Normal cranial sutures with measurement of HC below the normal limit (-2SD) according to GA	Normal cranial sutures with normal measurement of HC according to GA	
Isolated eye blinking		Not fluent (0-5 times of blinking)	Fluency (> 5 times of blinking)	
Facial alteration (grimace or tongue expulsion)		Not fluent (0-5 times of alteration)	Fluency (> 5 times of alteration)	
Mouth opening (yawning or mouthing)		Not fluent (0-3 times of alteration)	Fluency (> 3 times of alteration)	
Isolated hand movement	Cramped	Poor repertoire	Variable and complex	
Isolated leg movement	Cramped	Poor repertoire	Variable and complex	

Contd....

Contd....

Hand to face movements	Abrupt	Small range (0-5 movements)	Variable in full range, many alternation (>6 movements)
Fingers movements	Unilateral or bilateral clenched fist, (neurological thumb)	Cramped invariable finger movements	Smooth and complex, variable finger movements
Gestalt perception of GMs	Definitely abnormal	Borderline	Normal
			Total score

That was a preliminary study that has already been continued in several collaborative centers. Future database formed using this new score for fetal neurological assessment will help in distinguishing fetal neurobehavioral impairments due to the early brain damage occurring in utero. It is assumed that the study of a large population will hopefully validate the value of the new test as a predictive marker for fetal neurodevelopmental outcome in both low- and high-risk populations.

MULTICENTRIC STUDY

In our recent paper,[37] the potential of the test was investigated at four university departments after appropriate training by the authors of the test. We are reporting here on the preliminary results obtained in the high-risk group of patients, trying to distinguish normal fetal brain and neurodevelopmental alterations due to the early brain impairment occurring in utero.

The study participants were singleton pregnant women in the second and the third trimester of pregnancy (between 20 and 38 weeks of gestation), recruited in out- and inpatient clinics of University Departments of Obstetrics and Gynecology from four centers: General Hospital "Sveti Duh", Zagreb, Croatia; Marmara University Hospital, Istanbul, Turkey; University Hospital, Bucharest, Romania; and Hamad Medical Center, Doha, Qatar.

This was a multicenter, prospective cohort study, 288 pregnant women meeting the inclusion criteria given in the Table 17.2, who were found eligible to be included in the study. Distribution of study participants throughout four centers is presented in the Table 17.2.

TABLE 17.2: Inclusion criteria

Family history	Previous child with cerebral palsy
Maternal condition	Diabetes mellitus type 1 and 2, thyroid disease, pre-existent hypertension, drug abuse, thrombophilia, anemia, epilepsy
Pregnancy-related disorders	Gestational diabetes, Rh immunization, threatened preterm labor, pre-eclampsia, intrauterine infections, viral illness, cholestasis
Fetal condition	Structural and chromosomal abnormalities, polyhydramnion, intrauterine growth restriction, pathological findings in electrical fetal heart monitoring or Doppler findings.

The study was conducted after the approvals of local ethics committees of four above mentioned institutions. Each participant signed informed consent form.

Fetal behavior was assessed by 4D US. All 4D US examinations were performed by experienced operators using either the Voluson 730 Expert 11 (General Electric, USA) or Sonoline Antares (Siemens AG, Issaquah, USA) with transabdominal 5 MHz transducer. Methods of assessment have been described elsewhere.

The Kurjak's Antenatal Neurological Assessment (KANET) was used to assess fetal neurobehavior. The test has already been described elsewhere, but in this study we used a slightly modified version with the same descriptions of the parameters and the different scoring scale, which was for all parameters from 0 to 2, while in the originally published scoring test the scale was from 1 to 3. The used KANET form is illustrated on the Table 17.1. Table 17.3 was constructed arbitrary, representing allocation of fetuses

TABLE 17.3: Allocation of fetuses according to Kurjak's antenatal neurological screening Test

Total Score	Interpretation
0-5	Abnormal
6-13	Borderline
14-19	Normal

into three separate groups after KANET assessment: 0-5 points were considered abnormal; 5-13 borderline; ≥14 normal.

All neonates underwent postnatal neurological screening assessment according to Amiel-Tison at the postnatal age of one to three days. After the assessment infants were assigned as normal, borderline or abnormal. Infants from the borderline and abnormal group were assigned to the high-risk group for the development of neurological impairment. In this group of infants, for the purpose of this preliminary study, Prechtl's general movements were evaluated at the premature (28 to 36 postmenstrual weeks) and term (37 to 46 postmenstrual weeks) age. It is planned to repeat the GM assessment at the writhing age (46 to 52 postmenstrual weeks) and fidgety age (54 to 60 postmenstrual weeks). After any assessment of GM infant was classified to one of the groups according to Hadders Algra: normal optimal, normal suboptimal, abnormal and definitely abnormal. To simplify the analysis, the infants who were assigned to normal optimal and normal suboptimal group were considered as "normal" while the infants who were abnormal were considered as borderline, while those who were definitely abnormal were considered as abnormal.

All infants have been planed to be assessed by ATNAT screening test at 1, 3, 6, 9, 12 and 18 months of corrected age, while final assessment was planned to be at the corrected age of 24 months. All infants who needed additional assessments like neuroimaging, electrophysiological, ophthalmologic, orthopedic or any other examination were supposed to get it according to the local availability. It was intended to make the final diagnosis of disabling or nondisabling cerebral palsy at the corrected age of 24 months on the basis of child's ability to walk. Figure 17.4 presenting postnatal assessment flow chart.

The primary outcome was the usefulness of KANET to identify the fetuses from high-risk pregnancies at neurological risk. Due to relatively small sample size statistical analysis is at the moment not possible.

The number of fetuses assessed in four centers with the results of the KANET score are given in Table 17.4, while outcome of fetuses after KANET assessment is presented in Table 17.5. Combined results from the KANET, ATNAT

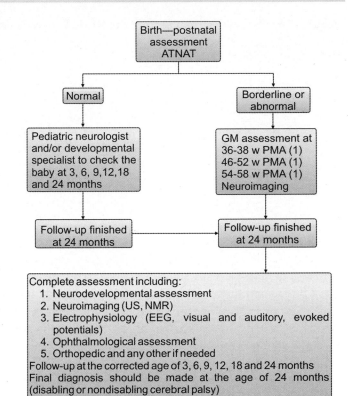

FIGURE 17.4: Postnatal assessment (Flow chart)

and general movement of the survivors are presented in Table 17.6.

TABLE 17.4: The number of fetuses assessed in four centers with the results of the KANET score

Center	Number of fetuses	Prenatal neurological assessment (KANET)		
		Normal	Borderline	Abnormal
Doha	58	39	11	8
Bucharest	68	62	5	1
Istanbul	45	34	5	6
Zagreb	117	105	9	3
Total	288	240	30	18

KANET = Kurjak antenatal neurodevelopmental test

TABLE 17.5: Outcome of fetuses after KANET assessment

KANET score	Terminated	Died	Alive	Total
0-5	5	6	7	18
6-13	2	3	25	30
≥ 14	6	0	234	240
Total	13	9	266	288

KANET = Kurjak antenatal neurodevelopmental test

TABLE 17.6: Combined results from the KANET, ATNAT and general movement assessment

Results of postnatal general movements (GMs)		Postnatal neonatal neurological assessment (ATNAT)			Prenatal assessment (KANET)	
		Normal	Borderline	Abnormal	Borderline	Abnormal
Normal optimal	4	3	1	0	4	0
Normal suboptimal	20	4	16	0	20	0
Abnormal	6	0	5	1	1	5
Definitely abnormal	2	0	0	2	0	2
Total	32	7	22	3	25	7

KANET = Kurjak antenatal neurodevelopmental test, ATNAT = Amiel-Tison's neurological assessment at term

As shown in Table 17.6, a total of 7 fetuses had abnormal KANET scores and 25 fetuses were borderline, for 32 fetuses at neurological risk. Of the seven fetuses with an abnormal KANET, postnatal neurological assessment by ATNAT revealed three newborns (arthrogryposis, vermis aplasia and neonate of the mother with the previous child with cerebral palsy out of seven fetuses to be abnormal, while four were considered normal (ventriculomegaly, pre-eclampsia, thrombophylia, oligohydramnios). Out of the 25 borderline KANET fetuses there were 22 borderline newborns by ATNAT, while 3 were normal (ventriculomegaly, syndrome of intra-amniotic infection, maternal thrombocytopenia). Those who were abnormal prenatally and normal postnatally had following prenatal risk factors: ventriculomegaly, Dandy Walker syndrome, skeletal dysplasia, polihydramnios, hydrocephaly, diabetes in pregnancy, nonimmune fetal hydrops, syndrome of intra-amniotic infection, intrauterine growth restriction (IUGR), trisomy 21, thrombocytopenia, thrombophylia, pre-eclampsia, achondroplasia, oligohydramnios. Out of the three abnormal neonates after ATNAT assessment, two had definitely abnormal Prechtl's premature general movements (arthrogryposis and vermis aplasia) and additional six were considered abnormal (neonate of the mother with the previous child with CP, Dandy-Walker syndrome, hydrocephaly, trisomy 21, ventriculomegaly, nonimmune hydrops). Rest of 24 children had normal optimal or normal suboptimal GMs.

DISCUSSION

Despite medical reports from 100 years ago and 25 years of systematic research initiated by Prechtl and DeVries, the study of fetal neurobehavior is still in its infancy. There were attempts to develop a prenatal neurological screening test based on 2D ultrasound. The test was based on quantifying the fetal movements and did not take into account the quality and variability of the movements. The facial expressions were not included in these tests since they can only be clearly visualized by 4D ultrasound. The duration of the test was from 30 to 60 minutes and was not practical for daily use. The most comprehensive review article on fetal behavior included 109 papers, the authors conclusion was that the future studies of fetal behavior have to focus on spontaneous fetal movements and general movements. It was stressed that the new 4D ultrasound technology could be the tool enabling new insight to fetal neurobehavior. The implementation of this new diagnostic data has raised our knowledge about central nervous system development. Furthermore, the traditional concept that the brain damage is caused during birth or early neonatal period has been challenged, antenatal and unclassifiable factors are now considered as most important etiological factors.

The three illustrative cases with abnormal KANET scoring that we would like to present are arthrogryposis, vermis aplasia and fetus whose previous sibling had verified CP. The fetuses in these three cases had especially reduced facial movements, the faces were like mask during repeated scans. Fetuses with vermis aplasia and arthrogryposis had normal cranial sutures but the isolated head flexion was small in range for both cases. Isolated hand movements, hand to face and leg movements were poor in repertoire for all three cases. The finger movements were cramped and invariable in all three cases. The Gestalt perception of general movements was abnormal in all three cases. We also followed longitudinally the behavior of a fetus with acranius. The mother decided not to terminate the pregnancy due to religious reasons. It has been clearly documented that the fetus at 20 weeks of gestation had hypertonic cramped movements with high amplitude and high speed. The movements emerged abruptly with burst-paused patterns, the variability of head movements was missing, without changes of facial expressions. As the gestational age advanced and the motor control was shifting from lower to upper control center, the movement patterns changed as well. At the gestational age of 32 weeks, the fetus had no facial expressions (face as a mask) and hand movement repertoire was very poor. At 36 weeks, the absence of both the facial expressions and limb movements was observed. The neonate died during labor.

It seems that some of the prenatal conditions are temporarily affecting fetal neurological status (ventriculomegaly, SIAI, thrombocytopenia, thrombophylia, polihydramnios, pre-eclampsia, IUGR, achondroplasia), having tendency for improvement in neurological status after birth. On the basis of our preliminary results, we can only speculate why this happened after delivery. It is known that birthing process is affecting neonates neurologically, but it seems like some fetuses got liberated after birth due to numerous intrauterine constraints.

Our study shows that the new test might be useful in the standardization of neurobehavioral assessments. Furthermore, there is a potential for antenatal detection of serious neurological problems. At this stage, test easily separates serious structural anomalies associated with brain impairment (arthrogryposis, vermis aplasia, anencephaly). Most of the high-risk cases have been found with normal neurobehavior and that has been proven by experienced neonatologist. Understandable serious abnormalities with brain impairment and abnormal test have been detected earlier and terminated.

This is work in progress and four collaborating centers are continuing investigation. In some of the centers (Doha, Zagreb) preliminary results are already obtained after one year of life. It is our belief that the new test is a promising tool for the assessment of integrity of young central nervous system. However, the test requires further studies before recommended for wider clinical practice. In the mean time, the potential of antenatal scoring system should not be neither overestimated nor underestimated.

CONCLUSION

One of the most promising advances in the unknown field of prenatal behavior has been the new 3D/4D-US technology. Its advance has been completed in giving visualizations in almost real-time and production of standards for different movement patterns to appear and develop. The 4D study of fetal is offering a great possibility of understanding the hidden function of the developmental pathway of the fetal CNS and the potentialities of originating a neurological investigation in utero. By 4D technology, we might be able to visualize an intrauterine neurological condition that would enable to identify, which

fetus is at risk and which is not. Existence of motoric competence in the newborn, even extremely, preterm infants is assumed to have its origins in prenatal life. Behavioral perinatology assessed by 4D sonography should be an interdisciplinary area of research involving concepts and conducting studies of the dynamic interplay between behavioral processes in fetal, neonatal and infant life. The ultimate clinical application of fetal neurobehavioral assessment will be to identify functional characteristics of the fetus that predict a range of subsequent developmental dysfunction. Establishing this link will require the demonstration of positive and negative predictability to outcomes significantly beyond the immediate perinatal period. After standardization of valid reference ranges of movements appropriate for the gestational age, attempts have been made to produce a new scoring system for fetal neurobehavior based on prenatal assessment by 3D/4D sonography. That preliminary work may help in detecting fetal brain and neurodevelopmental alterations due to in utero brain impairment that is inaccessible by any other method.

REFERENCES

1. Prechtl HFR. Qualitative changes of spontaneous movements in fetus and preterm infant are a marker of neurological dysfunction. Early Hum Dev 1990;23(3):151-8.
2. Nijhuis JG (Ed). Fetal Behaviour: Developmental and Perinatal Aspects. Oxford: Oxford University Press 1992.
3. Lee A. Four-dimensional ultrasound in prenatal diagnosis: leading edge in imaging technology. Ultrasound Rev Obstet Gynecol 2001;1:194-8.
4. Kozuma S, Baba K, Okai T, et al. Dynamic observation of the fetal face by three-dimensional ultrasound. Ultrasound Obstet Gynecol 1998;13:282-4.
5. Campbell S. 4D, or not 4D: that is the question. Ultrasound Obstet Gynecol 2002;19(1):1-4.
6. Azumendi G, Kurjak A. Three-dimensional and four-dimensional sonography in the study of the fetal face. Ultrasound Rev Obstet Gynecol 2003;3:1-10.
7. Kurjak A, Carrera J, Medic M, et al. The antenatal development of fetal behavioral patterns assessed by four-dimensional sonography. J Matern Fetal Neonatal Med 2005;17(6):401-16.
8. Kurjak A, Pooh RK, Merce LT, et al. Structural and functional early human development assessed by three-dimensional and four-dimensional sonography. Fertil Steril 2005;84(5):1285-99.
9. de Vries JIP, Visser GH, Prechtl HF. The emergence of fetal behavior, I. Qualitative aspect. Early Hum Dev 1982;7:301-22.
10. de Vries JI, Visser GH, Prechtl HF. The emergence of fetal behaviour. II. Quantitative aspects. Early Hum Dev 1985;12(2): 99-120.

11. Andonotopo W, A Kurjak, MI Kosuta: Behavioral of anencephalic fetus studied by 4D sonography. J Matern Fetal Neonatal Med 2005;17(2):165-8.

12. Andonotopo W, Stanojevic M, Kurjak A, et al. Assessment of fetal behavior and general movements by four-dimensional sonography. Ultrasound Rev Obstet Gynecol 2004;4:103.

13. Kurjak A, Kupesic S, Banovic I, et al. The study of morphology and circulation of early embryo by three-dimensional ultrasound and Power Doppler. J Perinat Med 1999;27(3):145-57.

14. Kurjak A, Chervenak F, Carrera JM, Andonotopo W, et al. Behavioral Perinatology Assessed by Four-Dimensional Sonography. In: Textbook of Perinatal Medicine, Kurjak A, (Ed). New Delhi: Informa Healthcare, 2006.

15. Kurjak A, Vecek N, Hafner T, et al. Prenatal diagnosis: what does four-dimensional ultrasound add? J Perinat Med 2002;30:57-62.

16. Kurjak A, Carrera JM, Stanojevic M, et al. The role of 4D sonography in the neurological assessment of early human development. Ultrasound Rev Obstet Gynecol 2004;4:148-59.

17. Andonotopo W, Medic M, Salihagic-Kadic A, et al. The assessment of fetal behavior in early pregnancy: comparison between 2D and 4D sonographic scanning. J Perinat Med 2005;33(5):406-14.

18. Pooh RK, Ogura T. Normal and abnormal fetal hand position and movement in early pregnancy detected by three- and four-dimensional ultrasound. Ultrasound Rev Obstet Gynecol 2004;4(1):46-51.

19. Yigiter AB, Kavak ZN. Normal standards of fetal behavior assessed by four-dimensional sonography. J Matern Fetal Neonatal Med 2006;19(11):707-21.

20. Kuno A, Akiyama M, Yamashiro C, et al. Three-dimensional sonographic assessment of fetal behavior in the early second trimester of pregnancy. J Ultrasound Med 2001;20(12):1271-5.

21. Sparling JW, Van Tol J, Chescheir NC. Fetal and neonatal hand movement. Phys Ther 1999;79(1):24-39.

22. Roodenburg PJ, Wladimiroff JW, van Es A, et al. Classification and quantitative aspects of fetal movements during the second half of normal pregnancy. Early Hum Dev 1991;25(1):19-35.

23. Kurjak A, Azumendi G, Vecek N, et al. Fetal hand movements and facial expression in normal pregnancy studied by four-dimensional sonography. J Perinat Med 2003;31(6):496-508.

24. Kurjak A, Stanojevic M, Andonotopo W, et al. Fetal behavior assessed in all three trimesters of normal pregnancy by four-dimensional ultrasonography. Croat Med J 2005;46(5):772-80.

25. Kurjak A, Andonotopo W, Hafner T, et al. Normal standards for fetal neurobehavioral developments—longitudinal quantification by four-dimensional sonography. J Perinat Med 2006;34(1):56-65.

26. Prechtl HF, Fargel JW, Weinmann HM, et al. Postures, motility and respiration of low-risk pre-term infants. Dev Med Child Neurol 1979;21(1):3-27.

27. Nijhuis JG, Prechtl HF, Martin CB, et al. Are there behavioural states in the human fetus? Early Hum Dev 1982;6:177-95.

28. Prechtl FR, Weinmann H, Akiyama Y. Organization of physiological parameters in normal and neurologically abnormal infants. Neuropaediatric 1969;1:101-29.

29. Kurjak A, Azumendi G, Andonotopo W, et al. Three- and four-dimensional ultrasonography for the structural and functional evaluation of the fetal face. Am J Obstet Gynecol 2007;196:16-28.

30. Kurjak A, Stanojevic M, Azumendi G, et al. The potential of four-dimensional (4D) ultrasonography in the assessment of fetal awareness. J Perinat Med 2005;33(1):46-53.

31. DeMeyer V, W Zemen, CG Palmer. The face predicts the brain: diagnostic significance of medial facial anomalies for holoprosencephaly (arhinencephaly). Pediatrics 1964;34:256-63.

32. Yan F, Dai SY, Akther N, et al. Four-dimensional sonographic assessment of fetal facial expression early in the third trimester. Int J Gynaecol Obstet 2006;94(2):108-13.

33. Kurjak A, Miskovic B, Stanojevic M, et al. New scoring system for fetal neurobehavior assessed by three- and four-dimensional sonography. J Perinat Med 2008;36(1):73-81.

34. Amiel-Tison C. Neurological assessment of the neonate revisited: a personal view. Dev Med Child Neurol 1990;32(12):1105-13.

35. Amiel-Tison C, Gosselin J, Kurjak A. Neurosonography in the second half of fetal life: a neonatologist's point of view. J Perinat Med 2006;34(6):437-46.

36. DiPietro JA, Costigan KA, Pressman EK. Fetal state concordance predicts infant state regulation. Early Hum Dev 2002;68(1):1-13.

37. Kurjak A, Abo-Yaqoub S, Stanojevic M, et al. The potential of 4D sonography in the assessment of fetal neurobehavior–multicentric study in high-risk pregnancies. J Perinat Med 2010;38(1):77-82.

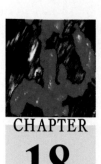

CHAPTER

18

Gestational Trophoblastic Disease

S Kupesic Plavsic, A Kurjak, K Baston

Gestational trophoblastic disease (GTD) is a group of disorders caused by the abnormal development of placental tissue.[1,2] It includes hydatidiform mole (complete and partial), placental site trophoblastic tumor, invasive mole and choriocarcinoma. Trophoblastic cells produce human chorionic gonadotropin (hCG), the hormone that serves as a marker for trophoblastic tissue.

Gestational trophoblastic disease is fortunately an infrequent complication of gestation. The incidence varies from 1:1,500-2,000 pregnancies in Central Europe and the USA, to 1:150 pregnancies in Asia.[3,4] The reported risk for invasive mole in the Western hemisphere is from 1:40,000 to 70,000 pregnancies. Gestational trophoblastic disease is considered to be highly treatable with the cure rate approaching 100%.[5,6] During the last decades, the survival of the patients has been improved as a result of better knowledge of the biological behavior and advances in chemotherapeutic treatments of these diseases.[7]

Pelvic angiographic evaluation of the patients affected with GTD documents the presence of enlarged spiral arteries feeding vesicular spaces with prominent arteriovenous shunting.[4] Several diagnostic modalities have been introduced to replace this invasive procedure; these include real time B-mode ultrasound, magnetic resonance imaging (MRI), transvaginal color and pulsed Doppler, as well as serum levels of chorionic gonadotropin measured by sensitive beta-subunit assays.

B-mode real time ultrasonography shows a characteristic "snow storm" sonographic pattern for a complete hydatidiform mole,[8,9] but there has been no ultrasonic method, which could accurately and reliably distinguish between noninvasive and invasive mole, as well as choriocarcinoma. In 1991, Flam and coworkers[4] compared the results of color Doppler examination and angiography in 10 patients with trophoblastic tumors and in all of the cases there was concurrence between color Doppler and pelvic angiography.

HYDATIDIFORM MOLE

Hydatidiform mole is characterized by the abnormalities of the chorionic villi, varying degrees of trophoblastic proliferations and edema of the villous stroma. Grossly the tumor is composed of multiple grapelike structures that occupy the uterine cavity. Rarely, it is located in the fallopian tube or the ovary.

Complete hydatidiform mole is characterized by generalized swelling of the villous tissue, trophoblastic hyperplasia and no evidence of embryonic or fetal tissue.[10] Complete hydatidiform moles are almost always diploid in karyotype and all chromosomes are paternally derived with a 46 XX chromosomal constitution in 82% to 86% of cases.[11] In most cases of complete mole, a haploid (23 X) sperm fertilizes an anuclear ovum and then reduplicates its own chromosomes. Approximately, 8% of patients with complete mole will develop a malignant tumor after evacuation.[12] Apart from the uterine cavity being filled with multiple sonolucent areas of various sizes, the ultrasonographer should carefully observe the ovaries. About 20% of patients with complete hydatidiform mole will have theca luteinic cysts exceeding 4 to 6 cm.[11]

The sonographic appearance of molar pregnancy varies with the gestational age.[13] A typical ultrasound B-mode real time scan of a complete hydatidiform mole shows a characteristic "snow storm" appearance (Figure 18.1). In the first trimester of pregnancy, hydatidiform mole can mimic blighted ovum, missed abortion, incomplete abortion

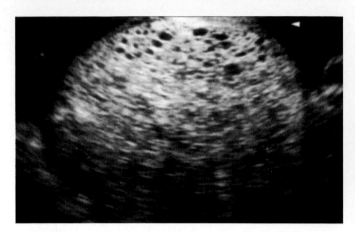

FIGURE 18.1: Transvaginal sonogram demonstrating a lacunar type of invasive mole.

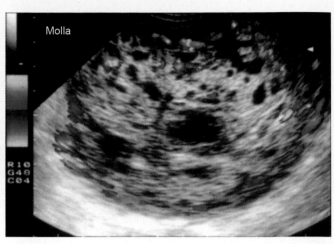

FIGURE 18.2: Color Doppler ultrasound of invasive mole. Color-coded zones represent trophoblastic invasion into the myometrial tissue.

or hydropic changes of the placenta. Lazarus[14] et al., examined the ultrasonographic appearance of early complete molar pregnancies. Out of 21 histologically diagnosed complete molar pregnancies with a mean gestational age of 10.5 weeks, the diagnosis of molar pregnancy was made on ultrasonography in 12 (57%) cases. No theca-lutein cysts were identified. They concluded that the classic appearance of a complete mole on ultrasonography is seen in less than two-thirds of cases and that typical findings are less common during the first trimester.

Partial hydatidiform moles are characterized by focal swelling of the villous tissue, focal trophoblastic hyperplasia and the presence of embryonic or fetal tissue.[11] Partial hydatidiform moles are usually triploid, having two sets of chromosomes from paternal origin and one from maternal origin.[12] Most have a 69 XXX or 69 XXY genotype derived from a haploid ovum with either reduplication of the paternal haploid set from a single sperm, or, less frequently, from dispermic fertilization.[2] The fetus usually presents severe intrauterine growth retardation and major congenital defects in approximately 90% of cases.

Sebire[15] et al, found that only 16 out of 91 cases (17%) of histologically proven partial moles were detected with sonography. The majority of partial molar pregnancies present as missed abortion and/or anembryonic pregnancy which highlights the importance of histological examination to diagnose gestational trophoblastic disease.

Using color Doppler ultrasound, zones of vascularization are seen inside the uterine cavity and peritrophoblastic area, superimposed on the characteristic "snow storm" ultrasonic appearance (Figure 18.2). These

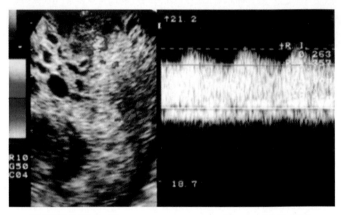

FIGURE 18.3: The same case as in Figure 18.2. Note reduced vascular resistance of the uterine artery (RI = 0.26).

blood vessels coded by color are enlarged spiral arteries, while in some cases of invasive mole and all cases of choriocarcinoma these signals represent neovascularization due to myometrial invasion by the trophoblastic tissue. Using the transvaginal color Doppler technique, the uterine, arcuate, radial and spiral arteries can be separated by their anatomical location, as well as by their typical pulsed wave Doppler signals (Figure 18.3).[16]

In some cases, real time B-mode scan may not be able to identify small molar changes in early first trimester pregnancy, or to distinguish an early mole from degenerating villi,[17] or may give a wrong impression of a blighted ovum. In these cases, color and pulsed Doppler ultrasound reveals highly vascularized areas in a close proximity to the gestational sac with low-resistance (RI) and pulsatility index (PI) values compared to normal pregnancy of the same gestational age.

Jauniaux et al.[18] found that triploids presenting with partial hydatidiform moles are associated with an increased umbilical artery resistance to flow and decreased umbilical vein pH, indicating an impairment of the villous circulation development and trophoblast functions. In these cases, abnormal umbilical artery flow velocity waveforms have been reported as early as 12 weeks of gestation. The combined use of ultrasound features, maternal serum proteins and fetal cytogenetic findings should enable early differential diagnosis *in utero* and the perinatal management of partial molar pregnancies presenting with an anatomically normal fetus.

Another entity that should be differentiated from molar pregnancy is pseudopartial hydatidiform mole that may occur in patients with missed abortion, independent of chromosomal abnormality. The progressive disappearance of the villous vasculature after embryonic death leads to villous hydrops, which does not, however, herald a true partial hydatidiform mole. Focal villous hydatidiform changes may also be detected in pregnancies presenting with trisomy or monosomy. These are probably related to insufficient development of the villous vasculature in some regions of the placenta as a part of larger vascular maldevelopment involving the fetal circulation or villous degeneration in case of placental retention after embryonic/fetal demise.[19,20]

INVASIVE MOLE

The invasive mole could be described as a hydatidiform mole that invades the myometrium and/or adjacent structures.[21] Its incidence is 10 to 15% of patients with primary molar pregnancy.[22] Improvement in chemotherapy of the invasive mole has resulted in a cure rate of up to 95%.[4,7,23,24]

B-mode real time scan is insufficient for the diagnosis of invasive mole and estimation of the myometrial invasion. Using transvaginal color Doppler technique, trophoblastic invasion into myometrial tissue is recognized as prominent color-coded zones in the myometrium and high velocity and low impedance blood flow pattern displayed by pulsed Doppler waveform analysis (Figure 18.4).

The latest findings of Tepper and coworkers[25] indicate that measured Doppler flow indices and beta-hCG levels during chemotherapy may serve for monitoring and follow-up of the patients' response to medical treatment. Good response to chemotherapy is predicted by a significant fall

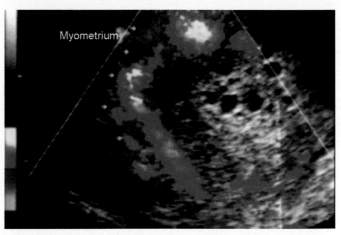

FIGURE 18.4: Transvaginal color Doppler scan of an invasive mole. The uterine cavity demonstrates typical "snow storm" appearance. Prominent blood flow signals detected within the myometrial portion of the uterus are pathognomonic for invasive mole.

in beta-hCG levels and elevation of the resistance index, while tumors resistant to chemotherapy have unchanged or decreased RI, as well as rising levels of beta-hCG. Bright signals on color Doppler scan in patients with invasive mole arise from pre-existing uteroplacental blood vessels (spiral, radial and arcuate arteries), which undergo changes, resulting from the trophoblastic invasion. Neovascularization located deep within the myometrium is conclusive of an invasive mole.

According to Shimamoto and coworkers,[26] the invasive mole is the best indication for color Doppler flow mapping because of the absence of false-negative results. Some authors reported a decrease in the diameter of color-coded blood flow areas detected by color Doppler sonography, following chemotherapy.[21,27]

In their recent observations on gestational trophoblastic tumors, Hsieh and coworkers[27] described and categorized these neoplasms using transvaginal color Doppler ultrasound according to the uterine vascular destruction patterns and correlated them with the serum beta-hCG levels, uterine hemodynamic, clinical response to chemotherapy and histopathologic diagnosis. Destruction of the uterine vasculature is a common characteristic of gestational trophoblastic tumors.[28] According to the vascular patterns showed by color Doppler ultrasound, gestational trophoblastic disease (GTD) could be categorized as diffuse, lacunar and compact types. In patients with diffuse lesions, beta-hCG is significantly lower than in the lacunar and compact type. Similarly, the uterine artery resistance index is significantly lower in lacunar type than in diffuse or compact type.[27,28] All types have significantly higher peak systolic velocity than normal pregnancy group but without significant difference among them. Patients with diffuse lesions are characterized with better response to chemotherapy than those with lacunar and compact lesions. In 11 out of 28 cases with histopathologic confirmation, lacunar vascular patterns correlated with invasive mole, whereas compact type represented choriocarcinoma.[27] Since morphologic patterns of GTD correlate well with color Doppler ultrasound parameters, this method can be potentially used for classification, staging and follow up of the GTD.

Kohorn[29] et al., showed that lesions are detectable by imaging modalities at relatively high levels of hCG, but may not be visualized at lower levels of hCG, when chemotherapy[30] is indicated and the diagnosis of neoplasia is fully justified. At lower levels of hCG (< 700 mIU7 mL), intramyometrial lesions may not be visualized by either color Doppler ultrasound or MRI. In cases with low beta-hCG levels, the sensitivity of imaging is no better than 70% and the specificity is even lower. Therefore, weekly serial assessment of serum hCG remains the most accurate, reliable and definitive arbiter of treatment management.

CHORIOCARCINOMA

Choriocarcinoma is one of the most malignant neoplasms affecting women.[27] This epithelial tumor is composed of highly anaplastic strands of interlacing syncytiotrophoblastic and cytotrophoblastic elements. The risk of developing choriocarcinoma is significantly greater after a molar pregnancy, but it can also follow an abortion, whether artificial or spontaneous, normal pregnancy or even an ectopic pregnancy.[31] Genomic imprinting is believed to play a pivotal role in the pathogenesis of hydatidiform moles. Hydatidiform mole carries a potential of a malignant transformation. Similar to other human cancers, malignant transformation in gestational trophoblastic tumors is likely a multistep process that involves multiple genetic alterations, including activation of oncogenes and inactivation of tumor suppressor genes. In addition, expression of telomerase activity, altered expression of cell-to-cell adhesion molecules and abnormal expression of matrix metalloproteinases has also been reported in GTD.[32]

Choriocarcinoma is a highly malignant tumor that arises from the trophoblastic epithelium and metastasizes readily to the lungs, liver and brain.[33] Thus, many women will present with dyspnea, neurologic symptoms and abdominal

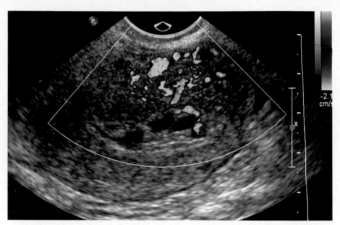

FIGURE 18.5A: Transvaginal color Doppler scan of a choriocarcinoma.

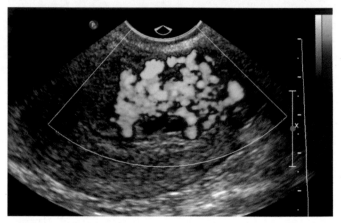

FIGURE 18.5B: Transvaginal power Doppler scan of the same case. Note the numerous randomly dispersed vessels suggestive of a malignant tumor.

pain a few weeks or months and sometimes up to 10 to 15 years after their last pregnancy.[33]

Treatment of malignant GTD includes chemotherapy.[27] The precise diagnosis requires histological evaluation, but due to its location some GTD are inaccessible to sampling by currettage. The next diagnostic criterion is based on the extremely high-level of gonadotropins. However, some highly anaplastic or necrotic choriocarcinomas may produce very little gonadotropin and yield a negative or weakly positive test.[34]

Prior to chemotherapy, ultrasound reveals hypoechoic areas surrounded by irregular echogenic areas with intramyometrial flow signals and low pulsatility index.[35-37] On color Doppler ultrasound, choriocarcinoma displays a typical color-coded "hot" area representing the pre-existing and newly formed blood vessels (Figures 18.5A and B). Neovascularization is characterized with high velocity and

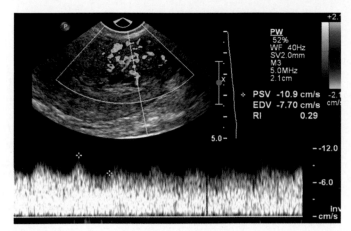

FIGURE 18.6: The same patient as in Figure 18.5. Low-vascular resistance (RI = 0.29) is obtained from bright color-coded zones within the uterus. Histopathology confirmed choriocarcinoma.

low impedance blood flow signals[35] (Figure 18.6). Color Doppler flow imaging and pulsed Doppler can also be used for follow-up of the chemotherapeutic results.[30]

Zanetta et al,[38] evaluated 25 patients with trophoblastic tumors. Uterine morphology was described by transvaginal ultrasound and the hemodynamics of intratumoral vessels was assessed by color Doppler. Sonographic findings were correlated with clinical outcome (local resolution or persistence). Transvaginal color Doppler ultrasound had 100% accuracy in predicting local resolution or local persistence. Resolution was predicted 8 weeks before the disappearance of beta-hCG, whereas indication for persistence was obtained 1 to 3 weeks before the increase of beta-hCG. The negative ultrasound and color Doppler findings in the presence of rising beta-hCG, in one patient were associated with extrauterine metastases. In patients with complete local resolution, there was a progressive reduction of the vascularization demonstrated by increasing PI and decreasing peak systolic velocities. There was a linear association between regression of beta-hCG titers and rising PI of the neovascular areas.

Lindholm et al,[39] presented three patients with choriocarcinoma whose hCG levels and clinical course were suggestive of a trophoblastic disease, but color Doppler findings were negative. Myometrial biopsy performed by hysteroscopy revealed small dark-red lesions typical of choriocarcinoma.

PLACENTAL SITE TROPHOBLASTIC TUMOR

Placental site trophoblastic tumor (PSTT) is the least common form of GTD. The tumor represents a neoplastic transformation of intermediate trophoblastic cells that normally play a critical role in implantation. PSTT can occur after a normal pregnancy, spontaneous abortion, termination of pregnancy, ectopic pregnancy or molar pregnancy. It displays a wide spectrum of behavior, and when metastatic, can be difficult to control even with surgery and chemotherapy. Because of PSTT's rarity, limited information is known about its natural history. Mitotic index is an important prognostic indicator and advances in chemotherapeutic regimens have improved clinical response in patients with metastatic disease.[40]

Color and pulsed Doppler ultrasound can be potentially used for the detection of the placental-site trophoblastic tumor. This tumor produces prominent vascularization characterized with high velocity and low vascular resistance, similar to that of choriocarcinoma.

ZAGREB EXPERIENCE

In our recent study, 30 patients with gestational trophoblastic disease were analyzed by transvaginal color Doppler.[34] The objective of the study was to test whether color and pulsed Doppler ultrasound may differentiate between noninvasive mole and gestational trophoblastic neoplasia.

The investigated group consisted of 20 complete hydatidiform moles, two partial moles, two invasive moles and six choriocarcinomas. A control group (n = 23) was established by the matched pairs according to the gestational age. The mean duration of pregnancy was 10.6 ± 0.4 weeks with a range of 8 to 12 weeks in both observed groups. The pulsed repetition frequency ranged from 1.2 to 22 kHz. Both RI and PI demonstrated a decrease of the blood flow impedance from the uterine artery to the spiral artery and/ or intratumoral blood flow. Resistance and pulsatility index values of the uterine arteries were progressively lower in patients with molar pregnancy and gestational trophoblastic neoplasia, when compared to normal pregnancies (Graphs 18.1 and 18.2). The RI reflected hemodynamic changes more reliably in the distal part of the uterine circulation (i.e. the spiral artery, Graphs 18.1A to D), while the PI was more predictive for analysis of the proximal portion of the uterine vasculature (i.e. the uterine artery, Graphs 18.2A to D). There was no statistically significant difference in the uterine, arcuate, radial and spiral artery RI and the PI in partial and complete hydatidiform moles. However, B-mode ultrasound provides valuable information in the terms of visualization of the fetal parts. The uterine artery vascular impedance in two cases of invasive hydatidiform mole, was significantly lower compared to normal pregnancy and the hydatidiform mole (Table 18.1). In both cases myometrial invasion was seen as prominent color-coded zones within the distal portion of the myometrium. Resistance and pulsatility indices obtained from these highly

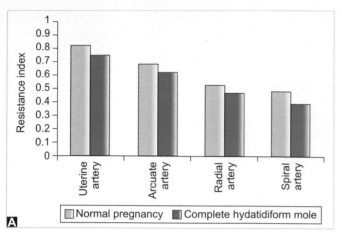

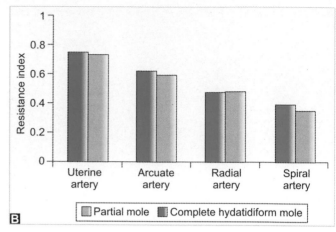

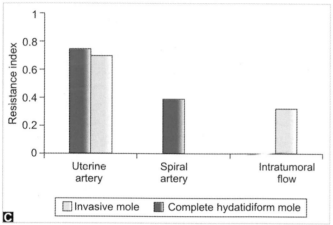

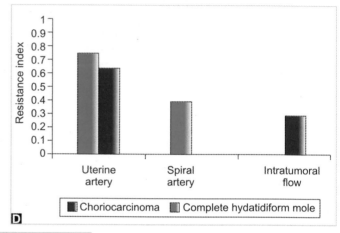

From reference 31, with permission

GRAPHS 18.1A to D: Comparison of obtained resistance index (RI) values among investigated groups of patients: (A) Normal pregnancy compared to hydatidiform mole; (B) Hydatidiform mole and partial mole; (C) Hydatidiform mole and invasive mole; (D) Hydatidiform mole and choriocarcinoma

TABLE 18.1: The resistance index (RI) and pulsatility index (PI) obtained from the uterine, arcuate, radial and spiral arteries in patients with GTD.

Patients	n	Uterine artery RI	Uterine artery PI	Arcuate artery RI	Arcuate artery PI	Radial artery RI	Radial artery PI	Spiral artery RI	Spiral artery PI	Peritumoral flow RI	Peritumoral flow PI
Complete hydatidiform mole	20	0.75* (0.03)	1.71* (0.41)	0.62* (0.08)	1.15* (0.35)	0.47* (0.07)	0.81* (0.23)	0.39* (0.05)	0.54* (0.18)	– –	– –
Partial mole	2	0.73 0.75	1.64 1.69	0.60 0.61	1.19 1.28	0.48 0.49	0.88 0.69	0.35 0.38	0.53 0.60	– –	– –
Invasive mole	2	0.70 0.71	1.24 1.26	– –	– –	– –	– –	– –	– –	0.33 0.30	0.48 0.53
Choriocarcinoma	6	0.64* (0.05)	1.23* (0.21)	– –	– –	– –	– –	– –	– –	0.29 (0.05)	0.43 (0.27)
Control group	23	0.82* (0.04)	2.18* (0.55)	0.68* (0.05)	1.46* (0.52)	0.52* (0.06)	0.92* (0.38)	0.48* (0.04)	0.58* (0.29)	– –	– –

( ) = 2 SD; * = statistical significance (p < 0.01)

From reference 31, with permission

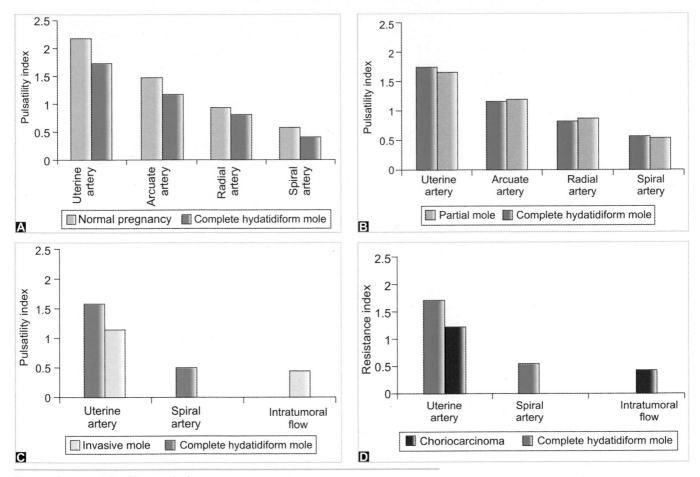

From reference 31, with permission

GRAPHS 18.2A to D: Comparison of pulsatility index (PI) values among investigated groups of patients: (A) Normal pregnancy compared to hydatidiform mole; (B) Hydatidiform mole and partial mole; (C) Hydatidiform mole and invasive mole; (D) Hydatidiform mole and choriocarcinoma.

vascularized areas revealed lower values compared to that of the uterine arteries.

Six cases of choriocarcinoma were correctly diagnosed by transvaginal color and pulsed Doppler ultrasound. Fluctuating colored zones representing blood vessels inside the uterine cavity and within the myometrium were easily displayed by color and power Doppler technique. In all the cases, vascular resistance of the intratumoral blood flow was significantly lower compared to the values obtained from spiral arteries in the patients with hydatidiform mole.

In conclusion, high-velocity and low-resistance blood flow are pathognomonic for gestational choriocarcinoma and predictive of its metastatic potential.

THREE-DIMENSIONAL POWER DOPPLER (3D PD)

The 3D power Doppler findings of gestational trophoblastic tumors are quite intriguing. The vasculature of diffuse and lacunar types appears quite similar on 3D rendering.[41] Their original uterine vasculature is disrupted and replaced by the abundant new vessels that are randomly arranged. The compact type of GTD is usually displayed as a solitary mass with an outer vascular ring. Choriocarcinoma may lack blood flow signals in the central portion but pulsed Doppler analysis of the uterine vasculature demonstrates a significant reduction in vascular impedance.

CONCLUSION

In patients with GTD, lower resistance and pulsatility index values are demonstrated in uteroplacental blood compared to normal early pregnancy. There is a correlation between the type of gestational trophoblastic neoplasia and peripheral resistance of the uteroplacental circulation expressed by Doppler indices (lower impedance values are detected in more "malignant" forms of the GTD). Color Doppler can assist the sonographer in detection of the persistent GTD and in follow-up of the patients receiving chemotherapy. It is hoped that 3D power Doppler angiography will further improve our diagnostic potential for the detection of gestational trophoblastic disease.

REFERENCES

1. Jaffe, R. Uteroplacental blood flow assessment in early pregnancy failure. In: Jaffe R and Warsof SL (Eds). Color Doppler Imaging in Obstetrics and Gynecology. New York: McGraw-Hill Inc 1992;73-84.
2. Jauniaux E and Campbell S. Ultrasonic assessment of placental abnormalities. Am J Obstet Gynecol 1990;163,1650-8.
3. Sherer DM, Allen T, Woods T. Transvaginal sonographic diagnosis of hydatidiform mole occuring two weeks after curettage for an incomplete abortion. J Clin Ultrasound 19(4):224-6.
4. Flam F, Lindhole H, Bui TH, et al. Color Doppler studies in trophoblastic tumors: A preliminary report. Ultrasound Obstet Gynecol 1991;1(5):349-52.
5. Howard HW. Gestational trophoblastic disease. In: Kase NG, Wiengold AB (Eds). Principles and Practice of Clinical Gynecology. New York: John Wiley and Sons 1983;907-26.
6. Single agent chemotherapy for non-metastatic gestational trophoblastic neoplasia. Perspectives for the 21st century after three decades of use. J Reprod Med 1991;36:49-55.
7. Newlands ES, Baghawe KD, Begent RHJ, et al. Developments in chemotherapy for medium- and high-risk patients with gestational trophoblastic tumors (1979-1984). Br J Obstet Gynecol 1986;93(1):63-9.
8. Timor-Tritsch IE, Rottem S. Pathology of the early intrauterine pregnancy. In: Timor-Tritsch IE, Rottem S (Eds.). Transvaginal Sonography, 2nd edn. New York: Elsevier; 1991;299-325.
9. Kurjak A, Crvenkovic G, Takeuchi H. Assessment of early pregnancy. In: Kurjak A (Ed). Transvaginal Color Doppler, Carnforth, UK, New Jersey: Parthenon Publishing 1991;41-52.
10. Szulman AE, Surti U. The syndromes of hydatidiform mole. II. Morphology evolution of the complete and partial mole. Am J Obstet Gynecol 1978;132:22-7.
11. Jauniaux E, Gavriil, Nicolaides K. Ultrasonographic assessment of early pregnancy complications. In: Jurkovic D, Jauniaux E. (Eds). Ultrasound and Early Pregnancy. London-New York: Parthenon Publishing 1996;53-64.
12. Fisher RA, Newlands ES. Rapid diagnosis and classification of hydatidiform moles with polymerase chain reaction. Am J Obstet Gynecol 1993;168(2):563-9.
13. Nyberg DA, Laing FC. Threatened abortion and abnormal first trimester intrauterine pregnancy. In: Nyberg DA, Hill LM, Bohm-Velez M, et al (Eds). Transvaginal Ultrasound. Boston, London: Mosby Year Book 1992;85-105.
14. Lazarus E, Hulka CA, Siewert B, et al. Sonographic appearance of early complete molar pregnancies. J Ultrasound Med 1999; 18(9):589-93.
15. Sebire NJ, Rees H, Paradinas F, et al. The diagnostic implications of routine ultrasound examination in histologically confirmed early molar pregnancies. Ultrasound Obstet Gynecol 2001;18(6):662-5.
16. Jurkovic D, Jauniaux E, Kurjak A. Transvaginal color Doppler assessment of the uteroplacental circulation in early pregnancy Obstet Gynecol 1991;77(3):365-9.
17. Berkowitz RS, Goldstein DP, Bernstein MR. Evolving concepts of molar pregnancy. J Reprod Med 36(1):40-4.
18. Jauniaux E, Bersinger NA, Gulbis B, et al. The contribution of maternal serum markers in the early prenatal diagnosis of molar pregnancies. Hum Reprod 14(3):842-6.
19. Jauniaux E, Halder A, Partington C. A case of partial mole associated with trisomy 13. Ultrasound Obstet Gynecol 1998; 11(1):62-4.
20. Astner A, Schwinger E, Caliebe A, et al. Sonographically detected fetal and placental abnormalities associated with trisomy 16 confined to the placenta. A case report and review of the literature. Prenat Diagn 1998;18(12):1308-15.
21. Aoki S, Hata H, Hata K, et al. Doppler color flow mapping on an invasive mole. Gynecol Obstet Invest 1989;27(1):52-4.
22. O'Quinn AG, Barnard DE. Trophoblastic disease. In: Benson H (Eds.) Current Obstetrics and Gynecologic Diagnosis and Treatment. Los Altos: Lange Medical Publications 1984;43.
23. Bracken MB, Brinton LA, Hayashi K. Epidemiology of hydatidiform mole and choriocarcinoma. Epidemiol Rev 1984; 6:52-75.
24. Cunningham FG, MacDonald PC, Gant NF. Disease and abnormalities of the placenta and fetal membranes. In: Williams E (Eds). Obstetrics, 18th Edition. Norwalk, San Mateo: Appleton & Lange 1991;533-53.
25. Tepper R, Shulman A, Altaras M, et al. The role of color Doppler flow in the management of nonmetastatic gestational trophoblastic disease. Gynecol Obstet Invest 1994;38(1):14-7.
26. Shimamoto K, Sakuma S, Ihigaki T, et al. Intratumoral blood flow: evaluating with color Doppler Echography. Radiology 1987;165(3):683-5.
27. Hsieh FJ, Wu CC, Lee CN, et al. Vascular patterns of gestational trophoblastic tumors by color Doppler ultrasound. 1994. Cancer 4(8):2361-5.
28. Mazur MT, Kurman RJ. Gestational trophoblastic disease. In: Kurman RJ (Eds.). Blaustein's pathology of the female-genital tract. 3rd Edition. New York: Springer-Verlag 1987;836-75.

29. Kohorn EI, McCarthy SM, Taylor KJW. Nonmetastatic gestational trophoblastic neoplasia. Role of ultrasonography and magnetic resonance imaging. J Reprod Med 1998;43(1):14-20.

30. Greenhill JP, Friedman EA. Biological Principles and Modern Practice of Obstetrics. Philadelphia, London, Toronto: WB Saunder Co 1976;556.

31. Kurjak A, Matijevic R, Kupesic S, et al. Gestational trophoblastic disease. In: Kurjak A (Ed.). An Atlas of Transvaginal Color Doppler. London-New York: Parthenon Publishing 1994;125-37.

32. Li HW, Tsao SW, Cheung AN. Current understanding of the molecular genetics of gestational trophoblastic diseases. Placenta 2002;23(1):20-31.

33. Todd A, Newlands E, Palazzo M. Unusual case of choriocarcinoma occurring 12 months after delivery. B Medical J 1998;316:532-4.

34. Matijevic R, Kurjak A, Shalan H. Predicting malignancy in gestational trophoblastic disease by transvaginal color and pulsed Doppler sonography. Ultrasound Obstet Gynecol 1992; 1:133.

35. Feng C, Lei X, Liu J. Diagnostic value of color Doppler flow imaging in gestational trophoblastic diseases (Chinese). Chinese Journal of Obstetrics and Gynecology 1996;31(4),209-11.

36. Kawano M, Mauzaki H, Ihimaru T. Transvaginal color Doppler studies in gestational trophoblastic disease. Ultrasound Obstet Gynecol 1996;7(3):197-200.

37. Flam F. Colour flow Doppler for gestational trophoblastic neoplasia. European J of Gynecol Oncol 1994;15(6):443-8.

38. Zanetta G, Lisoni A, Colombo M, et al. Detection of abnormal intrauterine vascularization by color Doppler imaging: a possible additional aid for the follow-up of patients with gestational trophoblastic tumors. Ultrasound Obstet Gynecol 1996;7(1):32-7.

39. Lindholm H, Radestad A, Flam F. Hysteroscopy provides proof of trophoblastic tumors in three cases with negative color Doppler images. Ultrasound Obstet Gynecol 1997; 9(1):59-61.

40. Feltmate CM, Genest DR, Goldstein DP, et al. Advances in the understanding of placental site trophoblastic tumor. J Reprod Med 2002;47(5):337-41.

41. Shih JC, Cheng SP, Hsieh FJ. Assessment of uterine neoplasms with three-dimensional power Doppler ultrasonography. In: Kurjak A (Ed.). Three-dimensional power Doppler in obstetrics and gynecology. New York, London: The Parthenon Publishing Group 2000;53-64.

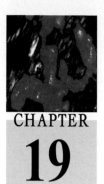

19

Clinical Sonographic Pearls

INTRODUCTION

"Clinical Sonographic Pearls" are developed to assist in performing a well-structured study of pregnant and nonpregnant female pelvis. To better serve the clinical needs, this chapter is organized section-wise according to the most common indications in the clinical practice:

PELVIC ULTRASOUND PEARLS

1. Amenorrhea.
2. Abnormal genital tract bleeding in reproductive age patients.
3. Menopause.
4. Peri- and postmenopausal bleeding.
5. Pelvic floor relaxation and urinary incontinence.
6. Evaluation, monitoring and treatment of female infertility.
7. Localization of an intrauterine contraceptive device and follow-up of the patients using birth control pills.
8. Signs and symptoms of pelvic inflammatory disease
9. Pelvic pain.
10. Abnormal Pap smear and cervical mass.
11. Uterine mass.
12. Adnexal mass.
13. Breast lump.

OBSTETRIC ULTRASOUND PEARLS

1. First Trimester Ultrasound Scan (Early pregnancy and Nuchal Translucency Scan).
2. Second and Third Trimester Ultrasound Examination (Fetal Anatomy Scan).
3. Bleeding in Pregnancy.

Because ultrasound findings may be difficult to explain, the author of "Clinical Sonographic Pearls" believes that the most efficient way of teaching ultrasound is to provide the medical illustrations. Graphics provided by Drs Patham and Subramanya exactly demonstrate what and why the sonographers and physicians should look for.

Second part of this manual provides the information how to enhance the skills in creating an ultrasound report. Although, "one picture is worth more than a thousand words", ultrasound report is the way how sonographers communicate their thoughts with referring physicians. Although, easy reading is difficult to write, I believe that brief explanations of the ultrasound images and graphics are self-explanatory guide to your everyday practice.

"Clinical Sonographic Pearls" are organized according to indication for ultrasound examination.[1-13] A brief clinical history of the patient (including Ob Gyn history, previous surgeries and the date of the last menstrual period) should be written in the introduction section. Before and during the course of ultrasound examination, the sonographer should ask clinically relevant questions and look for the patient's clinical findings that may help in performing an accurate diagnosis. Also, the sonographer should be aware of the investigations that were or have to be performed for each indication. The information on ultrasound findings may help the sonographers/physicians in pattern recognition, but also may assist in writing a systematic ultrasound report.

Finally, at the end of each section, there is a list of the differential diagnoses that have to be considered for each clinical presentation.

First part of the guide for practicing sonographers consists of 13 most common presentations for nonpregnant patients. Second part of the guide is dedicated to sonographic examinations during the first, second and third trimesters of pregnancy.

PELVIC ULTRASOUND PEARLS

Text and images by: S Kupesic Plavsic
Medical illustrations by: Bhargavi Patham and Sandesh Subramanya

Before you start an ultrasound examination make sure that you are provided with sufficient information about the patient and the indication for the ultrasound exam.

Pelvic ultrasound examination consists of transabdominal and transvaginal ultrasound exam. Transabdominal ultrasound is usually performed with a 3.5 MHz frequency transducer, while transvaginal scans are performed using frequencies of 5 MHz or higher. For a complete transabdominal pelvic sonogram, the patient's bladder should be appropriately distended. For transvaginal sonogram, the urinary bladder should be empty. The transvaginal transducer is introduced by the physician, the sonographer or the patient. Depending on the local policies, patient may consider to have a chaperone present during the pelvic ultrasound exam.[2,3]

UTERUS

The first structure to be evaluated during the pelvic exam is the uterus. The sonographer should always evaluate the size, shape and orientation (ante- or retroversion) of the uterus using standard (longitudinal and transverse) planes.[4-6]

Uterine Measurements

- Uterine length is measured in longitudinal plane (long axis) from the cervix to the fundus (from the external cervical os to the fundal serosa)
- Using the same plane (long axis) the sonographer measures the anteroposterior dimension of the uterus (the uterine thickness measurement is perpendicular to the line measuring the uterine length)
- The maximum width of the uterus is measured in a transverse plane (short axis).

Uterine Contours

- The sonographer should note any abnormality of the uterine contours (for example, fundal cleft suggestive of a bicornuate uterus).

Uterine Orientation

- Anteversion
- Retroversion.

Myometrium Assessment

- Define myometrial echogenicity (homogeneous/heterogeneous)

- Assess the myometrial masses
  - Each mass should be measured in 2 to 3 diameters
  - Specify the uterine mass echogenicity
  - Define the uterine mass borders (well-defined/ill-defined)
  - Assess the uterine mass location
- Identify myometrial cysts (specify the dimension and location of the cysts (inner, medial or deep myometrial layer)
  - Each cyst should be measured in 2 to 3 diameters
  - Define the location of the cyst (inner, medcal or deep myometrial layer).

Endometrial Assessment

- Thickness (double layer in long axis)[*,**]
- Echogenicity (triple layer/hyperechogenic)
- Focal abnormalities (yes/no)
- Presence of intracavitary fluid (yes/no)
- In menstruating patients, the endometrium should be correlated with the phase of the menstrual cycle:
  - Postmenstrual phase
  - Early proliferative phase
  - Late proliferative phase
  - Periovulatory phase
  - Early secretory phase
  - Late secretory phase.
- If endometrium cannot be clearly delineated or is poorly defined, the sonographer should report that endometrium is ill-defined.

* The endometrial measurement should include the anterior and posterior portions of the endometrium.

** Intracavitary fluid should be excluded from the measurement.

Apply Color and/or Power Doppler Ultrasound

To assess localization (peripheral/central vessels), penetrating (penetrating/nonpenetrating pattern) and branching pattern of the vessels (regular/irregular) of myometrial and/or endometrial lesions.

Perform Pulsed Doppler Analysis

To quantitatively analyze blood flow parameters (resistance index, pulsatility index) and differentiate physiologic angiogenesis from neovascularization.

Adnexa/Ovaries

- **Ovarian Measurements**
  Measure the ovarian length, width and thickness (cm) using two orthogonal planes
- In menstruating patients, you may visualize the follicles or corpus luteum. In this case correlate the ovarian and uterine/endometrial findings in respect to the phase of the menstrual cycle
- In infertile patients, you may be asked to monitor the follicular growth. In this case measure each follicle in two orthogonal planes. Measure and report the endometrial thickness and echogenicity
- **Document every intraovarian and/or adnexal lesion and describe its sonographic characteristics**
- Echogenicity (sonolucent/mixed echogenicity/hyperechogenic)
- Wall (thin/thick, regular/irregular wall thickening)
- Intracystic growths (papillary protrusions: solitary or multiple)
- Solid parts
- Shadowing echodensity
- Septations (thin/thick)
- Presence of free fluid in the cul-de-sac
- **Apply Color and/or Power Doppler Ultrasound**
  - To assess localization (peripheral/central vessels), penetrating (penetrating/nonpenetrating pattern) and branching pattern of the intraovarian vessels (regular/irregular)
- **Perform Pulsed Doppler Analysis**
  - To quantitatively analyze blood flow parameters (resistance index, pulsatility index) and differentiate physiologic angiogenesis from neovascularization.

TUBES

- The fallopian tubes are usually not identified by ultrasound, unless there is tubal pathology or free fluid in the cul-de-sac
- The area between the uterus and the ovaries should be carefully evaluated for tubular and complex structures
- Look for:
  - Distended tubes with incomplete septations
  - Pseudopapillary protrusions
  - Cogwheel sign
- Apply color and pulsed Doppler ultrasound to assess blood flow parameters.

CUL-DE-SAC

- Cul-de-sac should be evaluated for the presence of free fluid and/or a mass

- In case you find a mass in the cul-de-sac, define its position (in relation to the uterus and the ovaries), dimension and sonographic characteristics (refer to the sonographic characteristics of the adnexal masses).

WRITING AN ULTRASOUND REPORT

Ultrasound report is a permanent record of the ultrasound observations and impressions. It is also an integral component of the patient's permanent health record. Name of the ultrasound facility and date of the ultrasound examination should be provided on every image. Images of all the pelvic structures and organs should be stored, together with all the measurements.

The standard ultrasound report is organized according to the following structure:[13]

- **Preliminary Information: Patient's History and Indication**
  - Patient's full name, medical record number, date of birth and date when ultrasound study was performed
  - Clinical history
  - Indication
- **Findings**
  - Provide a step-by-step information about the
    - Uterine
    - Adnexal
    - Cul-de-sac findings
  - Provide the measurements for pelvic organs/structures
  - List the specific projections/planes of your studies
  - Describe your observations objectively in a paragraph-form report
- **Impression**
  - Summary of the most important ultrasound findings
  - The impressions should be numbered in decreasing order of importance
- **Recommendation (optional)**
  - Inform the referring physician about the necessity and time of the follow-up exam (if needed)
  - Provide clinical and/or therapeutic recommendations to the referring physician
- **Signature**
  - Every report has to be reviewed and signed by the author (interpreting physician).

Be aware that your report may serve different purposes. It is not only a communication tool with other health care professionals, but also a permanent record that may be utilized for medico-legal purposes. The ultrasound report is a valuable document in expediting the treatment of your patient and is an important step in formulating an accurate and precise diagnosis.[13]

The ultrasound report is as important as your clinical knowledge and scanning technique, so make sure that you always write a well-documented and precise ultrasound report.

REFERENCES

1. Kupesic S, Plavsic BM. Normal Anatomy of the Female Pelvis. In: Stephenson S (Ed). Diagnostic Medical Sonography in Obstetrics and Gynecology: A Guide to Clinical Practice, 3rd edition. Philadelphia: Lippincott Williams & Wilkins, 2000.
2. AIUM. (2009). Practice Guideline for the Performance of Pelvic Ultrasound Examinations. [online] by the American Institute of Ultrasound in Medicine. Available from http://www.aium.org/publications/guidelines/pelvis.pdf.
3. Stagno SJ, Forster H, Belinson J. Medical and osteopathic boards' positions on chaperones during gynecologic examinations. Obstet Gynecol 1999;94(3):352-4.
4. Kupesic S, de Ziegler D. Ultrasound and infertility. New York/London: Parthenon Publishing, 2000.
5. Kupesic S, Kurjak A. Normal Gynecologic Anatomy (Uterus, Tubes, Ovaries) Donald School Textbook of Ultrasound in Obstetrics and Gynecology. In: Kurjak A, Chervenak F (Eds). New Delhi:Jaypee Brothers Medical Publishers 2008;783-90.
6. Kupesic S, Kurjak A. Uterine Lesions: Advances in Ultrasound Diagnosis. Donald School Textbook of Ultrasound in Obstetrics and Gynecology. In: Kurjak A, Chervenak F (Eds). New Delhi: Jaypee Brothers Medical Publishers 2008;791-802.
7. Kupesic S, Kurjak A. Fallopian Tube. Donald School Textbook of Ultrasound in Obstetrics and Gynecology. In: Kurjak A, Chervenak F (Eds). New Delhi: Jaypee Brothers Medical Publishers 2008;855-64.
8. Kupesic S. Sonographic Imaging in Infertility. Donald School Textbook of Ultrasound in Obstetrics and Gynecology. In: Kurjak A, Chervenak F (Eds). New Delhi: Jaypee Brothers Medical Publishers 2008;865-86.
9. Kupesic S, Plavsic BM. Hystero-sono-salpingography: A Text-atlas of Normal and Abnormal Findings. Donald School Textbook of Ultrasound in Obstetrics and Gynecology. In: Kurjak A, Chervenak F (Eds). New Delhi: Jaypee Brothers Medical Publishers 2008;899-912.
10. Kupesic S, Kurjak A. Guided Procedures using Transvaginal Sonography. Donald School Textbook of Ultrasound in Obstetrics and Gynecology. In: Kurjak A, Chervenak F (Eds). New Delhi: Jaypee Brothers Medical Publishers; 2008;913-22.
11. Kupesic S, Plavsic BM. Sonographic Evaluation of Gynecologic and Obstetric Causes of Acute Pelvic Pain. Donald School Textbook of Ultrasound in Obstetrics and Gynecology. In: Kurjak A, Chervenak F (Eds). New Delhi: Jaypee Brothers Medical Publishers 2008;939-50.
12. Kupesic S. Ectopic pregnancy. Donald School Textbook of Ultrasound in Obstetrics and Gynecology. In: Kurjak A, Chervenak F (Eds). New Delhi: Jaypee Brothers Medical Publishers 2008;230-43.
13. Taylor JAM. Writing radiology reports. Journal of the CCA. 1990; 34(1):30-4.

19.1: AMENORRHEA

Text and images by: S Kupesic Plavsic
Medical illustrations by: Bhargavi Patham and Sandesh Subramanya

Amenorrhea is the absence of menstrual bleeding (Flow chart 19.1.1). It may indicate an anatomic, genetic, biochemical, physiologic or even psychological abnormality. Physiologic amenorrhea is the absence of the menstrual bleeding during pregnancy, lactation and after menopause. It is not a disease and does not need to be evaluated. Teenage girls may experience intervals of amenorrhea lasting 2 to 12 months during the first two years after menarche.

Pathologic amenorrhea is suspected in the following clinical situations:

(a) At 14 years of age, in the absence of menstruation and secondary sexual characteristics.

(b) At 16 years of age, regardless of whether there are secondary sexual characteristics.

(c) At any age when menstrual bleeding has ceased in a women who previously had normal menstrual function.

Oligomenorrhea is defined as a reduction in number of the menstrual periods and/or amount of menstrual flow.

Clinical Clues

- **Ask about:**
  - Age of the patient
  - Presence or absence of secondary sexual characteristics
  - Time of onset of amenorrhea
  - Use of medication
  - History of weight gain or loss, poor eating habits or strenuous exercise program
  - History of emotional stress
  - Body hair growth
  - Galactorrhea
  - Symptoms suggestive of thyroid disease
  - Symptoms suggestive of adrenal disease
  - Cyclic pelvic pain
- **Look for:**
  - Secondary sexual characteristics
  - Hirsutism
  - Acne
  - Defeminization
  - Masculinization
  - Somatic abnormalities
  - Thyroid and adrenal dysfunction
  - Presence or absence of a functional vagina
  - Presence or absence of a palpable pelvic mass on rectal examination.

Investigations

- Physical examination
- Laboratory studies:

Flow chart 19.1.1: Inductive reasoning scheme for diagnostic evaluation of patients presenting with amenorrhea (*Courtesy:* Paul L. Foster School of Medicine, Texas Tech University at El Paso, TX, USA). Ultrasound may assist in detection of gonadal failure, pregnancy, anovulation, and anatomical abnormalities, such as nonfunctional endometrium and abnormal outflow tract.

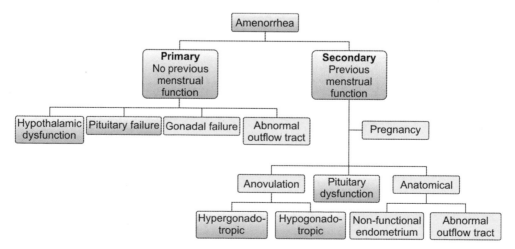

- Serum beta human chorionic gonadotropin levels (beta hCG to rule out pregnancy)
- Prolactin levels
- Thyroid stimulating hormone levels (TSH)
- Triiodothyronine (T3) and thyroxine (T4)
- Plasma testosterone and dehydroepiandrosterone sulfate (DHEAS)
- Cortisol levels (morning and evening)
- Glucose tolerance test
- Progesterone challenge test (medroxyprogesterone 10 mg daily for 5 days)
- In patients with negative progesterone challenge test evaluate the endometrial potential (sequential use of estrogen and progesterone: conjugated estrogen 2.5 mg daily for 21 days, with medroxyprogesterone 20 mg daily for the last 5 days of estrogen therapy)
- In case of hyperprolactinemia perform:
  - Computed axial tomography (CT) scan or magnetic resonance imaging (MRI) of the pituitary gland
- Laparoscopy (if indicated).

Ultrasound Findings

- Physiologic amenorrhea (menopause): small ovaries and thin endometrium (<5 mm) Premature ovarian failure: small ovaries and thin endometrium (<5 mm)
- Intrauterine pregnancy
- Anovulation/ovarian dysfunction: polycystic ovaries (enlarged ovaries (>10 cc, more than 10 follicles measuring from 2 to 9 mm, and enlarged and hyperechogenic stroma)
- Intrauterine adhesions (synechiae): irregular endometrium with hyperechogenic and avascular bridges, suggestive of intrauterine adhesions
- Imperforate hymen: muco/hematocolpos, muco/hematometra, muco/hematosalpynx and free fluid in the cul-de-sac.

Diagnoses to Consider

- Pregnancy
- Breastfeeding (lactation)
- Anovulation
  - Hypergonadotropic hypogonadism
  - Hypogonadotropic hypogonadism

- Ovarian dysfunction
  - Polycystic ovary syndrome
- Hypothalamic
  - Functional
  - Inflammatory/infiltrative disease
  - Hypothalamic tumors (e.g. craniopharyngioma)
  - Pituitary stalk dissection or compression
  - Brain injury
- Pituitary dysfunction
  - Hyperprolactinemia
  - Pituitary tumors
  - Meningioma, germinoma, glioma
  - Empty sella syndrome
  - Pituitary infarct
- Other endocrinological disorders
  - Hyper/hypothyroidism
  - Diabetes mellitus
  - Exogenous androgens
- Anatomic
  - Nonfunctioning endometrium (e.g. intrauterine adhesions)
  - Abnormal outflow tract

Some case studies related to amenorrhea are depicted in Figures 19.1.1 to 19.1.16.

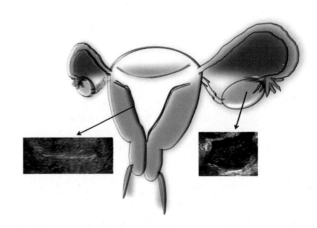

FIGURE 19.1.1: Thin endometrium and small ovaries are normal ultrasound finding in postmenopausal patients. Similar sonographic features are visualized in patients with premature ovarian failure. Note thin and hyperechoic endometrium on the left and small ovary with no evidence of follicular growth on the right.

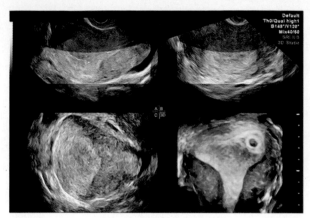

FIGURE 19.1.2: Three-dimensional ultrasound (multiplanar view and surface rendering) of an early gestational sac. Note the triangular shape of the uterine cavity and eccentric position of the gestational sac at 5 weeks gestation on the right low image.

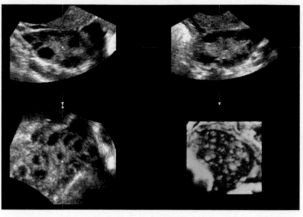

FIGURE 19.1.5: Multiplanar and surface rendering of an ovary in a patient presenting with amenorrhea. Note more than ten follicles at the periphery of enlarged ovarian stroma. This sonographic finding is typical of anovulation associated with polycystic ovarian syndrome.

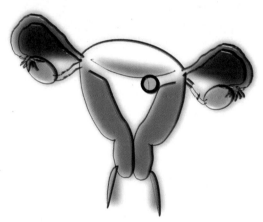

FIGURE 19.1.3: Intrauterine pregnancy is the most common finding in reproductive age patients presenting with amenorrhea. Therefore, beta hCG and ultrasound are the first investigations to be performed in this group of patients.

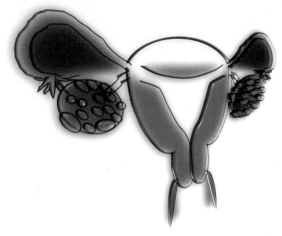

FIGURE 19.1.6: Sonographic criteria for polycystic ovaries are the following: enlarged ovaries (>10 cc), and 10 or more cystic structures (follicles measuring from 2 to 9 mm) arranged peripherally or scattered throughout the enlarged echo dense stroma.

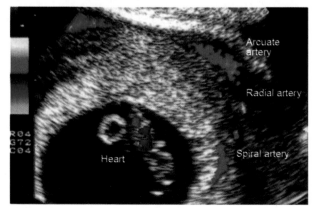

FIGURE 19.1.4: Color Doppler ultrasound of an early gestational sac containing yolk sac and embryo. Color signals are obtained from the maternal vessels (arcuate, radial and spiral arteries) and fetal heart.

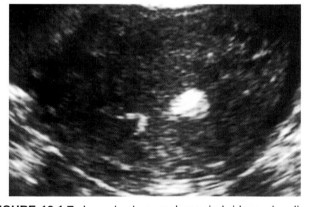

FIGURE 19.1.7: Irregular hyperechogenic bridges visualized within the central part of the uterine cavity in a patient with secondary amenorrhea following dilatation and curettage.

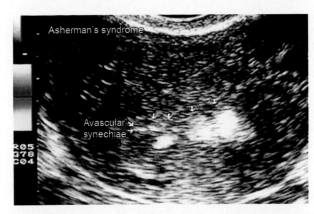

FIGURE 19.1.8: Color Doppler does not reveal any blood flow signals from the irregular hyperechogenic bridges within the uterine cavity. Hysteroscopy revealed intrauterine adhesions (Asherman syndrome).

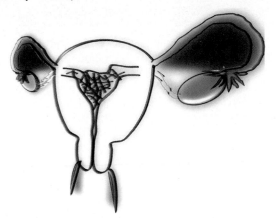

FIGURE 19.1.9: Intrauterine adhesions are scar tissue that can partially or completely obliterate the uterine cavity. Most commonly intrauterine adhesions are caused by instrumental procedures (curettage) after pregnancy (due to retained placenta or hemorrhage) or dilatation, evacuation and curettage for a miscarriage. Also, adhesions may develop following the uterine infections (for example, PID after abortion) and pelvic tuberculosis.

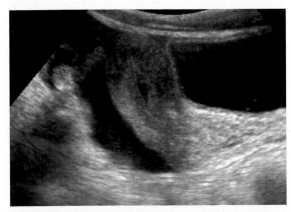

FIGURE 19.1.10: Distended uterine cavity and free fluid in the cul-de-sac in a 14-year-old patient with primary amenorrhea and cyclic abdominal and pelvic pain.

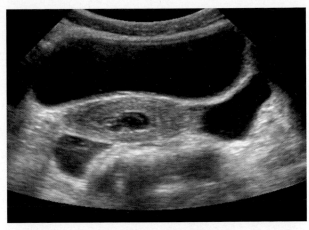

FIGURE 19.1.11: The same patient as in Figure 19.1.10. Note distended uterine cavity and free fluid in the cul-de-sac.

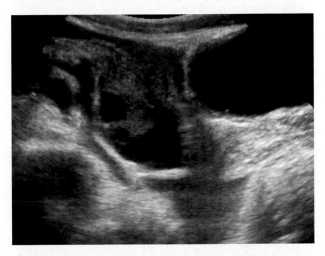

FIGURE 19.1.12: The same patient. Normal sized right ovary and hematosalpinx.

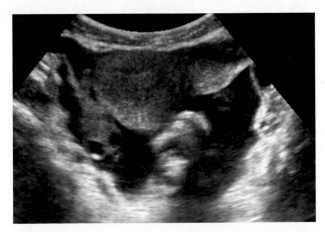

FIGURE 19.1.13: The same patient as in Figures 19.1.10 to 19.1.12. Bilateral hematosalpinx and free fluid in the cul-de-sac in a patient with primary amenorrhea and imperforate hymen.

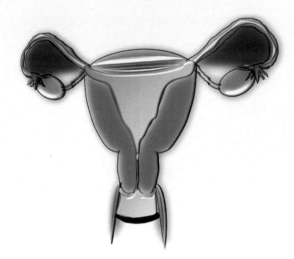

FIGURE 19.1.14: Imperforate hymen is the most common form of vaginal outflow obstruction. Normal hymen is visualized as ring-like structure at the level of the vaginal vestibule. Absence of the central portion of the hymenal membrane allows free drainage of the uterine and vaginal secretions. An imperforate hymen leads to entrapment of the mucus and/or blood and may lead to formation of the mucocolpos, hematocolpos, mucometra, hematometra, mucosalpinx and/or hematosalpinx.

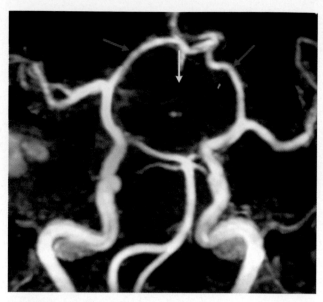

FIGURE 19.1.16: Pituitary macroadenoma in a patient with secondary amenorrhea. MR Angiography of the circle of Willis demonstrate the marked mass effect produced by the pituitary macroadenoma (yellow arrow) with dorsal displacement of bilateral A1 segments of the anterior cerebral arteries (red arrows). Contribution of Dr. J. Gavito (*Courtesy:* Medical Image Library, Eds. S. Kupesic Plavsic and B Patham, Paul L Foster School of Medicine, Texas Tech University at El Paso, TX, USA).

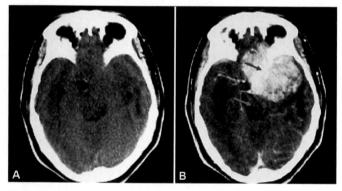

FIGURE 19.1.15: Sphenoid wing meningioma in a patient with secondary amenorrhea. CT scan A) without and B) with contrast, demonstrate a large intracranial mass attached to the left sphenoid wing (red arrow), producing marked mass effect with displacement of the adjacent brain parenchyma and brainstem (blue arrow). Contribution of Dr J Gavito (*Courtesy:* Medical Image Library, Eds S Kupesic Plavsic and B Patham, Paul L Foster School of Medicine, Texas, Tech University at El Paso, TX, USA).

BIBLIOGRAPHY

1. Beck WW. Obstetrics & Gynecology, 4th Edition. Philadelphia: Williams and Wilkins 1997.
2. Kupesic S, de Ziegler D. Ultrasound and infertility. New York/London: Parthenon Publishing 2000.
3. Kupesic S, Kurjak A. Normal Gynecologic Anatomy (Uterus, Tubes, Ovaries) Donald School Textbook of Ultrasound in Obstetrics and Gynecology. In: Kurjak A, Chervenak F (Eds). New Delhi: Jaypee Brothers Medical Publishers 2008;783-90.
4. Popat V, Prodanov T, Verma S, et al. Primary amenorrhea. http://emedicine.medscape.com/article/252928-overview
5. Speroff L, Glass RH, Kase NG. Clinical gynecologic endocrinology and infertility, 6th Edition. Philadelphia: Lippincott Williams and Wilkins 1999.

19.2: ABNORMAL GENITAL TRACT BLEEDING (REPRODUCTIVE AGE)

Text and images by: S Kupesic Plavsic
Medical illustrations by: Bhargavi Patham and Sandesh Subramanya

Vaginal bleeding is considered abnormal when it occurs at an unexpected time (before menarche or after menopause), when it varies from the normal amount or pattern, or when the pattern itself is abnormal (vaginal bleeding lasting more than 7 days, flow >80 ml, usually in clots and interval < 24 days) (Flow chart 19.2.1).

Menorrhagia is excessive uterine bleeding occurring at the expected intervals of menstrual periods. Metrorrhagia is uterine bleeding occurring at irregular intervals, particularly between the expected menstrual periods. Enometrorrhagia is excessive uterine bleeding both at the usual time of menstrual periods and at other irregular intervals (Flow chart 19.2.2).

Abnormal genital tract bleeding may arise from the lesion or disease at any anatomic site in the lower genital tract (vulva, vagina or cervix) or upper genital tract (uterine corpus or fallopian tubes). The source of bleeding may simulate vaginal bleeding but be of nongynecologic origin, such as the urethra, bladder or bowel.

During the reproductive age, genital tract bleeding usually reflects a disturbance in normal ovulatory function, but may also be associated with pregnancy complications. The sonographer should also look for uterine masses (fibroids, adenomyosis) and endometrial lesions (hyperplasia, polyps and carcinoma) (Flow chart 19.2.3).

Clinical Clues

- **Ask about:**
  - Menstrual periods: cyclic menses ± molimina (periodic symptoms associated with the physiological changes preceding or accompanying menstruation)
  - Irregular bleeding, bleeding after straining or heavy lifting (suggestive of polyps)
  - Postcoital bleeding (suggestive of cervical lesions)
  - Heavy or prolonged bleeding (suggestive of intramural and/or submucosal fibroids distorting the endometrial cavity)
  - Prolonged, heavy, painful menstrual periods associated with a diffusely enlarged uterus (suggestive of adenomyosis)
  - Use of hormonal contraceptives, intrauterine contraception and progestin-only contraceptives (for example, breakthrough bleeding)

Flow chart 19.2.1: Inductive reasoning scheme for diagnostic evaluation of the patients presenting with abnormal genital tract bleeding during reproductive age (*Courtesy:* Paul L. Foster School of Medicine, Texas Tech University at El Paso, TX, USA). Ultrasound and laboratory findings can distinguish between pregnant and nonpregnant patients, who can be further divided into the ovulatory and anovulatory subjects.

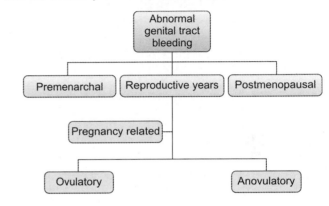

Flow chart 19.2.2: Menorrhagia can be a symptom of benign or malignant uterine tumors and can lead to anemia. Ultrasound imaging is the method of choice for visualization of the uterine tumors / lesions causing abnormally heavy or extensive menstrual flow.

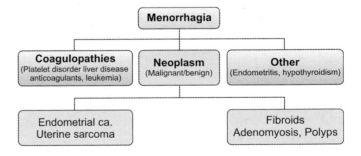

Flow chart 19.2.3: Using ultrasound, clinician can diagnose different causes of intermenstrual bleeding (such as endometrial and cervical polyps) and menorrhagia.

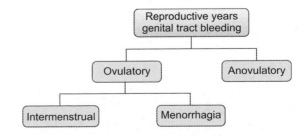

- Vaginal itching
- Trauma
- Urinary symptoms
- Weight gain and/or loss
- Endocrine disorders
- Systemic disease
- Coagulation disorder
- **Look for:**
  - Lower genital tract disorders (for example, cervical lesions)
  - Uterine dimension:
    - Endometrial polyps: uterus is normal on bimanual examination
    - Adenomyosis: diffusely enlarged uterus (associated with prolonged, heavy, painful menstrual periods)
    - Uterine fibroids: uterine enlargement, irregular uterine contour
- Adnexal mass
- Endocrine disorders (for example, hypothyroidism or hyperthyroidism)
- Severe organ disease, such as renal failure or liver failure
- Genital injury or a foreign object
- Coagulation defects (for example, von Willebrand's disease).

Investigations

- **Clinical history:**
  - Current bleeding history
  - Menstrual history
  - Use of oral contraception
  - Medical history with emphasis to coagulation disorders
  - Medication history
- **Physical examination:**
  - General physical examination
  - Pelvic examination
  - Rectal exam (if indicated)
- **Laboratory tests:**
  - Complete blood count (hemoglobin, hematocrit)
  - Thyroid stimulating hormone (TSH)
  - Coagulation profile (PT, PTT, BT)
  - Pregnancy test (if indicated)
- **Diagnostic studies:**
  - Pap smear, if indicated
  - Pelvic ultrasound
  - Colposcopy and biopsy, if appropriate (in adolescent patients)

- Follicle-stimulating hormone (FSH), Luteinizing hormone (LH) and E2 on day 3 of the menstrual cycle, if indicated
- Serum progesterone on day LH+7
- Thyroid stimulating hormone (TSH)
- Prolactin
- Androgen profile (testosterone, dehydroepiandrosterone, hydroxyprogesterone).

Ultrasound Findings

Uterus

- Look for enlarged uterus (look for uterine fibroids and adenomyosis)
- Evaluate myometrium
  - Heterogeneous myometrium: look for uterine fibroids and adenomyosis
  - Assess focal myometrial masses
    - Each mass should be measured in 2-3 diameters
    - Specify the uterine mass echogenicity
    - Define the uterine mass location (submucosal/intramural/subserosal)
    - Define the uterine mass borders (well-defined/ill-defined)
    - Identify myometrial cysts (specify the dimension and location of the cyst(s): inner, medial or deep myometrial layer, suggestive of adenomyosis)
    - Each cyst should be measured in 2-3 diameters
    - Define the location of the cysts (superficial, medial or deep myometrial layer)
    - Evaluate the regularity/irregularity of the endometrial-subendometrial layer
- Ill-defined, fast growing myometrial lesions with irregular blood flow pattern and low vascular impedance are suggestive of myometrial malignancy.
- Assess the **endometrium**
  - Thickness (double layer in a long axis)
  - Echogenicity (triple layer/hyperechogenic)
  - Look for focal abnormalities (yes/no)–suggestive of endometrial polyp(s)
  - Presence of intracavitary fluid (yes/no)
  - Correlate the endometrial appearance with the ovarian findings
  - If endometrium cannot be clearly delineated or is poorly defined, the sonographer should report that endometrium is ill-defined
  - In nonpregnant patients with unclear endometrial finding on ultrasound, saline infusion sonography should be performed.

- Ill-defined, abnormally thickened endometrium with penetrating vessels, irregular course and low vascular impedance is suggestive or endometrial malignancy.

Adnexa

- Perform ovarian measurements
- Rule out polycystic ovaries (volume > 10-12 ml, more than 10 follicles measuring from 2 to 8.2 mm)
- Document every intraovarian and/or adnexal lesion and describe its sonographic characteristics (in patients with dysfunctional bleeding rule out unruptured follicle and/or functional cyst)
- If adnexal lesion is visualized refer to clinical pearl on adnexal mass.

Cul-de-sac

- Evaluate cul-de-sac for the presence of free fluid.

Diagnoses to Consider

- Early postmenarche
  - Anovulation (hypothalamic immaturity)
  - Coagulation disorders
  - Stress (psychogenic, exercise-induced)
  - Pregnancy
  - Infection
  - Trauma
- Reproductive age
  - Lower genital tract disorders:
    - Vulva
  - Benign
    - Skin tags
    - Sebaceous cyst
    - Condylomata
- Cancer
- Infection: STD
- Trauma
- Vagina
- Benign
  - Gartner's duct cysts
  - Polyps
- Cancer
- Vaginitis/infection (bacterial, STD, atrophic vaginitis)
- Trauma
- Cervix
- Benign
  - Polyps
  - Ectropion
- Malignant

- Invasive and noninvasive carcinoma
- Metastatic tumors (rare)
- Infection: cervicitis
- Trauma
  - Upper genital tract disorders:
    - Uterus
  - Benign
  - Polyps
  - Endometrial hyperplasia
  - Adenomyosis
  - Leiomyomas (fibroids)
  - Malignant
  - Adenocarcinoma
  - Sarcoma
  - Fallopian tube lesions
  - Benign lesions
  - PID
  - Malignant lesions
  - Ovarian lesions
  - Benign
  - Malignant
  - Other
- Medications
- Systemic disease
- Pregnancy complications
- Ectopic pregnancy
- Threatened or impending miscarriage
- Implantation bleeding.

Some case studies related to abnormal genital tract bleeding (reproductive age) are depicted in Figures 19.2.1 to 19.2.30.

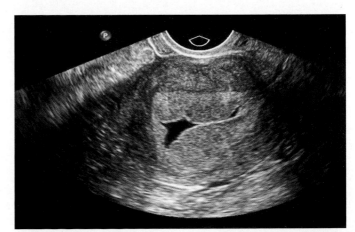

FIGURE 19.2.1: Distended uterine cavity filled with sonolucent fluid in a 17-year-old patient presenting with abnormal uterine bleeding. Note thickened hyperechogenic endometrium measuring 20 mm.

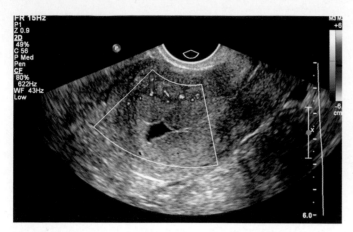

FIGURE 19.2.2: The same patient as in previous figure. Note color signals at the periphery of the thickened endometrium.

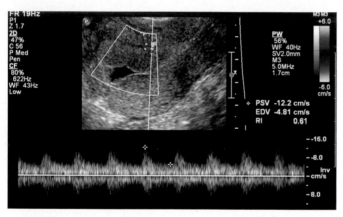

FIGURE 19.2.3: The same patient as in previous figures. Pulsed Doppler waveform analysis reveals moderate to high vascular impedance (RI = 0.61).

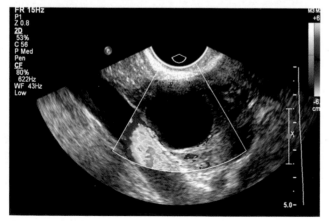

FIGURE 19.2.4: Transvaginal sonography reveals unruptured follicle measuring 25 x 27 mm. Color Doppler depicts iliac vessels and perifollicular capillaries.

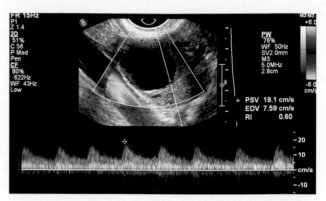

FIGURE 19.2.5: Pulsed Doppler analysis depicts moderate to high vascular impedance signals (RI = 0.60) from the periphery of unruptured follicle.

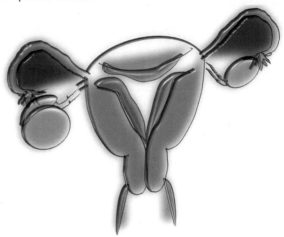

FIGURE 19.2.6: In patients with dysfunctional uterine bleeding sonographer should evaluate the endometrial thickness, echogenicity and vascularity, and compare it to the ovarian findings. Estrogen, produced by unruptured follicle causes abnormal thickening of the endometrium, that can no longer be sustained by its blood supply. Due to the absence of progesterone, the endometrium does not strip completely as during normal menstrual period, but demonstrates a prolonged and heavy bleeding.

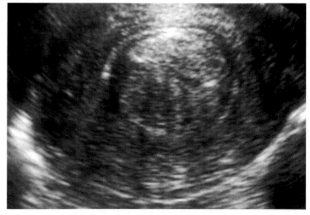

FIGURE 19.2.7: Transvaginal ultrasound of a submucosal uterine fibroid. Uterine fibroid capsule is clearly visualized at its periphery.

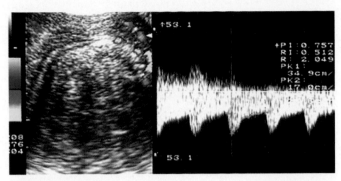

FIGURE 19.2.8: Transvaginal color Doppler scan of the same patient. Moderate-to-high vascular impedance (RI = 0.76) is typical of the uterine fibroid.

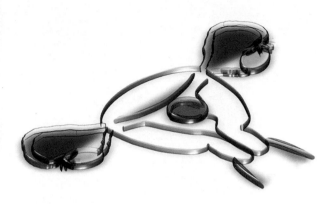

FIGURE 19.2.11: Fibroids located within the uterine cavity are called intracavitary fibroids. These tumors may be associated with abnormal uterine bleeding and infertility.

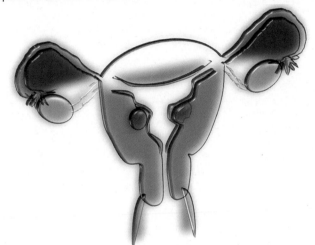

FIGURE 19.2.9: Submucosal fibroids are the fibroids that are located just below the endometrium. While they are the most infrequent type of fibroid, they often cause prolonged menstrual periods and excessive heavy bleeding (menorrhagia).

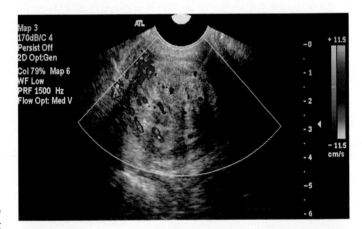

FIGURE 19.2.12: Color Doppler scan of an intramural fibroid.

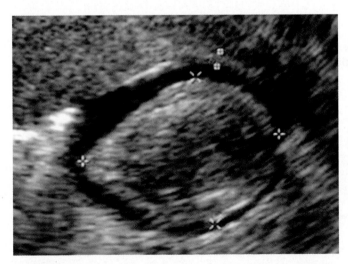

FIGURE 19.2.10: Saline infusion sonography (hysterosonography) enables clear visualization of the intracavitary fibroid.

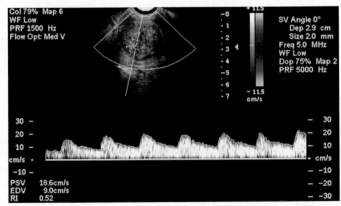

FIGURE 19.2.13: Pulsed Doppler waveform analysis demonstrates moderate vascular impedance blood flow signals (RI = 0.52) at the periphery of the uterine fibroid, typical of a benign uterine lesion.

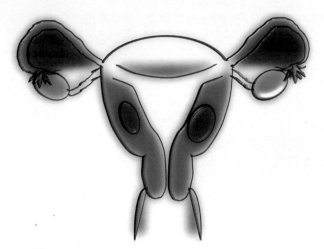

FIGURE 19.2.14: Intramural fibroids are the fibroids visualized within the uterine wall.

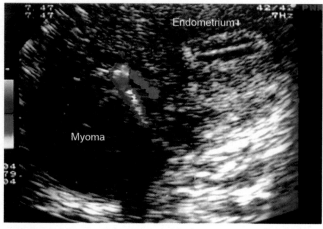

FIGURE 19.2.15: Transvaginal color Doppler scan of a subserosal, intraligamentary fibroid. Note the peripheral feeding vessels, derived from the arcuate arteries.

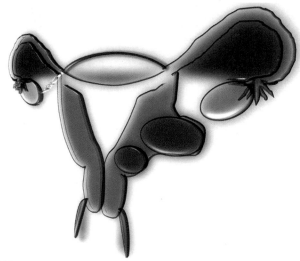

FIGURE 19.2.16: Subserosal fibroids grow on the outer wall of the uterus and usually cause no symptoms until they grow large to interfere with the neighboring organs.

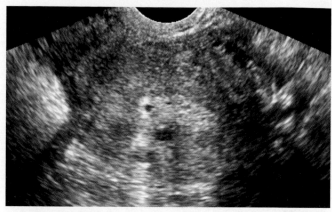

FIGURE 19.2.17: Enlarged uterus with heterogeneous myometrium. Note irregular junctional zone and a few cystic lesions within the endometrium and proximal layer of the myometrium in a patient with superficial adenomyosis.

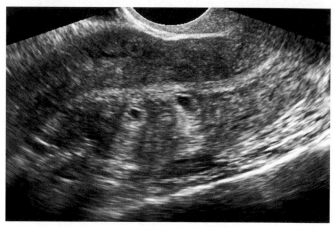

FIGURE 19.2.18: Longitudinal plane of the uterus in a patient with superficial adenomyosis.

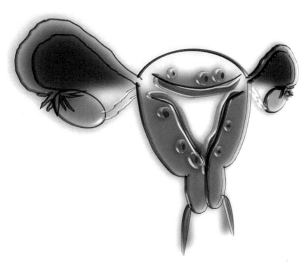

FIGURE 19.2.19: Superficial adenomyosis is the presence of endometrial foci within the proximal (inner third) myometrial layer.

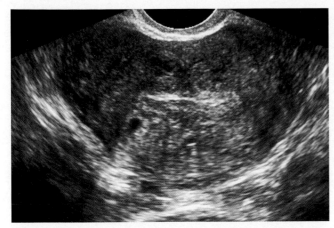

FIGURE 19.2.20: Heterogenicity of the myometrial echo-texture, myometrial cysts visualized deep within the myometrium and poorly defined endometrial-myometrial junction are typical features of deep adenomyosis.

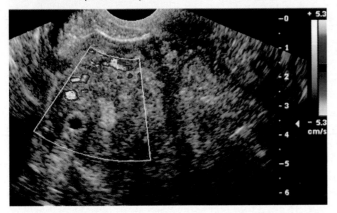

FIGURE 19.2.21: The same patient as in previous figure. Color Doppler reveals increased vascularity at the periphery of the heterotopic endometrial lesion.

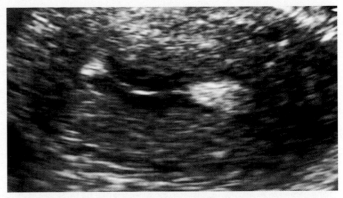

FIGURE 19.2.23: Transvaginal scan of the uterus in peri-ovulatory phase of the menstrual cycle. Focal areas of increased echogenicity (bigger to the right and smaller to the left) are typical of two endometrial polyps.

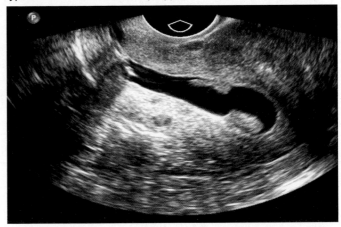

FIGURE 19.2.24: Saline infusion sonography (hysterosonography) in a patient with endometrial polyps. Note two endometrial polyps protruding into the uterine cavity.

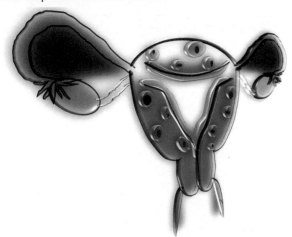

FIGURE 19.2.22: Deep adenomyosis is defined as penetration of the endometrial glands and stroma into the middle and deep myometrial layers (middle and outer third of the myometrium). It is an important cause of dysmenorrhea, menorrhagia and possibly subfertility.

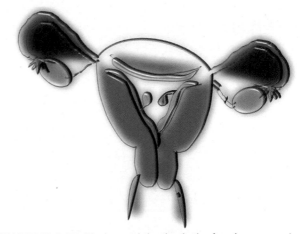

FIGURE 19.2.25: Endometrial polyp is the focal mass protruding from the inner lining of the endometrium. Endometrial polyps may be sessile or pedunculated. They may range in size from a few millimeters to several centimeters, and may protrude through the cervix into the vagina.

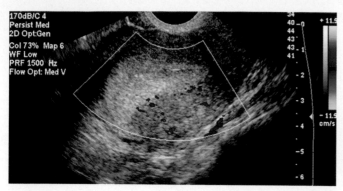

FIGURE 19.2.26: Diffusely thickened and hyperechogenic endometrium in a postmenopausal patient presenting with abnormal uterine bleeding. Color Doppler displays peripheral blood flow signals. Histology revealed endometrial hyperplasia.

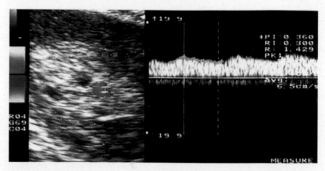

FIGURE 19.2.29: The same patient as in Figure 19.2.20. Low resistance obtained from the intratumoral vessels (RI = 0.30) is suggestive of endometrial malignancy.

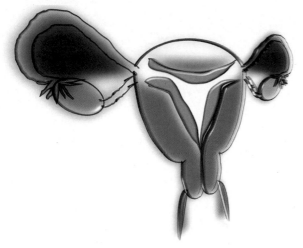

FIGURE 19.2.27: Endometrial hyperplasia is excessive and diffuse proliferation of the endometrium. In majority of the cases endometrial hyperplasia results from high-levels of estrogen.

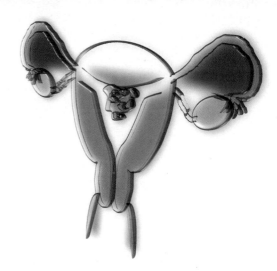

FIGURE 19.2.30: Endometrial carcinoma, the cancer that forms in the endometrium is among the most common pelvic malignancies. Multiple risk factors include conditions associated with disorders of menstruation, late menopause, long time period between menarche and menopause, use of estrogen replacement therapy and tamoxifen therapy for breast cancer, history of endometrial hyperplasia, obesity, nulliparity, diabetes mellitus and hypertension.

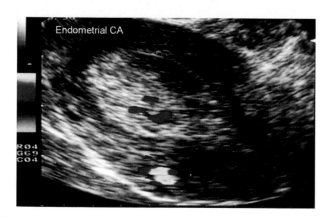

FIGURE 19.2.28: Transvaginal color Doppler scan of a 45-year-old patient with abnormal uterine bleeding and thickened endometrium. Patient was previously diagnosed with polycystic ovarian syndrome. Blood flow signals were obtained from the central portion of the lesion.

BIBLIOGRAPHY

1. Campbell S, Bourne T, Crayford T, et al. The early detection of endometrial cancer by transvaginal color Doppler ultrasonography. Eur J Obstet Gynecol Reprod Biol 1993;49 (1-2):44-5.
2. Kurjak A, Kupesic-Urek S, Miric D. The benign uterine tumor vascularization assessed by transvaginal color Doppler. J Ultrasound Med Biol 1992;18:645-9.
3. Kurjak A, Kupesic S, Shalan H, et al. Uterine sarcoma: A report of 10 cases studied by transvaginal color and pulsed Doppler sonography. Gynecol Oncol 1995;59(3):342-6.

4. Kurjak A, Shalan H, Sosic A, et al. Endometrial carcinoma in postmenopausal women: Evaluation by transvaginal color Doppler ultrasound. Obstet Gynecol 1993; 169(6):1597-603.

5. Kupesic S, Kurjak A, Zodan T. Staging of endometrial carcinoma by 3D power Doppler. Gynaecol Perinatol 1999; 8:1-521.

6. Kurjak A, Kupesic S. Three-dimensional power Doppler ultrasound examination of uterine lesions. In: Kurjak A (Ed). Three-dimensional power Doppler in obstetrics and gynecology. New York-London: Parthenon Publishing 1999;39-53.

7. Kupesic S, Kurjak A. Color Doppler assessment of uterine leiomyoma and sarcoma. In: Kurjak A, Kupesic S (Eds). An Atlas of transvaginal color Doppler. London-New York: Parthenon Publishing 2000;179.

8. Kupesic S, Kurjak A, Bjelos D. The assessment of uterine lesions. In: Kurjak A, Kupesic S (Eds). Clinical application of 3D sonography. London-New York: Parthenon Publishing 2000;55.

9. Kupesic S, Kurjak A, Bjelos D. Color Doppler and Three-Dimensional Ultrasound of the Uterine Lesions. In: Kupesic S (Ed). Color Doppler and three-dimensional ultrasound in gynecology, infertility and obstetrics. New Delhi: Jaypee Brothers 2003;29-43.

10. Kurjak A, Kupesic S. Transvaginal color Doppler and pulsed Doppler diagnosis of benign changes in the uterine myometrium. In: Schmidt W, Kurjak A (Eds). Color Doppler sonography in Gynecology and Obstetrics. Stuttgart, New York: Thieme Verlag 2005;274-8.

11. Kupesic S, Plavsic BM. Sonography of uterine leiomyomata. U: I. Brosens (ur): Uterine fibroids: Pathogenesis and management. London, New York: Taylor & Francis 2006; 139-51.

12. Kupesic S, Kurjak A. Normal Gynecologic Anatomy (Uterus, Tubes, Ovaries) Donald School Textbook of Ultrasound in Obstetrics and Gynecology. Kurjak A, Chervenak F (Eds). New Delhi: Jaypee Brothers Medical Publishers 2008;783-90.

13. Kupesic S, Kurjak A. Uterine Lesions: Advances in Ultrasound Diagnosis. Donald School Textbook of Ultrasound in Obstetrics and Gynecology. In: Kurjak A, Chervenak F (Eds). New Delhi: Jaypee Brothers Medical Publishers 2008;791-802.

19.3: MENOPAUSE

Text and images by: S Kupesic Plavsic
Medical illustrations by: Bhargavi Patham and Sandesh Subramanya

Women cease to have menstrual periods at about 50 years of age (physiologic menopause), although ovarian function declines earlier. Spontaneous cessation of menses before the age of 40 years is called premature menopause or premature ovarian failure. The reasons for premature ovarian failure are unknown. Chronic disease, infections or tumors of the reproductive tract can occasionally damage the ovarian follicular structures so severely as to precipitate the menopause. The menopause can also be hastened by excessive exposure to ionizing radiation, chemotherapeutic drugs, particularly alkylating agents and surgical procedures that impair ovarian blood supply. The permanent cessation of the ovarian function following the surgical removal of the ovaries or by radiation therapy is called an artificial menopause (Flow chart 19.3.1).

Clinical Clues

- **Ask about:**
  - Climacteric syndrome: Hot flashes, insomnia, weight gain and bloating, mood changes, irregular menses, mastodynia and headache
  - Vasomotor flush: Described as a feeling of warmth or heat that begins at the umbilical level and moves upward toward the head, followed by sweating of the head and upper body
  - Cardiovascular/neurologic symptoms: Palpitations, dizziness, light-headedness and vertigo with or without flushing
  - Vaginal pressure, lower back pressure or bulging at the vaginal introitus, suggestive of prolapse caused by loss of tone of pelvic floor after menopause, suggestive of a rectocele, cystocele or uterine prolapse
  - Urinary frequency, urgency and incontinence suggestive of atrophic cystitis.
- **Look for:**
  - Redder vaginal epithelium in early menopause (because of thinning of the epithelial layer and increased visibility of the small capillaries below the surface).
  - Pale vaginal epithelium in late menopause (further atrophy of the endometrium because of reduced number of capillaries).

Flow chart 19.3.1: Inductive reasoning scheme for diagnostic evaluation of the patients presenting with menopause *(Courtesy:* Paul L. Foster School of Medicine, Texas Tech University at El Paso, TX, USA). In addition to hormonal assays, ultrasound is widely used for evaluation of the patients with physiologic, premature and artificial menopause (yellow). Three-dimensional ultrasound may be used for the assessment of the ovarian reserve, based on the ovarian volume measurements and antral follicle count. Sonographic monitoring and hormonal assessment are necessary to distinguish between reversible and irreversible menopause.

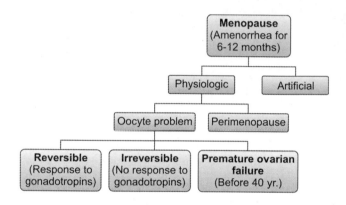

- Vulvar pruritus and malodorous discharge (decrease urine pH → change in bacterial flora)
- Rugation of the vaginal wall diminishes and the vaginal wall becomes smooth
- Smaller uterus (Fibroids, if present, become less symptomatic and may shrink so they can no longer be palpated on pelvic examination. Endometriosis and adenomyosis are also alleviated, so many patients with pelvic pain with the onset of menopause finally achieve a permanent pain relief)
- Small ovaries that may no longer be palpable during gynecologic examination (A palpable ovary on pelvic examination warrants a full evaluation in all women who are menopausal or postmenopausal)
- General loss of pelvic tone (manifesting as prolapse of reproductive or urinary tract organs. On examination, cystocele, rectocele and uterine prolapse may be found)
- Loss of skin elasticity
- Decline in bone mineral density

– Replacement of dense breast tissue by adipose tissue (making mammographic evaluation easier).

Investigations

- General physical examination
- Pelvic examination
- Serum FSH, LH and estradiol.

Ultrasound Findings

- Visualization of the small ovaries and thin endometrium (< 5 mm)
- In postmenopausal patients presenting with vaginal bleeding, every abnormal endometrial thickening (>/ = 5 mm) requires further evaluation (endometrial biopsy)
- B-mode ultrasound reveals an inverse relationship between the uterine size and the time since menopause: the uterine size and volume progressively decrease as the duration of the postmenopausal period increases
- There is an inverse relationship between the ovarian size and the time since menopause: ovarian size progressively decreases as the duration of the postmenopause increases
- B-mode and color Doppler ultrasound is used to distinguish benign and malignant uterine and ovarian lesions (refer to the Clinical Sonographic Pearls on Uterine and Adnexal Masses).

Diagnoses to Consider

- Amenorrhea associated with:
  - Extreme weight loss in anorexia nervosa
  - Hyperprolactinemia (look for galactorrhea)
  - Polycystic ovarian disease (look for hirsutism and obesity)
- Hot flushes should be differentiated from sensations of flushing in:
  - Hyperthyroidism
  - Pheochromocytoma
  - Carcinoid syndrome
  - Tuberculosis
  - Chronic infections
  - Emotional lability.
- Abnormal peri- and postmenopausal bleeding may occur in patients with
  - Atrophic endometrium
  - Endometrial hypereplasia
  - Endometrial polyp
  - Endometrial cancer.
- Atrophic vaginitis due to the lack of estrogen should be differentiated from

- Vulvar and vaginal diseases (e.g. trichomoniasis and candidiasis)
- Urinary tract infection.
- Back pain in postmenopausal patients with vertebral compression from osteoporosis may mimic:
  - Renal colic and pyelonephritis
  - Pancreatitis
  - Spondylolisthesis
  - Acute back strain
  - Herniated intervertebral disk.

Some case studies related to menopause are depicted in Figures 19.3.1 to 19.3.7.

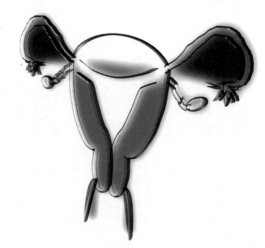

FIGURE 19.3.1: In patients presenting with menopause ultrasound reveals thin endometrium (less than 5 mm) and small ovaries with no evidence of follicular growth.

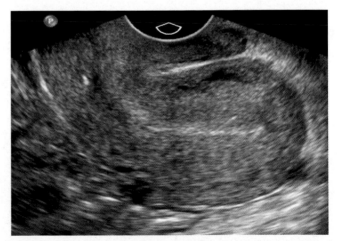

FIGURE 19.3.2: Transvaginal scan of a thin hyperechogenic endometrium in a postmenopausal patient. The cut-off value for endometrial thickness is 5 mm.

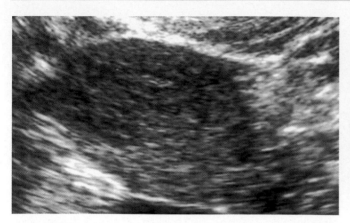

FIGURE 19.3.3: Transvaginal scan of a postmenopausal ovary with no evidence of follicular growth.

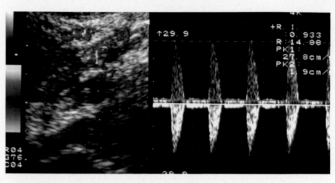

FIGURE 19.3.6: Uterine blood flow demonstrates high vascular impedance blood flow signals in the uterine artery (RI of 0.93). This is a typical finding in postmenopausal patients.

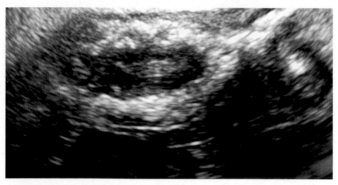

FIGURE 19.3.4: Diffused peripheral uterine calcifications in a patient with arteriosclerosis. Bright signals indicate vessel hardening and calcium deposits within the vessels' walls.

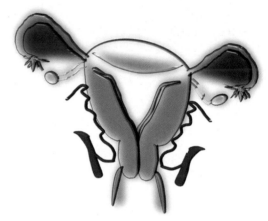

FIGURE 19.3.7: In addition to thin and hyperechogenic endometrium, postmenopausal patients present with increased vascular impedance in the uterine arteries (RI from 0.90 to 1.0). Uterine arteries are typically visualized laterally from the cervix, at the level of the cervicocorporeal junction.

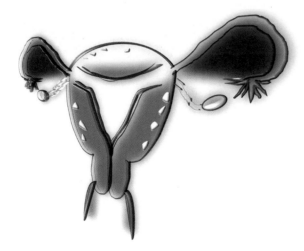

FIGURE 19.3.5: Aterosclerotic changes of the arcuate arteries in postmenopausal patient.

BIBLIOGRAPHY

1. Anderson GL, Limacher M, Assaf AR, et al. Effects of conjugated equine estrogen in postmenopausal women with hysterectomy: The Women's Health Initiative randomized controlled trial. JAMA 2004;291(14):1701-12.
2. Armstrong K, Eisen A, Weber B. Assessing the risk of breast cancer. N Engl J Med 2000;342(8):564-71.
3. Bekavac I, Kupesic S, Mihaljevic D, et al. Vascular impedance of uterine, inferior vesicle, and ophthalmic arteries in postmenopausal women receiving hormonal replacement therapy: Comparative Doppler study. Croat Med J 2000; 41(3):235-9.
4. Beck WW. Obstetrics & Gynecology, 4th edition. Philadelphia: Williams & Wilkins 1997.

5. Cramer DW, Harlow BL, Xu H, et al. Cross-sectional and case-controlled analyses of the association between smoking and early menopause. Maturitas 1995;22(2):79-87.

6. Curran D, Bachman G. Menopause. E-Medicine 2006.

7. Cohen LS, Soares CN, Poitras JR. Short-term use of estradiol for depression in perimenopausal and postmenopausal women: A preliminary report. Am J Psychiatry. 2003;160(8):1519-22.

8. Grady D, Cummings SR. Postmenopausal hormone therapy for prevention of fractures: How good is the evidence? JAMA 2001;285(22):2909-10.

9. Grady D, Applegate W, Bush T, et al. Heart and Estrogen/progestin Replacement Study (HERS): Design, methods, and baseline characteristics. Control Clin Trials 1998;19(4):314-35.

10. Kim C, Kwok YS. Decision analysis of hormone replacement therapy after the Women's Health Initiative. Am J Obstet Gynecol 2003;189(5):1228-33.

11. Kupesic S, Kurjak A. Uterine lesions: Advances in ultrasound diagnosis. Donald School Textbook of Ultrasound in Obstetrics and Gynecology. In: Kurjak A, Chervenak F (Eds). New Delhi: Jaypee Brothers Medical Publishers 2008;791-802.

12. Kurjak A, Kupesic S, Simunic V. Ultrasonic assessment of the peri-and postmenopausal ovary. Maturitas 2002;41(4):245-54.

13. Kupesic S, Kurjak A, Hajder E. Ultrasonic assessment of the postmenopausal uterus. Maturitas 2002;41(4):255-67.

14. Kurjak A, Shalan H, Sosic A, et al. Endometrial carcinoma in postmenopausal women: Evaluation by transvaginal color Doppler ultrasound. Am J Obstet Gynecol 1993;169(6):1597-603.

15. Kupesic S, Kurjak A, Babic MM. Uterine and ovarian perfusion changes from reproductive maturity to menopause. ACDS 1996;12:79-87.

16. Speroff L, Glass RH, Kase NG. Clinical gynecologic endocrinology and infertility. Menopause and perimenopausal transition, Philadelphia: Lippincott Williams & Wilkins 1999; 643-724.

17. Williams JK, Anthony MS, Herrington DM. Interactive effects of soy protein and estradiol on coronary artery reactivity in atherosclerotic, ovariectomized monkeys. Menopause 2001;8(5):307-13.

19.4: PERI- AND POSTMENOPAUSAL BLEEDING

Text and images by: S Kupesic Plavsic
Medical illustrations by: Bhargavi Patham and Sandesh Subramanya

Similar to reproductive age, postmenopausal bleeding may arise from the lesions at any anatomic site in the lower genital tract (vulva, vagina or cervix) or upper genital tract (uterine corpus or fallopian tubes). Clinicians should always differentiate nongynecological bleeding from the urethra, bladder or bowel. Abnormal genital tract bleeding during the perimenopausal period usually reflects a gradual decline of ovarian function. Perimenopause refers to the period of time just before and after the menopause. Menopause is that point in time when there is a permanent cessation of menstrual bleeding because of a loss of ovarian activity. Menopause is a retrospective diagnosis and occurs after menstrual bleeding was absent for 12 months in a woman older than 45 years (Flow chart 19.4.1).

Postmenopausal bleeding requires thorough investigation, during which ultrasound imaging plays an important role.

Clinical Clues

- **Ask about:**
  - Last menstrual period
  - Duration of bleeding

Flow chart 19.4.1: Inductive reasoning scheme for diagnostic evaluation of the patients presenting with peri- and postmenopausal bleeding (*Courtesy:* Paul L. Foster School of Medicine, Texas Tech University at El Paso, TX, USA). Ultrasound and endometrial biopsy are mandatory for evaluation of the postmenopausal patients presenting with bleeding from the upper genital tract (yellow).

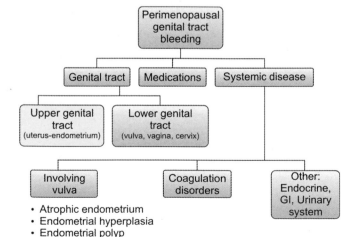

- Associated symptoms (for example, pain)
- Use of hormonal replacement therapy
- Duration of the menstrual cycle (perimenopausal patients: shortening of cycle length: usually associated with shortened follicular phase and elevated FSH level)
- Hot flushes
- Headaches
- Sleep disturbances
- **Look for:**
  - Lower genital tract abnormalities
  - Cervical lesions
  - Uterine enlargement
  - Abnormal endometrial thickening on ultrasound
  - Adnexal masses
  - Gastrointestinal or urinary origin of bleeding.

Investigations

- Medical history:
  - Coagulation disorders
  - Medication history (ask about the use of hormonal replacement therapy and anticoagulants)
  - Ask about liver, renal, endocrine and systemic disease
- Complete physical examination:
  - General physical examination
  - Pelvic examination
  - Rectovaginal examinaton (if indicated)
- Laboratory tests:
  - Pregnancy test (in perimenopausal patients)
  - Complete blood count (hemoglobin, hematocrit)
  - Thyroid stimulating hormone (TSH), if indicated
  - Coagulation profile (PT, PTT, BT)
- Diagnostic studies:
  - Pap smear
  - Colposcopy and biopsy, if appropriate
  - Ultrasound (TAS/TVS/saline infusion sonography, if indicated)
  - Endometrial biopsy
  - Hysteroscopy, if indicated
  - FSH, LH and E2 on day 3 of the menstrual cycle (in perimenopausal patients, if indicated)

– Serum progesterone on day LH+7 (in perimenopausal patients, if indicated)
– Thyroid stimulating hormone (TSH) and prolactin, if indicated
– Androgen profile, if indicated (testosterone, dehydroepiandrosterone).

Ultrasound Findings

Endometrial Lesions

- Endometrial thickness measurement
  – < 5 mm: atrophic endometrium
  – > or = to 5 mm: endometrial polyp, endometrial hyperplasia or endometrial carcinoma (perform endometrial biopsy)
- Endometrial – myometrial halo:
  – Regular: Benign endometrial lesions or localized/ early stage endometrial carcinoma
  – Irregular: Endometrial carcinoma invasion
- Color Doppler studies:
  – Moderate to high vascular impedance blood flow signals (RI > 0.50) at the periphery of endometrial lining: benign endometrial lesions
  – Low impedance blood flow signals (RI < 0.45): Increased risk of endometrial malignancy
  – Irregular vessels with low vascular impedance within the proximal myometrial layer: invasion of the endometrial carcinoma into the proximal half of the myometrium
  – Irregular vessels with low vascular impedance within the superficial, middle or deep myometrial portion and decreased resistance index in the uterine artery: deep invasion by endometrial carcinoma.
- 3D power Doppler studies:
  – Linear vessel arrangement and simple branching pattern: benign endometrial lesions
  – Chaotic vessel arrangement and complex branching pattern: malignant endometrial lesions.

Myometrial Lesions

- B-mode studies
  – Uterine enlargement associated with distortion of the uterine contour: intramural and/or subserosal leiomyoma
  – Uterine enlargement with distortion of the uterine cavity: submucosal leiomyoma
  – Heterogeneous uterine tumor with calcifications and anechoic areas: uterine leiomyoma with secondary degenerative changes

– "Swiss cheese" appearance of the myometrium: adenomyosis
  – Disordered echogenicity and intramural cystic lesions within the proximal layer of the endometrium: mild adenomyosis
  – Disordered echogenicity and cystic lesions within the middle layer of the myometrium: severe adenomyosis
  – Solid or solid-cystic fast growing myometrial lesion in menopausal patient: rule out uterine sarcoma
- Color Doppler studies
  – Moderate vascular impedance to blood flow (RI > 0.50): uterine leiomyoma and adenomyosis
  – High blood velocity and low impedance to blood flow (RI > 0.45): uterine sarcoma
- 3D power Doppler studies:
  – Linear vessel arrangement and simple branching pattern: benign myometrial lesions
  – Chaotic vessel arrangement and complex branching pattern: malignant myometrial lesions

Diagnoses to Consider

Lower Genital Tract Disorders:

- Vulva
  – Benign
  – Skin tags
  – Sebaceous cyst
  – Condylomata
  – Angiokeratoma
  – Cancer
  – Infection: STD
  – Trauma
- Vagina
  – Benign
  – Gartner's duct cysts
  – Polyps
  – Cancer
  – Vaginitis/infection (bacterial, STD, atrophic vaginitis)
  – Trauma
- Cervix
  – Benign lesions
  – Polyps
  – Ectropion
  – Malignant lesions
  – Invasive and noninvasive carcinoma
  – Metastatic tumors
  – Infection: cervicitis
  – Trauma

Upper Genital Tract Disorders:

- Uterus
  - Benign
  - Endometrial atrophy
  - Polyps
  - Endometrial hyperplasia
  - Adenomyosis
  - Leiomyomas (fibroids)
  - Malignant
  - Adenocarcinoma
  - Sarcoma
- Fallopian tube lesions
  - Benign
  - Malignant
  - PID
- Ovarian lesions
  - Benign
  - Malignant

Other

- Medications (for example, anticoagulants)
- Endocrine disorders
  - Thyroid disease
  - Adrenal tumor
  - Ovarian tumor
- GI bleeding
- Bleeding from the urethra and urinary system
- Systemic disease

Some case studies related to peri- and postmenopausal bleeding are depicted in Flow charts 19.4.2 to 19.4.5 and Figures 19.4.1 to 19.4.15.

Flow chart 19.4.2: Diagnostic algorithm for evaluation of the postmenopausal patients with upper genital tract bleeding and thin endometrium. Patients with thin (less than 5 mm) endometrium are considered to bleed due to the atrophic endometrium.

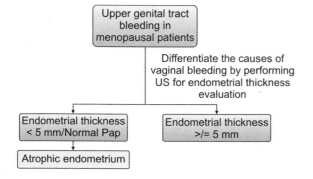

Flow chart 19.4.3: Diagnostic algorithm (I) for postmenopausal patients with upper genital tract bleeding and endometrial thickness equal to or above 5 mm.

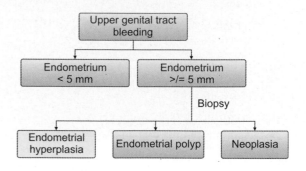

Flow chart 19.4.4: Diagnostic algorithm (II) for postmenopausal patients with upper genital tract bleeding and endometrial thickness equal to or above 5 mm.

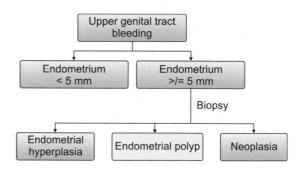

Flow chart 19.4.5: Diagnostic algorithm (III) for postmenopausal patients with upper genital tract bleeding and endometrial thickness equal to or above 5 mm.

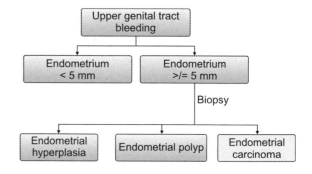

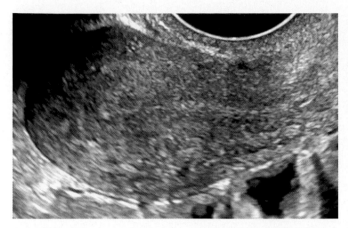

FIGURE 19.4.1: Transvaginal scan of a thin and hyperechoic endometrium in a postmenopausal patient.

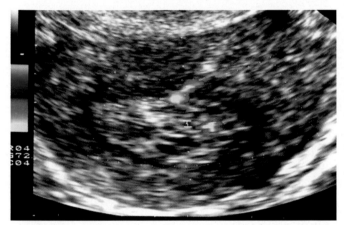

FIGURE 19.4.2: Thickened and hyperechogenic endometrium in a postmenopausal patient presenting with abnormal uterine bleeding.

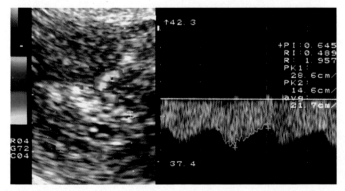

FIGURE 19.4.3: The same patient as in previous figure. Pulsed Doppler waveform analysis demonstrates moderate vascular impedance blood flow signals and resistance index of 0.64.

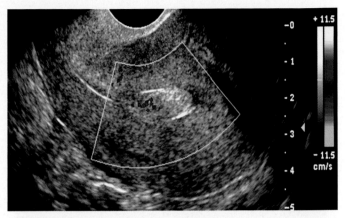

FIGURE 19.4.4: Focal endometrial thickening in a post-menopausal patient with abnormal uterine bleeding. Color Doppler depicts blood flow vessels within the stalk. Histology revealed an endometrial polyp.

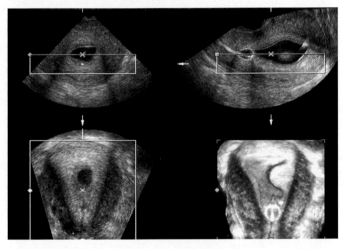

FIGURE 19.4.5: Multiplanar view demonstrating saline infusion sonography in a patient with postmenopausal bleeding. Surface rendering view (right low image) clearly demonstrates an endometrial polyp.

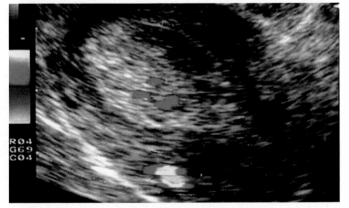

FIGURE 19.4.6: Transvaginal color Doppler scan of a postmenopausal patient with abnormal uterine bleeding and thickened endometrium. Blood flow signals are obtained from the central part of the endometrial lesion.

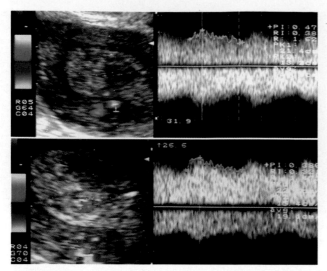

FIGURE 19.4.7: Pulsed Doppler waveform analysis of the same postmenopausal patient. Peritumoral vessels demonstrate high velocity and low resistance, suggestive of an endometrial cancer. Similar characteristics are observed in myometrial vessels.

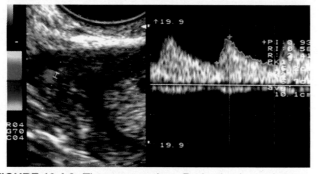

FIGURE 19.4.8: The same patient. Reduction in uterine artery resistance (RI = 0.58) indicates deep myometrial invasion by endometrial carcinoma. Invasive endometrial carcinoma was confirmed by histology.

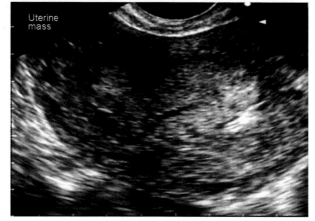

FIGURE 19.4.9: Transvaginal scan of a postmenopausal patient with enlarged and heterogeneous uterus. Transvaginal ultrasound could not delineate the endometrial lining.

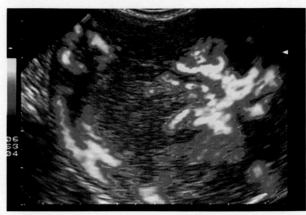

FIGURE 19.4.10: The same patient. Power Doppler imaging demonstrates neovascular areas within the myometrium. Such a finding suggests deep myometrial invasion by endometrial carcinoma.

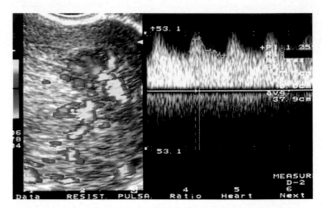

FIGURE 19.4.11: The same patient. Low vascular impedance (RI = 0.35) and high velocity of the blood flow (47.7 cm/s) are suggestive of neovascularization within the deep myometrial layer. Histopathology revealed deep myometrial invasion.

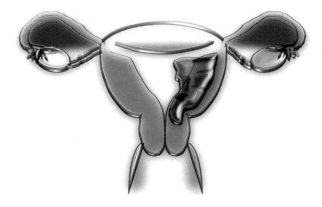

FIGURE 19.4.12: Invasive endometrial carcinoma is visualized as thickened heterogeneous endometrium with irregular sub-endometrial halo.

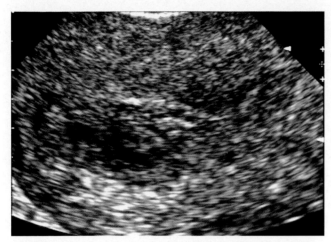

FIGURE 19.4.13: Solid uterine tumor demonstrated sudden growth in a postmenopausal patient presenting with vaginal bleeding.

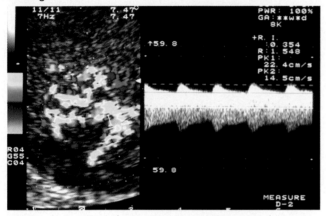

FIGURE 19.4.14: Low vascular impedance blood flow signals obtained from area of neovascularization indicate uterine malignancy. Uterine sarcoma was confirmed by histology.

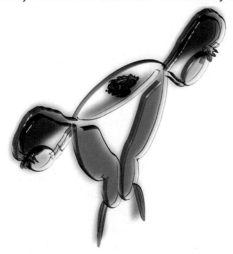

FIGURE 19.4.15: Uterine sarcoma is a malignant tumor that arises from the smooth muscle or connective tissue of the uterus.

BIBLIOGRAPHY

1. Anderson GL, Limacher M, Assaf AR, et al. Effects of conjugated equine estrogen in postmenopausal women with hysterectomy: The Women's Health Initiative randomized controlled trial. JAMA 2004;291(14):1701-2.
2. Armstrong K, Eisen A, Weber B. Assessing the risk of breast cancer. N Engl J Med 2000;342(8):564-71.
3. Beck WW Jr. Obstetrics & Gynecology, 4th edition. Philadelphia: Williams & Wilkins 1997.
4. Bekavac I, Kupesic S, Mihaljevic D, et al. Vascular impedance of uterine, inferior vesicle, and ophthalmic arteries in postmenopausal women receiving hormonal replacement therapy: Comparative Doppler study. Croat Med J 2000;41(3): 235-9.
5. Cohen LS, Soares CN, Poitras JR. Short-term use of estradiol for depression in perimenopausal and postmenopausal women: A preliminary report. Am J Psychiatry 2003;160(8):1519-22.
6. Cramer DW, Harlow BL, Xu H, et al. Cross-sectional and case-controlled analyses of the association between smoking and early menopause. Maturitas 1995;22(2):79-87.
7. Curran D, Bachman G. Menopause. E-Medicine 2006.
8. Grady D, Applegate W, Bush T, et al. Heart and Estrogen/ progestin Replacement Study (HERS): Design, methods, and baseline characteristics. Control Clin Trials 1998;19(4):314-35.
9. Grady D, Cummings SR. Postmenopausal hormone therapy for prevention of fractures: how good is the evidence? JAMA 2001;285(22):2909-10.
10. Kim C, Kwok YS. Decision analysis of hormone replacement therapy after the Women's Health Initiative. Am J Obstet Gynecol 2003;189(5):1228-33.
11. Kupesic S, Kurjak A, Babic MM. Uterine and ovarian perfusion changes from reproductive maturity to menopause. ACDS 1996;12:79-87.
12. Kupesic S, Kurjak A, Hajder E. Ultrasonic assessment of the postmenopausal uterus. Maturitas 2002;41(4):255-67.
13. Kupesic S, Kurjak A. Uterine Lesions: Advances in Ultrasound Diagnosis. Donald School Textbook of Ultrasound in Obstetrics and Gynecology, In: Kurjak A, Chervenak F (Eds). New Delhi. Jaypee Brothers Medical Publishers 2008;791-802.
14. Kurjak A, Kupesic S, Simunic V. Ultrasonic assessment of the peri- and postmenopausal ovary. Maturitas 2002;41(4):245-54.
15. Kurjak A, Shalan H, Sosic A, et al. Endometrial carcinoma in postmenopausal women: Evaluation by transvaginal color Doppler ultrasound. Am J Obstet Gynecol 1993;169(6):1597-603.
16. Speroff L, Glass RH, Kase N.G. Clinical gynecologic endocrinology and infertility. Menopause and perimenopausal transition, Philadelphia: Lippincott Williams & Wilkins 1999; 643-724.
17. Williams JK, Anthony MS, Herrington DM. Interactive effects of soy protein and estradiol on coronary artery reactivity in atherosclerotic, ovariectomized monkeys. Menopause 2001;8(5):307-13.

19.5: PROLAPSE AND PELVIC FLOOR RELAXATION

Text and images by: S Kupesic Plavsic
Medical illustrations by: Bhargavi Patham and Sandesh Subramanya

Pelvic organ prolapse occurs with descent of one or more pelvic structures: the uterine cervix or vaginal apex, anterior vagina (usually with bladder, cystocele), posterior vagina (usually with rectum - rectocele) or peritoneum of the cul-de-sac (usually with intestine - enterocele). Possible risk factors for pelvic organ prolapse include genetic predisposition, parity (particularly vaginal birth) and advanced age (Flow chart 19.5.1).

Symptoms of prolapse and pelvic relaxation include vaginal fullness and pressure. A prolapsed uterus is graded based on the level of descent: to the upper vagina (1st degree), to the introitus (2nd degree) or external to the introitus (3rd degree). Treatment includes behavioral modification, pelvic floor muscle rehabilitation, use of pessaries and surgical treatment (hysteropexy and round ligament suspension).

Flow chart 19.5.1: Inductive reasoning scheme for diagnostic evaluation of the patients presenting with pelvic floor relaxation and/or urogynecological problems (*Courtesy:* Paul L. Foster School of Medicine, Texas Tech University at El Paso, TX, USA). Pelvic ultrasound may be used to assess the volume of the residual urine, evaluate the bladder wall thickness, study cervical descent on straining, analyze bladder neck position, and measure the anterior urethral angle, posterior urethro-vesical angle, urethral and anal sphincters. Due to its non-invasiveness, ultrasound is among first diagnostic methods for the evaluation of the patients with urogynecologic problems.

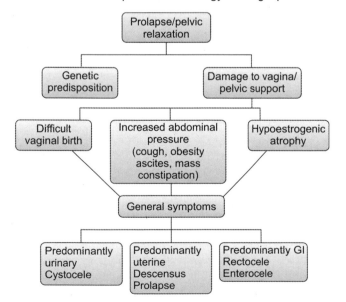

Clinical Clues

- **Ask about:**
  - Parity (particularly vaginal birth)
  - History of instrumental deliveries
  - Previous surgery
  - Last menstrual period (postmenopause)
  - Pelvic discomfort
  - Recurrent urinary tract infections
  - Voiding problems
  - Incomplete bladder emptying
  - A lump at the opening of the vagina
  - Urinary and bowel dysfunction
  - Chronic constipation
  - Neurologic conditions (e.g. spina bifida)
  - Respiratory problems
  - Sexual dysfunction
  - Dyspareunia
  - Back pain
  - Certain occupations (involving heavy lifting or exertion)
  - Use of medications, such as diuretics
  - Caffeine use
  - Back or pelvic fractures during falls
  - Motor vehicle accidents
  - Connective tissue disorders
  - Previous irradiation.
- **Look for:**
  - Obesity
  - Chronic constipation with excessive straining
  - Menopause and advancing age.

Investigations

- Bimanual pelvic examination
- Blood tests, urinalysis or urine culture (to rule out urinary tract infection)
- Abdominal, transvaginal and/or transperineal ultrasound
- Assessment of the efficiency of bladder emptying (by measuring the patient's voided volume when she has a comfortably full bladder, followed by the assessment of postvoid residual urine volume by bladder ultrasonography or catheterization)
- Urodynamic studies (tests to measure the pressure and urine flow):

– Urinary postvoid residual to measure how much urine remains in the bladder after urination

– Urinary stress test (checks for urine loss when bladder muscles are stressed usually by coughing, lifting or exercise)

• Cystourethroscopy
• X-ray with urotropic radiographic contrast medium
• MRI scan.

Ultrasound Findings

• Transperineal approach using a curved sector transducer (3.5 MHz), and transvaginal transducer (5-10 MHz) frequency to visualize the symphysis pubis, bladder base, measure the residual volume of the urine, and assess the urethra and urethra-pubic ligaments, vaginal vault, anorectal junction, postanal space, and internal and external anal sphincters.

• Technique for sonography of the female pelvic floor is described on www.pelviperineology.org and includes the assessment of the following structures:
  – Bladder neck position (at rest and on straining) in relation to the symphysis as a reference point (measured in mm above/below)
  – Anterior urethral angle (alpha): Angle formed between the proximal urethra and X axis of the pubic bone (normal from 60° to 110°)
  – Posterior urethrovesical angle (beta): Angle formed between the proximal urethra and a line tangent the lowermost back aspect of the bladder base.
  – Urethral sphincter: Width (15–20 mm) and thickness (8-10 mm).
  – Bladder wall thickness: When less than 20 ml of residual urine is detected, normal bladder wall thickness is < 5 mm.
  – Internal and external anal sphincters: Normal 2.5–7 mm (mean 5 mm).
  – Cervical descent on straining: Dislocation in relation to pubic bone (X axis).

Diagnoses to Consider

• Genetic predisposition for prolapse and pelvic relaxation
• Damage to vagina/pelvic support:
  – Difficult vaginal delivery
  – Obesity
  – Increased abdominal pressure (e.g. cough)
  – Severe constipation
  – Hypoestrogenic atrophy (menopause)

• Cystocele
• Enterocele
• Rectocele
• Pelvic organs prolapse
• Fistulas:
  – Vesicovaginal (bladder – vagina)
  – Vesicouterine (bladder – uterus)
  – Vesicocutaneous (bladder – abdominal wall)
  – Rectovaginal (rectum – vagina).

Some case studies related to prolapse and pelvic floor relaxation are depicted in Figures 19.5.1 to 19.5.16.

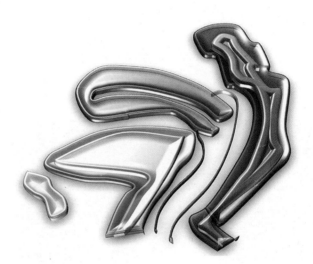

FIGURE 19.5.1: Normal anatomy of the pelvis organs: yellow– pubic bone, blue – urinary bladder and urethra, brown – uterus and vagina, and pink rectum.

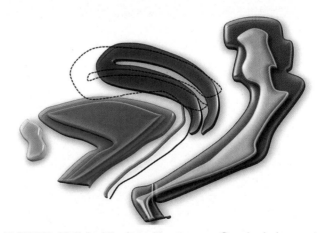

FIGURE 19.5.2: Uterine descensus. Cervical descent on straining represents dislocation in relation to the pubic bone. Normal position of the uterus is demonstrated with red dotted line.

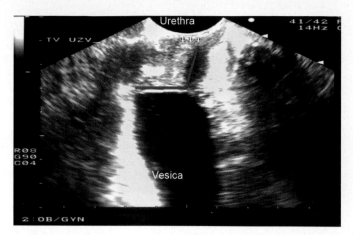

FIGURE 19.5.3: Normal angle between the urethra and posterior part of the urinary bladder measures between 100 and 110 degrees.

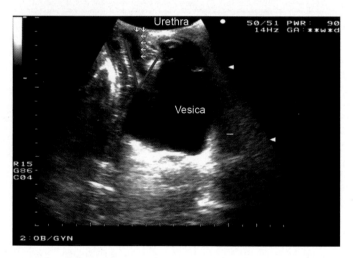

FIGURE 19.5.4: Measurement of an abnormal angle between the urethra and posterior part of the urinary bladder (45 degrees) is typical for stress incontinence. Dynamic evaluation of passive opening of the vesical neck and the proximal urethra by increasing of the intra-abdominal pressure should be performed. Descensus of the vesical neck for more than 1 cm by increasing intra-abdominal pressure is associated with stress incontinence.

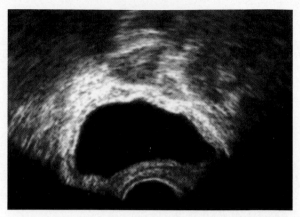

Figure 19.5.5: Evaluation of the urinary bladder includes estimation of the residual urine volume and measurement of the urinary bladder wall thickness. Volume of the residual urine is measured using a formula for an ellipsoid (D1 x D2 x D3 x 0.52). Wall thickness >5 mm is associated with detrusor insufficiency.

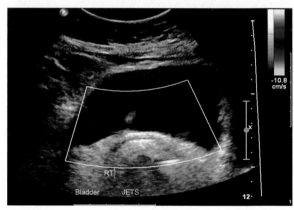

FIGURE 19.5.6: Color Doppler enables visualization of the ureteric jets that represent the inflow of the urine from the ureters into the bladder.

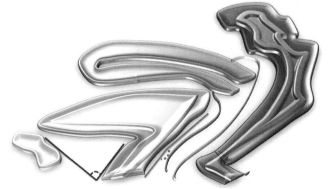

FIGURE 19.5.7: Anterior urethral angle (red): angle formed between the proximal urethra and X-axis of the pubic bone (normal from 60 to 110°). Posterior urethrovesical angle (green): angle formed between the proximal urethra and a line tangent the lowermost back aspect of the bladder base.

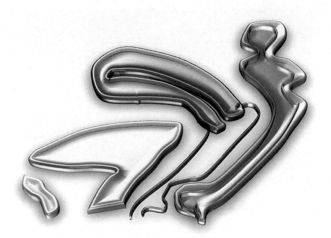

FIGURE 19.5.8: A rectocele occurs when the end or large intestine (rectum) pushes against and moves the back wall of the vagina.

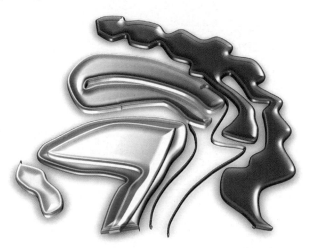

FIGURE 19.5.9: An enterocele is a small bowel prolapse when the small bowel presses against and moves the upper wall of the vagina.

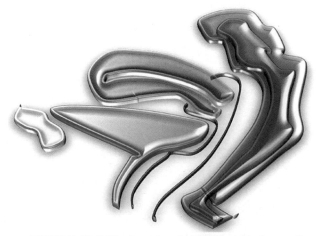

FIGURE 19.5.10: A cystocele is the protrusion or the prolapse of the urinary bladder into the vagina.

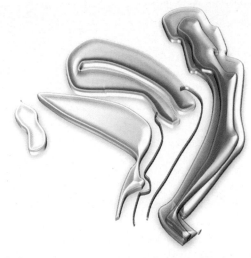

FIGURE 19.5.11: An urethrocele occurs in the urethra and surrounding tissue sags downward into the vagina.

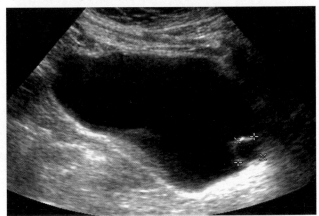

FIGURE 19.5.12: A sac-like pouch in prevoid bladder is suggestive of an ureterocele. Ureterocele is swelling in one of the ureters that carry urine from the kidney to the bladder. The swelling can block the flow of the urine. Most common symptoms are urgency, frequency, hematuria, urinary incontinence and abdominal/pelvic pain.

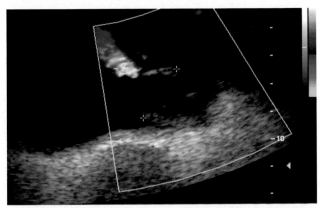

FIGURE 19.5.13: Color signals demonstrating urine jet in a patient with ureterocele.

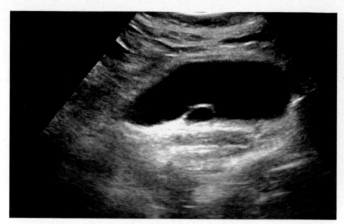

FIGURE 19.5.14: Another case of sonolucent sac-like structure in the urinary bladder, suggestive of an ureterocele.

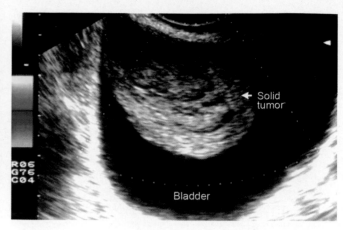

FIGURE 19.5.16: Transvaginal sonogram of the solid tumor of the urinary bladder. Histology revealed carcinoma of the urinary bladder.

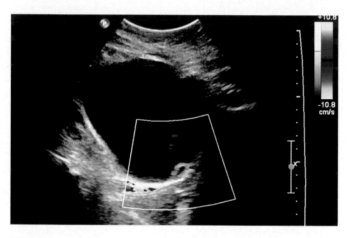

FIGURE 19.5.15: Color Doppler signals demonstrate ureteric jet in a patient with ureterocele.

BIBLIOGRAPHY

1. ACOG Committee on Practice Bulletins-Gynecology. ACOG Practice bulletin No. 85: Pelvic organ prolapse 2007;110 (3):717-29.
2. Beckmann RBC, Ling FW, Smith RP, et al. Obstetrics and Gynecology, 5th edition. Philadelphia: Lippincott Williams and Wilkins; 2002; 291-3.
3. Bekavac I, Kupesic S, Kurjak A. Three-dimensional ultrasound in urogynecology. In: Kurjak A, Kupesic S (Eds). Clinical application of 3D sonography. London-New York: Parthenon Publishing 2000; 103.
4. Technique for sonography of the female pelvic floor www.pelviperineology.org.

19.6: CONTRACEPTION

Text and images by: S Kupesic Plavsic
Medical illustrations by: Bhargavi Patham and Sandesh Subramanya

The prevention of an unwanted pregnancy should be directed at the education of male and female patients, preferably before their first sexual contact. Contraceptive efficacy is assessed by measuring the number of unplanned pregnancies that occurred during a specified period of exposure and use of a contraceptive method (Flow chart 19.6.1).

Clinical Clues

- **Ask about:**
  - Female/Male age
  - Near-term and long-term desire for children
  - Frequency of sexual activity
  - Prior pregnancies (including ectopic and miscarriages)
  - Risk for sexually transmitted infections
  - Family history
  - Personal health risks
  - Medical and surgical history
  - Patient's compliance (discipline for the use of different methods of contraception)
  - Cultural and moral concerns that may influence the ability to use a contraceptive method
- **Look for:**
  - Health risks (candidates for oral contraception):
    - History of arterial cardiovascular, ischemic heart and valvular heart diseases, elevated blood pressure, and current deep vein thrombosis or pulmonary embolism.
    - Diabetes mellitus with related eye, liver and nerve diseases.
    - Gallbladder disease
    - History of smoking
    - Headaches with auras
    - Liver disease: acute viral hepatitis, cirrhosis, liver tumors
    - Uterine anomalies or submucosal fibroids, which are absolute contraindications for the use of intrauterine contraception
    - History of ectopic pregnancy (relative contraindication for the use of intrauterine contraception)

- Previous pregnancies of the female partner (some methods like intrauterine device are not recommended for a woman who did not give the birth)
- Type of relationship patient is involved (casual sex, new relationship, established partnership, completed reproduction)
- Reliability (for example, is the patient reliable at taking pills regularly or undergoing injections?)

Flow chart 19.6.1: Inductive reasoning scheme for contraception counseling (*Courtesy:* Paul L. Foster School of Medicine, Texas Tech University at El Paso, TX, USA). Candidates for intrauterine device (IUD) should be scanned by transvaginal ultrasound prior to the insertion of an IUD to rule out uterine abnormalities (such as congenital uterine anomalies and submucosal fibroids). It is recommended that patients are re-scanned one week after the placement of an IUD to monitor the position of an IUD. Patients with intrauterine contraception who present with abnormal genital tract bleeding or pelvic pain should be referred for ultrasound evaluation to check whether the IUD has become displaced, expelled or has perforated through the uterus. Ultrasound may also be used for evaluation of patients receiving birth control pills who present with spotting and/or amenorrhea. In these patients sonographer should pay attention to endometrial thickness of presence of the ovarian follicles and/or cysts.

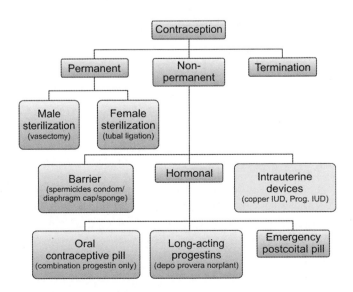

Investigations

- Clinical history and general physical examination
- Pelvic examination
- Pap smear
- In patients with higher risk of sexually transmitted disease (STD) perform testing for Chlamydia trachomatis and *Nesseria gonorrhoeae*, especially prior to the IUD placement
- Laboratory tests:
  - CBC, including glucose and cholesterol
  - Coagulation tests
  - Liver function tests
  - Urine analysis.

Ultrasound Findings

- In patients using hormonal contraception ultrasound may be used to visualize quiescent ovaries and thin endometrium.
- Candidates for intrauterine device (IUD) should be scanned by transvaginal ultrasound prior to the insertion of an IUD to rule out uterine abnormalities (such as congenital uterine anomalies and submucosal fibroids). It is recommended that patients are rescanned one week after the placement of an IUD to monitor the position of an IUD.
- Patients with intrauterine contraception who present with abnormal genital tract bleeding or pelvic pain should be referred for ultrasound evaluation to check whether the IUD has become displaced, expelled or has perforated through the uterus. Also, be aware that patients with intrauterine contraception are at increased risk of pelvic inflammatory disease (PID).

Diagnoses to Consider

- IUD dislocation
- Pelvic inflammatory disease
- Uterine perforation
- Dysmenorrhea
- Dysfunctional menstrual bleeding
- Pregnancy
- Functional cysts.

Some case studies related to contraception are depicted in Figures 19.6.1 to 19.6.18.

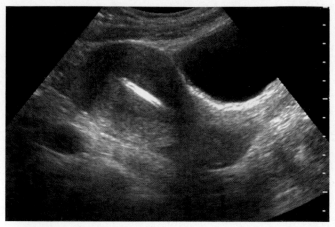

FIGURE 19.6.1: Transabdominal ultrasound–longitudinal scan of the uterus with normal position of IUD.

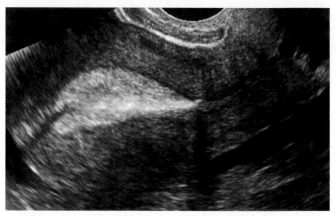

FIGURE 19.6.2: Transvaginal scan of an intrauterine device. IUD should always be visualized in a longitudinal plane of the uterus.

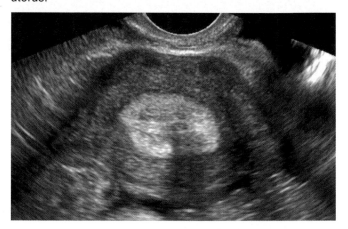

FIGURE 19.6.3: Transvaginal scan of an intrauterine device in a transverse plane.

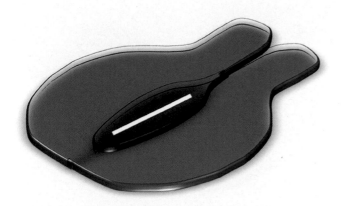

FIGURE 19.6.4: Pelvic ultrasound may be efficiently used for monitoring of the position of an IUD.

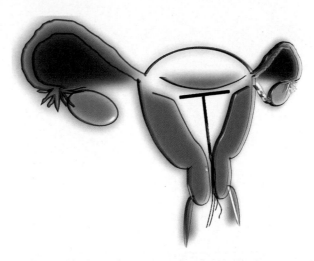

FIGURE 19.6.7: Frontal reformatted section of the uterus demonstrating normal position of an IUD.

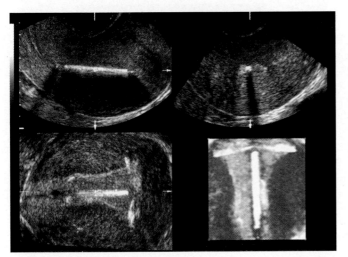

FIGURE 19.6.5: Three-dimensional ultrasound and multiplanar imaging of an intrauterine device. Note the correct placement of the copper T device at the highest possible position within the uterine cavity.

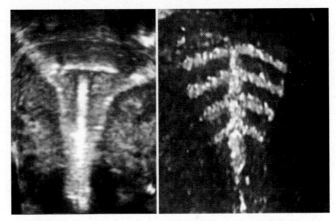

FIGURE 19.6.8: Frontal reformatted section of the uterus demonstrating normal position of the different types of IUD (Copper T on the left, and Dalkon Shield on the right).

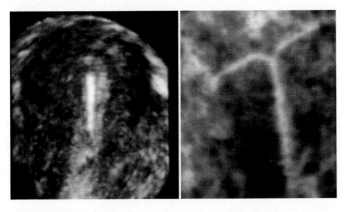

FIGURE 19.6.6: 2D (left) and 3D ultrasound (right) images of an intrauterine device in a normal position.

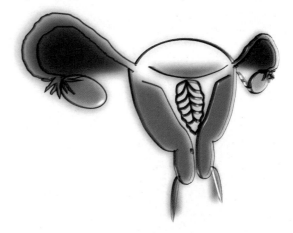

FIGURE 19.6.9: Frontal reformatted section of a correctly positioned Dalkon Shield IUD.

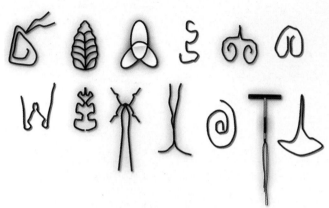

FIGURE 19.6.10: Ultrasound can be used for visualization of the different types of IUD.

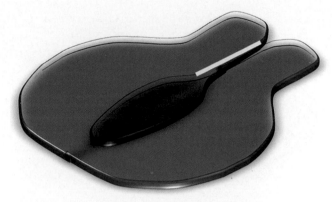

FIGURE 19.6.13: Displaced IUS should always be visualized in a longitudinal plane. This section allows visualization of the endometrium, above the position of a displaced IUD.

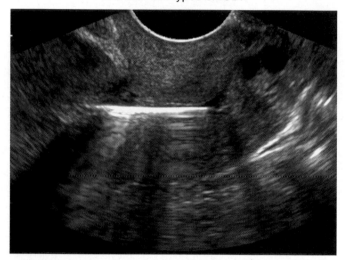

FIGURE 19.6.11: Longitudinal scan of the uterus and cervix demonstrating a displaced IUD. The IUD is visualized within the cervix. Patient presented with irregular menstrual bleeding and pelvic pain.

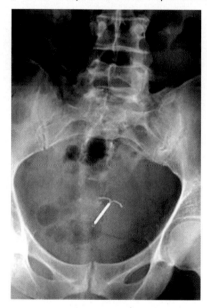

FIGURE 19.6.14: Abdominal X-ray of the patient presenting with low abdominal pain. An intrauterine device is visualized within the abdominal cavity. Laparoscopy revealed perforation of the uterus.

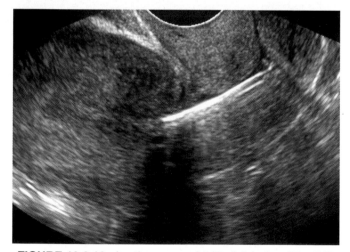

FIGURE 19.6.12: Another case of IUD dislocation. The IUD is clearly visualized within the cervical canal.

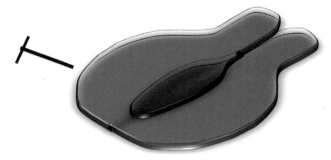

FIGURE 19.6.15: A displaced IUD that has perforated the uterus. In most cases this type of complication cannot be demonstrated by ultrasound.

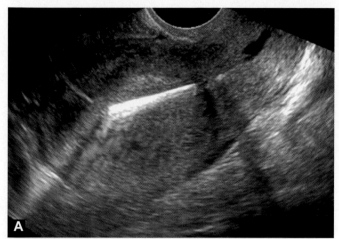

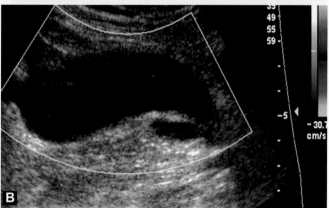

FIGURES 19.6.16A and B: Transvaginal sonogram of a complex adnexal mass containing a folded dilated tube and enlarged ovary in a patient with acute pelvic pain. The patient has IUD for 6 years. Medical history revealed a high risk sexual behavior.

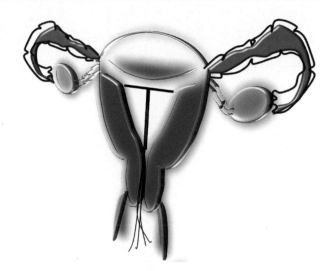

FIGURE 19.6.17: Patients with intrauterine contraception who present with abnormal vaginal discharge, abnormal uterine bleeding and pelvic pain should be referred for ultrasound evaluation to rule out pelvic inflammatory disease.

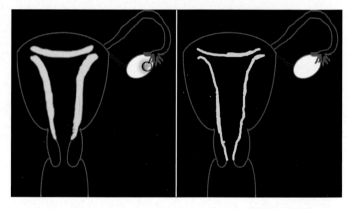

FIGURE 18.6.18: In patients using hormonal contraception ultrasound may be used for follow-up, particularly in patients with breakthrough bleeding. Left image demonstrates follicular growth and thickened endometrium in a patient with ovulatory menstrual cycle. Right image demonstrates quiescent ovaries and thin endometrium in a patient using birth control pills.

BIBLIOGRAPHY

1. Beck WW. Obstetrics and Gynecology, 4 th edition. Baltimore: Williams & Wilkins 1997.
2. Beckmann RBC, Ling FW, Smith RP, et al. Obstetrics and Gynecology, 5th edition. Philadelphia: Lippincott Williams and Wilkins 2002.
3. Grimes DA, Kaunitz AM, Nelson AL (2009). Female contraception: Reducing the rate of unintended pregnancy. Medscape CME. Available from http://cme.medscape.com/viewprogram/18691.
4. Kurjak A, Kupesic S. Color Doppler and 3D Ultrasound in Obstetrics, Gynecology and Infertility. London, New York: Parthenon Publishing 2000.
5. Samra-Latiff OM (2009). Contraception. E-medicine. Available from http://emedicine.medscape.com/article/258507-overview.
6. Speroff L, Glass RH, Kase NG. Clinical gynecologic endocrinology and infertility. Philadelphia: Lippincott Williams & Wilkins 2006.

19.7: INFERTILITY

Text and images by: S Kupesic Plavsic
Medical illustrations by: Bhargavi Patham and Sandesh Subramanya

Infertility, meaning the inability to conceive after one year of intercourse without contraception, affects about 15% of couples. Since male-associated factors account for approximately half of the infertility cases, both partners should be thoroughly investigated. Female infertility problems may be divided into the ovarian, tubal and uterine causes (Flow charts 19.7.1 and 19.7.2).

Clinical Clues

- **Ask about:**
  - Duration of infertility
  - Prior pregnancies (including ectopic and miscarriages), fertility in other relationships (to distinguish primary from secondary infertility)
  - Frequency of intercourse and use of lubricants
  - Previous infertility testing and therapies
  - Family history of birth defects, mental retardation and reproductive failure
  - In men, medical and surgical history, including testicular surgery and history of mumps, medications, chemotherapy or radiation, cigarette smoking, alcohol, marijuana and other drug use; environmental and occupational exposures, sexual dysfunction or impotence, frequency of intercourse, use of lubricants, previous infertility testing and therapies, family history of birth defects, mental retardation and reproductive failure.
  - In women, menstrual history (age at menarche, cycle length and regularity)
  - Presence of molimina or vasomotor symptoms (hot flashes) to determine whether menstrual cycles are anovulatory or normal.
- **Look for:**
  - Body mass index (BMI)
  - Abnormalities of the thyroid gland
  - Galactorrhea
  - Signs of androgen excess (hirsutism, acne, male pattern baldness)
  - Changes in the basal body temperature
  - Changes in the cervical mucus quality
  - Tenderness or masses in the adnexal region or cul-de-sac
  - Vaginal/cervical abnormalities

- Uterine enlargement, irregularity or lack of mobility
- Adnexal mass

Investigations

- Semen analysis to detect male factor infertility
- BBT graph
- Day 21 to 23 serum progesterone
- FSH, LH, E2 and Prolactin (PRL) between 3rd and 5th day of the menstrual cycle
- Saline infusion sonography (hystero-contrast-salpingography or X ray HSG) to rule out uterine abnormalities or tubal occlusion, if indicated
- Endometrial biopsy (2-3 days before the expected menstrual period), if indicated
- Hysteroscopy, if indicated
- Diagnostic laparoscopy to visualize the fallopian tubes, identify tubal abnormalities and peritubal adhesions, if indicated.

Flow chart 19.7.1: Inductive reasoning scheme for diagnostic evaluation of the patients presenting with infertility (*Courtesy:* Paul L. Foster School of Medicine, Texas Tech University at El Paso, TX, USA). Ultrasound assists in detection of ovulation and anovulatory disorders (yellow).

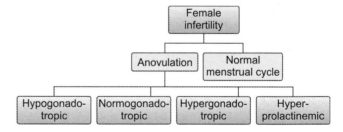

Flow chart 19.7.2: Inductive reasoning scheme for diagnostic evaluation of the patients presenting with infertility (*Courtesy:* Paul L. Foster School of Medicine, Texas Tech University at El Paso, TX, USA). Ultrasound may assist in detection of the uterine, tubal and ovarian causes of infertility (yellow).

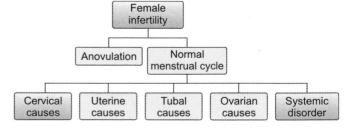

Ultrasound Findings

- Ultrasound monitoring of the follicles and endometrial changes
- Ultrasound examination to rule out ovarian, tubal and uterine causes of infertility
- Saline infusion ultrasound (hysterosonosalpingography, HSSG) to visualize the uterine cavity and assess tubal patency and function.

Diagnoses to Consider

- Cervical factors
  - Abnormalities of the cervix
  - Abnormalities of the cervical mucus
- Uterine factors
  - Uterine anomalies
  - Intrauterine adhesions
  - Submucosal fibroids
- Tubal factors
  - Pelvic inflammatory disease
  - Endometriosis
- Ovarian factors
  - Anovulation
    - Hypothalamic causes
    - Hyperprolactinemia due to a pituitary adenoma
    - Premature ovarian failure
    - Polycystic ovarian syndrome
    - Ovarian cysts
  - Luteal phase defect
  - Ovarian endometrioma
- Systemic disorders
  - SLE
  - Rheumatoid disease
  - Chronic renal failure
  - Diabetes mellitus.

Some case studies related to infertility are depicted in Figures 19.7.1 to 19.7.49.

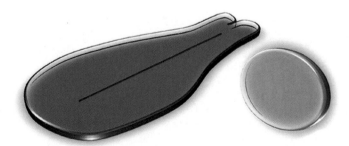

FIGURE 19.7.1: Postmenstrual endometrium. During the postmenstrual phase the endometrium is thin (about 2 mm) and ovary does not contain a growing follicle.

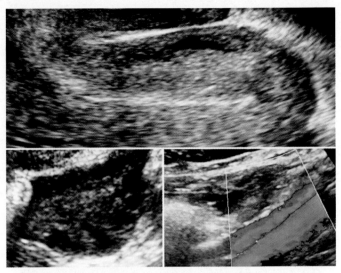

FIGURE 19.7.2: Transvaginal scan of the endometrium immediately after completion of the menstrual bleeding. At this stage there is no evidence of growing follicles.

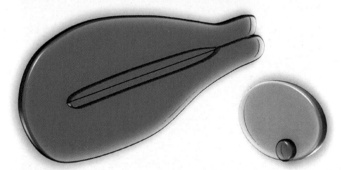

FIGURE 19.7.3: During an early proliferative phase due to edema of the superficial cells the endometrium becomes thicker with a looser texture. On ultrasound there is evidence of a narrow hyperechoic border and a thin high level central echo separated by a hypoechoic zone.

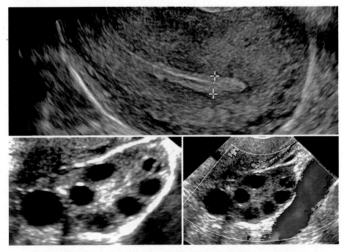

FIGURE 19.7.4: Early proliferative endometrium and dominant follicle during early follicular phase.

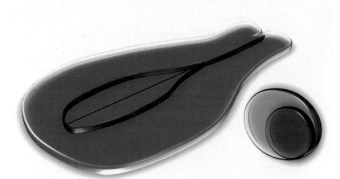

FIGURE 19.7.5: Triple line endometrium during the periovulatory phase. The endometrium reaches a thickness of 10 to 14 mm when preovulatory follicle measures about 20 mm.

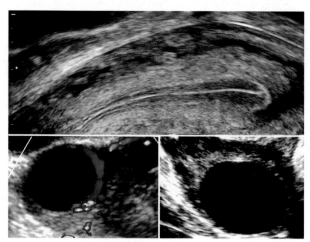

FIGURE 19.7.6: During the periovulatory phase the dominant follicle reaches about 20 mm. Careful exploration of its inner wall may depict a cumulus oophorus. Color Doppler reveals a rim of angiogenesis at the periphery of the follicle. At this time the endometrium is thick with hyperechoic border and bright central echo.

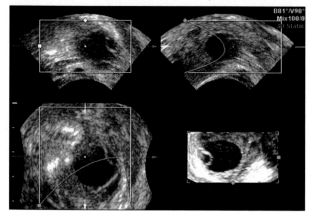

FIGURE 19.7.7: Three-dimensional ultrasound of a preovulatory follicle. Careful exploration of its inner wall depicts a cumulus oophorus.

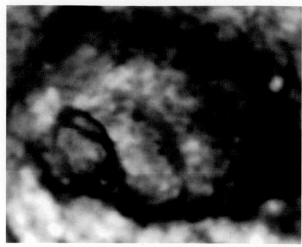

FIGURE 19.7.8: Surface rendering of the preovulatory follicle. Cumulus oophorus is bulging from the inner wall of the follicle.

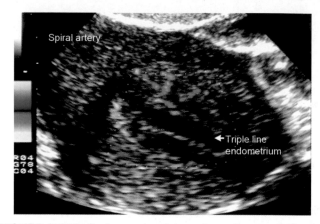

FIGURE 19.7.9: During periovulatory phase transvaginal color Doppler may depict subendometrial blood signals, the spiral arteries.

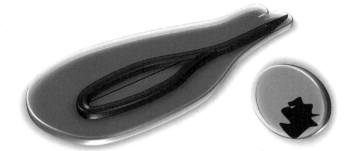

FIGURE 19.7.10: During the early luteal phase the endometrium shows a slight decrease in thickness due to the regression of the stromal edema. As a result of secretory transformation, the endometrium becomes increasingly dense and echogenic, starting from the basal layers. At this time, the follicle is no longer visualized. Collapsed follicle and minimal amount of free fluid in the cul-de-sac are typical features of ovulation.

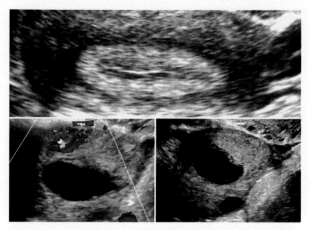

FIGURE 19.7.11: Note the hyperechoic basal layers of the endometrium (ring sign), fading of the central echo and collapsed follicle. Color Doppler starts to demonstrate marked peripheral vascularization of the corpus luteum.

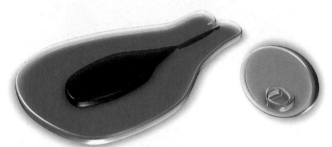

FIGURE 19.7.12: During the late secretory phase, the endometrium is homogeneously hyperechoic. Shortly before menstruation, there is a marked decline of the endometrial thickness. During the process of luteolysis the corpus luteum is being broken down by macrophages and fibroblasts and regresses to the corpus albicans.

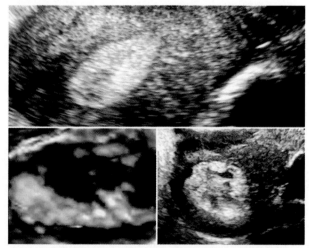

FIGURE 19.7.13: Secretory changed endometrium is homogeneously hyperechoic. Corpus luteum and/or albicans is visualized as echogenic structure within the ovary, with prominent peripheral vascularization.

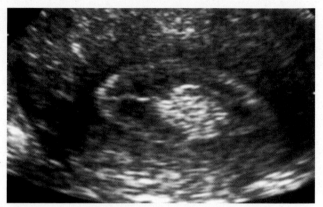

FIGURE 19.7.14: Focal endometrial thickening typical of an endometrial polyp in a patient with secondary infertility.

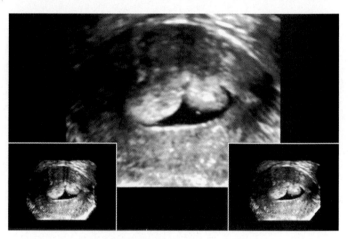

FIGURE 19.7.15: Three-dimensional ultrasound of two endometrial polyps in a patient with secondary infertility.

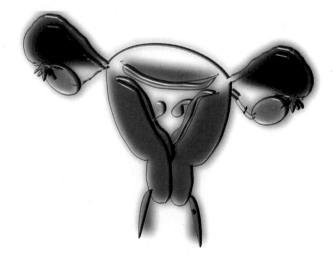

FIGURE 19.7.16: Uterine polyps, benign growths that protrude from the interior lining of the uterus, may sometimes cause infertility.

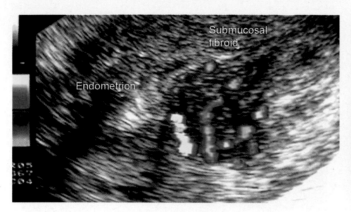

FIGURE 19.7.17: Color Doppler ultrasound of submucosal fibroid in a patient with metrorrhagia and primary infertility.

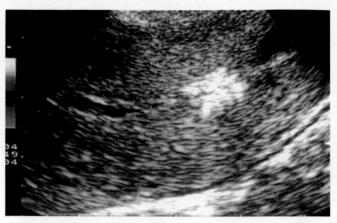

FIGURE 19.7.20: Hyperechogenic bridges visualized within the endometrial cavity in a patient with secondary amenorrhea and infertility are suggestive of intrauterine adhesions.

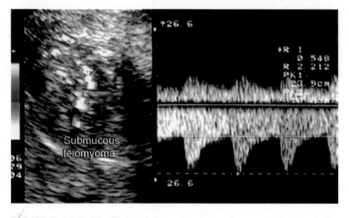

FIGURE 19.7.18: Pulsed Doppler waveform analysis of the fibroid feeding vessels. Moderate vascular impedance blood flow signals and resistance index of 0.55 are isolated from the vessels within the capsule of the fibroid.

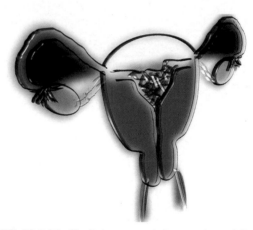

FIGURE 19.7.21: Partial or complete scarring of the uterine cavity causes partial or complete obliteration of the uterine cavity and may cause infertility or miscarriage.

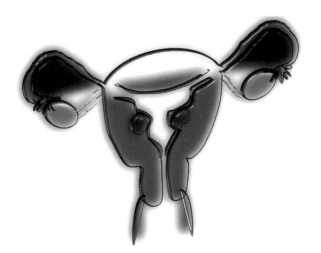

FIGURE 19.7.19: Submucosal fibroids which grow below the endometrium may interfere with implantation.

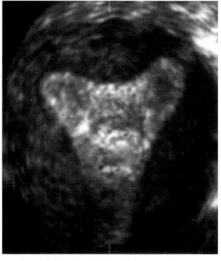

FIGURE 19.7.22: Three dimensional ultrasound and frontal reformatted section of an arcuate uterus.

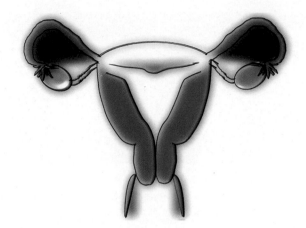

FIGURE 19.7.23: Arcuate uterus. Note a slight indentation of the uterine cavity. Arcuate uterus develops due to the failure of resorption of the midline uterine septum.

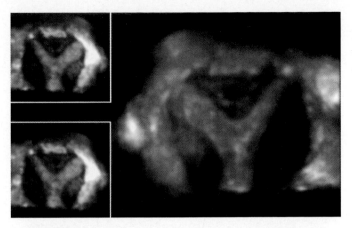

FIGURE 19.7.26: Three-dimensional ultrasound (frontal reformatted section) of a partial septate uterus.

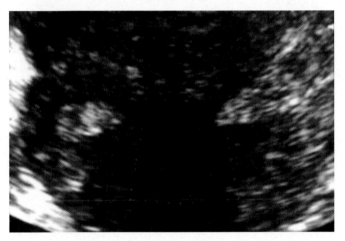

FIGURE 19.7.24: Transvaginal two-dimensional ultrasound of the endometrium in a patient with uterine septum. In a transvers plane there is evidence of clear separation of the endometrial lining.

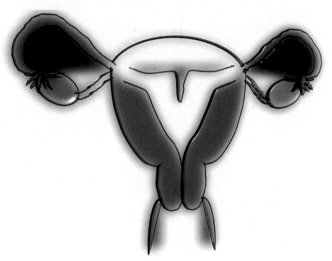

FIGURE 19.7.27: Septate uterus is the most common Müllerian duct anomaly and composes approximately 55% of the uterine anomalies. Partial septate uterus results from the partial failure of resorption of the uterovaginal septum after the fusion of the paramesonephric ducts.

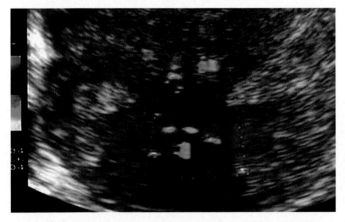

FIGURE 19.7.25: Color Doppler ultrasound of a septate uterus. Note rich vascular perfusion of the thick septum.

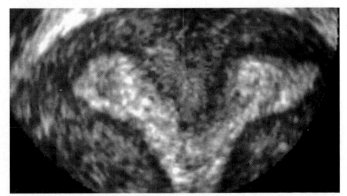

FIGURE 19.7.28: Frontal reformatted section of a septate uterus. Note clear division of the uterine cavity in the upper half of the uterine cavity.

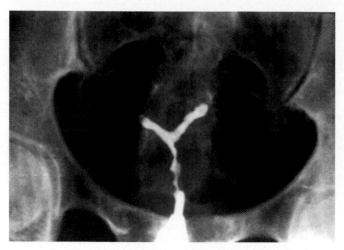

FIGURE 19.7.29: X-ray hysterosalpingography of a septate uterus.

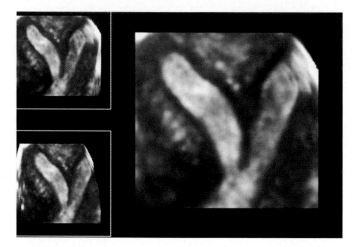

FIGURE 19.7.30: Three-dimensional ultrasound and frontal reformatted section of a complete septate uterus. Note clear division of the entire uterine cavity.

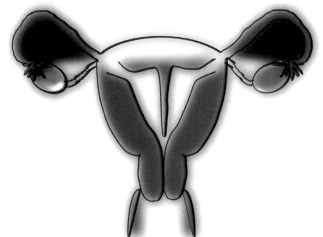

FIGURE 19.7.31: Complete septate uterus results from failure of resorption of the uterovaginal septum after fusion of the paramesonephric ducts.

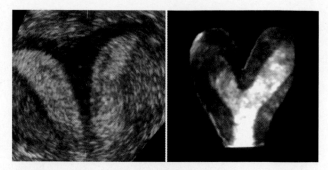

FIGURE 19.7.32: Three-dimensional ultrasound and frontal reformatted section of a bicornuate uterus. Note clear separation of the uterine cavity and fundal indentation exceeding 1 cm.

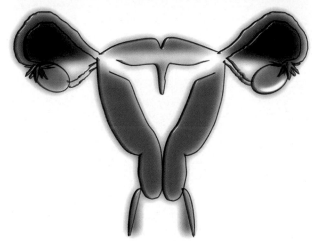

FIGURE 19.7.33: A bicornuate uterus (commonly referred as "heart-shaped" uterus) results from a partial nonfusion of the Müllerian ducts.

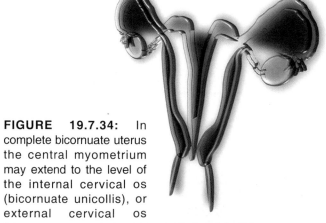

FIGURE 19.7.34: In complete bicornuate uterus the central myometrium may extend to the level of the internal cervical os (bicornuate unicollis), or external cervical os (bicornuate bicollis). The latter is distinguished from the uterus didelphys because it demonstrates some degree of fusion between the two horns, while in classic didelphys uterus, the two horns and cervices are completely separated. Another difference between dydelphys and bicornuate uterus is that the horns of the bicornuate uteri are not fully developed; typically, they are smaller than those of didelphys uteri.

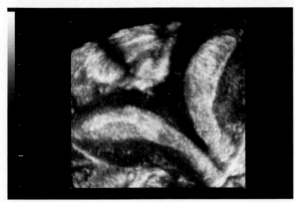

FIGURE 19.7.35: Three-dimensional ultrasound of a didelpys uterus. Duplication of the cervix and the vagina is clearly visualized.

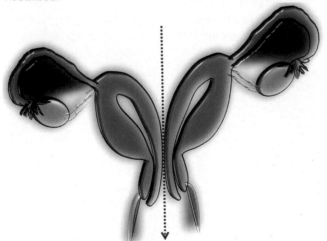

FIGURE 19.7.36: Didelphys uterus results from a complete nonfusion of both Müllerian ducts. The individual horns are fully developed and almost normal in size. Two cervices are inevitably present. A longitudinal or transverse vaginal septum may also be noted. Didelphys uteri have the highest association with transverse vaginal septa but septa also may be observed in other anomalies.

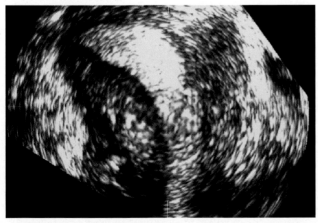

FIGURE 19.7.37: Three-dimensional ultrasound of an unicornuate uterus.

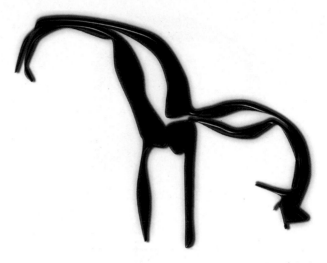

FIGURE 19.7.38: Unicornuate uterus. Note only the right horn of the uterus and communicating rudimentary horn containing the functional endometrium. Unicornuate uterus develops due to the unilateral Mullerian duct agenesis. Laparoscopy and hysteroscopy are required to differentiate between the different types of unicornuate uterus.

FIGURE 19.7.39: Unicornuate uterus with non-communicating rudimentary horn containing the functional endometrium.

FIGURE 19.7.40: Unicornuate uterus with non-communicating rudimentary horn containing the nonfunctional endometrium.

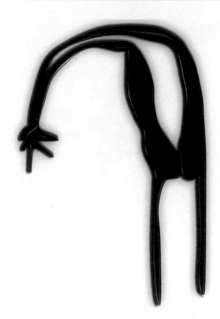

FIGURE 19.7.41: Unicornuate uterus with no evidence of rudimentary horn.

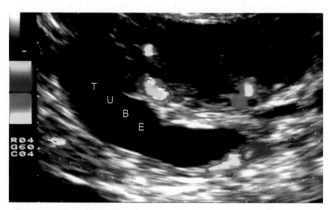

FIGURE 19.7.42: Dilated and fluid filled tube in an infertile patient with tubal cause of infertility.

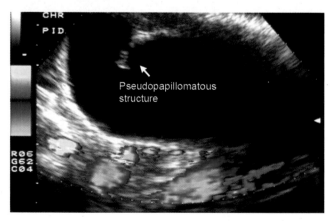

FIGURE 19.7.43: Dilated and fluid filled tube in an infertile patient, caused by a previous pelvic infection.

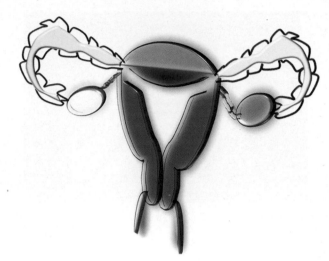

FIGURE 19.7.44: Hydrosalpinx is a blocked, fluid filled fallopian tube. In mild cases fertility may be restored by opening the tube surgically, otherwise IVF is the method of choice.

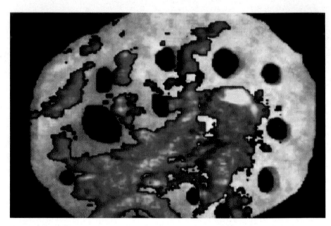

FIGURE 19.7.45: "Swiss cheese" appearance of the polycystic ovary obtained by 3D ultrasound. Power Doppler depicts dilated intraovarian vessels.

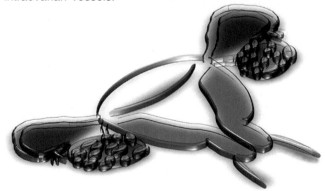

FIGURE 19.7.46: Polycystic ovaries are defined as presence of 10 or more follicles measuring from 2 to 9 mm in diameter, and increased ovarian volume (>10 ml). These patients present with oligo- or anovulation (irregular periods) and clinical or biochemical signs of hyperandrogenism.

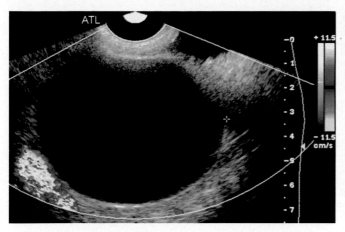

FIGURE 19.7.47: Simple ovarian cyst in a patient with secondary infertility and anovulation.

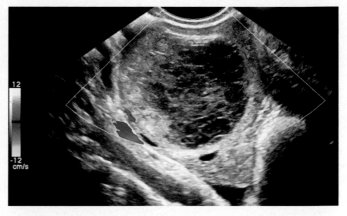

FIGURE 19.7.48: Complex ovarian (corpus luteum) cyst in a patient with secondary infertility and anovulation. Note blood clot appearance, peripheral vascularization and presence of a small amount of free fluid.

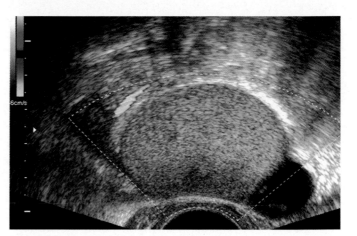

FIGURE 19.7.49: Ovarian endometrioma in a patient with primary infertility, chronic pelvic pain and dysmenorrhea. Homogeneously echogenic (chocolate paste) fluid, clear demarcation from the ovary and peripheral vascularization are typical findings of ovarian endometriosis.

BIBLIOGRAPHY

1. Beck WW Jr. Obstetrics & Gynecology, 4th edition. Philadelphia: Williams & Wilkins 1997.
2. Kupesic S, de Ziegler D. Ultrasound and infertility. New York/London: Parthenon Publishing 2000.
3. Kupesic S. Ultrasound, color Doppler and 3D ultrasound in Obstetrics, Gynecology and Infertility New York/London: Parthenon Publishing 2005.
4. Kupesic-Urek S, Kurjak A. Transvaginal color Doppler in the assessment of uterine perfusion in infertile patients. Gynaecol Perinatol 1992;3:123-7.
5. Kupesic S, Kurjak A. The assessment of uterine and ovarian perfusion in infertile patients. Eur J Obstet Gynecol Reprod Biol 1997;71(2):151-4.
6. Kupesic S, Bjelos D, Kurjak A. Three-dimensional ultrasound in the assessment of infertility. Ultrasound Rev Obstet Gynecol 2001;2:149-67.
7. Kupesic S, Kurjak A. Transvaginal color Doppler in the assessment of infertility. In: Kurjak A, Kupesic S (Eds). An Atlas of transvaginal color Doppler. London-New York: Parthenon Publishing 2000;83.
8. Kupesic S, Kurjak A. The assessment of female infertility. In: Kurjak A, Kupesic S (Eds.). Clinical application of 3D sonography. London-New York: Parthenon Publishing 2000; 67.
9. Kupesic S, Kurjak A, Bjelos D. Color Doppler and three-dimensional sonographic imaging in infertility. In: Kupesic S. (Ed). Color Doppler and three-dimensional ultrasound in gynecology, infertility and obstetrics. New Delhi: Jaypee Brothers Medical Publishers Pvt Ltd 2003;112-40.
10. Kupesic S, Kurjak A, Bjelos D. Color Doppler and 3D power Doppler hysterosalpingography (sonohysterosalpingography). In: Kupesic S (Ed). Color Doppler and three-dimensional ultrasound in gynecology, infertility and obstetrics. New Delhi: Jaypee Brothers Medical Publishers Pvt Ltd 2003;141-56.
11. Kupesic S. Sonographic Imaging in Infertility. Donald School Textbook of Ultrasound in Obstetrics and Gynecology. In: Kurjak A, Chervenak F (Eds). New Delhi: Jaypee Brothers Medical Publishers 2008;865-86.
12. Laparosc 2001;8(1):111-6.
13. Speroff L, Glass RH, Kase NG. Clinical gynecologic endocrinology and infertility, 6th edition. Philadelphia: Lippincott Williams & Wilkins 1999.

19.8: PELVIC INFLAMMATORY DISEASE

Text and images by: S Kupesic Plavsic
Medical illustrations by: Bhargavi Patham and Sandesh Subramanya

Pelvic inflammatory disease (PID) is the inflammation of the uterus (endometritis), fallopian tubes (salpingitis) and/or the ovaries (oophoritis). If untreated PID may progress to formation of adhesions with nearby tissues and organs (Flow chart 19.8.1).

Clinical Clues

- **Ask about:**
  - Hygiene practices
  - Sexual history
  - Purulent discharge
  - Vulvovaginal irritation
  - Abnormal genital tract bleeding (usually associated with endometritis)
  - Postcoital bleeding (cervicitis)
  - Dysmenorrhea
  - Abdominal and/or pelvic pain
  - Fever (upper genital tract disease (PID) or herpes simplex)
  - Dysuria
  - Urinary frequency (typically due to concomitant chlamydial urethral infection)
  - Suprapubic pain (suggestive of cystitis)
  - Pruritus, irritation and burning
  - Soreness
  - Odor
  - Specific symptoms:
    - *Candidiasis* may present with scant curd-like discharge, significant symptoms of inflammation (pruritus, soreness, dyspareunia). It is frequently premenstrual in occurrence.
    - *Bacterial vaginosis* (BV) may present with malodorous discharge and no signs or symptoms of inflammation. Sometimes BV is asymptomatic.
    - *Trichomoniasis* is presented with malodorous, purulent discharge and dyspareunia. It often occurs during or immediately after menses.
  - History of diabetes mellitus
  - Dyspareunia (may be insertional, deep or both and thus can be the result of a localized vaginitis or cervicitis or an upper genital tract problem, such as

pelvic inflammatory disease (PID), endometriosis or other uterine pathology)
  - Medications, prescriptions and nonprescriptions.
    - Antibiotics may disturb normal vaginal flora, creating an opportunity for the growth of opportunistic organisms, such as *Gardnerella vaginalis*, *Escherichia coli*, group B streptococci, genital mycoplasma and *Candida albicans*.
    - Exogenous estrogen, often as oral contraceptives, may induce superphysiologic discharge as well.
- **Look for:**
  - Degree of vulvovaginal inflammation
    - Vulva usually appears normal with BV
    - Erythema, edema, fissure suggest candidiasis, trichomoniasis or dermatitis
  - Characteristics of vaginal discharge
    - *Bacterial vaginosis*: Thin, gray, homogeneous with "fishy" odor discharge

Flow chart 19.8.1: Inductive reasoning scheme for diagnostic evaluation of the patients presenting with vaginal discharge, sexually transmitted disease and pelvic inflammatory disease (*Courtesy:* Paul L. Foster School of Medicine, Texas Tech University at El Paso, TX, USA). Patients with pelvic discomfort due pelvic inflammatory disease should always be evaluated by ultrasound, which can be efficiently used for staging and monitoring of the PID.

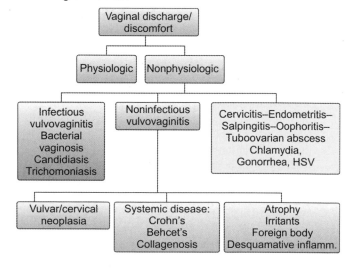

- *Candidiasis:* Thick, white, adherent, "cottage cheese-like" discharge
- *Trichomoniasis*: Greenish-yellow purulent discharge
- Presence of cervical inflammation
- Suggestive of cervicitis not vaginitis
- If cervicitis, expect friablility with mucopurulent discharge
- Distinguish cervicitis from normal ectropion (normal physiologic presence of endocervical glandular tissue on the ectocervix)
- Abdominal or cervical motion tenderness, suggestive of PID
  - Cervical motion tenderness associated with purulent/mucopurulent discharge, cervical friability (easy bleeding with culture swab, Pap smear, etc.) and cervical edema, suggestive of cervical infection with *Chlamydia or Gonorrhoeae.*
  - *HSV:* Diffuse vesicular lesions/ulcerations on cervix
  - *Trichomonas:* Punctate hemorrhages (strawberry cervix).

Investigations

- Pelvic exam
- Wet mount
- Pap smear
- Laboratory examination of the vaginal discharge:
  - Vaginal pH:
    - pH > 4.5 in premenopausal female suggests infections, such as BV or trichomoniasis (pH 5-6) and excludes candidiasis (pH 4-4.5).
    - pH subject to alteration by lubricating gels, semen, douches and intravaginal medications.
    - pH is not useful parameter in premenarchal and postmenopausal females where normal values are ≥ 4.7.
  - Microscopy:
    - *Bacterial vaginosis:* clue cells (epithelial cells studded with adherent coccobacilli) on "wet mount" (sample of vaginal discharge suspended in normal saline).
      - "Whiff test": smelling a slide immediately after putting vaginal secretions from a patient with BV in KOH will yield a fishy (amine) odor.

- *Candidiasis*: Candidal buds and/or hyphae, especially noticeable if sample of vaginal discharge is suspended in 10% potassium hydroxide (KOH) solution.
- *Trichomoniasis*: Motile trichomonads.
- Cervicitis: abundant leukocytes (WBCs) without evidence of any of the above. Note: microscopy has very low sensitivity for BV and trichomoniasis.
- Cervical culture:
  - In patients with mucopurulent discharge, cervicitis, fever, cervical motion and/or abdominal tenderness. Consider cervical culture for *Chlamydia trachomatis* and/or *Neisseria gonorrhoeae.*
  - In patient with risky sexual behavior (e.g. new or multiple partners, symptomatic partner, partner who is or has been engaged in high risk behavior, sexually active adolescents) culture the cervix and test for *syphilis, hepatitis B, and HIV.*
  - Perform endocervical swab for nucleic acid amplification testing (*Chlamydia/Gonorrhoea*).
  - *Trichomonas:* Sensitivity of microscopy (wet prep) depends on the experience of the examiner. Therefore, symptomatic females with cervicitis and negative microscopy should undergo cervical culture.
  - *HSV*: Viral culture, PCR (most expensive), direct flourescence antibody, type-specific serologic tests.
- In patients with pelvic and/or abdominal pain, suggestive of upper genital tract problem perform ultrasound.

Ultrasound Findings

- Abnormally thickened and vascularized endometrium, suggestive of endometritis.
- Fluid filled tortuous tubes with thickened walls and free fluid in the cul-de-sac, suggestive of salpingitis.
- Enlarged ovaries with echogenic cysts–inflamed follicles and free fluid in the cul-de-sac, suggestive of oophoritis.
- Tubular fluid filled tubes with thin walls, incomplete septations and pseudopapillomatous protrusions, suggestive of hydrosalpinx.
- Complex adnexal mass (usually multilocular cystic structure with echogenic fluid and thick septations) and free fluid in the cul-de-sac, suggestive of tuboovarian abscess.

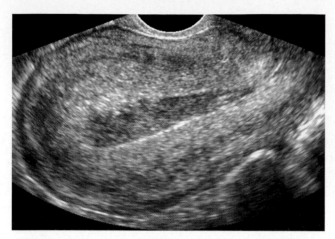

FIGURE 19.8.1: Distended uterine cavity in a patient with endometritis.

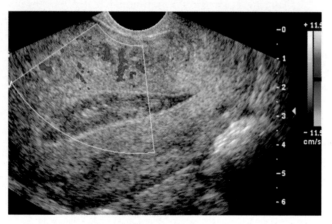

FIGURE 19.8.2: The same patient. Note vascularized endometrium in a patient with endometritis.

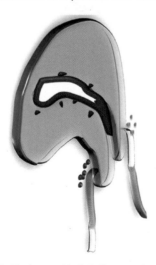

FIGURE 19.8.3: Endometritis is inflammation of the endometrial lining of the uterus. In acute phase, endometritis is characterized by the presence of neutrophils within the endometrial glands. Most common presenting symptoms are pelvic and/or abdominal pain, vaginal discharge, bleeding and fever.

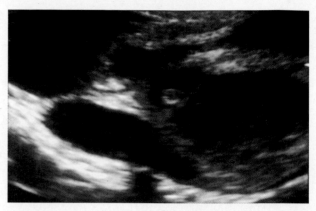

FIGURE 19.8.4: Complex adnexal mass occupying the pouch of Douglas in the patient with acute pelvic inflammation. Note typical signs of acute salpingitis: Fluid filled tubes with thickened walls and free fluid in the cul-de-sac.

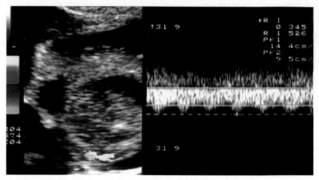

FIGURE 19.8.5: Complex adnexal mass occupying the pouch of Douglas in a patient with acute pelvic inflammation. Increased vascularity indicates a response to various bacterial antigens and inflammatory products and is easily detectable using color Doppler ultrasound. Pulsed Doppler waveform analysis obtained low impedance blood flow signals (RI = 0.35) from tiny tubal arteries.

Diagnoses to Consider

- Physiologic leukorrhea
- Nonphysiologic vaginal discharge
  - Vaginitis
  - Vulvovaginal candidiasis
  - Bacterial vaginosis
  - Trichomoniasis
    - Endometritis
    - Salpingitis
    - Oophoritis
    - Tubo-ovarian abscess
    - Hydrosalpinx

Some case studies related to pelvic inflammatory disease are depicted in Figures 19.8.1 to 19.8.20.

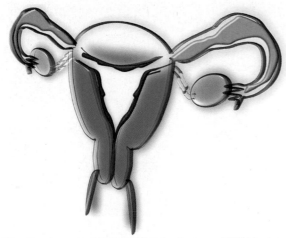

FIGURE 19.8.6: Pelvic inflammatory disease (PID) is spread of the severe inflammation from the vagina and cervix towards the uterus and the fallopian tubes. Salpingitis is inflammation of the fallopian tubes.

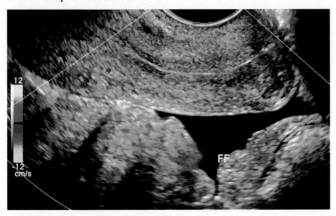

FIGURE 19.8.7: In patients with acute pelvic inflammation, ultrasound may visualize free fluid in the posterior cul-de-sac (due to peritonitis).

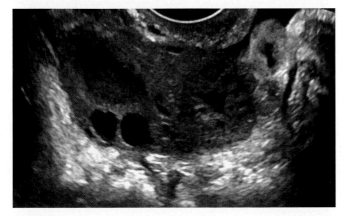

FIGURE 19.8.8: Transvaginal sonogram of a patient with oophoritis (inflammation of the ovaries). Note enlarged ovary with echogenic cysts (inflamed follicles) and free fluid in the cul-de-sac.

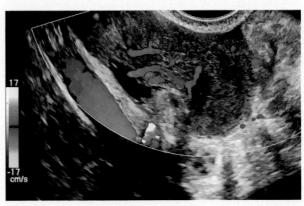

FIGURE 19.8.9: Color Doppler ultrasound of a patient with tuboovarian abscess. Note complex adnexal mass (usually multilocular cystic structure with echogenic fluid and thick septations) and free fluid in the cul-de-sac. Dilated vessels indicate increased angiogenesis.

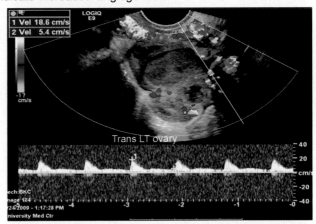

FIGURE 19.8.10: Tubo-ovarian abscess (TOA) is a late complication of PID. It is recognized by a complete breakdown of the normal structure of the fallopian tubes and the ovaries.

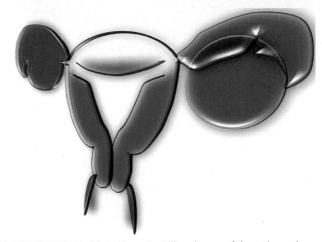

FIGURE 19.8.11: Note the retort like shape of the adnexal mass in a patient with chronic pelvic pain and infertility. Echoucent tubular structure with complete and incomplete septations is typical of hydrosalpinx.

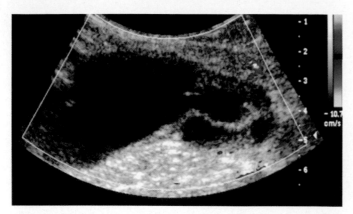

FIGURE 19.8.12: Note the retort like shape of the adnexal mass in a patient with chronic pelvic pain and infertility. Echoucent tubular structure with complete and incomplete septations is typical of hydrosalpinx.

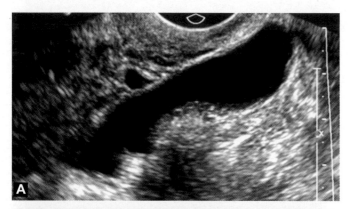

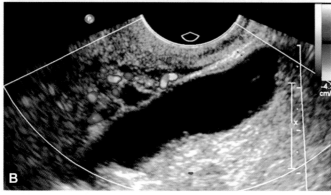

FIGURES 19.8.13A AND B: Sausage-like, dilated fluid filled tube in a patient with hydrosalpinx. Note discrete vascularization at the periphery of the fluid filled dilated fallopian tube. Color Doppler clearly differentiates hydrosalpinx from dilated pelvic veins.

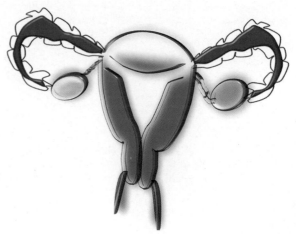

FIGURE 19.8.14: Hydrosalpinx represents a distally blocked fallopian tube, filled with serous or clear fluid. This condition is usually bilateral and in majority of the patients affected tubes measure several centimeters in diameter. The blocked tubes may cause infertility.

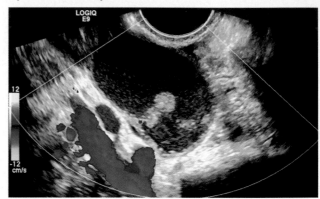

FIGURE 19.8.15: Complex adnexal mass in a patient with chronic pelvic inflammatory disease. Hypovascularized papillary protrusion represents tubal mucosal fold.

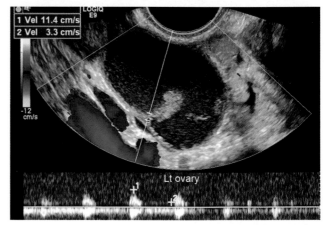

FIGURE 19.8.16: The same patient. Moderate to high vascular impedance blood flow signals are obtained from the base of the papillary like structure. Laparoscopy confirmed hydrosalpinx (tubal cause of infertility).

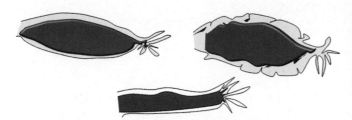

FIGURE 19.8.17: Hydrosalpinx develops as a consequence of the fusion of the fimbrial end of the tube and the subsequent accumulation of the tubal secretions and tubal distention. Chronic salpingitis is characterized with formation of intratubal adhesions. The tubal plicae, denuded of epithelium, adhere to one another and slowly fuse in a reparative, scarring process that forms blind pouches. Abnormalities of the fallopian tube lumen may result in infertility or ectopic pregnancy.

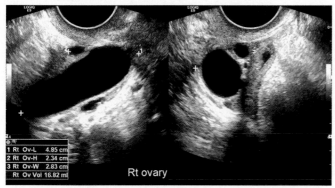

FIGURE 19.8.18: Transvaginal sonogram of a patient with hydrosalpinx in two different planes. Note the importance of performing different planes because hydrosalpinx may sometimes be misinterpreted as ovarian or paraovarian cyst.

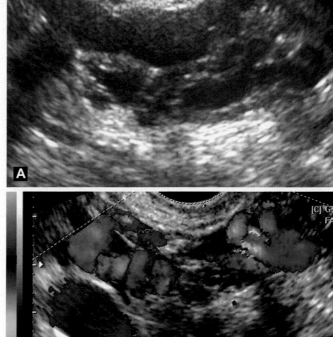

FIGURES 19.8.20A AND B: Every adnexal mass should be evaluated with B-mode and color Doppler ultrasound to differentiate between the fluid filled tubes and pelvic congestion syndrome.

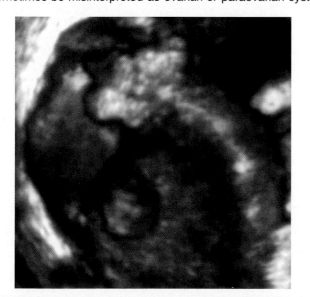

FIGURE 19.8.19: Three-dimensional ultrasound of salpingitis. Note thickened fallopian tube with irregular appearance of the fimbrial end.

BIBLIOGRAPHY

1. Beckmann RBC, Ling FW, Smith RP, et al. Obstetrics and Gynecology, 5th Edition. Philadelphia: Lippincott Williams and Wilkins 2002;273-88.
2. Beck WW. Obstetrics and Gynecology, 4th Edition. Baltimore: Williams & Wilkins 1997;325-39.
3. Kupesic A, Kurjak D, Bjelos. Pelvic inflammatory disease. In: Kupesic S (Ed). Color Doppler and three-dimensional ultrasound in gynecology, infertility and obstetrics. New Delhi: Jaypee Brothers 2003;94-103.
4. Kupesic S, Kurjak A, Pasalic L, et al. The value of transvaginal color Doppler in the assessment of pelvic inflammatory disease. J Ultrasound Med Biol 1995;6:733-8.

19.9: PELVIC PAIN

Text and images by: S Kupesic Plavsic
Medical illustrations by: Bhargavi Patham and Sandesh Subramanya

Pelvic pain may be acute or chronic. Chronic pelvic pain (CPP) is of 6 months duration, occurs below the umbilicus and is severe enough to cause functional disability or require treatment. Approximately 10% of referrals to a gynecologist are for CPP (Flow chart 19.9.1).

Acute pelvic pain is associated with a broad range of conditions involving the reproductive, gastrointestinal, genitourinary and musculoskeletal systems. It may also be a symptom of infection, ovarian cysts, ectopic pregnancy, appendicitis or neoplasia.

Clinical Clues

- **Ask about:**
  – Pain location, radiation, intensity (with menstrual cycle, urination, defecation and physical activity), timing (especially, if only during the course of the period or with intercourse) and quality.
  – Reproductive, urological and gastrointestinal systems.
  – Phase of the menstrual cycle (in reproductive age patients)
  – Pregnancy test (in reproductive age patients)
  – Screening questionnaires for depression, sexual and physical abuse and somatization.
  – Past history: Ask about history of endometriosis, PID, GI disease (especially irritable bowel syndrome (IBS)), urinary disease (especially interstitial nephritis/painful bladder syndrome), musculoskeletal disease, psychiatric disease, history of previous diagnostic tests/treatments for pain.)
  – Sexual history: Assessment of the risk factors for sexually transmitted disease.
  – Missed/delayed period, nausea, vomiting, breast tenderness, suggestive of pregnancy.
  – Sudden, severe pain, suggestive of a ruptured ectopic pregnancy, acute degeneration of a uterine fibroid, adnexal torsion and cystic rupture.
  – Triad of amenorrhea, abnormal vaginal bleeding and pelvic pain, suggestive of ectopic pregnancy.
- **Look for:**
  – Results of a detailed abdominal and pelvic examination
  – Abdominal scars, site and degree of tenderness

– Atypical discharge, cervical lesions, bulky uterus, unilateral tenderness or generalized tenderness
– Type, duration (constant or intermittent), location and severity of the pain
– Onset of the pain (pain that first develops prior to menarche is unlikely to have a gynecologic etiology)
– Associated symptoms (for example, weight loss may occur in association with malignancy)
– Quality of the pain
  - Aching pain perceived to be near the surface of the body, suggestive of a referred pain.
  - Dull, diffuse pain whose location is difficult to determine, suggestive of a visceral pain. In contrast, the specific location of somatic pain can be accurately described.
– Alleviating and aggravating factors
– Relevant system symptoms (GU, GI and musculoskeletal)
– Effect of pain on patient's daily life

Investigations

- History and physical examination
- Pelvic examination

Flow chart 19.9.1: Inductive reasoning scheme for diagnostic evaluation of patients presenting with pelvic pain (*Courtesy:* Paul L. Foster School of Medicine, Texas Tech University at El Paso, TX, USA). Ultrasound can precisely differentiate gynecologic (uterine, ovarian and tubal), and nongynecologic causes of pelvic pain.

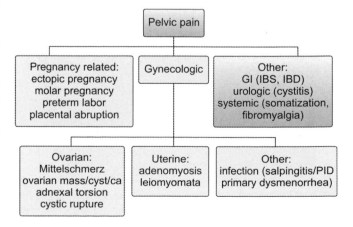

- Pregnancy test (if indicated)
- CBS, differential, CRP and ESR
- Urinalysis
- Testing for Chlamydia and Gonorrhea infections
- Pelvic ultrasound
- CT of the abdomen and pelvis

Ultrasound Findings

- Retroverted uterus, bilateral echogenic ovarian cysts, free fluid in the cul-de-sac, all suggestive of endometriosis.
- Enlarged, globular, tender uterus with myometrial cystic lesions, suggestive of adenomyosis.
- Enlarged, mobile uterus with irregular contour and solitary or multiple submucosal, intramural or subserosal fibroids.
- Uterine tenderness and/or cervical motion tenderness during transvaginal ultrasound exam, thickened and vascularized endometrium, suggestive of endometritis related to PID (refer to "Clinical Sonographic Pearls" on PID).
- Adnexal enlargement in patients with ovarian cysts, endometrioma or neoplasm.
- Fever, cervical motion tenderness, tenderness of the adnexa, leukocytosis, mucopurulent cervicovaginal discharge, associated with tubular tubal masses, suggestive of PID.
- Complex adnexal mass, irregular branching and penetrating pattern of intratumoral vessels, abdominal swelling, pallor, weight loss, lymphadenopathy and ascites, suggestive of ovarian malignancy.
- Varicosities within the uterus, suggestive of intraparenchymatous type of pelvic congestion syndrome.
- Varicosities of periuterine and periovarian vessels, suggestive of extraparenchymatous type of pelvic congestion syndrome.
- Lack of mobility of the pelvic organs, suggestive of pelvic pain caused by adhesions, endometriosis, previous surgery or infection. This finding is commonly associated with infertility and chronic pelvic pain.

Diagnoses to Consider

- Gynecologic pain
  - Ovarian:
    - Ovarian cyst/mass/torsion
    - Endometriosis
    - PID/Tubo-ovarian abscess
    - Ovarian remnant/Residual ovary
  - Uterine:
    - Adenomyosis
    - Endometritis
    - Leiomyoma
  - Other
    - Mittelschmerz (unilateral lower abdominal pain that occurs around the time of ovulation)
    - Pelvic adhesions
    - Pelvic congestion syndrome (varicosities)
- Pregnancy-related pain
  - Abnormal early pregnancy (missed abortion, anembryonic pregnancy)
  - Ectopic pregnancy
  - Gestational trophoblastic disease (GTD)
  - Preterm labor
  - Placental abruption
- Gastrointestinal tract related pain
  - Appendicitis
  - Irritable bowel syndrome (IBS) or irritable bowel disease (IBD)
  - Diverticulitis
  - Neoplasia
  - Obstruction
  - Constipation
  - Sprue
- Urinary tract related pain
  - Cystitis, urinary tract infection
  - Neoplasia
  - Urethral diverticulum
  - Chronic urethral syndrome
- MSK/Neuro/Mental health-related pain
  - Musculoskeletal pain
    - Myalgia
    - Piriformis syndrome
    - Coccydynia
    - Hernia
    - Myofascial syndrome
    - Figromyalgia
  - Neurological pain
    - Neuralgia
    - Herniated nucleus pulposus
    - Neoplasia
    - Abdominal epilepsy/migraine
  - Mental health-related pain
    - Somatization disorder
    - Substance abuse
    - Depression

Some case studies related to pelvic pain are depicted in Figures 19.9.1 to 19.9.29.

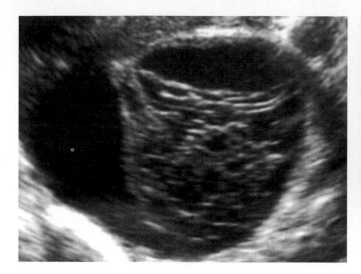

FIGURE 19.9.1: Corpus luteum cyst may occur after an oocyte has been released from a follicle. In nonpregnant patients the corpus luteum usually breaks down and disappears. In some patients corpus luteum may fill with fluid or blood and persist for a few months. Due to internal hemorrhage these cysts usually appear as a complex mass with central blood clot ("spider net" like image)and echogenic septations.

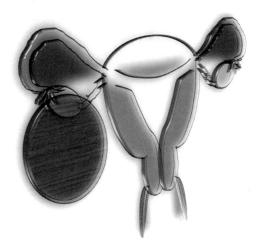

FIGURE 19.9.2: Abdominal and/or pelvic pain on one side may be associated with postovulatory formation of the corpus luteum cyst. The persistent corpus luteum cyst may cause pain, tenderness, and delayed menstruation.

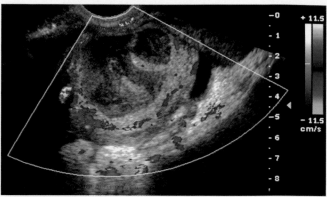

FIGURE 19.9.3: Color Doppler image of a hemorrhagic cyst of the right ovary. The internal appearance is created by a retracting clot which does not show increased vascularity. Peripheral vessels are clearly displayed by color Doppler ultrasound.

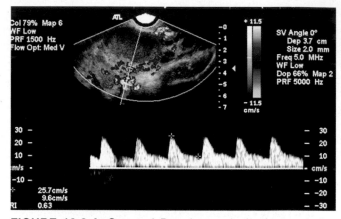

FIGURE 19.9.4: Spectral Doppler analysis demonstrates moderate vascular impedance blood flow signals with resistive index (RI) of 0.63.

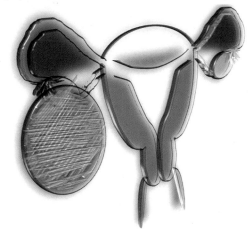

FIGURE 19.9.5: Hemorrhagic cyst of the ovary is a functional cyst which occurs when bleeding occurs within a cyst. Patient presents with symptoms such as unilateral abdominal and/or back pain.

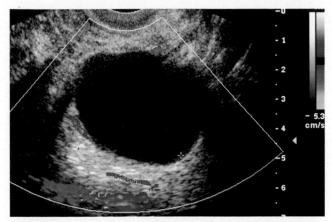

FIGURE 19.9.6: Partial adnexal torsion of a simple ovarian cyst. Discrete blood flow signals are detected at the periphery of the ovarian cyst.

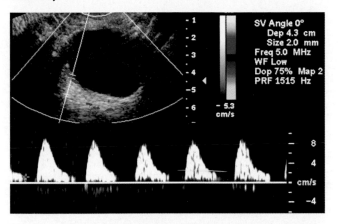

FIGURE 19.9.7: The same patient. Pulsed Doppler waveform analysis demonstrates arterial type of blood flow signals with absence of diastolic flow. Sonographic and Doppler findings are suggestive of partial adnexal torsion. Note that venous type of blood flow signals was not obtained.

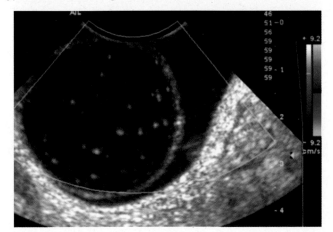

FIGURE 19.9.8: Color Doppler scan of a complete adnexal torsion. Note the absence of both the venous and arterial blood flow signals.

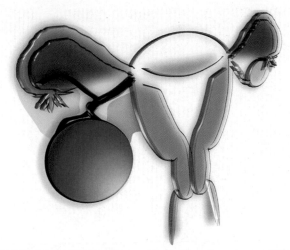

FIGURE 19.9.9: Two-dimensional color Doppler and 3D power Doppler US are useful in early diagnosis of a complete adnexal torsion and follow up of the ovarian reperfusion after detorsion of the partially twisted adnexa.

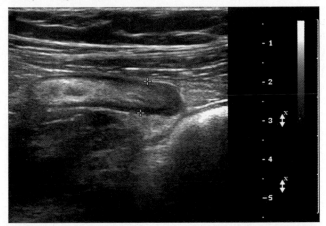

FIGURE 19.9.10: Ultrasound image of the right low abdominal quadrant in a patient presenting with right sided pelvic pain. Note longitudinal scan of an inflammed appendix.

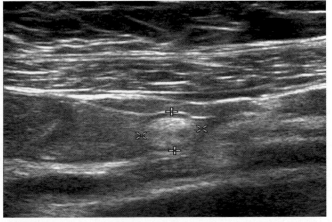

FIGURE 19.9.11: The same patient. Note transverse section of an inflamed apendix with an appendicolyth.

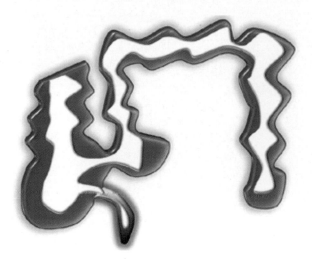

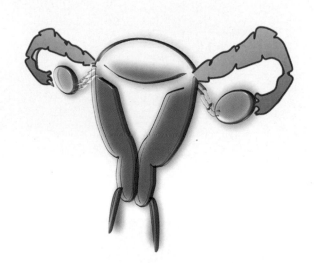

FIGURE 19.9.12: Ultrasound is very useful in differentiation of acute appendicitis from other acute conditions in female pelvis. Using graded compression technique (uniform pressure applied to the right low quadrant by a hand holding ultrasound transducer). Normal and gas-filled loops of intestine are either displaced or compressed between the anterior and posterior abdominal walls. Inflamed appendix remains incompressible and is optimally visualized as a blind ended tubular structure with laminated wall arising from the base of the cecum. It is aperistaltic, noncompressible blind ended echogenic lesion, with diameter >6 mm. Demonstration of an apendicolith, visualized as bright echogenic foci with distal acoustic shadowing is additional confirmatory finding.

FIGURE 19.9.14: Many patients with hydrosalpinx have chronic or recurrent pelvic pain, while others are asymptomatic. Patients with hydrosalpinx may experience repeated acute tubal infections, which may cause fever and pain.

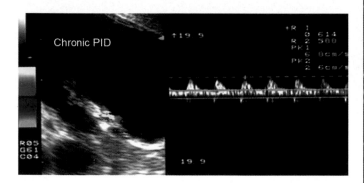

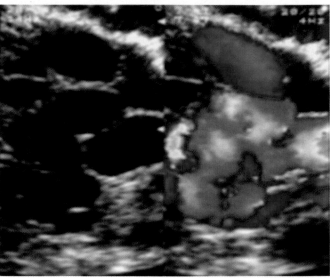

FIGURE 19.9.13: Pelvic pain may also be present in patients with acute and/or chronic PID. Hydrosalpinx is blocked, dilated, fluid-filled fallopian tube usually caused by a previous tubal infection. Pelvic infections that cause hydrosalpinx formation are usually caused by sexually transmitted diseases, namely Chlamydia trachomatis and Neisseriae gonorrhea.

FIGURE 19.9.15: In a patient presenting with pelvic pain ultrasound has revealed tortuous structures around the right ovary and the uterus. Color Doppler ultrasound demonstrated dilated and tortuous vessels with prominent venous flow. Laparoscopy confirmed pelvic congestion syndrome.

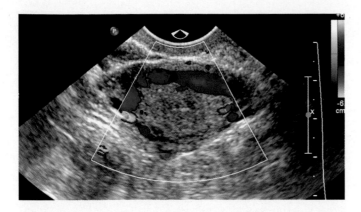

FIGURE 19.9.16: Dilated veins may also be observed within the uterus. Note dilated arcuate veins within the distal portion of the myometrium.

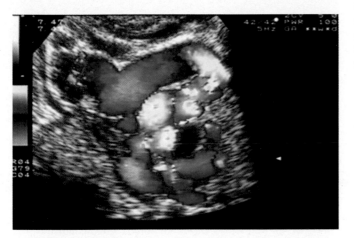

FIGURE 19.9.17: Tortuous and dilated pelvic venous plexuses may mimic complex adnexal mass.

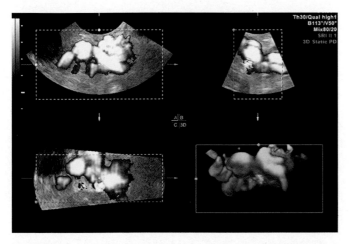

FIGURE 19.9.18: Three-dimensional power Doppler ultrasound of pelvic varicosities in a patient with chronic pelvic pain.

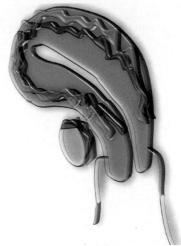

FIGURE 19.9.19: Color Doppler ultrasound is a feasible noninvasive technique for the detection of pelvic congestion syndrome in patients presenting with chronic pelvic pain. The same modality may be used for the detection of the patients who may benefit from selective ovarian venography and embolization procedures.

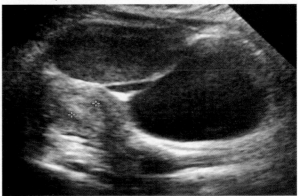

FIGURE 19.9.20: Bilateral echogenic cystic structures in a patient presenting with pelvic pain. Parenchymatous texture of the "chocolate" paste-like fluid is typical of ovarian endometrioma.

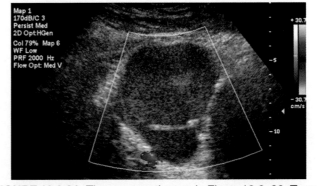

FIGURE 19.9.21: The same patient as in Figure19.9. 20. Transabdominal color Doppler ultrasound of ovarian endometrioma. Homogeneous mid-level internal echoes and peripheral vascularization are typical of ovarian endometriosis.

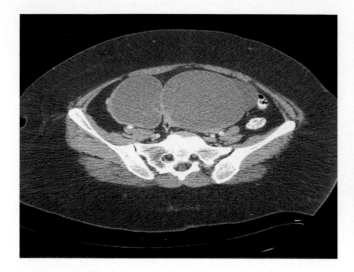

FIGURE 19.9.22: Multidetector CT of bilateral ovarian endometriosis in the same patient. Abdominal CT is advantageous for visualization of the bilateral ovarian endometriotic cysts.

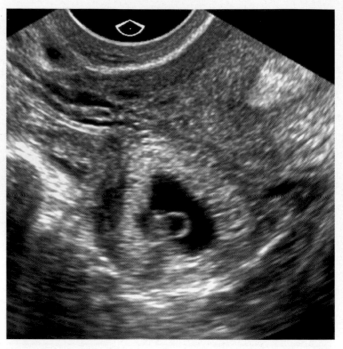

FIGURE 19.9.24: In every reproductive age patient presenting with pelvic pain sonographer has to exclude pregnancy related caused of pelvic pain. Key to the diagnosis of ectopic pregnancy is the determination of the presence or absence of an intrauterine gestational sac correlated with quantitative serum beta-subunit hCG (ß-hCG) levels. An ectopic pregnancy should be suspected, if transvaginal ultrasonography does not show an intrauterine gestational sac when the beta hCG level is higher than 1.500 mIU per ml. In this case an experienced sonographer may demonstrate an ectopic gestational sac with or without a yolk sac or an embryonic pole.

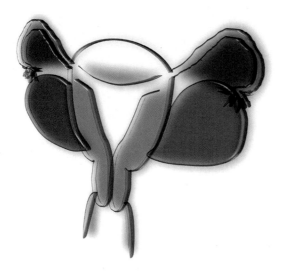

FIGURE 19.9.23: Ultrasonographic examination is the most common imaging modality used to evaluate women suspected of having endometriosis. It is particularly helpful for detection of the endometriotic cysts but has a limited role in the diagnosis of adhesions or superficial peritoneal implants.

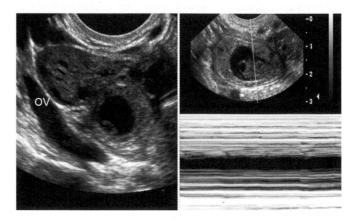

FIGURE 19.9.25: The same patient. Note a concentric gestational ring in close proximity to the ovary. M-mode reveals absence of the embryonic heart tones.

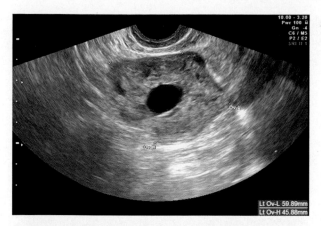

FIGURE 19.9.26: Two-dimensional ultrasound of tubal ectopic pregnancy.

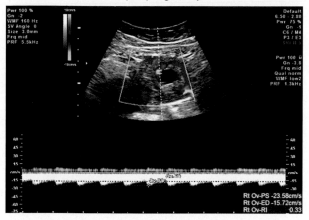

FIGURE 19.9.27: Color Doppler ultrasound of ectopic pregnancy. High velocity – low resistance blood flow signals obtained from the periphery of the ectopic gestational sac indicate vital trophoblast.

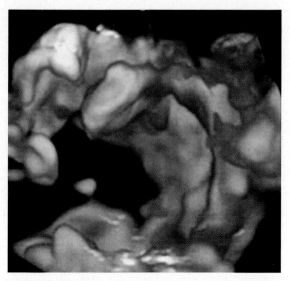

FIGURE 19.9.28: Three-dimensional power Doppler image of an ectopic gestational sac. "Ring of fire" guides the sonographer to the location of the ectopic pregnancy and shortens the diagnostic process.

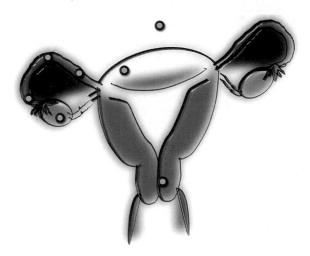

FIGURE 19.9.29: Transvaginal 2D and 3D ultrasound with addition of color/power Doppler improve early detection of tubal, isthmic, cervical, ovarian and abdominal pregnancy.

BIBLIOGRAPHY

1. Kurjak A, Kupesic S. Color Doppler and 3D ultrasound in Gynecology, Infertility and Obstetrics. London, New York: Parthenon Publishing 2000.
2. Kupesic S, Aksamija A. Acute pelvic pain. In: Kurjak A, Chervenak F (Eds). Donald School Textbook of Ultrasound in Obstetrics and Gynecology. New Delhi: Jaypee Brothers Medical Publishers 2003;747-63.
3. Kupesic S, Plavsic BM. Sonographic Evaluation of Gynecologic and Obstetric Causes of Acute Pelvic Pain. Donald School Textbook of Ultrasound in Obstetrics and Gynecology. In: Kurjak A, Chervenak F. New Delhi: Jaypee Brothers Medical Publishers 2008;939-50.
4. Lippincot Williams & Wilkins Emergency Medicine Book Collection, Ovid Internet (regularly updated).
5. Mattu A, Goyal D. Emergency Medicine. London-New York: Blackwell Publishing 2007.
6. Swartz MH. Textbook of Physical Diagnosis, 5th Edition. New York: Saunders 2006.

19.10: ABNORMAL PAP SMEAR AND CERVICAL MASS

Text and images by: S Kupesic Plavsic
Medical illustrations by: Bhargavi Patham and Sandesh Subramanya

Data from the literature indicate that carcinoma of the cervix is a preventable disease. Therefore, any female patient who visits a physician should have current screening guidelines applied and, if appropriate, a Pap smear performed. A Pap smear is done in conjunction with a pelvic examination. It has been suggested that the first Pap smear should be performed about three years after the first coitus or at age 21, whichever comes first. Annual Pap tests are recommended for patients between 21 and 29 years and every two to three years, if patient over 30 has had three negative tests in a row. If patient has certain risk factors, such as previous diagnosis of cervical cancer or a Pap smear that showed precancerous cells, HIV infection, weakened immune system (due to chemotherapy, chronic use of corticosteroids or organ transplantation), Pap test should be performed on annual basis. Patients after total hysterectomy following noncancerous condition and older age patients (>70 years with three negative tests during the last 10 years) may decide not to continue Pap testing (Flow chart 19.10.1).

Clinical Clues

Ask about:

– Menstrual cycle
– Symptoms of sexually transmitted disease, such as vaginal discharge
– Unprotected sex
– Multiple partners
– Age of first sexual intercourse
– Use of alcohol and illegal drugs
– Use of birth control pills as a sole form of contraception
– Previous Pap tests results
– Previous sexually transmitted disease

Look for:

– Vaginal discharge
– Painful intercourse
– Pain or discomfort in the lower abdomen and/or pelvis
– Swelling, blisters, open sores, rush or warts

Investigations

- Pelvic examination
- Pap smear
- Colposcopy
- Colposcopy directed biopsy
- Pelvic ultrasound
- CT of the abdomen and pelvis

Ultrasound Findings

- Describe sonographic characteristics of the cervix:
  – Dimension
  – Contours (regular/irregular)
  – Presence of sonolucent areas (typical for nabothian cysts)
  – Echogenicity (mixed echogenicity/hyperechogenic)
  – Presence of a solid or complex cervical mass
  – Distended uterine cavity (hematometra), suggestive of cervical obstruction

Flow chart 19.10.1: Inductive reasoning scheme for diagnostic evaluation of patients undergoing Pap smear screening (*Courtesy:* Paul L. Foster School of Medicine, Texas Tech University at El Paso, TX, USA). Although ultrasound is not an initial method for evaluation of the cervical lesions, transvaginal sonography with color and pulsed Doppler may be used for evaluation of patients with cervical mass.

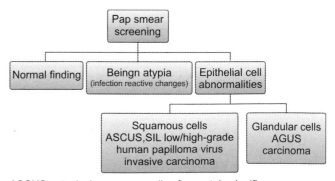

ASCUS= atypical squamous cells of uncertain significance
AGUS= atypical glandular cells of uncertain significance
SIL= squamous intraepithelial lesion

- Apply color and/or power Doppler ultrasound to assess cervical vasculature: vessels architecture (linear/chaotic), penetrating pattern (penetrating/nonpenetrating pattern) and branching pattern (simple/complex)
- Perform pulsed Doppler analysis of the cervical lesion to quantitatively analyze blood flow parameters (resistance index, pulsatility index): low vascular impedance blood flow signals suggest cervical malignancy
- Assess uterine artery blood flow (decreased vascular impedance in patients with cervical neoplasia)
- Assess lower uterine segment and parametria
- Evaluate pelvic lymph nodes
- Apply transrectal ultrasound, if indicated.

Diagnoses to Consider

- Normal finding
- Benign atypia (infection or reactive changes)
- Epithelial cells abnormalities:
  1. Atypical squamous cells of undetermined significance (ASCUS): Squamous cells are slightly abnormal but the changes do not suggest precancerous changes (recommendation: reanalyze the sample and check for the presence of human papilloma virus (HPV)).
  2. Squamous intraepithelial lesion (SIL): The cells collected from the Pap smear may be precancerous.
     - Low-grade SIL: Minimal changes of the size, shape and number of the cells that form the surface of the cervix (most of these lesions return to normal without treatment)
     - High-grade SIL: Cells in this category look very different from normal cells and are less likely to return to normal without treatment.
  3. Atypical glandular cells of undetermined significance (AGUS): Glandular cells are slightly abnormal, but the changes do not suggest precancerous changes (recommendation: reanalyze the sample and check for the presence of HPV).
  4. Carcinoma *in situ*: The cancer cells are confined to the surface of the cervix.
  5. Invasive cervical cancer: Look for local spread to the upper vagina, low uterine segment, and into the surrounding tissue (the parametria). Cervical cancer may grow toward the pelvic sidewall and may obstruct the ureters, and spread to the bladder and rectum. Cervical carcinoma invades the lymphatic system and spread to the lymph nodes around the vessels on the pelvic wall, iliac and aortic lymph nodes.

Some case studies related to abnormal pap smear and cervical mass are depicted in Figures 19.10.1 to 19.10.20.

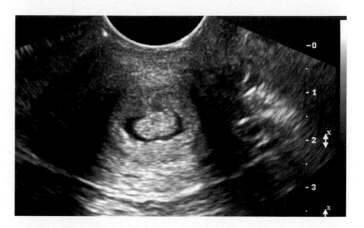

FIGURE 19.10.1: Transvaginal ultrasound of a polypous cervical mass. Note dilated cervical canal and sonolucent fluid surrounding the cervical lesion.

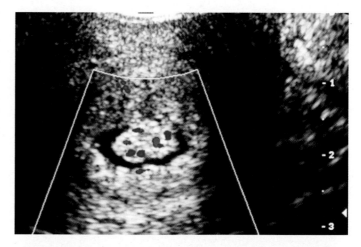

FIGURE 19.10.2: Color Doppler image of the polypous cervical mass.

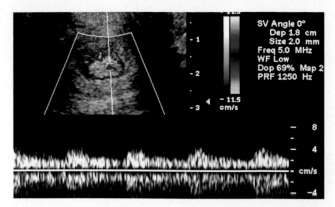

FIGURE 19.10.3: Pulsed Doppler waveform analysis demonstrates moderate vascular impedance blood flow signals with RI of 0.50. Sonographic and Doppler findings are typical for cervical polyp, which was confirmed by histology.

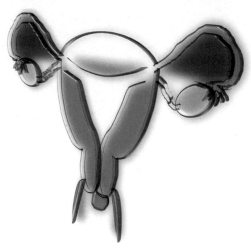

FIGURE 19.10.4: Cervical polyp is a benign lesion on the surface of the cervical canal. The most common presenting symptom is intermenstrual and/or postcoital bleeding. Often, cervical polyps show no symptoms. Treatment consists of a removal of the polyp. Because about 1% of cervical polyps show neoplastic changes histology should always be performed.

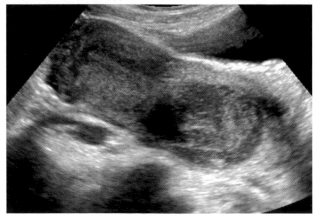

FIGURE 19.10.5: Longitudinal transvaginal scan demonstrating a solid heterogeneous cervical mass.

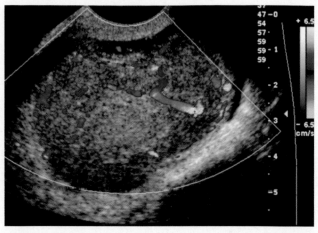

FIGURE 19.10.6: Color Doppler scan of a solid tumor in the posterior aspect of the cervix. Note randomly dispersed irregular vessels, suggestive of cervical carcinoma.

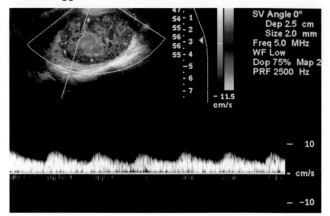

FIGURE 19.10.7: The same patient as in Figures 19.10.5 and 19.10.6. Pulsed Doppler waveform analysis demonstrates low to moderate vascular impedance blood flow signals obtained from the intratumoral vessels.

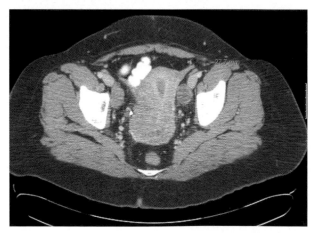

FIGURE 19.10.8: Computed tomography scan of a large, lobulated cervical mass showing nonuniform hypoattenuation. The central hypoattenuation in the uterine corpus is suggestive of minimal fluid in the cavity. Cervical cancer was confirmed by histology.

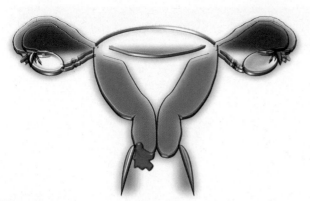

FIGURE 19.10.9: Cancer of the cervix typically originates from a dysplastic or premalignant lesion previously present at the active squamocolumnar junction. Carcinoma *in situ* precedes invasive cervical cancer. Progression to invasive carcinoma is considered irreversible once the malignant process extends through the basement membrane and invasion of the cervical stroma occurs.

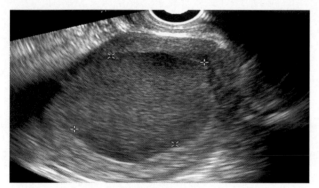

FIGURE 19.10.10: Transvaginal ultrasound of a distended uterine cavity filled with echogenic fluid in a patient presenting with pelvic midline pain. Sonographic finding is typical for muco-hematometra.

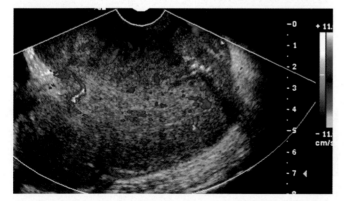

FIGURE 19.10.11: The same patient. Enlarged cervix with randomly dispersed vessels. Chaotic branching and irregular course of the vessels are suggestive of cervical carcinoma.

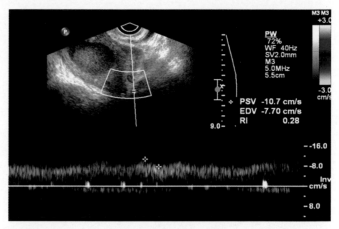

FIGURE 19.10.12: Pulsed Doppler ultrasound finding of the same patient. Note distended uterine cavity on the left. Low vascular impedance blood flow signals are obtained from the left parametrium, indicating cervical carcinoma invasion.

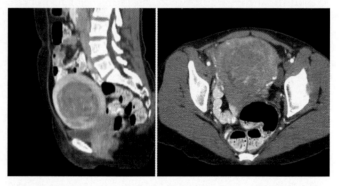

FIGURE 19.10.13: Computed tomography scan of a patient with cervical carcinoma. The uterine cavity is distended and filled with heterogeneous material and blood. CT finding indicates muco-hematometra caused by distal (cervical) obstruction.

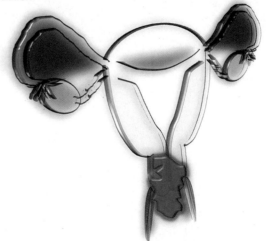

FIGURE 19.10.14: The exophytic type of cervical cancer arises from the exocervix and is often polypoid. On pelvic exam it is visualized as a large, friable, bulky mass, which has the tendency for excessive bleeding. On ultrasound cervical cancer is visualized as a solid or complex cervical mass.

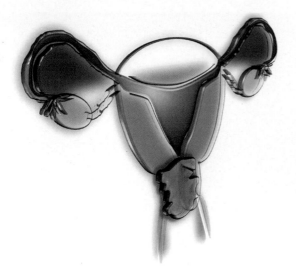

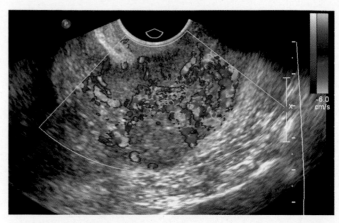

FIGURE 19.10.17: Color Doppler ultrasound of the same patient. Note numerous randomly dispersed vessels with chaotic branching, suggestive of a malignant cervical mass.

FIGURE 19.10.15: Large cervical masses may circumferentially involve the entire endocervical region. Infiltrative exocervical lesions tend to invade the vaginal fornices and the upper part of the vagina. Infiltrative endocervical lesions tend to extend into the corpus and the lateral parametria. They may also lead to distal obstruction and cause distension of the uterine cavity (muco- and/or hematometra).

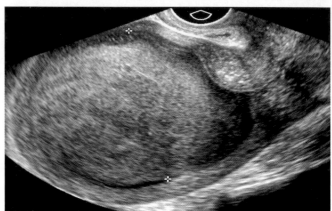

FIGURE 19.10.18: The same patient. Sagittal transvaginal ultrasound demonstrates distended uterine cavity filled with mobile low level echoes. Closed cervix is visualized on the right side of the image.

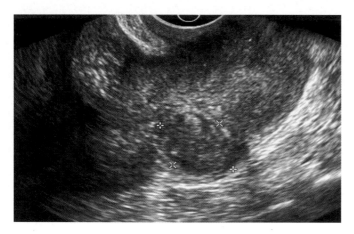

FIGURE 19.10.16: Transvaginal scan of the cervix in a 47 years old patient who presented to the emergency department with severe suprapubic pain. Ultrasound revealed a solid cervical mass measuring 2 × 2.2 cm.

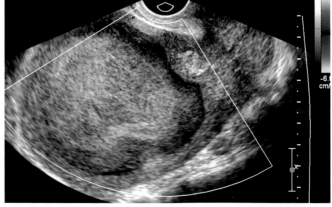

FIGURE 19.10.19: Color Doppler ultrasound demonstrates prominent vascularity of the uterine isthmus, indicating spread of the cervical carcinoma into direction of the uterine corpus.

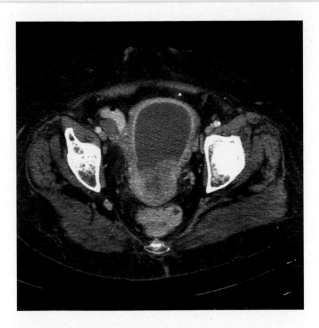

FIGURE 19.10.20: Computerized tomography scan of a cervical mass and distended uterine cavity. Sonographic finding indicates hematometra secondary to cervical cancer.

BIBLIOGRAPHY

1. Beckmann RBC, Ling FW, Smith RP, et al. Obstetrics and Gynecology, 5th Edition. Philadelphia: Lippincott Williams and Wilkins 2002;432-47.
2. Beck WW. Obstetrics and Gynecology. 4th Edition. Baltimore: Williams and Wilkins 1997;409-10.
3. Kurjak A, Kupesic S. Color Doppler evaluation of the uterine cervix. In: Kurjak A, Kupesic S (Eds). An Atlas of transvaginal color Doppler. London-New York: Parthenon Publishing 2000; 187.

19.11: UTERINE MASS

Text and images by: S Kupesic Plavsic
Medical illustrations by: Bhargavi Patham and Sandesh Subramanya

There are many causes of uterine enlargement and most of them are benign. Uterine masses may cause annoying symptoms, such as heavy and prolonged menstrual bleeding, anemia, abdominal pain and urinary problems (Flow chart 19.11.1).

Clinical Clues

- **Ask about:**
  - Heavy periods
  - Vaginal spotting
  - Breakthrough bleeding
  - Bleeding during intercourse
  - Abdominal pressure
  - Bloating
  - Abdominal pain
  - Dull ache in the lower back and thighs
  - Problems passing urine completely
  - Problems with defecation.

Flow chart 19.11.1: Inductive reasoning scheme for diagnostic evaluation of the patients presenting with pelvic (uterine and adnexal) mass (*Courtesy:* Paul L. Foster School of Medicine, Texas Tech University at El Paso, TX, USA).

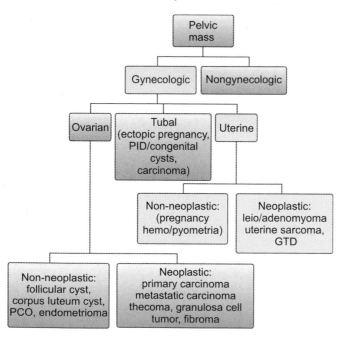

- **Look for:**
  - Enlarged uterus, breast changes, softening and enlargement of the cervix (suggestive of pregnancy)
  - Heavy menstrual bleeding, usually in clots, pain in the pelvis, pain during sexual intercourse, frequent urge to urinate, constipation and lower backache (suggestive of uterine fibroids)
  - Menstrual cramps, heavy bleeding during periods, passage of blood clots during menstruation (suggestive of adenomyosis)
  - Vaginal bleeding after menopause (suggestive of endometrial pathology)
  - Abdominal tenderness/mass, adnexal tenderness/mass and cervical motion tenderness (suggestive of PID).

Investigations

- Pelvic examination
- Pregnancy test (if indicated)
- Pelvic ultrasound
- Endometrial biopsy in patients with abnormal endometrial thickening.

Ultrasound Findings

- Enlarged uterus (look for uterine fibroids and adenomyosis)
- Heterogeneous myometrium (look for uterine fibroids and adenomyosis)
  - Assess the myometrial mass
    - Each mass should be measured in 2 to 3 diameters
    - Specify the uterine mass echogenicity
    - Define the uterine mass location (submucosal/intramural/subserosal)
    - Define the uterine mass borders (well-defined/ill-defined)
    - Assess the uterine mass location
  - Identify cysts (specify the dimension and location of the cyst(s): inner, medical or deep myometrial layer, suggestive of adenomyosis
    - Each cyst should be measured in 2 to 3 diameters
    - Define the location of the cyst (inner, medial or deep myometrial layer)

- Assess the endometrium
  - Thickness (double layer in long-axis)
  - Echogenicity (triple layer, hyperechogenic)
  - Look for focal abnormalities (suggestive of endometrial polyp)
  - Presence of intracavitary fluid (suggestive of uterine bleeding and/or distal obstruction)
  - If endometrium cannot be clearly delineated or is poorly defined, the sonographer should report that endometrium is ill-defined.
  - In patients with unclear endometrial findings saline infusion sonography should be performed.

Diagnoses to Consider

- Leiomyoma
- Adenomyosis
- Uterine sarcoma
- Endometrial hyperplasia
- Endometrial polyp
- Endometrial carcinoma
- Hematometra.

Some case studies related to uterine mass are depicted in Figures 19.11.1 to 19.11.28.

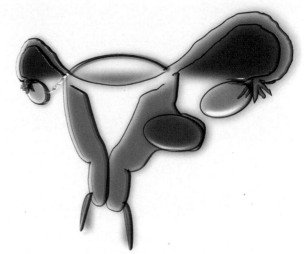

FIGURE 19.11.2: Homogeneous or heterogeneous (in case of degenerating fibroids) well-defined mass originating beneath the uterine serosa. Due to its location it may be misdiagnosed as ovarian neoplasm.

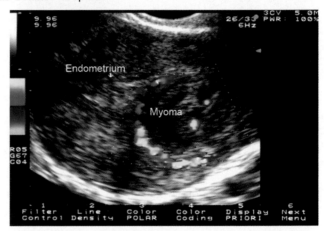

FIGURE 19.11.3: Color Doppler ultrasound of an intramural fibroid. Note color coded signals within the capsule of the uterine fibroid.

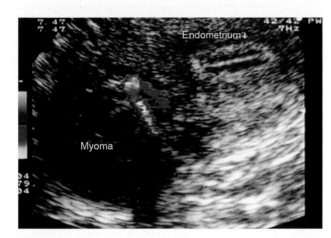

FIGURE 19.11.1: Transvaginal color Doppler scan of a subserosal, intraligamentary fibroid. Color Doppler reveals peripheral vessels or vessels within the stalk of a pedunculated fibroid.

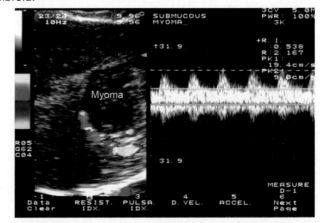

FIGURE 19.11.4: Pulsed Doppler waveform analysis obtained from the fibroid vessels demonstrates moderate vascular impedance (RI of 0.54).

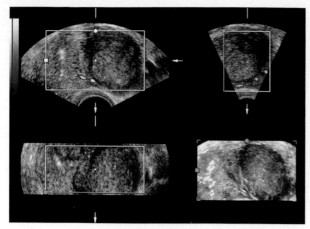

FIGURE 19.11.5: 3D power Doppler ultrasound of the uterine fibroid vessels.

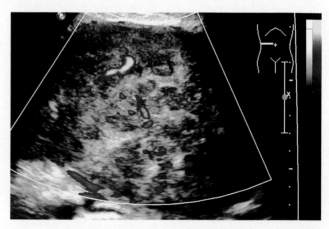

FIGURE 19.11.8: Power Doppler ultrasound of the degenerative fibroid vasculature. Prominent color/power signals are visualized within the central portion of the fibroid.

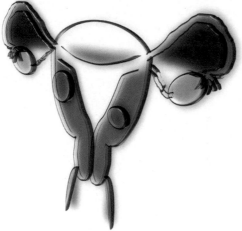

FIGURE 19.11.6: Intramural fibroid is a round, well-defined myometrial mass. It is the most common gynecologic tumor in women of reproductive age. Majority of intramural fibroids are asymptomatic. Abnormal uterine bleeding is the most common presenting symptom. Malignant transformation is extremely rare (0.1 to 0.3%).

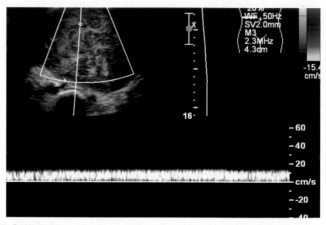

FIGURE 19.11.9: Pulsed Doppler ultrasound of a patient with degenerative fibroid. Note venous type of the blood flow signals obtained from the central portion of a degenerative fibroid.

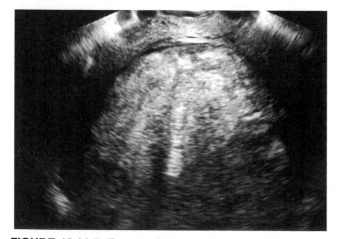

FIGURE 19.11.7: Transvaginal sonogram of a degenerative fibroid.

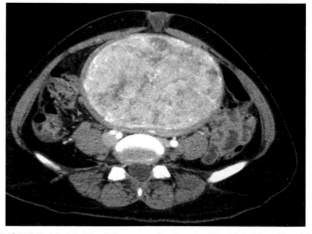

FIGURE 19.11.10: CT scan of a large degenerative fibroid.

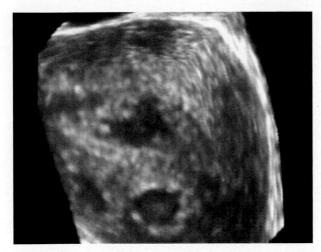

FIGURE 19.11.11: "Swiss cheese" appearance of the myometrium on three-dimensional ultrasound is typical of deep adenomyosis. Cystic lesions are visualized within the subserosal layer of the uterus.

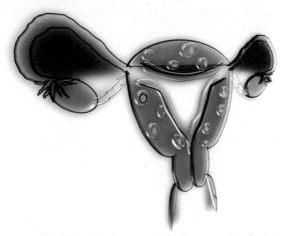

FIGURE 19.11.12: Adenomyosis represents heterotopic endometrial glands and stroma within the myometrial portion of the uterus. Transvaginal sonography demonstrates diffuse uterine enlargement and presence of the myometrial cysts and/or myometrial striations.

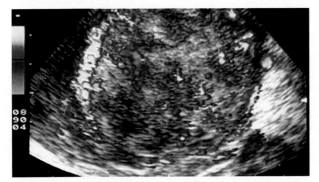

FIGURE 19.11.13: Fast growing uterine tumor in a postmenopausal patient shows highly vascularized areas. Randomly dispersed vessels with irregular course are suggestive of uterine malignancy.

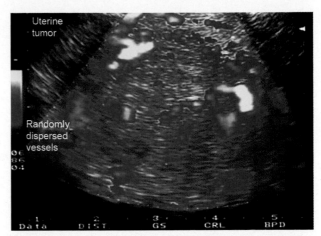

FIGURE 19.11.14: Power Doppler ultrasound facilitates detection of numerous, small, randomly dispersed vessels, typical of uterine malignancy.

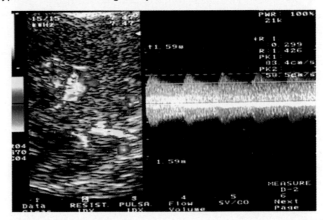

FIGURE 19.11.15: Pulsed Doppler waveform analysis demonstrates prominent flow with small systolic-to-diastolic variation and low vascular resistance (RI = 0.42), indicative of uterine malignancy. Uterine sarcoma was confirmed by histology.

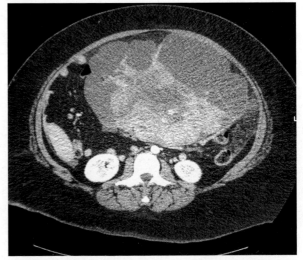

FIGURE 19.11.16: CT of a heterogeneous uterine mass. Histology revealed uterine leiomyosarcoma.

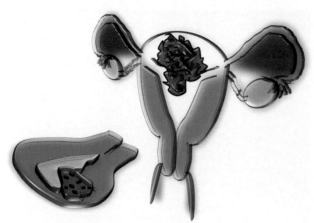

FIGURE 19.11.17: Leiomyosarcoma is visualized as a solitary, heterogeneous, poorly demarcated uterine mass with areas of hemorrhage and necrosis. By morphology, leiomyosarcoma may be indistinguishable from the uterine leiomyoma, but its rapid increase in size, poor demarcation and increased vascularity are suggestive of leiomyosarcoma.

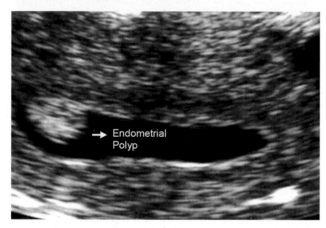

FIGURE 19.11.18: Saline infusion sonography (hysterosonography) outlines focal endometrial thickening. Finding is typical of an endometrial polyp.

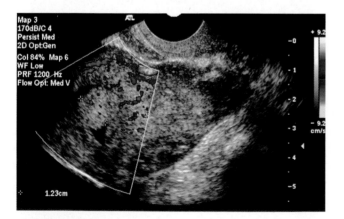

FIGURE 19.11.19: Focal endometrial thickening demonstrated by color Doppler ultrasound.

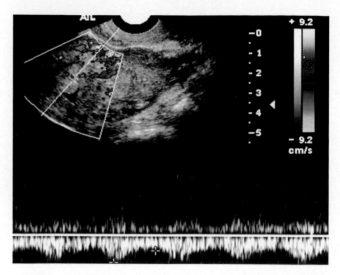

FIGURE 19.11.20: Pulsed Doppler waveform analysis demonstrates low-to-moderate vascular impedance blood flow signals (RI = 0.46) isolated from an endometrial polyp. Secondary degenerative changes were diagnosed by histology.

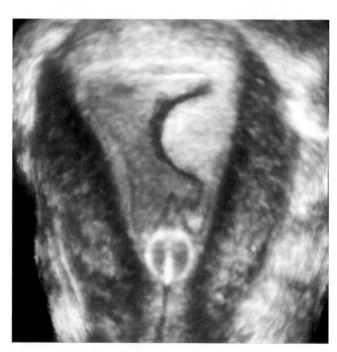

FIGURE 19.11.21: Saline infusion sonography (hysterosonography) by three-dimensional ultrasound. Focal endometrial lesion is clearly visualized on the right. Catheter with balloon is demonstrated within the isthmic portion of the uterus.

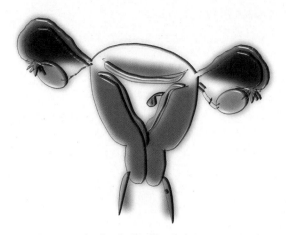

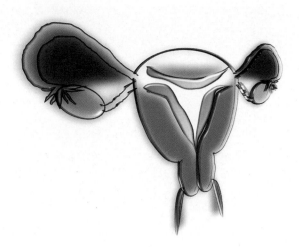

FIGURE 19.11.22: Endometrial polyps are visualized as intraluminal pedunculated endometrial lesions. Color Doppler usually demonstrates blood vessels within the stalk. Most common clinical presentation of the patients with endometrial polyps is postmenopausal bleeding, intermenstrual bleeding, menorrhagia or menometrorrhagia.

FIGURE 19.11.25: Endometrial hyperplasia is excessive proliferation of endometrial glands with an increased ratio of glands to stroma. Ultrasound reveals diffusely thickened hyperechoic endometrium. Color Doppler depicts moderate vascular impedance blood flow signals from the feeding vessels at the periphery of the endometrium. Most common presenting symptom is irregular uterine bleeding, postmenopausal bleeding, menorrhagia or menometrorrhagia.

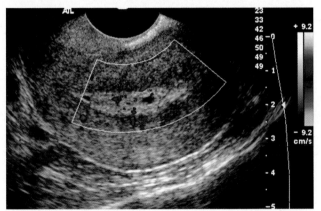

FIGURE 19.11.23: Transvaginal color Doppler scan of a 60-year-old patient with endometrial hyperplasia presenting with postmenopausal bleeding. Note increased vascularity at the periphery of the endometrium.

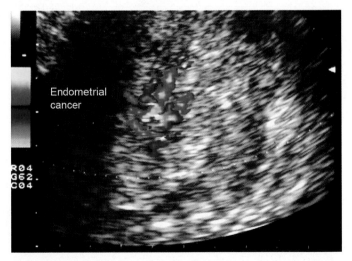

Endometrial cancer

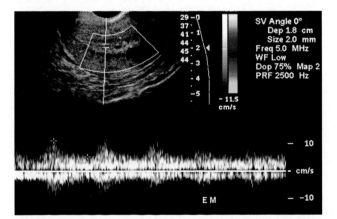

FIGURE 19.11.24: . Pulsed Doppler analysis reveals moderate vascular impedance blood flow signals, typical for endometrial hyperplasia.

FIGURE 19.11.26: Thick heterogeneous endometrium with stelate peripheral and intratumoral neovascularization demonstrated by color Doppler imaging.

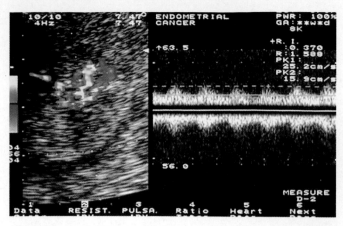

FIGURE 19.11.27: Color Doppler analysis shows low vascular resistance (RI = 0.37) blood flow signals obtained from the area of neovascularization. Endometrial malignancy was confirmed by histology.

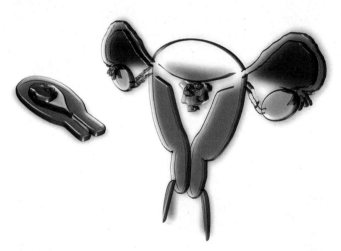

FIGURE 19.11.28: Endometrial carcinoma is visualized as a polypous or diffuse thickening of the endometrium. Disruption of the endometrial-subendometrial halo suggests myometrial invasion. Ultrasound is not considered the method of choice for evaluation of the endometrial carcinoma invasion towards the cervix, parametria and lymph nodes. The most common presenting symptom of endometrial carcinoma is abnormal uterine bleeding (in majority of the patients, postmenopausal bleeding). For more details please refer to clinical presentation on postmenopausal bleeding.

BIBLIOGRAPHY

1. Kupesic S, Kurjak A, Bjelos D. Color Doppler and Three-Dimensional Ultrasound of the Uterine Lesions. In: Kupesic S (Ed). Color Doppler and three-dimensional ultrasound in gynecology, infertility and obstetrics. New Delhi:Jaypee Brothers Medical Publishers 2003;29-43.
2. Kupesic S, Kurjak A, Bjelos D. The assessment of uterine lesions. In: Kurjak A, Kupesic S (Eds). Clinical application of 3D sonography. London-New York: Parthenon Publishing 2000;55.
3. Kupesic S, Kurjak A, Zodan T. Staging of endometrial carcinoma by 3-D power Doppler. Gynaecol Perinatol 1998; 8:1-5.
4. Kupesic S, Kurjak A. Color Doppler assessment of uterine leiomyoma and sarcoma. In: Kurjak A, Kupesic S (Eds). An Atlas of transvaginal color Doppler. London-New York: Parthenon Publishing 2000;179.
5. Kupesic S, Plavsic BM. Sonography of uterine leiomyomata. U: I. Brosens (ur): Uterine fibroids: Pathogenesis and management. London, New York: Taylor & Francis 2006;139-151.
6. Kupesic-Urek S, Shalan H, Kurjak A. Early detection of endometrial cancer by transvaginal color Doppler. Eur J Obstet Gynecol Reprod Biol 1993;49(1-2):46-9.
7. Kurjak A, Kupesic S, Shalan H, et al. Uterine sarcoma: A report of 10 cases studied by transvaginal color and pulsed Doppler sonography. Gynecol Oncol 1995;59(3):342-6.
8. Kurjak A, Kupesic S. Three-dimensional power Doppler ultrasound examination of uterine lesions. In: Kurjak A (Ed). Three-dimensional power Doppler in obstetrics and gynecology. New York-London: Parthenon Publishing 1999;39-53.
9. Kurjak A, Kupesic S. Transvaginal color Doppler and pulsed Doppler diagnosis of benign changes in the uterine myometrium. In: Schmidt W, Kurjak A. (Eds). Color oppler sonography in Gynecology and Obstetrics. Stuttgart, New York: Thieme Verlag 2005;274-8.
10. Kurjak A, Kupesic-Urek S, Miric D. The benign uterine tumor vascularization assessed by transvaginal color Doppler. J Ultrasound Med Biol 1992;18:645-9.
11. Kurjak A, Shalan H, Sosic A, et al. Endometrial carcinoma in postmenopausal women: evaluation by transvaginal color Doppler ultrasound. Am J Obstet Gynecol 1993;169(6):1597-603.

SECTION 19.12: ADNEXAL MASS

Text and images by: S Kupesic Plavsic
Medical illustrations by: Bhargavi Patham and Sandesh Subramanya

Adnexal masses may occur in any age group and on ultrasound may be cystic, complex or solid. Possible etiologies differ among the age groups and there is a need to diagnose them at an early stage because early detection may significantly affect the clinical outcome (Flow chart 19.12.1).

Clinical Clues

Ask about:

– Menstrual history
– Fertility
– Medical history (e.g. use of ovulation induction)
– Obstetrical history
– Symptoms:
  - Pain: Unless bleeding or torsion occurs, adnexal lesions are usually asymptomatic

Flow chart 19.12.1: Inductive reasoning scheme for diagnostic evaluation of patients presenting with pelvic mass (*Courtesy:* Paul L. Foster School of Medicine, Texas Tech University at El Paso, TX, USA).

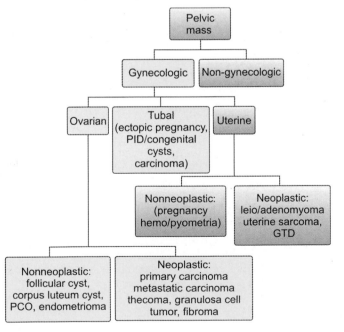

- Bloating
- Tenesmus
- Deep dyspareunia (suggestive of endometriosis)
- Delayed menstrual period followed by spotting, unilateral pelvic pain, suggestive of a follicular or luteal cyst.
– Associated symptoms, such as amenorrhea, hirsutism, obesity, (± acanthosis nigricans), suggestive of PCOS.
– Family history of ovarian cancer, bloating, urinary urgency, abdominal/pelvic pain, increased abdominal size, vaginal bleeding, change in bowel habit, suggestive of an ovarian neoplasm.

Look for:

– Pelvic examination findings:
  - Tender adnexal masses and irregular menstrual cycle are suggestive of follicular or luteal cysts.
  - Pelvic mass, ascites, pleural effusion, abdominal mass or bowel obstruction, suggestive of ovarian neoplasm.
  - Signs of androgenization (think of Sertoli Leyding cell tumor)
  - Signs of estrogenization and abnormal genital tract bleeding (think of granulosa cell tumor or thecoma).

Investigations

• General physical examination
• Pelvic examination
• Pregnancy test
• Blood tumor markers (e.g. CA-125)
• Diagnostic imaging: Ultrasound, CT, MRI

Ultrasound Findings

• Follicular cysts appear smooth, thin walled and unilocular.
• Corpus luteum cysts have complex appearance. Color Doppler reveals low to moderate vascular impedance blood flow signals, typical for luteal conversion. Patients with corpus luteum cysts have secretory transformed endometrium.

- Hemorrhagic cysts are characterized with numerous thin septations typical of a retracting clot. Color Doppler reveals low vascular impedance blood flow signals, typical for luteal conversion. Free fluid in the cul-de-sac and secretory transformed endometrium are additional findings in patients presenting with hemorrhagic cysts.
- Presence of 10 or more follicles in each ovary measuring 2 to 9 mm in diameter and/or increased ovarian volume (>10–12 mL; calculated using the formula 0.5 × length × width × thickness) is suggestive of polycystic ovaries (PCO).
- Ovarian dermoid is visualized as predominantly cystic structure, complex cystic lesion with internal solid component (mural nodule), cystic mass with multiple linear hyperechogenic echoes, fat, cystic mass with convolute of hair, or predominantly solid mass. Teeth, bone and calcification cause strong echogenicity and posterior shadowing. Color Doppler usually demonstrates regularly separated peripheral vessels and lack of any blood flow within the solid parts (hair, dermoid mesh, etc).
- Ovarian fibroma is visualized as a solid hypoechoic ovarian mass, similar to uterine leiomyoma. Since the mass is separate from the uterus and blood flow characteristics are different from the uterine vessels, the most likely diagnosis is solid ovarian stromal tumor (Brenner tumor, ovarian fibroma, thecoma or fibrothecoma).
- Cystadenomas are visualized as unilocular or multilocular adnexal masses filled with watery (serous cystadenomas) or thick, sticky gelatinous fluid (mucinous cystadenomas). Color Doppler usually demonstrates regularly separated vessels with moderate vascular impedance blood flow signals.
- Sonographic findings of concern include presence of a complex adnexal mass with thick and irregular internal septations, solid elements, internal echoes, papillary protrusions, presence of daughter cysts and free fluid in the cul-de-sac.
- Paraovarian cysts are usually asymptomatic, sonolucent unilateral cysts with thin and regular walls. They are visualized adjacent to the ovary. Depending on their size and location, paraovarian cysts may undergo torsion or may cause pelvic pain (e.g. dyspareunia).
- There are four types of tubal masses: hydrosalpinx, pyosalpynx, hematosalpinx and tubal neoplasm:
  - Hydrosalpinx is visualized as a fluid filled dilated tube with incomplete septations and longitudinal folds (pseudopapillomatous structures).
  - Pyosalpinx is visualized as dilated tube with thickened walls filled with echogenic fluid
  - Hematosalpinx represents blood within the distended tube in patients with tubal ectopic pregnancy.
  - In early stages, tubal neoplasm is visualized as a complex or solid mass within the dilated tube, clearly separated from the ovary. In late stage of the disease, tubal mass cannot be distinguished from the ipsilateral ovary. Color Doppler reveals neovascular signals, characterized with irregular vessels' arrangement, penetrating pattern and low vascular impedance blood flow signals.

Diagnoses to Consider

- Ovarian masses:
  - Ovarian cysts: follicular, luteal and hemorrhagic
  - Polycystic ovarian syndrome (PCOS)
  - Ovarian endometrioma
  - Cystic teratoma
  - Ovarian fibroma
  - Ovarian cystadenoma
  - Ovarian neoplasm
- Tubal masses:
  - Pelvic inflammatory disease (hydrosalpinx)
  - Tubo-ovarian abscess (pyosalpinx)
  - Periovarian/paratubal cysts
  - Ectopic pregnancy (hematosalpinx)
  - Tubal neoplasm.

Some case studies related to adnexal masses are depicted in Figures 19.12.1 to 19.12.61.

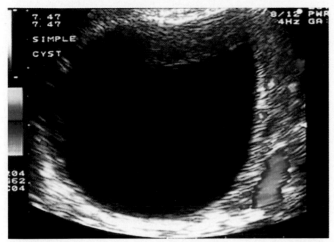

FIGURE 19.12.1: Transvaginal color Doppler scan of a unilocular cyst. Note the thin walls, clear fluid content and pericystic flow.

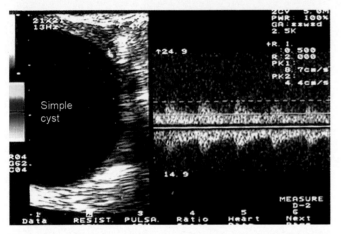

FIGURE 19.12.2: Moderate vascular impedance signals (RI = 0.50) are extracted from the pericystic vessels. Benign histology was obtained following laparoscopic surgery.

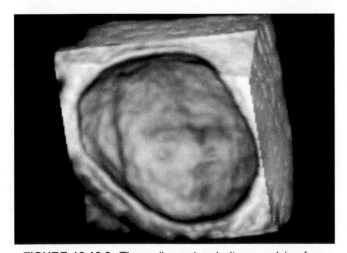

FIGURE 19.12.3: Three-dimensional ultrasound (surface rendering) of a simple ovarian cyst.

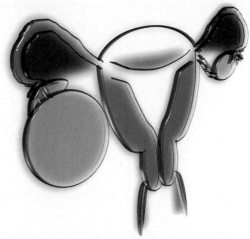

FIGURE 19.12.4: Follicular cyst is a smooth, thin walled, and unilocular cystic structure. Most simple cysts are asymptomatic and majority regress spontaneously in 2-3 months. Treatment is expectative and follow-up ultrasound should be performed in 6 weeks, preferentially during the postmenstruation period.

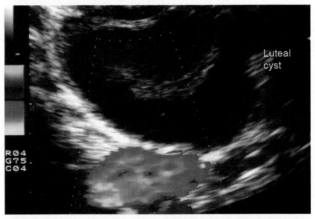

FIGURE 19.12.5: Transvaginal color Doppler scan of a patient with corpus luteum cyst. Note avascular retracting clot and thick walls of the cyst.

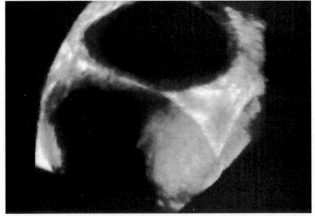

FIGURE 19.12.6: The same patient. Three-dimensional ultrasound (surface rendering) of the corpus luteum cyst. Retracting clot is visualized on the right.

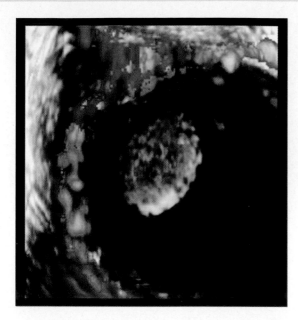

FIGURE 19.12.7: Power Doppler scan of a corpus luteum cyst. Note significant vascularity at the periphery of the cyst and absence of any color signals within the solid portion of the lesion.

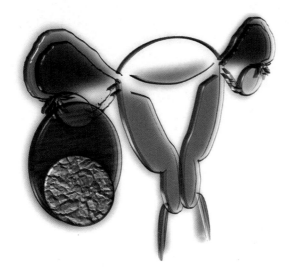

FIGURE 19.12.8: Corpus luteum cyst is visualized as a thick walled cyst with retracted clot. In some patients fluid level is observed, while in other patients spider-web-like content dominates. Most of the patients are asymptomatic, while other may be presenting with pain and/or adnexal mass. Treatment is expectative and follow-up ultrasound should be performed in 6 weeks, preferentially during the postmenstruation period.

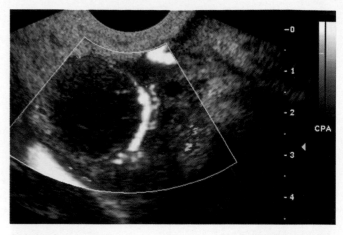

FIGURE 19.12.9: Power Doppler image of a hemorrhagic cyst. Note echogenic fluid and regularly separated vessels at the periphery, forming a "ring of fire".

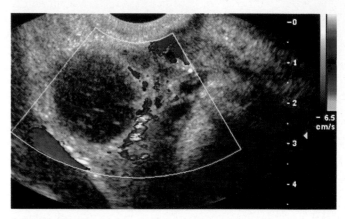

FIGURE 19.12.10: Color Doppler image of the same patient. Note echogenic fluid, web like content and peripheral vascularization. Careful observation of the posterior cul-de-sac reveals free fluid.

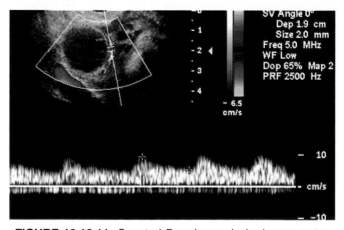

FIGURE 19.12.11: Spectral Doppler analysis demonstrates low vascular impedance blood flow signals.

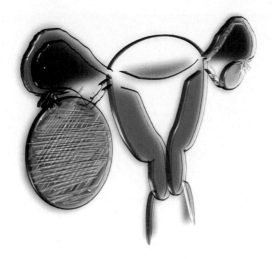

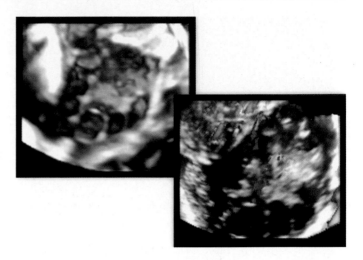

FIGURE 19.12.12: Hemorrhagic cysts are characterized with numerous thin septations typical of a retracting clot. Color Doppler reveals low vascular impedance blood flow signals at the periphery of the cystic lesion, typical for luteal conversion. Free fluid in the cul-de-sac and secretory transformed endometrium are additional findings in patients presenting with hemorrhagic cysts. Treatment is expectative and follow-up ultrasound should be performed in 6 weeks, preferentially during the postmenstruation period. Laparoscopy may be required for patients presenting with pain, significant intraabdominal bleeding and hemoperitoneum, which is an uncommon presentation.

FIGURE 19.12.14: Three dimensional ultrasound enables more precise volume assessment. Three dimensional power Doppler ultrasound demonstrates increased stromal vascularity.

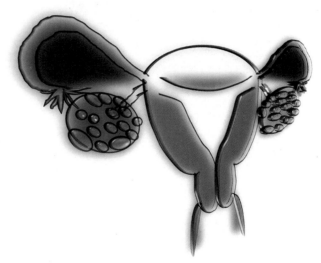

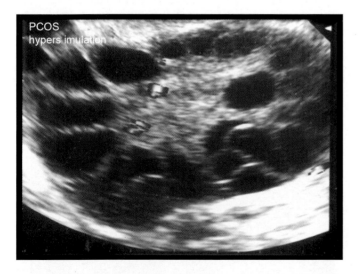

FIGURE 19.12.13: Polycystic ovaries are characterized by increased ovarian volume (>10 - 12 ml; calculated using the formula 0.5 x length x width x thickness) and presence of 10 or more follicles in each ovary measuring from 2 to 9 mm in diameter.

FIGURE 19.12.15: Patients with PCOS usually present with infertility, amenorrhea, or irregular menstrual cycles. Polycystic ovaries are commonly associated with obesity and insulin resistance. Sonographic criteria for polycystic ovaries are the following: bilaterally enlarged ovaries, multiple (>10) small follicles measuring from 2 to 9 mm and increased stromal echogenicity and vascularity. Sonographers should be aware that polycystic ovaries require hormonal assessment. The initial screening tests include determinations of the blood serum levels of TSH, FSH, LH and prolactin (PRL). In some patients, testosterone and dihydroepiandrosterone sulfate (DHEAS) levels and progesterone challenge tests are performed.

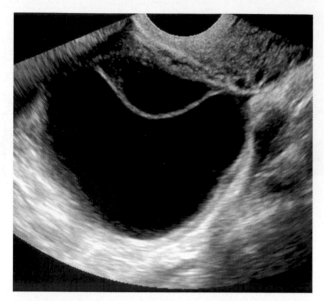

FIGURE 19.12.16: Transvaginal sonogram of a bilocular ovarian cyst.

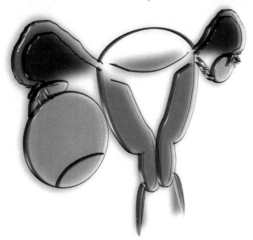

FIGURE 19.12.17: In every patient presenting with adnexal mass, sonographer should look for intracystic septations. Here is an example of a bilocular cystic structure.

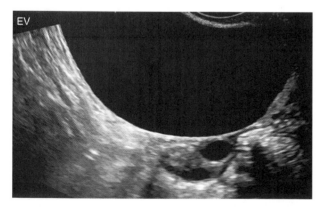

FIGURE 19.12.18: Transvaginal sonogram of a paraovarian cyst. Note normal morphology of the ipsilateral ovary.

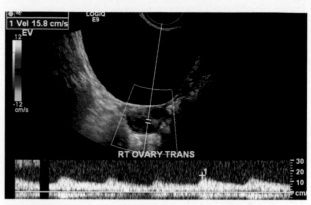

FIGURE 19.12.19: Transvaginal color Doppler image of the same patient. Moderate vascular impedance blood flow signals are obtained from the intraovarian vessels.

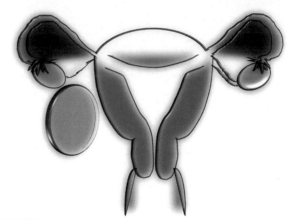

FIGURE 19.12.20: Paraovarian cyst is a sonolucent cystic mass with thin walls, near the ipsilateral round ligament, ovary and the uterus. Demonstration of a normal ipsilateral ovary close to, but separated from the cyst is an important ultrasound finding for the diagnosis of a paraovarian cyst. In patients presenting with pelvic pain color Doppler may be efficiently used to rule out adnexal torsion.

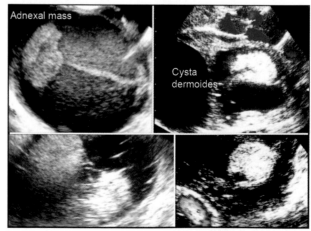

FIGURE 19.12.21: Transvaginal ultrasound of a dermoid cyst is characterized by the presence of a dermoid plug and visualization of the calcified elements with posterior shadowing. "Dermoid mesh" represents hyperechoic lines caused by hair.

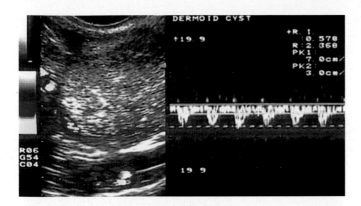

FIGURE 19.12.22: Transvaginal color Doppler scan of a dermoid cyst. Note echogenic nodule protruding into the cystic cavity. Color Doppler demonstrates regularly separated vessels with moderate to high vascular impedance (RI = 0.57).

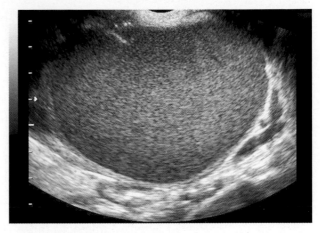

FIGURE 19.12.24: Transvaginal scan of an ovarian endometrioma. Note uniform low level echoes, typical of ovarian endometrioma.

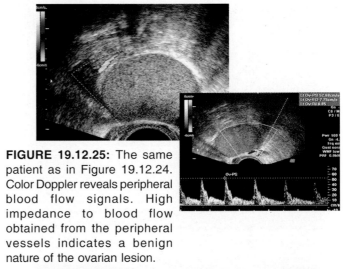

FIGURE 19.12.25: The same patient as in Figure 19.12.24. Color Doppler reveals peripheral blood flow signals. High impedance to blood flow obtained from the peripheral vessels indicates a benign nature of the ovarian lesion.

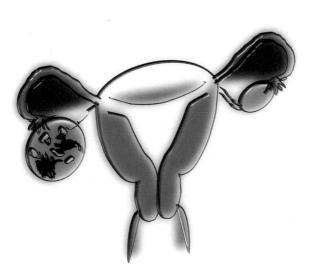

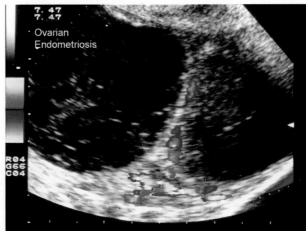

FIGURE 19.12.23: Dermoid cyst is visualized as a complex adnexal mass. Ultrasound appearance depends on the size of a dermoid plug, presence of hair and calcified elements and fatty component. The sonographer should look for multiple thin echogenic lines caused by the presence of hair in the cystic cavity ("dermoid mash") and/or presence of the echogenic nodule (dermoid plug or Rockitansky nodule). Shadowing caused by calcified structures, such as bone and teeth is another common feature of the dermoid cysts. Dermoid cysts are usually asymptomatic, and may be incidentally diagnosed. However, some patients may be presenting with acute pelvic pain due to adnexal torsion. Dermoids involved in torsion are larger and lack intracystic blood flow signals.

FIGURE 19.12.26: Color Doppler ultrasound of an ovarian endometrioma with multilocular appearance. Color Doppler depicts hilar vascularity, another typical feature of ovarian endometriosis.

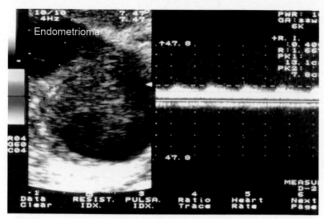

FIGURE 19.12.27: Pulsed Doppler waveform analysis demonstrates low vascular impedance blood flow signals, obtained during the early proliferative phase of the menstrual cycle.

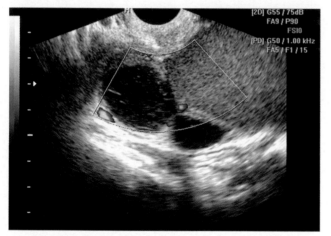

FIGURE 19.12.28: In majority of the patients, preserved ovarian tissue is visualized adjacent to the ovarian endometrioma.

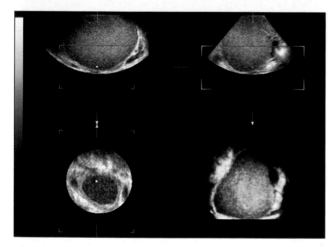

FIGURE 19.12.29: Multiplanar view and surface rendering of the ovarian endometrioma enable meticulous evaluation of the cystic walls and internal echoes.

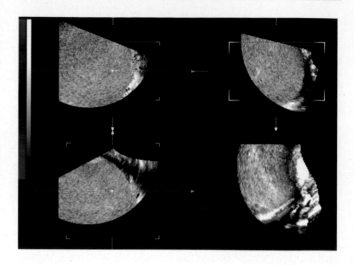

FIGURE 19.12.30: 3D color and power Doppler analysis demonstrates regular course of the peripheral vessels and absence of the penetrating vessels. Both vascular features are reassuring of a benign nature of the ovarian lesion.

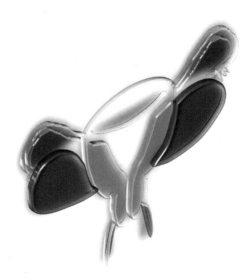

FIGURE 19.12.31: Ovarian endometriotic cysts (endometrioma) are usually bilateral, retrouterine, attached to the pelvic sidewall, uterosacral ligament or cul-de-sac. They are filled with homogeneous paste like fluid and may be associated with chronic pelvic pain, dyspareunia and infertility.

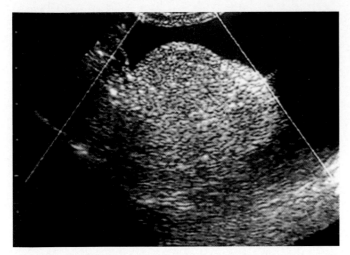

FIGURE 19.12.32: Transvaginal color Doppler scan demonstrates a case of avascular, solid ovarian tumor associated with ascites (Meig's syndrome). Brenner tumor was diagnosed by histology.

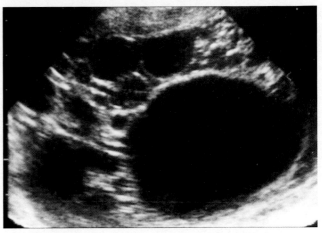

FIGURE 19.12.34: Transvaginal ultrasound scan of a multiloculated cystic mass. Hystology confirmed cystadenoma.

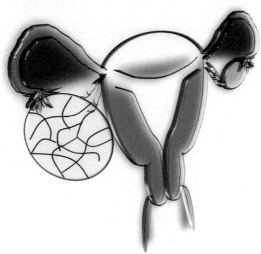

FIGURE 19.12.35: Mucinous cystadenoma is typically a multiloculated cystic mass. Loculations may show different echogenicity. Most common clinical presentation is palpable mass on pelvic exam. However, some patients may be presenting with pelvic pain and/or increased abdominal girtlh.

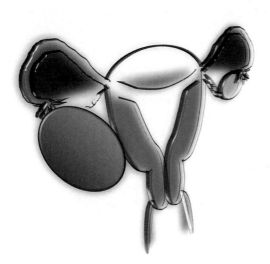

FIGURE 19.12.33: Most common solid adnexal masses are fibroma, thecoma, fibrothecoma, Brenner tumor and pedunculated uterine leiomyoma. Color Doppler may show a wide range of vascular impedance, depending on vascularity. In patients with thecoma, sonographer should report on the endometrial thickness (due to estrogen secretion). Some patients with thecoma may present with hirsuitism and amenorrhea (due to androgen secretion). Majority of the patients are asymptomatic and are evaluated by ultrasound because of the palpable adnexal mass. Rarely, patients with solid ovarian tumors may present with acute pelvic pain secondary to adnexal torsion.

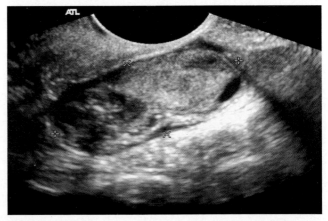

FIGURE 19.12.36: Transvaginal sonogram of a 4x3 cm ovary in an asymptomatic postmenopausal patient.

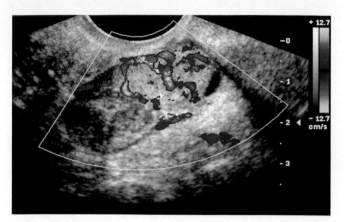

FIGURE 19.12.37: The same patient as in Figure 19.12.36. Penetraging pattern of the irregular vessels is suggestive of ovarian malignancy.

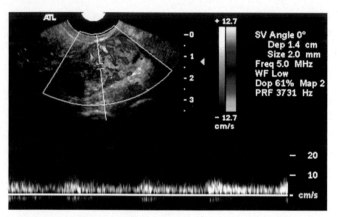

FIGURE 19.12.38: Pulsed Doppler analysis demonstrates low vascular impedance blood flow signals. Ovarian carcinoma was confirmed by histology.

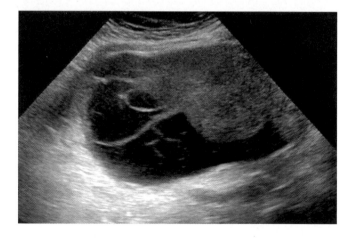

FIGURE 19.12.39: Transabdominal image of a complex adnexal mass. Note multiseptated complex adnexal mass with heterogeneous solid component.

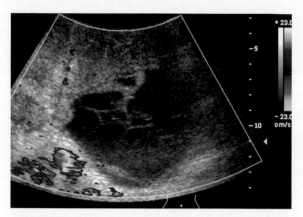

FIGURE 19.12.40: The same patient as in Figure 19.12.39. Tranvaginal color Doppler ultrasound demonstrates increased vascularity within the solid part.

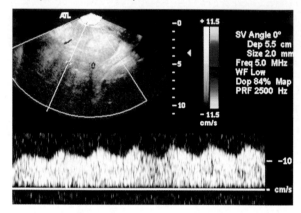

FIGURE 19.12.41: Pulsed Doppler analysis reveals low vascular impedance blood flow signals, typical for ovarian cystadenocarcinoma. Ovarian malignancy was confirmed by histology.

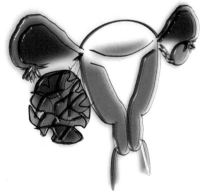

FIGURE 19.12.42: On grayscale ultrasound cystadenocarcinoma is visualized as a complex adnexal mass containing different echogenic patterns, thick walls, thick and irregular septations, nodules and/or papillary projections. Color Doppler demonstrates low vascular impedance blood flow signals obtained from the randomly dispersed vessels with irregular course. Majority of the patients are asymptomatic until an abdominal mass and/or ascites becomes evident.

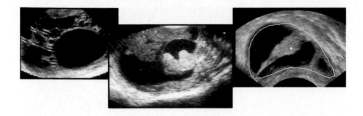

FIGURE 19.12.43: Typical features of ovarian malignancy are thick septations and presence of solid parts.

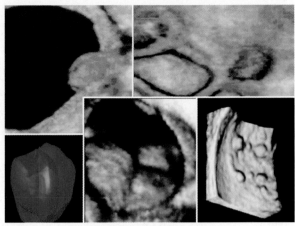

FIGURE 19.12.46: Three-dimensional ultrasound improves visualization of the papillary protrusions, septations, solid parts, wall irregularities, capsule infiltration and volume measurement. Improved demonstration of the ovarian tumor architecture may lead to improved diagnostic accuracy and earlier detection of ovarian cancer.

Peripheral Pattern

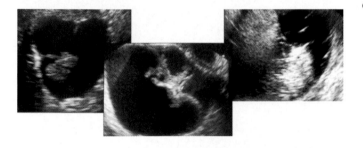

FIGURE 19.12.44: Another morphologic features of ovarian malignancy are presence of papillary irregularities and absence of the posterior shadowing from solid parts. Posterior shadowing from the calcified structures, such as bone and teeth is pathognomonic for the dermoid cysts.

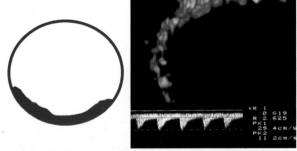

FIGURE 19.12.47: In benign ovarian lesions, blood vessels arise outside the lesion and surround it. Pulsed Doppler waveform analysis reveals moderate to high impedance blood flow signals.

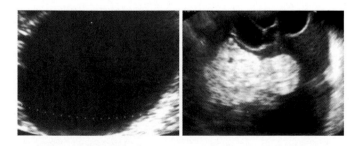

FIGURE 19.12.45: Mixed echogenicity and presence of free fluid (ascites) are additional signs of ovarian malignancy.

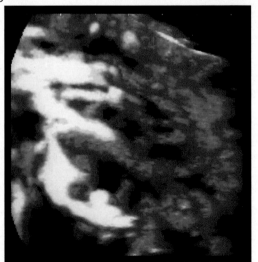

FIGURE 19.12.48: Penetrating pattern of irregular randomly dispersed vessels is suggestive of ovarian malignancy.

Penetrating pattern

Mixed
Penetrating and Peripheral

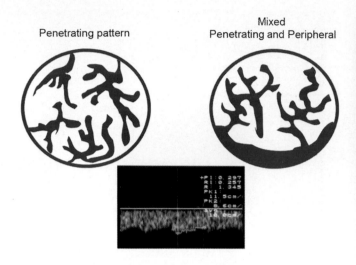

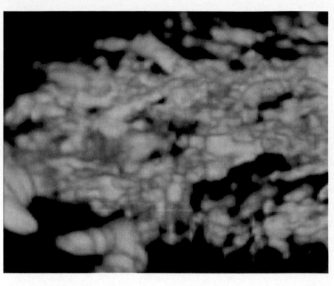

FIGURE 19.12.49: Color and pulsed Doppler sonography enables visualization of the pelvic mass vascularity and provides information regarding tumor neovascularization. Color and power Doppler features suggestive of ovarian malignancy are penetrating and mixed pattern (penetrating and peripheral) of the tumoral vessels. Pulsed Doppler analysis reveals high velocity and low impedance blood flow signals.

FIGURE 19.12.51: Randomly dispersed vessels within irregular course and branching demonstrated following the injection of an echo enhancing contrast.

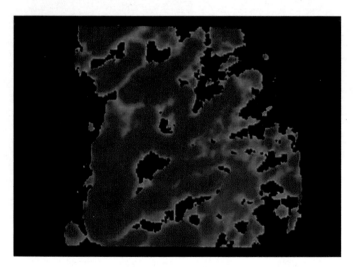

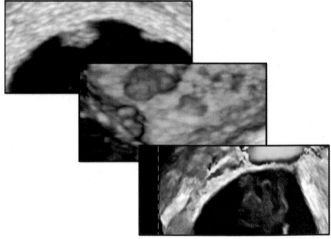

FIGURE 19.12.50: Echo enhancing contrast media may be efficiently used for the visualization of the pelvic tumor vasculature. Three-dimensional power Doppler scan of an ovarian carcinoma after injection of echo-enhancing contrast medium demonstrates irregular, thorn like vessels.

FIGURE 19.12.52: Three-dimensional ultrasound improves visualization of the cystic wall irregularities, while 3D power Doppler allows visualization of the peripheral vessels and irregular course of the vessels within the papilla (mixed pattern of the tumoral vascularity).

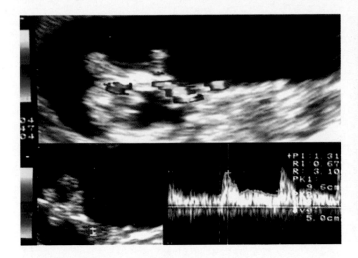

FIGURE 19.12.53: Complex adnexal mass containing a fluid-filled distended tube. Note a pseudopapillomatous vascularized structure protruding into the tubal lumen. Pulsed Doppler analysis demonstrates moderate to high vascular impedance blood flow signals (RI = 0.67).

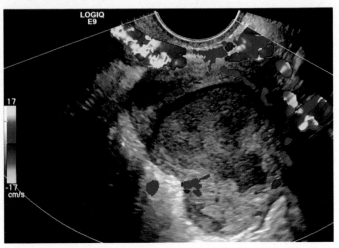

FIGURE 19.12.56: The same patient as in Figure 19.1.12.55. Color Doppler ultrasound reveals increased angiogenesis suggestive of a tuboovarian abscess. Acute pelvic inflammatory disease involving the left ovary and fallopian tube was confirmed by laparoscopy.

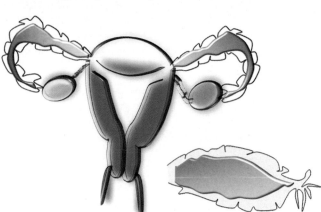

FIGURE 19.12.54: Hydrosalpinx is a distally blocked fallopian tube, filled with fluid. Finding is usually bilateral and patients may present with pelvic mass on pelvic exam. Incomplete septations and longitudinal folds are visualized as pseudopapillomatous protrusions and incomplete septations.

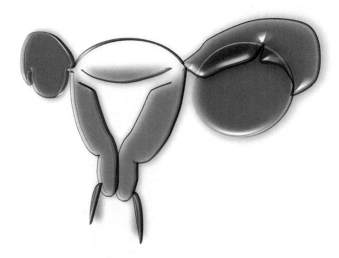

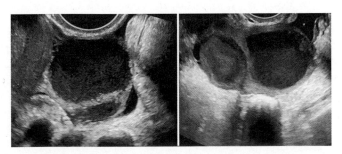

FIGURE 19.12.55: Complex adnexal mass in a patient presenting with low abdominal pain and fever.

FIGURE 19.12.57: Tubo-ovarian abscess is a severe form of PID. Patients usually present with low abdominal pain, vaginal dishcarge and fever. Additional signs are irregular bleeding and vomiting. Ultrasound demonstrates a complex adnexal mass with thick walls and echogenic fluid.

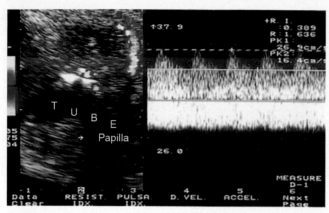

FIGURE 19.12.58: Transvaginal color Doppler scan of a sausage shaped adnexal mass. Note papillary projection with low vascular impedance blood flow signals (RI = 0.39) and presence of an arteriovenous shunt. Tubal malignancy was confirmed by histology.

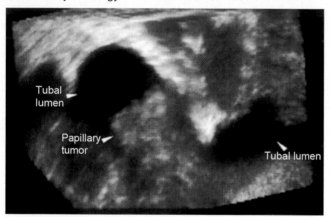

FIGURE 19.12.59: Three-dimensional ultrasound of a Fallopian tube carcinoma. Note distended tubal lumen and papillary protrusion.

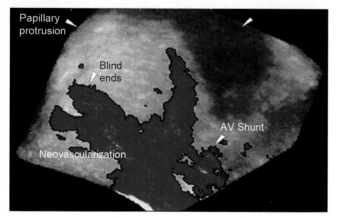

FIGURE 19.12.60: Three-dimensional power Doppler scan of the Fallopian tube carcinoma. Three-dimensional power Doppler ultrasound depicts typical features of the malignant tumor vessels: blind ends, tumoral lakes and arterio-venous shunting.

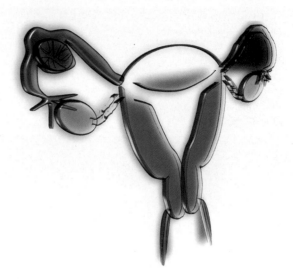

FIGURE 19.12.61: Primary fallopian tube carcinoma is an uncommon pelvic malignancy, usually occurring between the forth and sixth decades of life. The most common presenting symptoms are abnormal vaginal bleeding or spotting, palpable pelvic mass and/or ascites. Sonographic appearance of the fallopian tube carcinoma is nonspecific. In early stages, fallopian tube cancer is visualized as a sausage-shaped mass with papillomatous protrusions and/or solid parts. Color Doppler ultrasound demonstrates low impedance blood flow signals. Three-dimensional ultrasound can better demonstrate tubal wall irregularities (papillae and nodules). Three-dimensional power Doppler ultrasound depicts arteriovenous shunts, microaneurysms, tumor lakes, blind ends and dichotomous branching, typical of tubal malignancy.

BIBLIOGRAPHY

1. Kupesic S, Kurjak A. Contrast enhanced, three-dimensional power Doppler sonography for differentiation of adnexal lesions. Obstet Gynecol 2000;96(3):452-8.
2. Kupesic S, Plavsic M. Branko. (2009). Adnexal torsion: color Doppler and three-dimensional ultrasound. Abdominal Imaging; DOI: 10.1007/s00261-009-9573-0 (online).
3. Kurjak A, Kupesic S, Bekavac I. Adnexal masses. In: Kupesic S. (Ed). Color Doppler and three-dimensional ultrasound in gynecology, infertility and obstetrics. New Delhi: Jaypee Brothers Medical Publishers 2003;44-65.
4. Kurjak A, Kupesic S, Bekavac. Three- and three-dimensional power Doppler in the assessment of adnexal masses. In: Kurjak A, Jackson D. (Eds). An Atlas of three- and four-dimensional sonography in Obstetrics and Gynecology. London, New York: Taylor and Francis 2004;39-59.

5. Kurjak A, Kupesic S, Zodan T. Color Doppler assessment of malignant adnexal masses. In: Kurjak A, Kupesic S (Eds). An Atlas of transvaginal color Doppler. London-New York: Parthenon Publishing 2000;203.

6. Kurjak A, Kupesic S. Benign adnexal masses assessed by color and pulsed Doppler. In: Kurjak A, Fleischer A (Eds). Doppler ultrasound in gynecology. New York: Parthenon Publishing 1998;37-46.

7. Kurjak A, Predanic M, Kupesic S, et al. Adnexal masses: Malignant ovarian tumors. In: Kurjak A (Ed). Atlas of transvaginal color Doppler. London: Parthenon Publishing; 1994; 291-317.

8. Kurjak A, Sparac V, Kupesic S, et al. Three-dimensional ultrasound and three-dimensional power Doppler in the assessment of adnexal masses. Ultrasound Rev Obstet Gynecol 2001;2:167-184.

19.13: BREAST LUMPS

Text and images by: S Kupesic Plavsic
Medical illustrations by: Bhargavi Patham and Sandesh Subramanya

Breast lumps are common indication for ultrasound imaging. The vast majority of breast lumps is caused by a benign breast disease (cysts and fibroadenomas). However, breast cancer is found in about 10% of women complaining of a lump and 4% of women with any other breast complaint (Flow chart 19.13.1).

Clinical Clues

Ask about:

– How breast lump was discovered (by patient herself accidentally, during self-breast examination, during clinical periodic clinical breast examination or during screening mammography procedure)?
– Where the breast lump is precisely located?
– How long it has been present?
– Is lump associated with nipple discharge?
– Is there any change in size of the lump?
– Whether the lump waxes and wanes at the time of the menstrual cycle? (benign cysts may be more prominent during the premenstrual phase and regress in size during the follicular phase)
– Past history of breast cancer or breast biopsy.
– History of risk factors for breast cancer (e.g. age, family history of breast cancer, age of menarche, age at first pregnancy, age at menopause, alcohol use and hormonal replacement therapy)
– Breast feeding (reduced risk for breast cancer)
– Obstetrical history (≥5 pregnancies lowers the risk for breast cancer)
– Regular exercise and BMI (BMI < 23 reduces the risk of breast cancer)
– Aspirin (aspirin weekly for > 6 months reduces the risk of breast cancer)
– Oophorectomy (oophorectomy before age 35 years reduces the risk of breast cancer)
– No history of breast cancer in mother or sister (reduced risk of breast cancer)
– If patient is < 30 years of age (reduced risk of breast cancer)
– If patient had menarche at > 14 years of age (reduced risk of breast cancer)
– Had first baby before 20 years of age (reduced risk of breast cancer)
– Menopause before 45 years of age (reduced risk of breast cancer)
– Abstains from alcohol (reduced risk of breast cancer).

Look for:

– Changes in the shape of the breast
– Breast mass, which feels distinctly different from other breast tissue
– Scaly skin around the nipple
– Changes in the nipple (e.g. turning inward)
– Nipple discharge
– On palpation breast cancer is usually
– Hard
– Immovable
– With irregular borders
– Size ≥ 2 cm
– Axilary and supraclavicular lymph nodes involvement

Flow chart 19.13.1: Inductive reasoning scheme for diagnostic evaluation of patients presenting with breast disorders (lumps, pain or discharge) (*Courtesy:* Paul L. Foster School of Medicine, Texas Tech University at El Paso, TX, USA). Imaging (mammography, ultrasound and MRI) has significantly improved differentiation between benign and malignant breast lesions.

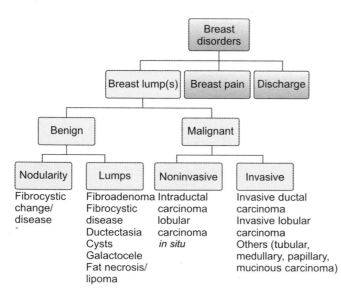

Investigations

- General physical examination
- Breast examination
- Mammography
- Ultrasound
- Ultrasound guided fine needle aspiration:
  - Nonbloody fluid
  - Bloody fluid
  - When no fluid is obtained (the mass turns out to be solid), cells should be aspirated for cytologic analysis with fine needle aspiration biopsy (FNAB).
- Ultrasound guided core needle biopsy (the "gold standard" is histology).

Ultrasound Findings

- Ultrasound is effective in delineating breast lesions
- Color Doppler increases the specificity of the diagnosis:
  - Breast cysts are avascular
  - Fibroadenomas are hypovascular
  - Breast abscess shows increased peripheral flow
  - Breast carcinoma demonstrates penetrating and irregular distribution of the newly formed vessels
- Fine needle aspiration under ultrasound guidance may be used for management of the breast cysts
- Core needle biopsy obtains tissue specimen suitable for histology
- Mammography is recommended in any woman age older than 35 who has a breast mass. The following mammographic features suggest breast malignancy:
  - Increased density
  - Irregular margins
  - Spiculation
  - Accompanying clustered irregular microcalcifications.

Diagnoses to Consider

- Diffuse changes:
  - Fibrocystic changes/disease
- Focal lesions:
  - Fibroadenoma
  - Cysts
  - Galactocele
  - Duct ectasia
  - Fat necrosis
  - Lipoma
  - Abscess
  - Carcinoma:
    - Noninvasive: Intraductal, lobular
    - Invasive: Ductal, lobular, tubular, medullary, papillary, mucinous

Some case studies related to breast lumps are depicted in Figures 19.13.1 to 19.13.25.

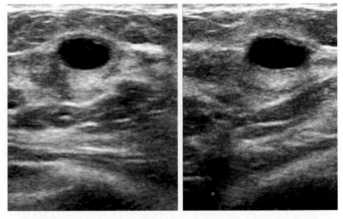

FIGURE 19.13.1: Two-dimensional ultrasound of a 5 mm breast cyst. Note completely smooth inner cyst wall.

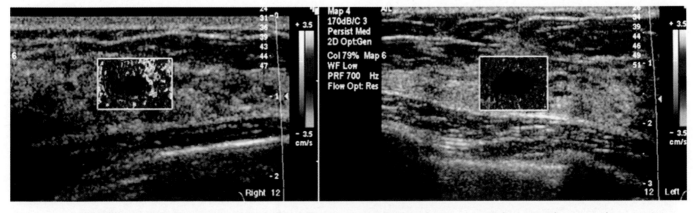

FIGURE 19.13.2: The same patient. Color Doppler examination does not reveal penetrating vessels.

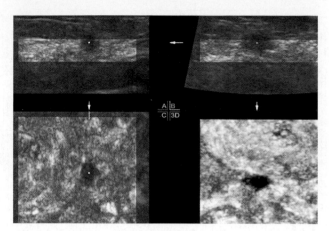

FIGURE 19.13.3: Multiplanar display and surface rendering of the same patient. Benign breast cysts were confirmed by histology.

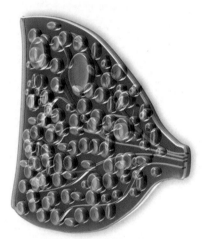

FIGURE 19.13.4: Benign breast cysts are visualized as sonolucent round or oval cystic structures with distinct edges. On palpation breast cysts feel like a smooth, nontender soft grape. Breast cysts require no treatment, unless the cysts are large and/or painful. In some cases fluid drainage from the breast cyst may relieve patient's symptoms.

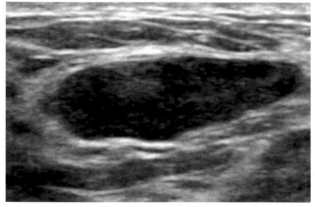

FIGURE 19.13.5: Two-dimensional ultrasound image of a fibroadenoma.

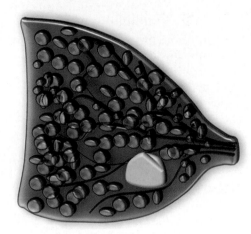

FIGURE 19.13.6: Fibroadenoma is the most common breast tumor among women between 15 and 35 years of age. On palpation they are mobile, nontender, well delineated rubbery lesions. The diagnosis has to be confirmed with fine needle aspiration or excisional biopsy.

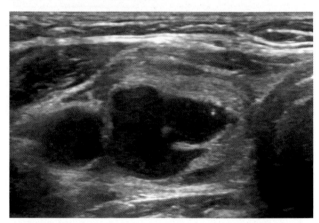

FIGURE 19.13.7: Complex mass in a lactating breast of a patient presenting with breast pain and fever.

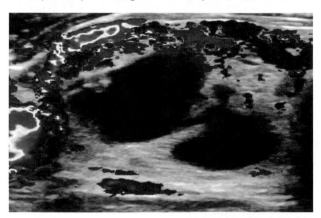

FIGURE 19.13.8: Color Doppler ultrasound of the same patient. Increased angiogenesis with no evidence of penetrating vessels is clearly demonstrated. Sonographic and Doppler findings indicate breast abscess.

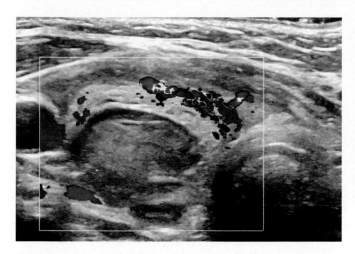

FIGURE 19.13.9: The same patient as in Figure 19.13.6 one week later. The patient was treated with antibiotics, with no success. Fine needle aspiration removed 130 cc of the purulent material.

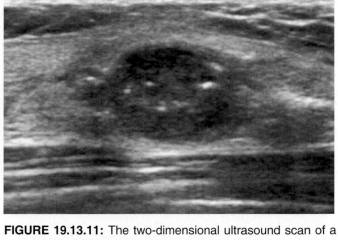

FIGURE 19.13.11: The two-dimensional ultrasound scan of a breast lesion showing no definite malignant criteria in sagittal section.

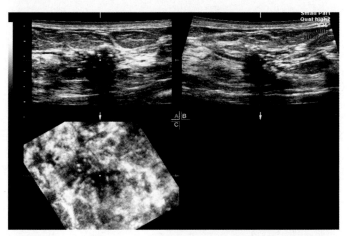

FIGURE 19.13.12: The same patient as in Figure 19.13.9 evaluated by 3D ultrasound. The coronal plane (low left image) demonstrates a stellate pattern suggestive of a malignancy. Histology revealed a tubular breast carcinoma.

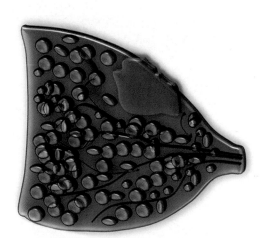

FIGURE 19.13.10: Breast abscess is a localized area of pus formation in the breast. Most frequently breast abscess is seen in lactating women with symptoms of mastitis who delay treatment for more than 24 hours. In untreated the pocket area filled with pus softens and abscess may reach the skin surface (induration). The abscess may rupture into the surrounding tissue and may lead to septicemia. Most common symptoms of mastitis complicated by abscess are fever, chills and headache. In case of septicemia, patient may also complain of the nausea, vomiting and diarrhea. On palpation breast feels ass tender and hard reddened area in the breast.

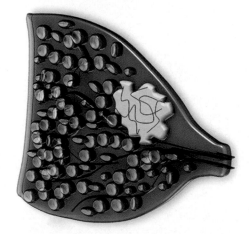

FIGURE 19.13.13: Breast carcinoma

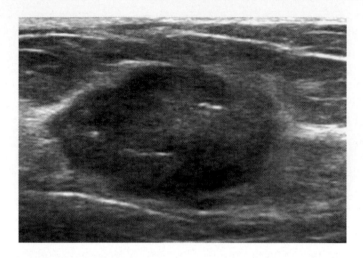

FIGURE 19.13.14: Two-dimensional ultrasound of an oval breast mass in a 45-year-old woman. The mass appear fairly innocuous in the sagittal plane.

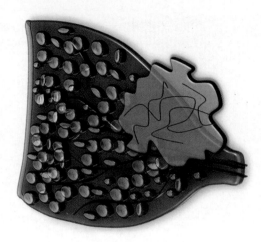

FIGURE 19.13.16: Breast carcinoma originates from the breast tissue (inner lining of the milk ducts – ductal carcinomas or the lobules – lobular carcinomas). There are many different types of malignant breast neoplasms, with different stages and aggressiveness. The most common presenting symptom is a breast lump and/or enlarged lymph nodes in the armpits. Sometimes patients may notice changes in breast size and shape, nipple inversion, nipple discharge or skin changes.

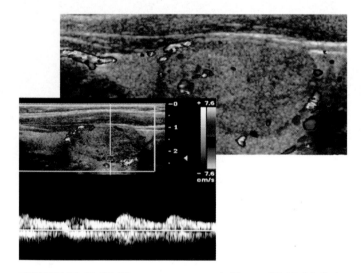

FIGURE 19.13.15: The same mass as in Figure 19.13.14. Color Doppler depicts penetrating vessels with low vascular impedance. Histology revealed breast carcinoma.

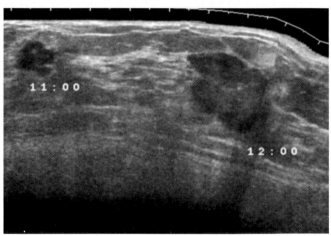

FIGURE 19.13.17: Two dimensional ultrasound of a multifocal breast lesion. Nonhomogeneous internal echo pattern and lobulated margins are suggestive of a breast cancer.

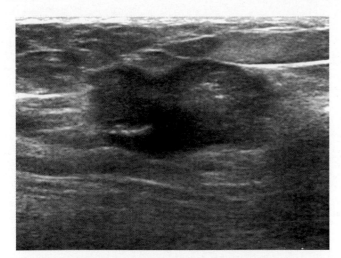

FIGURE 19.13.18: Another case of a lobulated breast mass on 2D ultrasound.

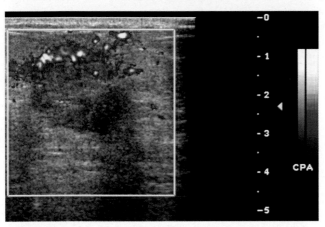

FIGURE 19.13.19: Power Doppler ultrasound of a lobulated breast mass demonstrates peripheral and penetrating pattern of the vessels.

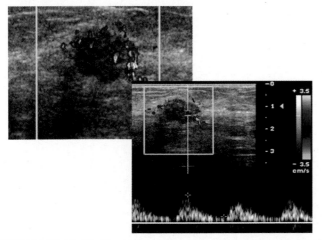

FIGURE 19.13.20: The same patient as in Figures 19.13.18 and 19.13.19. Color and pulsed Doppler ultrasound demonstrate abnormal, penetrating pattern of the vessels with moderate vascular impedance.

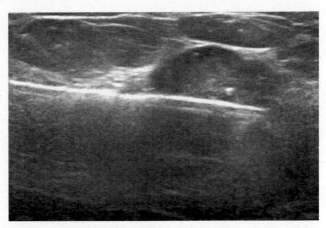

FIGURE 19.13.21: Two-dimensional ultrasound assessment of needle placement during a biopsy procedure. Despite peripheral position of the needle, it was possible to aspirate the cystic content for cytologic analysis. Medullary breast carcinoma was confirmed by histology.

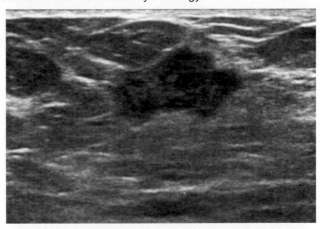

FIGURE 19.13.22: Two-dimensional ultrasound of an invasive ductal carcinoma.

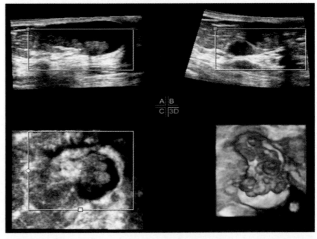

FIGURE 19.13.23: Multiplanar view and surface rendering of a complex breast mass. Note papillary protrusions and irregular contours of the solid mass. *Courtesy:* of GE Image Library.

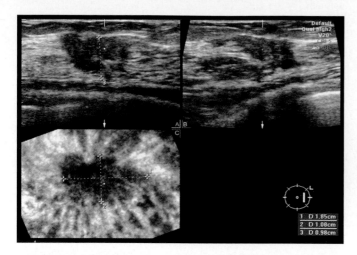

FIGURE 19.13.24: Multiplanar view of a breast carcinoma. Note retraction pattern in coronal plane, typical of invasive ductal breast carcinoma. Courtesy of GE Image Library.

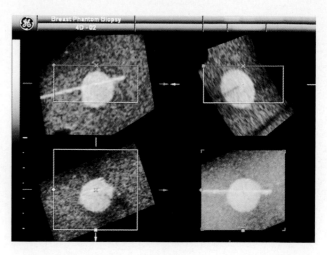

Figure 19.13.25: Three-dimensional assessment of needle placement during breast phantom biopsy. Courtesy of Kretztechnique / GE Image Library.

BIBLIOGRAPHY

1. Barton MB, Harris R, Fletcher SW. The rational clinical examination. Does this patient have breast cancer? The screening clinical breast examination: Should it be done? How? JAMA 1999;282(13):1270-80.
2. Millet AV, Dirbas FM. Clinical management of breast pain: a review. Obstet Gynecol Surv 2002;57(7):451-61.
3. Moy L, Slanetz PJ, Moore R. Specificity of mammography and ultrasound in the evaluation of palpable breast abnormality: A retrospective review. Radiology 2002;225:176-181.
4. Venta LA. Image guided biopsy of non-palpable breast lesions. In: Harris JR, Lippman ME, Morrow M, et al. (Eds). Diseases of the breast, 2nd Edition. Philadelphia: Lippincott Williams and Wilkins 2000;149-64.

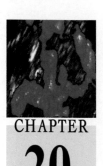

CHAPTER

20

Obstetric Ultrasound Pearls

Medical Illustrations by: B Patham and S Subramanya
Text by: S Kupesic Plavsic
Images by: V D'Addario, S Kupesic Plavsic, G Azumendi, K Gersak

Obstetric ultrasound pearls are developed to assist in performing a well-structured obstetrical ultrasound study during the first, second and third trimesters of pregnancy. Baseline ultrasound examination standards are best outlined in AIUM Practice Guideline for the Performance of Obstetric Ultrasound Examinations published by the American Institute of Ultrasound in Medicine in 2009.[1]

20.1: FIRST TRIMESTER ULTRASOUND EXAMINATION

- *Indications* for first trimester ultrasound examination are the following:[1]
  - Confirmation of an intrauterine pregnancy
  - Estimation of the gestational age
  - Diagnosis of multiple pregnancy/assessment of the chorionicity and amnionicity
  - Confirmation of the fetal viability (cardiac activity yes/no)
  - Evaluation of the pregnant patients, presenting with vaginal bleeding (rule out ectopic pregnancy, pregnancy complications, intrauterine hematoma, GTD, etc.)
  - Evaluation of the pregnant patients, presenting with pelvic pain (rule out ectopic pregnancy, pregnancy complications, intrauterine hematoma, GTD, etc.)
  - Evaluation of pelvic masses in pregnant patients
  - Ultrasound screening for nuchal translucency
  - Assessment of the fetal anomalies (for example, anencephaly) detectable in early pregnancy.

- **Report**
  - Size, shape, outer contours and orientation of the uterus
  - Presence/absence of the intrauterine gestational sac (record the three diameters of the gestational sac and compare the mean gestational sac diameter to the gestational (menstrual) age)
  - Presence/absence of the yolk sac
  - Presence/absence of the embryonic pole (when possible record crown rump length, CRL)
  - Presence/absence of the embryonic heart activity (fetal heart activity should be assessed when embryo's CRL is 5 mm)
  - Report the number of the gestational sacs/fetuses (chorionicity and amnionicity)
  - Look for intrauterine hematoma (define size, echogenicity and location of the intrauterine hematoma: supracervical or fundal)
  - Observe the cervix (define cervical shape (T, Y, U), evaluate the internal cervical os and cervical canal)
  - Rule out adnexal masses (define size, location and ultrasound appearance of the adnexal mass: cystic, cystic-solid, solid)
  - In patients with positive pregnancy test and absence of intrauterine gestational sac look for intracavitary fluid collection (pseudogestational sac of ectopic pregnancy) and search for adnexal findings suggestive of ectopic pregnancy
  - Presence/Absence of free fluid in the cul-de-sac.

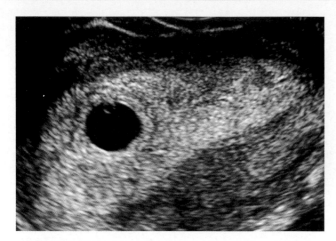

FIGURE 20.1.1: Gestational sac at 5 weeks gestation containing a yolk sac.

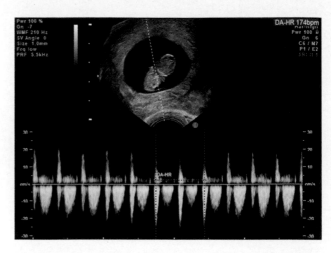

FIGURE 20.1.3: Pulsed Doppler waveform analysis of the fetal heart action at 8 weeks gestation.

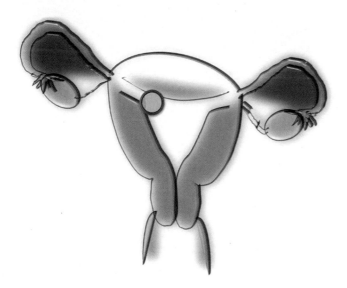

FIGURE 20.1.2: Eccentric position of the gestational sac at 5 weeks gestation. The yolk sac should always be visualized when a gestational sac measures greater than 10 mm.

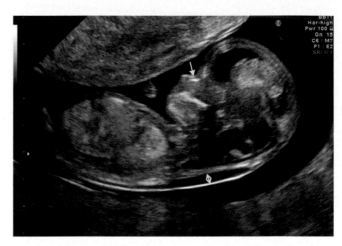

FIGURE 20.1.4: Nuchal translucency is visualized by transabdominal or transvaginal scanning in the longitudinal sagittal plane. The scan should be performed as we are measuring fetal crown rump length. The fetus should be in a neutral position, displayed on the monitor in the midsaggital section at the highest magnification. The nuchal translucency should be measured in its maximum thickness and should include only the echo free area.

NUCHAL TRANSLUCENCY MEASUREMENT (11 TO 13 WEEKS AND 6 DAYS)

- The gestational age: From 11 to 13 weeks and 6 days
- CRL: From 45 to 84 mm
- The fetus should be in midsagittal plane and neutral position
- The amnion should be clearly separated from the nuchal translucency
- The widest part of the nuchal translucency should be

measured by placing the calipers on the inner borders of the nuchal space (the calipers should be perpendicular to the long axis of the fetus).

Some cases related to early pregnancy and nuchal translucency scan are given in Figures 20.1.1 to 20.1.6.

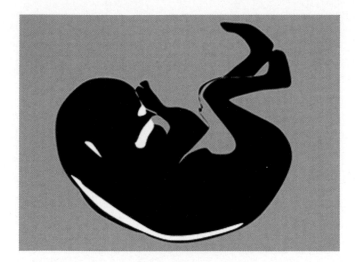

FIGURE 20.1.5: Nuchal translucency is an anechoic space reflecting a collection of fluid under the skin at the back of the fetal neck. It can be measured when fetus is between 11 weeks and 13 weeks plus six days.

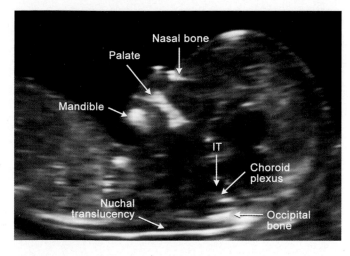

FIGURE 20.1.6: Nuchal translucency scan should also include the evaluation of the nasal bone and intracranial translucency (IT). The image of the nose includes three lines. The top line represents the nasal skin, in continuity with the skin is the tip of the nose and the bottom line, which is thicker and more echogenic, represents the nasal bone. Intracranial translucency is the assessment of the forth ventricle between the 11th and 14th week of gestation. It is presented parallel to NT and is delineated by two echogenic borders: the dorsal part of the brain stem anteriorly and the chorionic plexus of the fourth ventricle posteriorly.

20.2: SECOND AND THIRD TRIMESTER ULTRASOUND EXAMINATION (FETAL ANATOMY SCAN)

- **Indications** for second and third trimester ultrasound examination are the following:[1,2]
  - Estimation of the gestational age
  - Assessment of fetal anatomy
  - Evaluation of fetal growth
  - Cervical assessment (define cervical shape (T, Y, U), evaluate the internal cervical os and cervical canal)
  - Rule out multiple pregnancy/assess chorionicity and amnionicity
  - Rule out GTD
  - Rule out intrauterine death
  - Assess amniotic fluid index
  - Determine fetal position
  - Premature delivery assessment
  - Premature rupture of membranes
  - Abnormal biochemical markers
  - Rule out fetal anomalies/History of previous fetal anomaly
  - Uterine or adnexal masses
  - Uterine anomalies
  - Assessment of placental location/Rule out placenta previa
  - Suspected placental abruption
  - Evaluation of fetal well-being
  - Monitoring of invasive diagnostic procedures (CVS, amniocentesis, chordocentesis, etc.)
- **Report**

The following parameters of a standard fetal anatomy survey:

  - **Head, Face and Neck**
    - Measure the biparietal diameter, BPD (at the level of the thalami and cavum septi pelucidi)
    - Measure head circumference (at the same level as BPD)
    - Measure cerebellum, lateral cerebral ventricles and cisterna magna
    - Evaluate choroid plexus, midline falx and cavum septi pelucidi
    - Evaluate upper lip (nose-lip complex)
  - **Spine**

    Assess cervical, thoracic, lumbar and sacral spine in longitudinal and transverse planes

– **Chest**
  - Assessment of fetal heart: Four-chamber view and view of the outflow tracts
  - Using M-mode assess fetal heart activity (beats per minute)
  - Diaphragm
– **Abdomen**
  - Abdominal circumference (determined at the skin line of a true transverse view at the level of the junction of the umbilical vein, portal sinus and fetal stomach)—estimate fetal weight (rule out intrauterine growth restriction, IUGR and macrosomia)
  - Front abdominal wall (rule out gastroshisis and/or omphalocele)
  - Stomach (size and place)
  - Kidneys and bladder
– **Extremities**
  - Femoral length (measure the long axis of the femoral shaft excluding the distal femoral epiphysis)
  - Legs (presence/absence, position)
  - Arms (presence/absence, position)
– **Umbilical Cord**
  - Insertion site into the fetal abdomen
  - Number of the vessels in the umbilical cord (three vessels' cord: yes/no)
– **Placenta**
  - Location (anterior, fundal, posterior)
  - Appearance
  - Relationship to the internal cervical os
– **Amniotic Fluid**
  Amniotic fluid index or single deepest pocket
– **Cervix** (consider transperineal or transvaginal approach if indicated)
  - Length
  - Shape
  - Dynamic evaluation
– **Assess fetal movement**
– **Assess fetal position**
• Look for discrepancy between the gestational age and fetal biometry
• Observe scars from previous maternal surgeries (for example, Cesarean section scar)
• Report any technical problems (for example, imaging artifacts due to acoustic shadowing, low resolution due to maternal abdominal wall thickness, etc.)

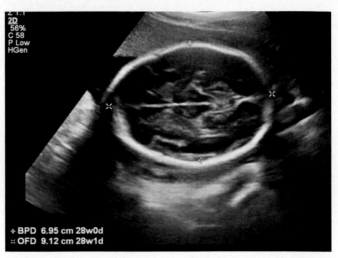

FIGURE 20.2.1: A fetal biometry assessment starts with the biparietal diameter, BPD, which is taken from the proximal outer wall of the fetal skull to the distal inner wall at the level of the occipitofrontal plane. Biparietal diameter, occipitofrontal diameter (OFD) and head circumference (HC) are usually measured simultaneously.

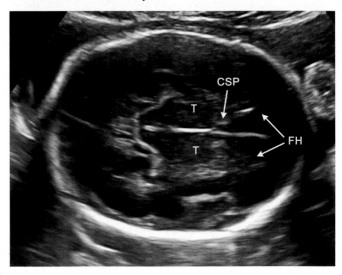

FIGURE 20.2.2: A trans-thalamic scan is used for the measurement of biparietal diameter and head circumference. In a transverse scan the midline echo is visualized as a hyperechoic line running along the fronto-occipital midline of the skull. Anteriorly and posteriorly it is formed by the falx cerebri and the interhemispheric fissure, and centrally by cavum septi pellucidi (CSP). Thalami are marked as "T" and frontal horns of the lateral ventricles are marked as "FH".

• In patients with inappropriate fetal growth perform follow-up ultrasound exam in two weeks.

Illustrative cases of fetal anatomy are given in Figures 20.2.1 to 20.2.62.

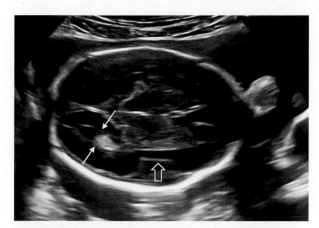

FIGURE 20.2.3: A transventricular scan is used for the measurement of the atrial width. Note arrows pointing to the atrium of the lateral ventricle. The arrowhead demonstrates the insula.

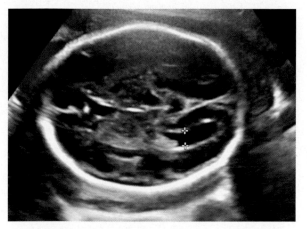

FIGURE 20.2.4: This image demonstrates a lateral ventricle measurement. Note the correct placement of the cursor.

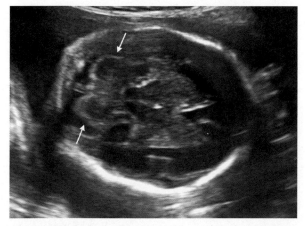

FIGURE 20.2.5: A transcerebellar scan is used for the measurement of the cerrebellum. Arrows are pointing the transverse cerebellar diameter. The cerebellum is contoured by the cisterna magna.

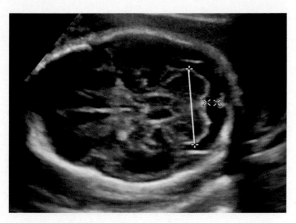

FIGURE 20.2.6: In transcerebellar view the precise measurement of the cerebellum (yellow) and cisterna magna (red) is performed.

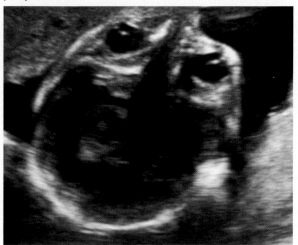

FIGURE 20.2.7: Transverse scan on the orbits enables assessment of the interorbital distance and the visualization of both lenses.

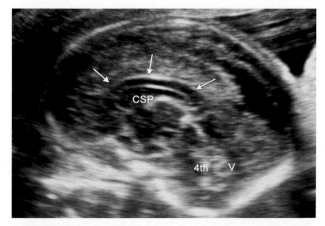

FIGURE 20.2.8: A midsagittal scan through the fetal brain is showing the corpus callosum (demonstrated by arrows), the cavum septi pellucidi (CSP), the posterior fossa with the cerebellar vermis (V) and the forth ventricle (4th V).

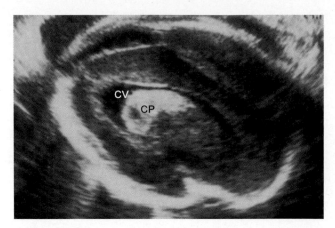

FIGURE 20.2.9: A parasagittal scan through the fetal brain showing the lateral ventricle (LV) with the choroid plexus (CP).

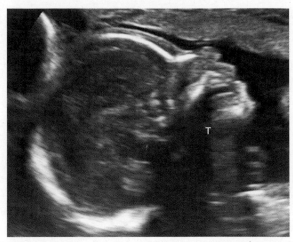

FIGURE 20.2.12: A midsagittal scan delineates fetal facial profile. The nasal bone is clearly visualized. The tongue (T) is demonstrated within the oral cavity.

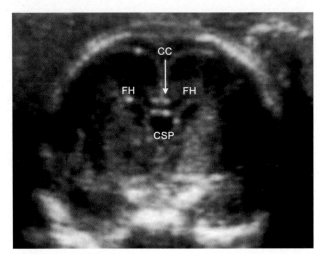

FIGURE 20.2.10: An anterior coronal scan of fetal brain demonstrates the frontal horns of the lateral ventricles (FH) divided by the corpus callosum (CC). Note that corpus callosum is located above the cavum septi pellucidi (CSP).

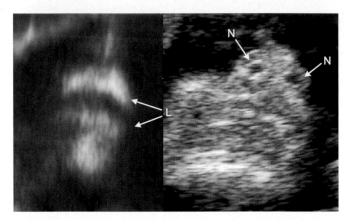

FIGURE 20.2.13: A coronal scan through the nasal tip and lower jaw. Note the lips (L) and the nostrils (N).

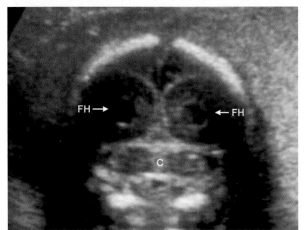

FIGURE 20.2.11: A posterior coronal scan of the brain showing the frontal horns of the lateral ventricles (FH). The cerebellum (C) is visible above the tentorium.

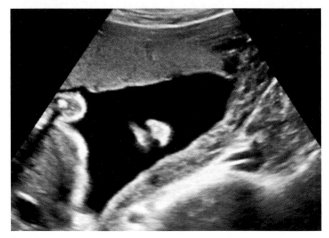

FIGURE 20.2.14: An angled coronal scan demonstrating the nose lips complex.

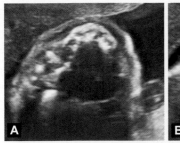 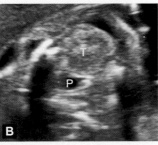

FIGURES 20.2.15A AND B: An axial scan of the mouth. At the upper section (A) the maxilla is clearly visualized;. At the lower level (B) the tongue (T) and the pharynx (P) are demonstrated.

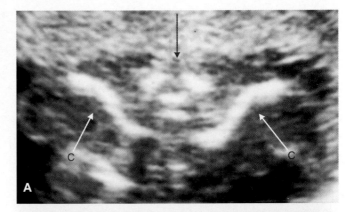

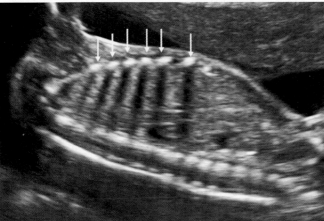

FIGURE 20.2.16: A full length view of the fetal spine at 22 weeks gestation. The ribs demonstrated by arrows produce sharp acoustic shadows.

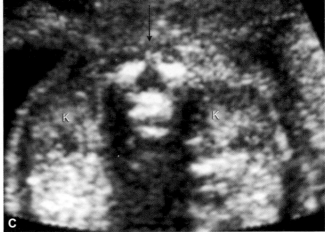

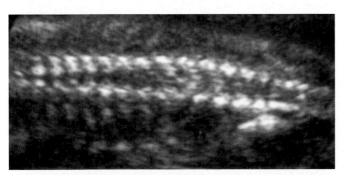

FIGURE 20.2.17: The spinal canal is demonstrated in the coronal scan of the spine passing trough the laminae.

FIGURES 20.2.18A TO C: The transverse scan of the vertebrae at different levels: (A) Cervical level, where the clavicles (C) are seen; (B) Thoracic level, where the ribs (R) are visualized; (C) Lumbar level where the kidneys (K) are demonstrated. Independently from the level of the vertebrae (black arrows) show to three ossification centers referring to the body and the laminae.

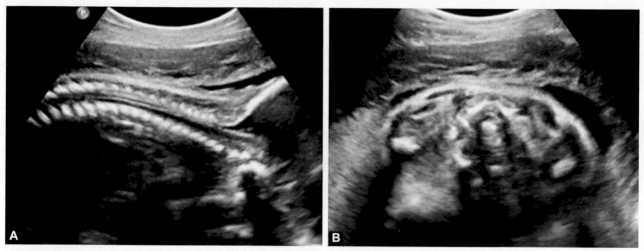

FIGURES 20.2.19A AND B: The longitudinal (A) and transverse (B) planes should be visualized for each segment of the cervical spine.

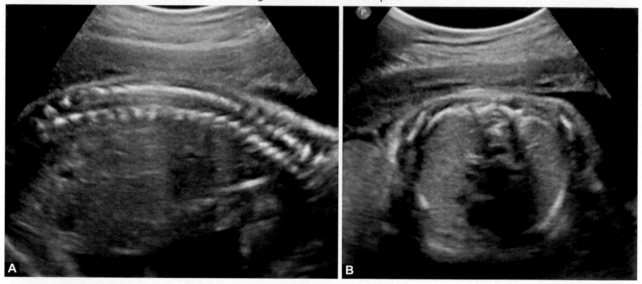

FIGURES 20.2.20A AND B: The longitudinal (A) and transverse (B) planes of the thoracic spine.

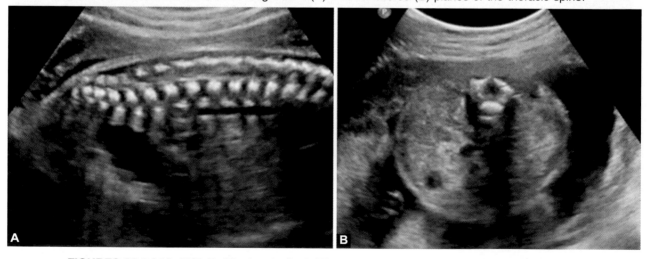

FIGURES 20.2.21A AND B: The longitudinal (A) and transverse (B) planes of the lumbar spine.

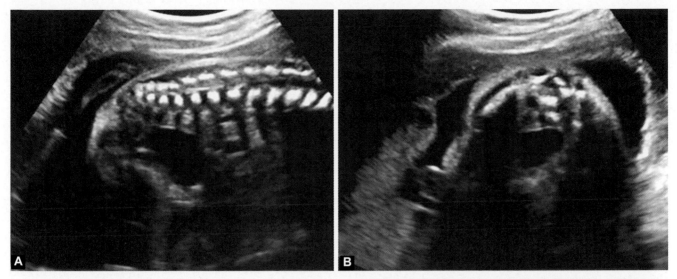

FIGURES 20.2.22A AND B: The longitudinal (A) and transverse (B) planes of the sacral spine.

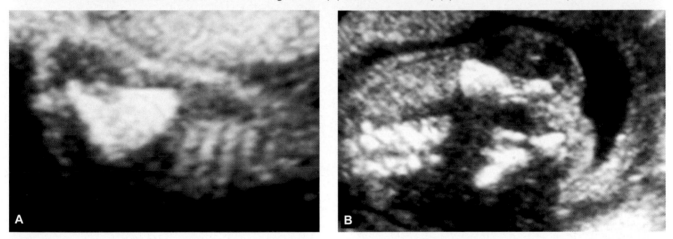

FIGURES 20.2.23A AND B: The scapula (A) and iliac wings (B) are visualized adjacent to the spinal canal. The echogenic iliac wing appears on each side of the fetal spine at the level of lumbosacral junction. Posterior shadowing from the upper iliac wing can mimic a defect of the spinal column.

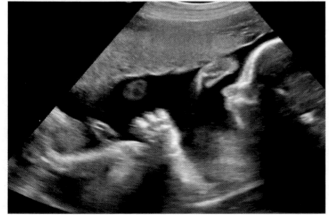

FIGURE 20.2.24: During a fetal anatomy survey the fetal extremities should be explored. This image demonstrates a fetal hand at 24 weeks gestation.

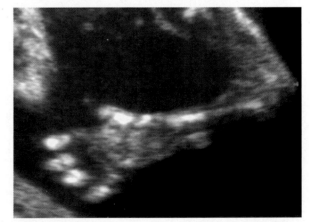

FIGURE 20.2.25: During sonographic assessment, the sonographer should evaluate the position and movement of the fetal extremities. Here is an example of the fetal hand at 25 weeks gestation.

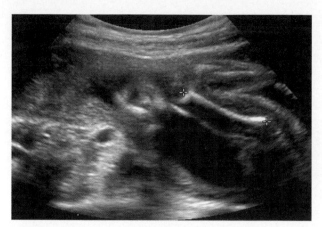

FIGURE 20.2.26: The routine ultrasound examination should asses femur length. The measurement should include the long axis of the femoral shaft excluding the distal femoral ephysis.

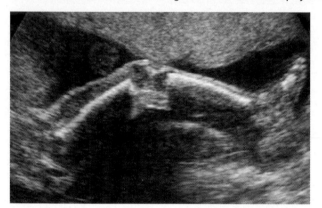

FIGURE 20.2.27: Extended fetal leg is visualized. Note fetal femur, tibia and foot.

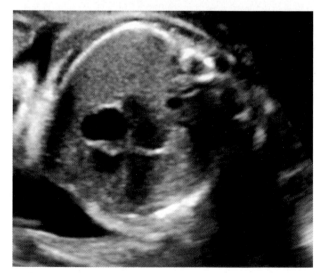

FIGURE 20.2.28: An apical four chamber view can be visualized in various fetal positions. It depicts both atria and ventricles, the interventricular and interatrial septum and the descending aorta.

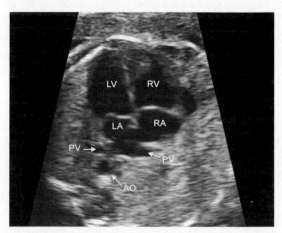

FIGURE 20.2.29: A "four chamber" apical view of the heart demonstrating left and right ventricles and atria, pulmonary veins and the descending aorta (LV = left ventricle; RV = right ventricle; LA = left atrium; RA = right atrium; PV = pulmonary veins; Ao = descending aorta).

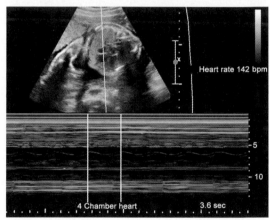

FIGURE 20.2.30: In every fetus, the fetal heart rate should be assessed by M-mode. In this fetus, M-mode demonstrates regular heart action with a frequency of 142 beats per minute.

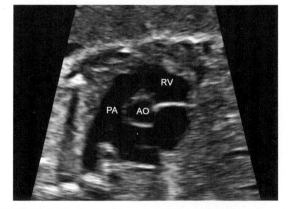

FIGURE 20.2.31: In the short-axis view, the aorta is encircled by the right ventricular inflow tract and the right outflow tract. Note the pulmonary artery (PA) emerging from the right ventricle and dividing into the right pulmonary artery and left pulmonary artery.

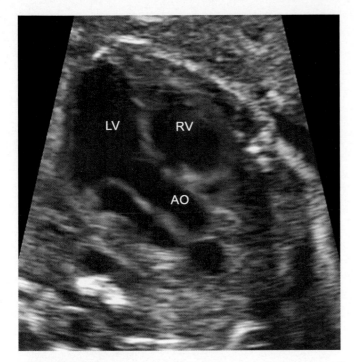

FIGURE 20.2.32: Left long-axis of the heart or "five chamber" view demonstrating the origin of the aorta from the left ventricle. (RV = right ventricle; LV = left ventricle; AO= aorta).

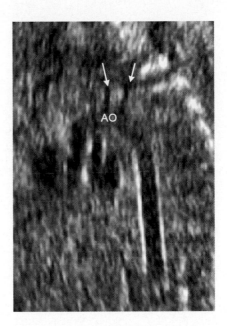

FIGURE 20.2.34: Longitudinal scan demonstrating the aortic arch (AO). The arrows point to the brachicephalic vessels.

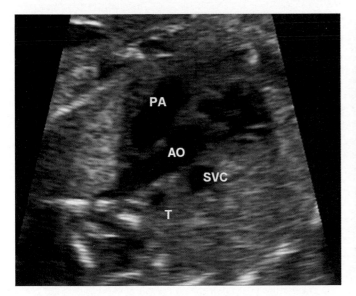

FIGURE 20.2.33: The three vessels-trachea view shows the superior vena cava (SVC), the aortic arch (AO), the pulmonary artery (PA) continuing in the ductal arch and the trachea (T).

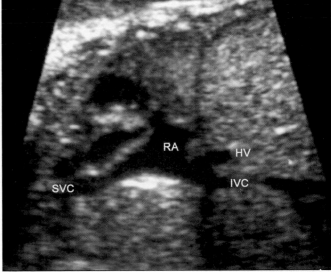

FIGURE 20.2.35: The longitudinal scan shows the superior (SVC) and inferior vena cava (IVC) opening in the right atrium (RA). HV represents the hepatic vein.

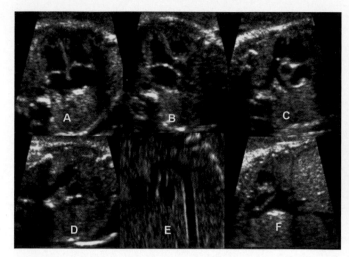

FIGURE 20.2.36: The fetal cardiac scan starts with "four chamber" view demonstrated in Figure A. Figure B shows the left ventricle outflow tract. The right ventricle outflow tract is demonstrated in figure C. The three vessels-trachea view in Figure D shows the pulmonary artery, aorta and superior vena cava. The aortic arch in longitudinal plane is demonstrated in Figure E, while Figure F illustrates the opening of the superior and inferior vena cava in the right atrium.

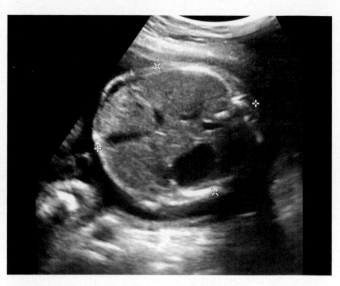

FIGURE 20.2.38: Abdominal circumference measurement is used for estimation of the fetal weight and detection of intrauterine growth restriction (IUGR) and macrosomia.

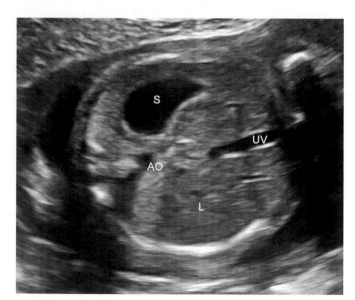

FIGURE 20.2.37: A transverse scan of the abdomen is used for the measurement of the abdominal circumference. Fetal abdominometry is performed in a transverse scan perpendicular to the long-axis, in which the liver (L), the stomach (S), the umbilical vein (UV) and the abdominal aorta (AO) are identified. Once the correct reference plane is identified the transverse and sagittal diameters are measured as outer-to-outer dimensions, and the abdominal circumference is calculated according to the formula for an ellipsoid. The abdominal circumference (AC) may also be measured electronically by tracing around it.

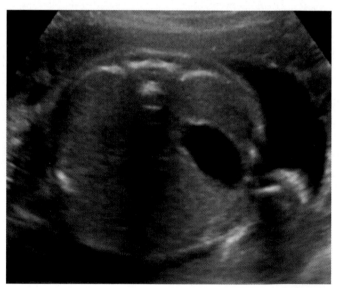

FIGURE 20.2.39: Transverse scan through the fetal abdomen demonstrates a stomach filled with fluid.

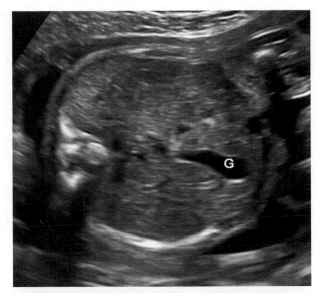

FIGURE 20.2.40: The gallbladder (G) appears as a pear-shaped anechoic structure on the right side of the liver.

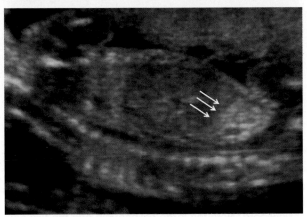

FIGURE 20.2.41: The bowel may be evaluated in both transverse and longitudinal planes. It appears as an echogenic area in the lower part of the abdomen as demonstrated by the arrows.

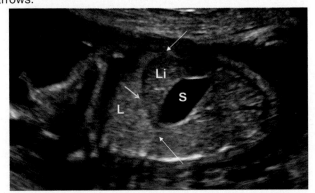

FIGURE 20.2.42: The fetal diaphragm appears as a thin curve hypoechoic line demonstrated by a yellow arrow dividing the liver (Li) from the lung (L). The stomach (S) is clearly seen adjacent to the liver.

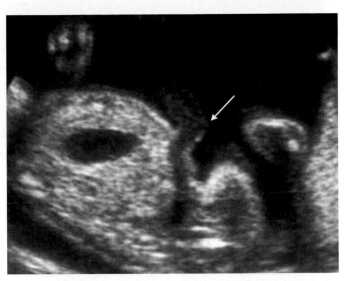

FIGURE 20.2.43: The abdominal insertion of the umbilical cord may be assessed in longitudinal plane.

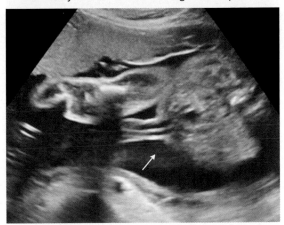

FIGURE 20.2.44: The transverse plane demonstrates abdominal insertion of the umbilical cord.

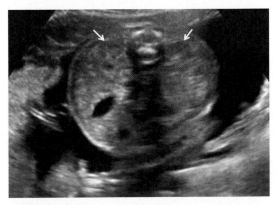

FIGURE 20.2.45: In transverse plane of the fetal abdomen kidneys are clearly visualized.

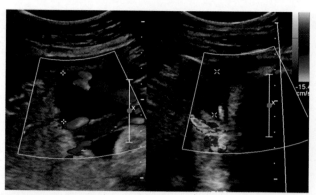

FIGURE 20.2.57: The umbilical cord occupies most of the fluid pocket. In this case, the umbilical vessels should be excluded from the measurement.

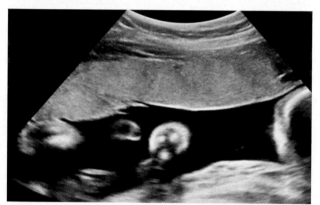

FIGURE 20.2.58: Placental ultrasound is an integral part of the obstetric ultrasound examination. The placenta is visualized as a homogeneous, moderately echogenic structure. In this image, the placenta is localized on the anterior uterine wall. It exhibits a smooth chorionic plate and has a homogeneous internal structure. The basal plate shows no echogenic areas. All of these features indicate grade 0 of placental maturity.

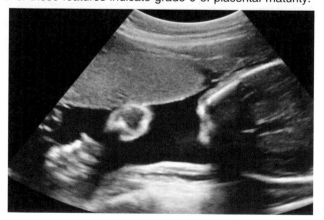

FIGURE 20.2.59: Vaginal bleeding in the second or third trimester is always suspicious for an abnormal placental location or marginal sinus hemorrhage. In these cases sonographer should measure the distance between the lower placental margin and the internal cervical os.

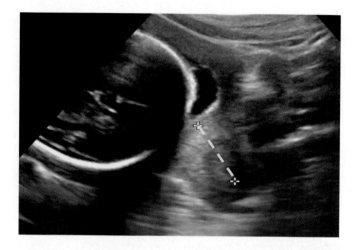

FIGURE 20.2.60: Cervical incompetence is one of the most common precipitating factors of late habitual abortion. Ultrasound examination of the cervix has become the standard method for diagnosing cervical incompetence. To better evaluate the cervical length and internal os, transabdominal ultrasound should be performed with a slightly distended urinary bladder. Here you can see a normal cervical length marked from cursor (*) to cursor (*).

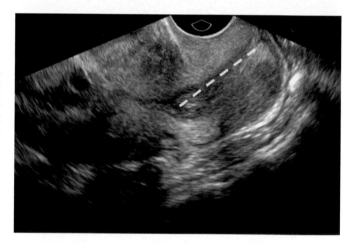

FIGURE 20.2.61: A transvaginal ultrasound enables precise noninvasive assessment of the cervical length and shape. Normally, the cervical length is always greater than the cervical thickness and the internal os is closed. Dashed yellow line demonstrates the cervical length from the inner to the outer cervical os.

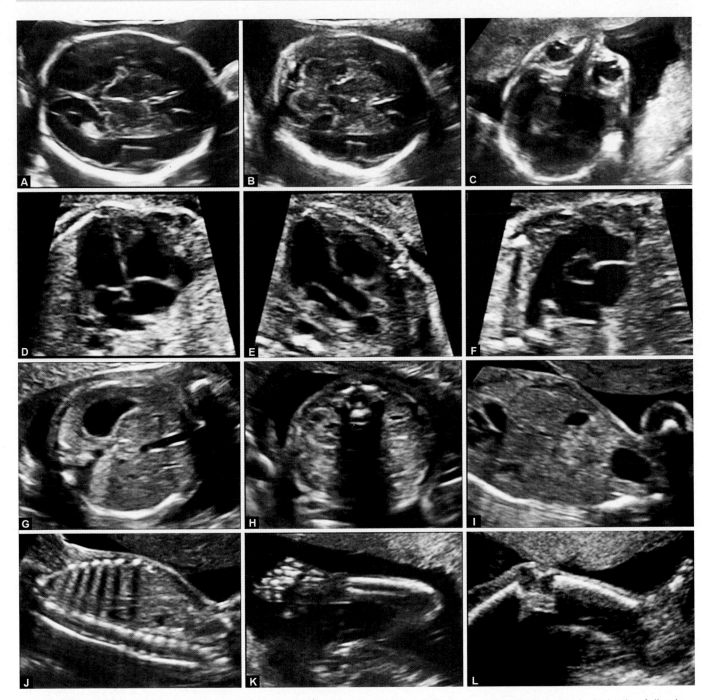

FIGURES 20.2.62A TO L: Minimal standards for fetal anatomical survey during the second trimester include the following: (A) transventricular view; (B) transcerebellar view; (C) transorbital view; (D) four chamber view; (E) left outflow tract; (F) right outflow tract; (G) transabdominal view with the stomach; (H) transverse view of the kidneys; (I) bladder; (J) longitudinal and transverse view of the fetal spine; (K) upper limb; (L) lower limb.

20.3: BLEEDING IN PREGNANCY

Illustrative cases of bleeding in pregnancy are given in Figures 20.3.1 to 20.3.28.

WRITING AN OBSTETRIC ULTRASOUND REPORT

The standard obstetrical ultrasound report is organized according to the following structure:[1]

- **Preliminary Information: Patient's History and Indication**
  - Patient's full name, medical record number, date of birth and date when ultrasound study was performed
  - Clinical history including the date of the last menstrual period (first day of LMP) and obstetric history
  - Indication for obstetric ultrasound
  - Results of the previous ultrasound examinations
  - Result of biochemical screening, if available
  - History of previous congenital anomalies
- **Findings**
  - Provide a step-by-step information about the following fetal structures:
    - Head, face and neck (intracranial structures)
    - Chest (heart: four-chamber view, outflow tracts, fetal heart frequency)
    - Diaphragm
    - Abdomen (stomach, kidneys, bladder and pyelectasis, if detected)
    - Front abdominal wall
    - Extremities (legs and arms)
  - Provide the following fetal biometry parameters: BPD, HC, FL and AC.
  - Provide information about the placental location, appearance and relationship to the internal cervical os.
  - Umbilical cord (insertion, number of umbilical cord vessels)
  - Report on the amount of amniotic fluid (AFI)
  - Provide information about fetal movement and position
  - Assess the cervix (length and shape)
  - In case of multiple pregnancy report on fetal number, chorionicity and amnionicity, assess fetal biometry and position for each embryo/fetus
  - When indicated, provide the measurements of the uterine and/or adnexal lesions.
  - Describe your observations objectively in a paragraph-form report
  - In patients with fetal anomalies provide detailed explanation.
- **Impression**
  - Summary of the most important ultrasound findings
  - The impressions should be numbered in the decreasing order of importance
- **Recommendation** (optional)
  - Inform the referring physician about the necessity and time of the ultrasound follow-up exam, if needed
  - Provide clinical and/or therapeutic recommendations to the referring physician.

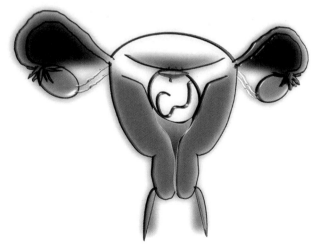

FIGURE 20.3.1: Threatened abortion describes any vaginal bleeding during pregnancy, which should be further evaluated. Clinical findings are consistent with closed cervix and no evidence of cervical motion tenderness or tissue passed.

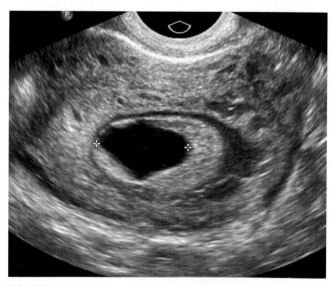

FIGURE 20.3.2: Transvaginal sonogram of anembryonic pregnancy (blighted ovum). Note that the diameter of the gestational sac was exceeding 1.5 cm.

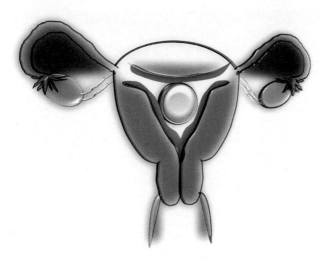

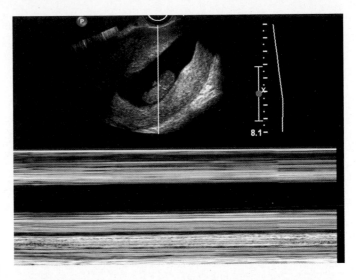

FIGURE 20.3.3: On transvaginal ultrasound the diagnosis of anembryonic pregnancy is certain when the mean gestational sac diameter exceeds 8 – 10 mm without the visualization of a yolk sac, or when there is no evidence of a living embryo when the mean diameter of the gestational sac exceeds 15 mm. In patients with no pain and/or bleeding the possibility of incorrect dates should be considered and ultrasound examination should be repeated in one week.

FIGURE 20.3.5: M-mode demonstrating the absence of the fetal heart activity in a patient presenting with vaginal bleeding and cramping pain.

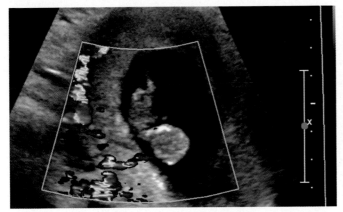

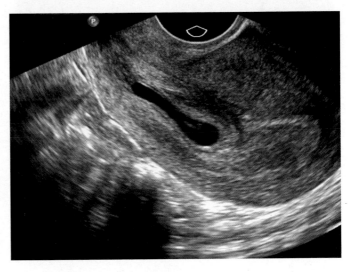

FIGURE 20.3.4: Transvaginal color Doppler scan of a missed abortion. Note the absence of the fetal heart activity. Ultrasound findings should always be correlated with the patient's symptoms, gestational age, and beta hCG values.

FIGURE 20.3.6: Transvaginal scan of an abortion in progress. Note irregular contours of the gestational sac and opening of the internal cervical os.

- **Signature**
  - Every report has to be reviewed and signed by the interpreting physician

Make sure that you are performing obstetric ultrasound examinations only when indicated. Ultrasound exam should be performed using the lowest possible ultrasonic exposure, according to the as low as reasonably achievable (ALARA) principle.[1,3]

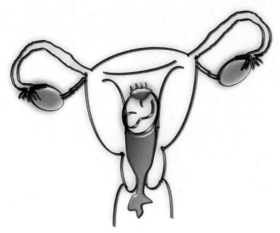

FIGURE 20.3.7: Inevitable abortion is characterized by severe vaginal bleeding, dilatation of the cervical canal, and commonly associated with cramping pain.

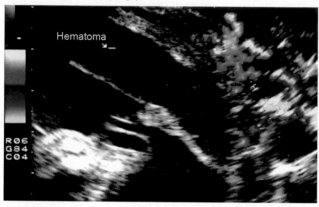

FIGURE 20.3.8: Transvaginal color Doppler scan of a fundal hematoma in a patient presenting with lower abdominal pain. Color signals are obtained from the adjacent spiral arteries.

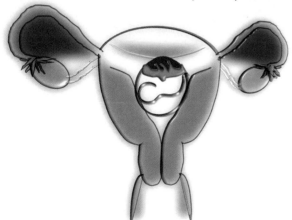

FIGURE 20.3.9: Subchorionic hematoma is bleeding that causes a marginal abruption with separation of the chorion from the endometrial lining. On ultrasound subchorionic hematoma is visualized as a hypoechoic or sonolucent area adjacent to the gestational sac. Fundal subchorionic hematoma is reported to have poor prognosis as compared with the hematoma in the lower uterine segment.

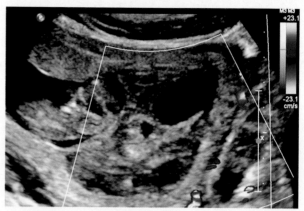

FIGURE 20.3.10: Transvaginal scan of a supracervical hematoma with septated appearance. Color signals adjacent to the hematoma site indicate normal uterine perfusion.

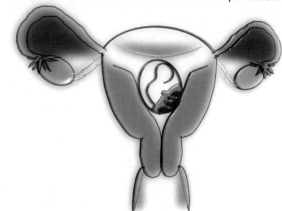

FIGURE 20.3.11: Supracervical subchorionic hematoma is reported to have better prognosis than fundal subchorionic hemorrhage.

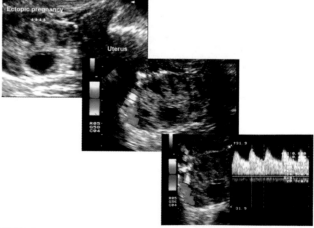

FIGURE 20.3.12: In every patient presenting with bleeding and/or pain during early pregnancy an ectopic pregnancy should be ruled out. Ectopic pregnancy may be visualized as an empty uterus, complex adnexal mass, tubal ring, ovarian cyst, or extrauterine fetus with or without heart activity and free fluid in the cul-de-sac. Ectopic active trophoblast enables demonstration of a "ring of fire" coupled with low vascular impedance on pulsed Doppler analysis.

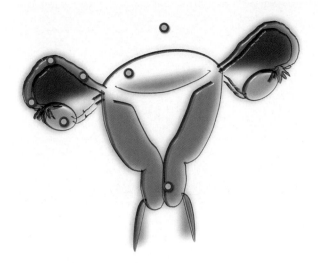

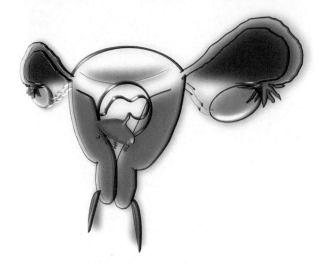

FIGURE 20.3.13: Ultrasound findings should always be correlated with beta hCG values. Failure to detect an intrauterine gestational sac by transvaginal ultrasound when beta hCG values exceed 1.500 mIU/ml indicate an increased-risk of ectopic pregnancy. Such a diagnostic approach improves early detection of tubal, isthmic, cervical, ovarian and abdominal pregnancy.

FIGURE 20.3.15: Bleeding during second and third trimesters areusually secondary to abnormal placental implantation. Therefore, in these patients the sonographer should evaluate placental location and differentiate total placenta previa from the partial, marginal or low lying placenta.

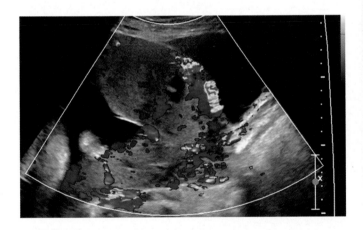

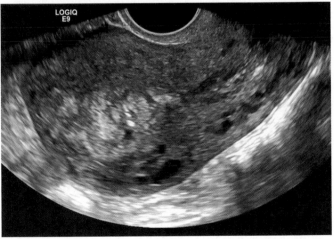

FIGURE 20.3.14: Placenta previa is one of the leading causes of vaginal bleeding in the second and third trimesters of pregnancy. Placenta previa can be visualized by transabdominal, transvaginal or transperineal sonography.

FIGURE 20.3.16: B-mode transvaginal ultrasound of a patient with incomplete abortion. Thickened endometrial lining greater than 8 mm, with or without hypoechoic material within the endometrial cavity are non-specific signs of residual products of conception.

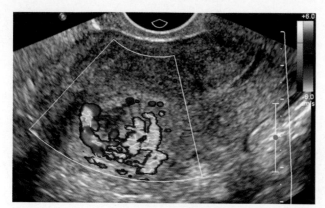

FIGURE 20.3.17: Transvaginal color Doppler image of an incomplete abortion. Note prominent vascularization within the uterine cavity confirming the diagnosis of retained products of conception and differentiating it from blood clots.

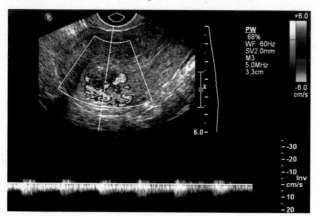

FIGURE 20.3.18: Pulsed Doppler waveform analysis demonstrates low vascular impedance blood flow signals indicative of active trophoblast.

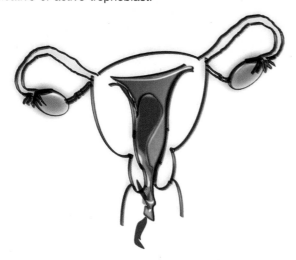

FIGURE 20.3.19: Persistent vaginal bleeding after an abortion may be due to retained products of conception. B-mode and color and pulsed Doppler analysis are methods of choice for detection of incomlete abortion.

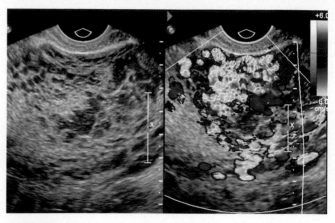

FIGURE 20.3.20: Transvaginal B-mode and color Doppler scan demonstrating a lacunar type of a complete mole.

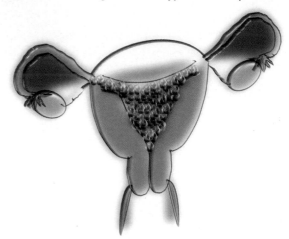

FIGURE 20.3.21: Hydatidiform mole is characterized by abnormalities of the chorionic villi, varying degrees of trophoblastic proliferations and edema of the villous stroma. Grossly the tumor is composed of multiple grapelike structures that occupy the uterine cavity.

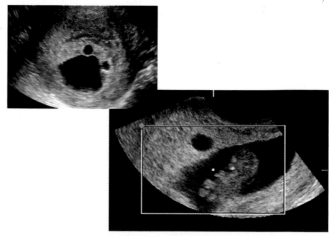

FIGURE 20.3.22: Hydropic changes of the chorionic tissue and presence of fetal parts are suggestive of a partial mole.

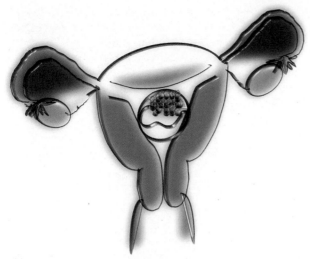

FIGURE 20.3.23: Partial hydatidiform mole is characterized by focal swelling of the villous tissue, focal trophoblastic hyperplasia and the presence of embryonic or fetal tissue.

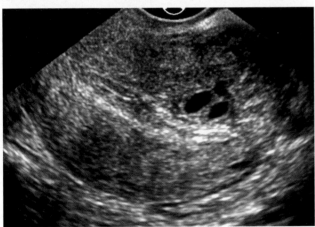

FIGURE 20.3.24: Transvaginal scan of a heterogeneous uterine mass in a patient with choriocarcinoma.

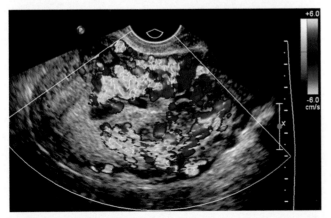

FIGURE 20.3.25: Transvaginal color Doppler scan of a choriocarcinoma. Note typical signs of neovascularization: bright signals from randomly dispersed vessels with irregular course.

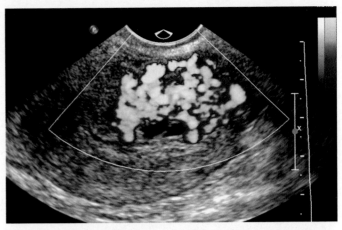

FIGURE 20.3.26: Power Doppler scan of a choriocarcinoma.

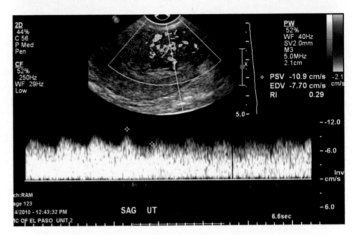

FIGURE 20.3.27: Low vascular resistance (RI = 0.29) obtained from color-coded zones within the uterus is typical for uterine malignancy. Choriocarcinoma was confirmed by histology.

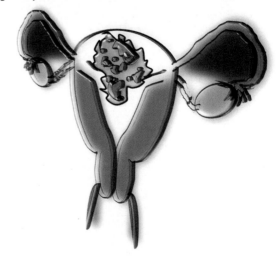

FIGURE 20.3.28: Choriocarcinoma is a malignant and aggressive cancer of the placenta. It is characterized by early hematogenous spread to the lungs. Patients usually present with vaginal bleeding and increased beta hCG values.

REFERENCES

1. AIUM Practice Guideline for the Performance of Obstetric Ultrasound Examinations. 2009. By the American Institute of Ultrasound in Medicine. Available from http://www.aium.org/publications/guidelines/obstetric.pdf.
2. D'Addario V, Pinto V, Di Cagno L, et al. Fetal anatomical survey during second trimester screening examination. In: Kurjak A, Chervenak F (Eds). Donald School Textbook of Ultrasound in Obstetrics and Gynecology. New Delhi: Jaypee Brothers Medical Publishers (P) Ltd 2008;258-68.
3. Sharma G, Chasen ST, Chervenak FA. Routine use of obstetric ultrasound. In: Kurjak A, Chervenak F (Eds). Donald School Textbook of Ultrasound in Obstetrics and Gynecology. New Delhi: Jaypee Brothers Medical Publishers (P) Ltd 2008;100-19.

Index